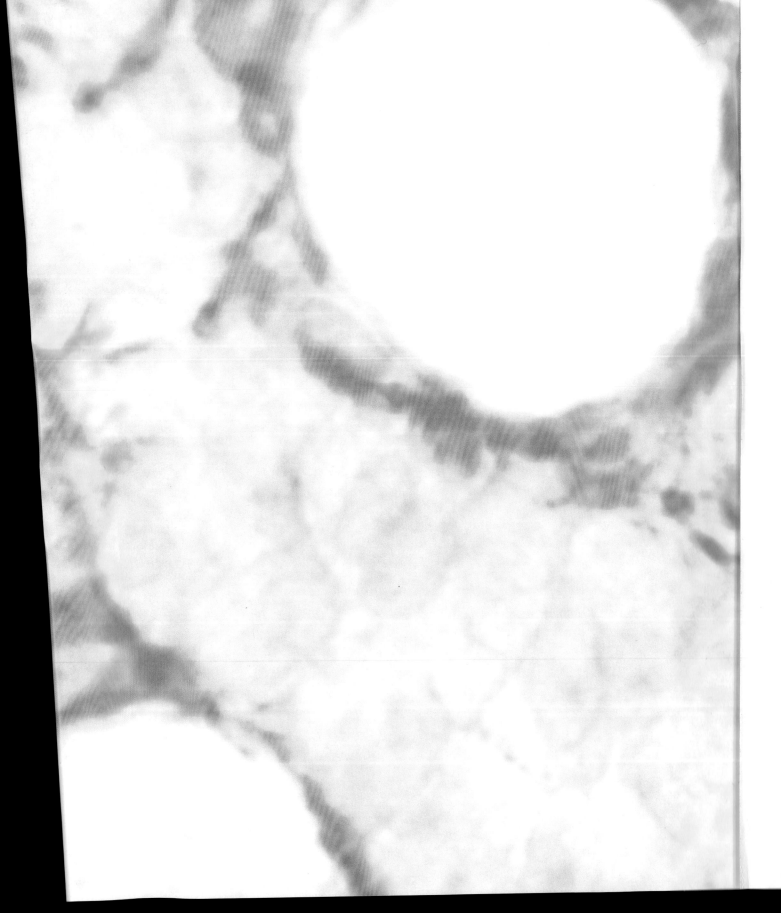

M Merchison

DIAGNOSTIC PATHOLOGY
BREAST

AMI

DIAGNOSTIC PATHOLOGY
BREAST

AMIRSYS®

David G. Hicks, MD
Professor of Pathology and Laboratory Medicine
Director of the Surgical Pathology Unit
University of Rochester Medical Center
Rochester, NY

Susan C. Lester, MD, PhD
Chief, Breast Pathology Services
Brigham and Women's Hospital
Assistant Professor, Harvard Medical School
Staff Pathologist, Dana Farber Cancer Institute
Boston, MA

AMIRSYS®

Names you know. Content you trust.®

First Edition

Printed in Canada by Friesens, Altona, Manitoba, Canada

ISBN: 978-1-931884-57-0

Notice and Disclaimer

Library of Congress Cataloging-in-Publication Data

Hicks, David G., 1957-
  Diagnostic pathology. Breast / David G. Hicks, Susan C. Lester.
    p. ; cm.
  Breast
  Includes bibliographical references and index.
   ISBN 978-1-931884-57-0 (hardback)
  1. Breast--Cancer--Atlases. 2. Breast--Cancer--Diagnosis--Atlases. 3. Breast--Cancer--Pathophysiology--Atlases. I. Lester, Susan Carole. II. Title. III. Title: Breast.
   [DNLM: 1. Breast Neoplasms--pathology--Atlases. 2. Neoplasm Staging--methods--Atlases. 3. Specimen Handling--methods--Atlases. WP 17]
   RC280.B8H55 2012
   616.99'449--dc23
                        2011015974

To my lovely wife, Patti—my best friend, companion, and golfing partner—and the amazing children we share. I will forever be grateful for all of your love and support.

And to my parents, Herman and Maralee, who were my first teachers. Your encouragement and unwavering belief in me has made all the difference.
DGH

To my wonderful former chairman, Ramzi Cotran, who stopped me in the hall one day when I was a senior resident, slapped his hands in his classic fashion, and said, "Susan, Susan, where can I find a breast pathologist?" I said, "I could be a breast pathologist." And only 20 years later, here is this book.
SCL

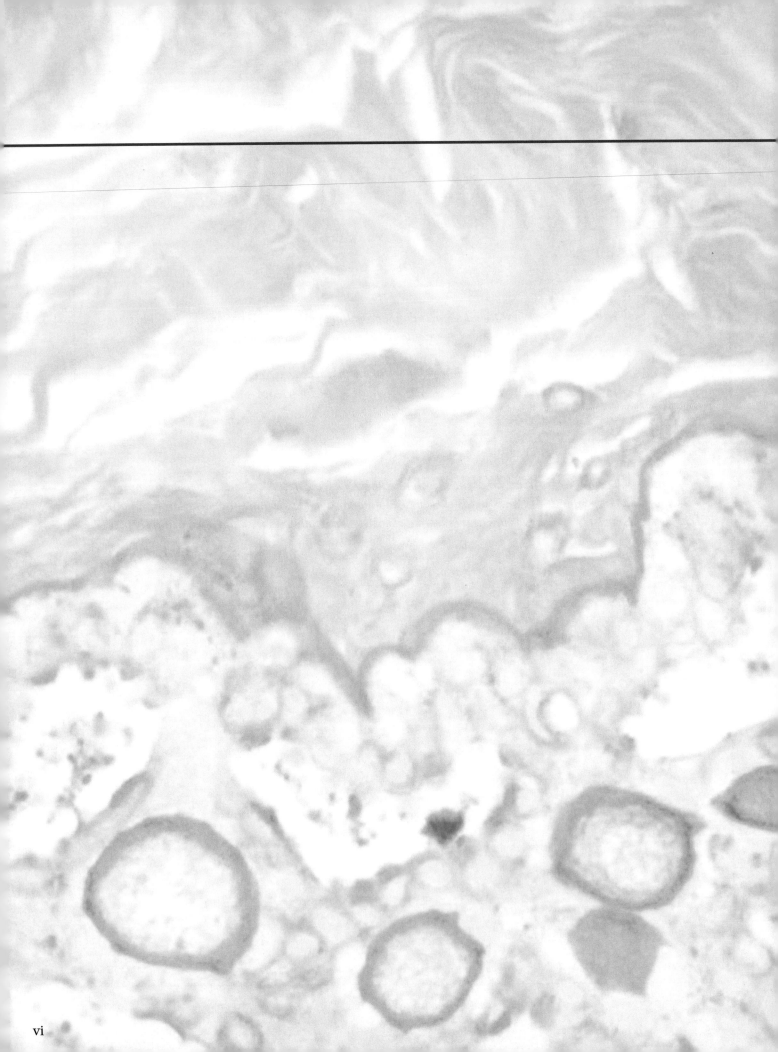

DIAGNOSTIC PATHOLOGY
BREAST

AMIRSYS®

Amirsys, creators of the highly acclaimed radiology series Diagnostic Imaging, proudly introduces its new Diagnostic Pathology series, designed as easy-to-use reference texts for the busy practicing surgical pathologist. Written by world-renowned experts, the series will consist of 15 titles in all the crucial diagnostic areas of surgical pathology.

The newest book in this series, *Diagnostic Pathology: Breast*, contains approximately 550 pages of comprehensive, yet concise, descriptions of more than 90 specific diagnoses. Amirsys's pioneering bulleted format distills pertinent information to the essentials. Each chapter has the same organization providing an easy-to-read reference for making rapid, efficient, and accurate diagnoses in a busy surgical pathology practice. A highlighted Key Facts box provides the essential features of each diagnosis. Detailed sections on Terminology, Etiology/Pathogenesis, Clinical Issues, Macroscopic and Microscopic Findings, and the all important Differential Diagnoses follow so you can find the information you need in the exact same place every time.

Most importantly, every diagnosis features numerous high-quality images, including gross pathology, H&E and immunohistochemical stains, correlative radiographic images, and richly colored graphics, all of which are fully annotated to maximize their illustrative potential.

We believe that this lavishly illustrated series, with its up-to-date information and practical focus, will become the core of your reference collection. Enjoy!

Elizabeth H. Hammond, MD
Executive Editor, Pathology
Amirsys, Inc.

Paula J. Woodward, MD
President
Amirsys Publishing, Inc.

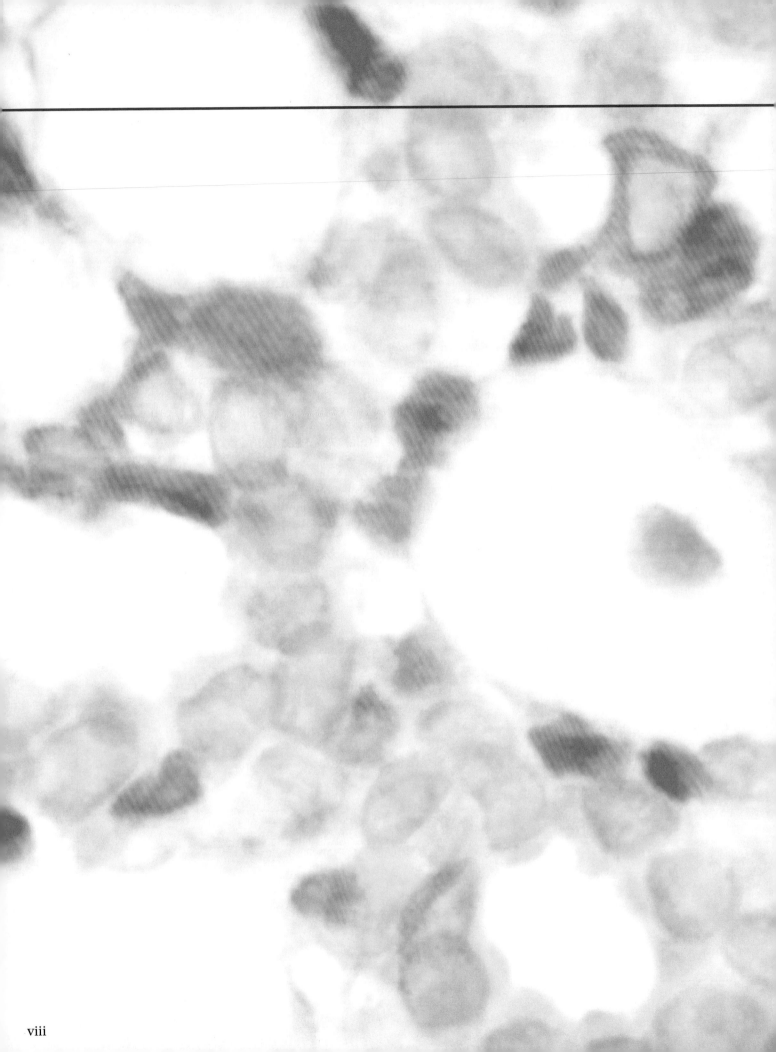

PREFACE

When asked to write a book about the breast as part of the Diagnostic Pathology series from Amirsys, the first question we asked ourselves was, "What can we contribute that hasn't already been done?" There are several breast pathology texts by excellent authors currently in print. As we thought about it, however, valuable resources specific to this project became evident. We both have many years of experience as surgical pathologists and have developed complementary specific areas of expertise. Two authors working closely together are able to maintain a consistent approach and style throughout.

Although we were both convinced we could produce a worthwhile textbook, what first inspired us was the knowledge that our breast pathology book will eventually become part of a larger online diagnostic support tool available to pathologists and clinicians alike—not just a paper book read off a computer screen, but part of a new generation of books that incorporate all the possibilities of computer technology. There is already a longer book with additional illustrations living in cyberspace, and it will be possible to update the eBook version almost instantaneously.

While working on the book, we integrated into almost every chapter the new technologies and molecular approaches rapidly making their way from the basic science laboratory into clinical diagnosis and therapeutic decision-making. We were supported by an excellent team of medical artists, and together we created unique illustrations to illuminate difficult areas in diagnosis and classification. Photographs of cases from both of our institutions and the vast array of images from the publisher's image bank were available.

Preparing this material has been a long and very challenging, but rewarding, process. Dr. Elizabeth Hammond, the executive pathology editor at Amirsys, played a major role in convincing us this was a project we could and should do. We would not have completed the book without the outstanding assistance of the Amirsys staff—especially Dave Chance, Laura Sesto, and Kellie Heap—who guided us through this complicated process with helping hands and gentle humor. We are also tremendously grateful to and would like to acknowledge and thank three extremely dedicated and skilled pathologists' assistants—Laurie Baxter, Lee Ann Kushner, and Kristi Gill who are primarily responsible for the remarkable gross photographs seen throughout the book. Finally, we are grateful to our families whose encouragement, patience, and support helped make this book a reality.

Like seeing a child off to college, it is with some wistfulness that we release our book out into the world at large. However, just as we hope for great things for our children, we trust that this book will live up to our expectations as one of an amazing new generation of textbooks.

David G. Hicks, MD
Professor of Pathology and Laboratory Medicine
Director of the Surgical Pathology Unit
University of Rochester Medical Center
Rochester, NY

Susan C. Lester, MD, PhD
Chief, Breast Pathology Services
Brigham and Women's Hospital
Assistant Professor, Harvard Medical School
Staff Pathologist, Dana Farber Cancer Institute
Boston, MA

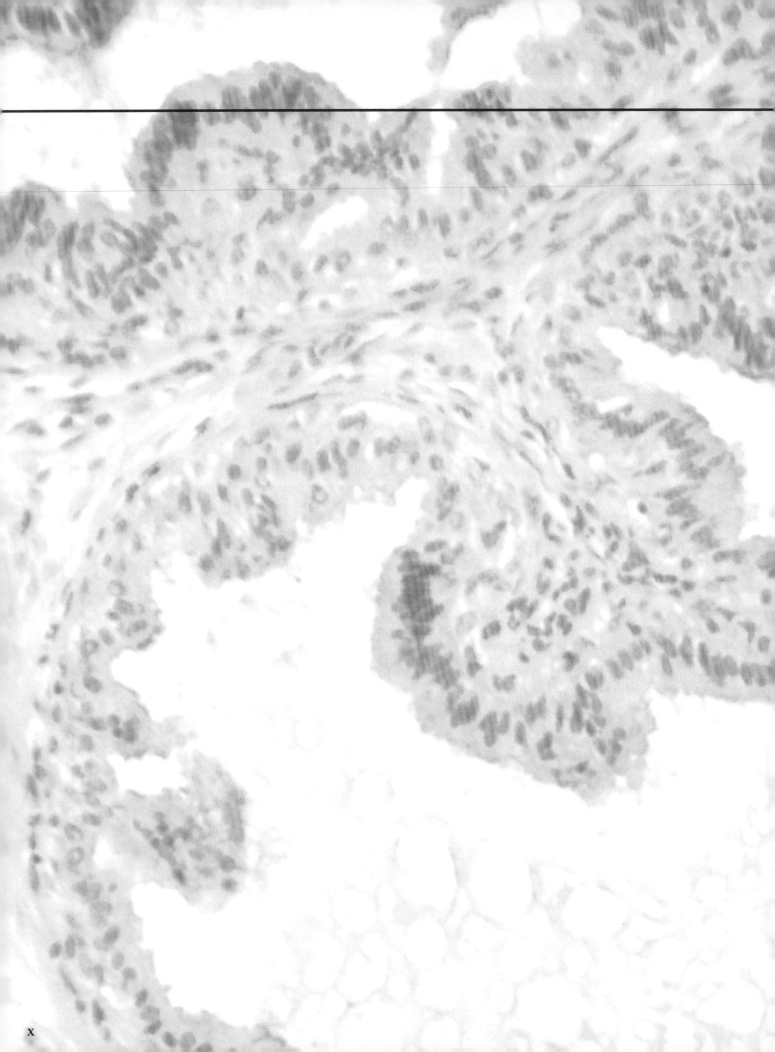

ACKNOWLEDGMENTS

Text Editing

Ashley R. Renlund, MA

Arthur G. Gelsinger, MA

Matthew R. Connelly, MA

Lorna Morring, MS

Alicia M. Moulton, BA

Rebecca L. Hutchinson, BA

Angela M. Green, BA

Image Editing

Jeffrey J. Marmorstone, BS

Lisa A. Magar, BS

Medical Text Editing

Dora M. Lam-Himlin, MD

Nicole Winkler, MD

Illustrations

Laura C. Sesto, MA

Lane R. Bennion, MS

Richard Coombs, MS

Brenda L. McArthur, MA

Art Direction and Design

Laura C. Sesto, MA

Mirjam Ravneng

Assistant Editor

Dave L. Chance, MA

Publishing Lead

Kellie J. Heap, BA

AMIRSYS®

Names you know. Content you trust.®

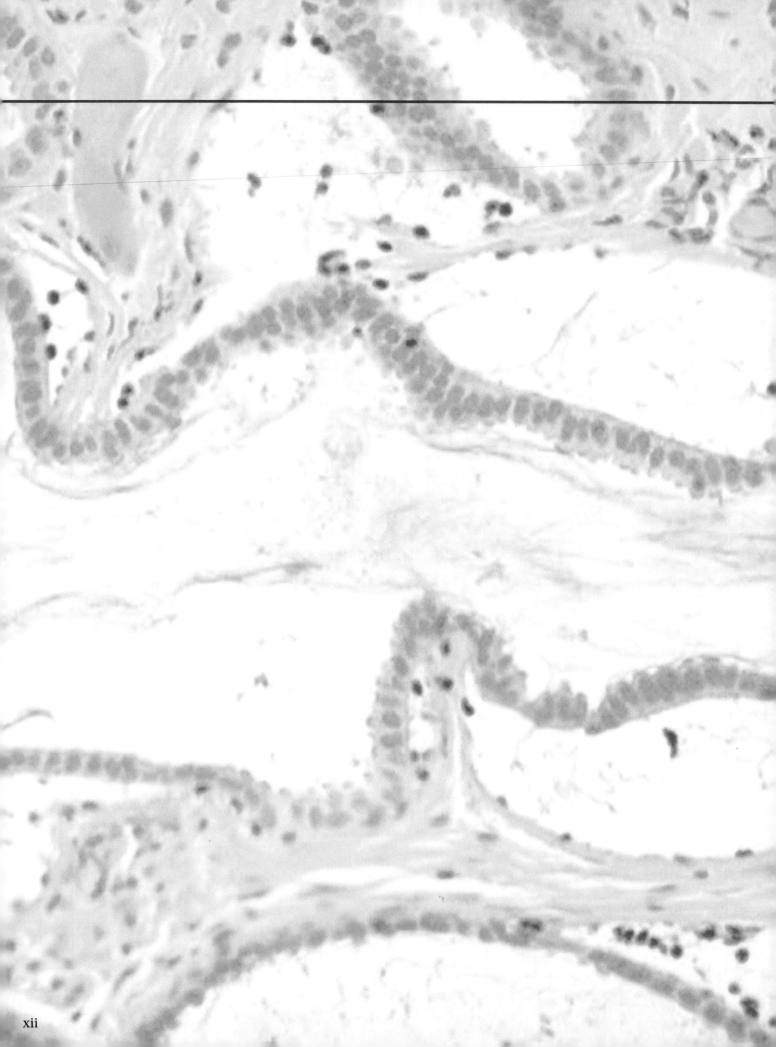

SECTIONS

Normal Breast

Breast Specimens, Processing

Disorders of Development

Benign Epithelial Lesions

Carcinomas

Stromal Lesions

Inflammatory Lesions

Other Types of Malignancies

Reference

TABLE OF CONTENTS

DIAGNOSTIC PATHOLOGY

BREAST

AMIRSYS®

Normal Breast

ANATOMIC STRUCTURE AND LIFECYCLE CHANGES

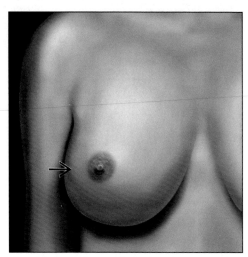

The adult female breast is located on the anterior chest wall, overlying the pectoralis muscles. The normal nipple-areolar complex ➡ is positioned slightly inferior to center.

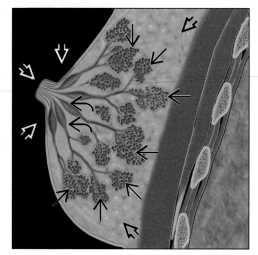

The major breast structures are the nipple-areolar complex ➡, the large duct system ➡, the terminal duct lobular units ➡, which are supported by intralobular stroma, and the interlobular stroma ➡.

NORMAL BREAST

Introduction
- Highly evolved modified skin appendage
  - Defining feature of class Mammalia
- Provides source of nourishment and immunologic protection for newborn
- Unlike other organs, changes over the lifecycle in response to menarche, pregnancy, lactation, and menopause

Embryologic Development
- Stroma differentiates first and induces downgrowth of overlying epithelium
- Milkline extends from axilla to groin
  - In primates, bats, elephants, and manatees, only 2 pectoral breasts normally develop
  - In rare cases, supernumerary nipples &/or breast tissue can develop in other areas along milkline
    - Can enlarge and produce milk during pregnancy and lactation

Gross Anatomy
- Breasts rest on anterior chest wall overlying pectoralis major and minor muscles
- Borders of breast
  - Superior border approximately at 2nd rib; inferior at 6th rib; lateral at mid axillary line; medial at edge of sternum
  - Breast tissue often extends into axilla (tail of Spence)
    - Lesions occurring in this tissue may be difficult to distinguish from diseases involving nodes
  - Deep margin of breast rests on fascia of pectoralis major muscle
- In some women, breast tissue is present in subcutaneous tissue and can extend beyond grossly evident breast borders
  - Mastectomies remove majority of breast tissue but may not remove all epithelial cells

- Suspensory (Cooper) ligaments are fascial attachments to skin and chest wall
  - Attached to both fascia of skin and pectoralis major muscle
  - Provide support and allow for mobility
  - Swelling of breast tissue around these ligaments causes orange peel appearance of skin ("peau d'orange")
  - Carcinoma involving these ligaments results in skin retraction &/or dimpling
- Lymphatic drainage
  - Majority of lymphatic drainage (~ 75%) passes to axilla and initially flows to 1 or 2 sentinel nodes
    - Injection of dye or radioactive tracer to identify these nodes can be performed either adjacent to the carcinoma or more superficially in the breast
    - For women with metastases to nodes, sentinel node is 1st to be involved in > 90% of patients
    - Intramammary nodes can also be involved by metastases but are rarely the sentinel node
  - Less commonly, flow goes to lymphatics, penetrating pectoralis muscles and chest wall
    - Internal mammary nodes or other nodal basins can harbor the sentinel node
    - Abnormal flow patterns may occur when axilla is obstructed by disease
  - Breast lymphatics are present preferentially in superficial location
    - Some, but not all, lymphatics connect with plexus of lymphatics at areola ("Sappey plexus")
    - Dermal lymph-vascular invasion is seen most commonly close to nipple
  - Cutaneous lymphatic anastomoses may account for rare cases of metastases to contralateral breast in absence of distant metastases

Microscopic Anatomy: Introduction
- Breast tissue consists of
  - 2 types of epithelial structures
    - Large ducts

ANATOMIC STRUCTURE AND LIFECYCLE CHANGES

- Terminal duct lobular units
  - 2 types of epithelial cells
    - Luminal cells
    - Myoepithelial cells
  - 2 types of stroma
    - Interlobular stroma
    - Intralobular stroma
- Specific lesions arise in each of these structures

Nipple

- Positioned slightly medial and inferior to center of breast
  - Located at 4th intercostal space in nonpendulous breast
  - Cone-shaped, average height 10-12 mm
- Covered by pigmented squamous epithelium
- May contain cytologically benign cells with clear or pale cytoplasm
  - Toker cells are similar to luminal cells in appearance and immunophenotype
    - Present in majority of nipples if identified by cytokeratin 7 studies
    - Most common next to nipple orifices
    - Must be distinguished from DCIS involving nipple skin (Paget disease)
  - Occasional squamous cells can also have cytoplasmic clearing
    - Intercellular bridges are usually evident
- Keratin-producing squamous cells extend into ducts 1-2 mm
  - Outside of lactation, keratin plug may be present in nipple orifice
- Abrupt transition from squamous cells to normal luminal/myoepithelial lining of ducts
  - If keratin-producing cells extend deeper into duct (squamous metaplasia of lactiferous ducts [SMOLD]), keratin can be trapped, creating an epidermal inclusion cyst
  - If ruptured, subareolar abscesses may result due to intense inflammatory response to keratin spilled into stroma
- Basement membrane of ducts is continuous with basement membrane of skin
  - Surrounds entire ductal/lobular system; separates epithelial cells from breast stroma
    - Consists of type IV collagen and laminin
  - In Paget disease, tumor cells can cross from ductal system into nipple skin without crossing basement membrane
  - Elastic fibers are normally present in varying amounts around mammary ducts, but not lobules
  - With age, supporting structures of major ducts can weaken and allow extravasation of nipple contents
    - Resulting chronic inflammation may cause nipple discharge and periductal fibrosis ("duct ectasia")
- Nipple-areolar complex is supported by a subdermal layer of circumferential smooth muscle
  - Facilitates nipple erection and function during nursing
  - Very rare leiomyomas can arise from this muscle
- Milk secretion occurs through 10-15 major duct orifices opening on surface of nipple
  - Arranged radially in nipple crevices

- Some major ducts may bifurcate beneath nipple
  - Ducts dilate to form lactiferous (milk) sinuses
    - Serve as reservoir for subareolar milk during nursing
    - Sinuses have serrated contour and are supported by smooth muscle, collagen, and elastic fibers
  - Some lesions are specific to nipple
    - Large duct papillomas
    - Duct ectasia
    - Squamous metaplasia of lactiferous ducts (SMOLD)
    - Paget disease of nipple
    - Syringomatous adenoma

Areola

- Lacks pilosebaceous units and hair except at periphery
- Contains numerous sebaceous glands
  - Open through small prominences at periphery of areola and are associated with lactiferous ducts (Montgomery tubercles)
- Numerous sensory nerve endings are present

Large Duct System

- 15-20 major ductal systems emptying at nipple
  - Additional smaller ductal systems open onto areola
- Ducts ramify until they form terminal duct lobular units (TDLUs)
- Ductal systems vary considerably in size and extent
  - Often overlap
  - Rarely confined to single quadrant
  - Size and extent vary greatly in different individuals; location of ductal system cannot be predicted
    - Some large ducts branch and fill widely separated areas of breast
  - Cannot be recognized grossly; requires duct injection or serial section reconstruction in 3 dimensions
  - Anastomoses between ductal systems were reported in 1 study
- Significance for carcinoma
  - DCIS is clonal population that involves a single ductal system
  - Distribution of DCIS generally follows the system
    - e.g., fan-shaped with apex toward nipple
  - Multiple duct systems could be involved in the following situations
    - 2 separate clonal populations of DCIS are present
    - DCIS grows into a 2nd ductal system via one of the reported anastomoses
    - DCIS grows into a 2nd ductal system by crossing into another duct orifice at the nipple

Lobules

- Formed when terminal duct branches into multiple rounded acini
  - Functional unit of breast for milk production
- Lobulocentric architecture (duct surrounded by multiple acini) is important in distinguishing benign lesions that maintain this structure from malignant lesions that do not
- Majority of breast lesions referred to as "ductal" arise from TDLU

ANATOMIC STRUCTURE AND LIFECYCLE CHANGES

○ TDLU can unfold with coalescence of acini to form structures resembling ducts
○ Cysts, epithelial hyperplasia, sclerosing adenosis, and majority of carcinomas are thought to arise from TDLU

Epithelial Cell Types

• 2 types of epithelial cells are present in both ducts and lobules: Luminal cells and myoepithelial cells
  ○ Precursor or stem cells may be present, but special techniques are required for recognition
  ○ Precursor cell is thought to give rise to both cell types
    ▪ Supported by occurrence of benign and malignant tumors composed of both cell types
• Normal ducts and lobules are lined by epithelium that consists of 2-cell layer
  ○ Recognition of normal 2-cell layer is important feature to distinguish benign lesions from invasive carcinoma
• **Luminal cells form innermost cell layer**
  ○ Produce milk in TDLU
    ▪ Luminal cells in large ducts do not undergo lactational changes and do not produce milk
  ○ Some luminal cells extend to basement membrane
  ○ Cuboidal to columnar in shape
    ▪ Nuclei are small, round to oval, and usually have inconspicuous nucleoli
    ▪ Cells have moderate amount of eosinophilic cytoplasm
  ○ Usually express "luminal" low molecular weight keratins 7, 8, 18, 19
    ▪ May also express "basal" keratins
  ○ Some, but not all, luminal cells are positive for ER-α &/or PR at any given time
    ▪ Receptors are not expressed in proliferating cells
    ▪ Positive cells are present in both large duct system and TDLU but may be more frequent in latter
  ○ Express E-cadherin and other catenins
  ○ Some cells are positive for mammaglobin &/or gross cystic disease fluid protein 15 (GCDFP-15)
  ○ Thought to be precursor cell for majority of carcinomas
• **Myoepithelial cells form outer layer on basement membrane**
  ○ Cells form a contractile meshwork that does not cover entire basement membrane
    ▪ In cross section, myoepithelial cell layer is incomplete
  ○ These cells have multiple functions
    ▪ Contract for milk ejection during breastfeeding
    ▪ Help maintain basement membrane
    ▪ Aid in luminal cell polarity
    ▪ Inhibit angiogenesis
  ○ Cells are often flattened with small, round, condensed nuclei
    ▪ Cytoplasm can be more abundant and clear; may mimic lobular neoplasia
    ▪ With age, cells can become prominent and spindled in shape ("myoepithelial atrophy")
  ○ Usually express "basal" high molecular weight keratins 5/6, 14, and 17

▪ May also express "luminal" keratins
○ Express contractile proteins: Actin-sm, calponin, SMHC
○ Also express p63, CD10, P-cadherin, mapsin, as well as other proteins not expressed by luminal cells
  ▪ Do not express ER or PR
○ Myoepithelial cells associated with carcinomas can diminish in number, become displaced from basement membrane, and fail to express some cell-specific markers
○ Complete loss of myoepithelial cells is useful diagnostic feature to recognize invasive carcinomas
  ▪ Microglandular adenosis is only "benign" lesion lacking myoepithelial cells
  ▪ Likely a nonmetastasizing form of invasive carcinoma

Stroma

• Composition depends on patient age, menstrual status, and history of pregnancy and lactation
  ○ Composed of varying amounts of fibroglandular breast tissue and adipose tissue
• **Interlobular stroma surrounds large ducts and TDLUs**
  ○ Responsible for majority of breast volume
  ○ 1/2 of fibroglandular tissue is located in upper outer quadrant
    ▪ Nearly 1/2 of all cancers occur in this area
  ○ Ratio of ductal/fibrous breast tissue to adipose tissue varies between individuals and changes over time
    ▪ Determines mammographic density of breast tissue
    ▪ Increased density makes detection of abnormalities during clinical exam and mammography more difficult
    ▪ Relative proportion of adipose tissue increases with age
  ○ Increase in breast size at puberty is primarily due to increase in interlobular stroma
    ▪ Therefore, there are hormonal influences on this stroma that are not well understood
    ▪ Juvenile hypertrophy is bilateral enlargement of breasts; possibly due to hormonal imbalance
  ○ Cellular components include fibroblasts, myofibroblasts, adipocytes, blood vessels, and lymphatics
    ▪ Majority of fibroblasts and myofibroblasts are CD34 positive
    ▪ Some myofibroblasts are positive for ER &/or PR
  ○ Large multinucleated stromal cells may be due to degenerative changes
  ○ Some lesions of this stroma also occur outside of breast
    ▪ Lipomas and angiolipomas
    ▪ Myofibroblastomas (but most common in breast)
    ▪ Nodular fasciitis (less common in breast)
    ▪ Desmoid fibromatosis
    ▪ Angiosarcomas (most common in breast, other types of sarcomas very rare)
  ○ Other stromal lesions are specific to breast
    ▪ Pseudoangiomatous stromal hyperplasia (PASH)
• **Intralobular stroma surrounds acini in TDLU**

- Looser, more cellular appearance compared to interlobular stroma
- Often has scattering of lymphocytes and plasma cells
- May be myxoid in appearance
- Lesions of this stroma are biphasic (include both stroma and epithelial cells)
  - Fibroadenomas
  - Phyllodes tumors

BREAST DEVELOPMENTAL CHANGES

Childhood and Puberty
- At birth, breast consists of nipple and large ducts
  - Infants, especially breastfed infants, can transiently produce milk under influence of maternal hormones ("witch's milk")
- At puberty in females, main mammary ducts branch, giving rise to terminal duct buds
  - Precursors of future TDLUs
- Connective tissue elements proliferate
  - Adipose cells proliferate and extend into subcutaneous tissue
  - Periductal stromal tissue and vascular supply proliferates
- Tanner phases of pubertal breast development
  - Phase 1
    - Nipple elevation but no palpable glandular tissue
  - Phase 2
    - Mound of nipple and breast tissue projects from chest wall
    - Palpable tissue present in subareolar region
  - Phase 3
    - Increased glandular tissue elements
    - Increased areolar size with development of pigmentation
  - Phase 4
    - Development of separate nipple-areolar complex and secondary mound anterior to breast tissue
  - Phase 5
    - Final adolescent development, smooth breast contour
- At puberty in males, breast usually does not develop beyond a rudimentary large duct system
  - Lobules are only very rarely present
  - 2/3 of males may experience some degree of breast enlargement (gynecomastia) that does not persist

Menstrual Cycle Changes
- Proliferative phase of menstrual cycle
  - Early breast changes prior to ovulation (days 3-14)
    - Increased in ovarian estrogen production
    - Mammary lobules are relatively quiescent
    - Decreased stromal density
    - Decreased breast volume and water content
    - Breast MR examination should be scheduled during early phase of cycle
- Secretory phase of menstrual cycle
  - Later breast changes after ovulation (days 15-28)
    - Due to estrogen production with increased progesterone levels (luteal phase)

- Proliferation of mammary ductal epithelium, increased number of acini
- Increased stromal density (edema)
- Increased breast volume and water content
- Some women may experience symptoms due to increased interlobular fluid and epithelial proliferation
- Menstruation
  - Decreasing estrogen and progesterone levels
    - Regression of lobules and disappearance of stromal edema

Pregnancy-related Changes
- With onset of pregnancy, breast tissue becomes fully mature and functional
  - Lobules progressively increase in number and size
- Early pregnancy changes
  - Generalized breast enlargement
    - Marked ductal and lobular proliferation
    - Increase in number of lobules and acinar units within each lobule
  - Increased nipple-areolar complex pigmentation
    - Montgomery tubercles (sebaceous glands of areola) become prominent; appear as rounded papules on skin surface
    - Function in nipple lubrication during breastfeeding
- Later pregnancy changes
  - Progressive stimulation of lobular proliferation
    - Cytoplasm of luminal cells becomes vacuolated
    - Stimulation of secretion into expanded TDLU acini
  - Increase in stromal fat elements

Lactation-related Changes
- Postpartum enlargement of breast due to distension of lobular acini and accumulation of colostrum
  - Luminal cells show cytoplasmic vacuolization with bulbous or "hobnail" projections into acini
  - Milk production occurs in TDLU and is transferred to nipple via large duct system
- Luminal cells of large ducts do not undergo secretory changes
- Milk ejection reflex ("let-down") is mediated by oxytocin, which causes myoepithelial cell contraction

Lesions Related to Pregnancy &/or Lactation
- Lactational change with psammoma body calcifications
  - Lobules can undergo sporadic lactational change in absence of pregnancy or other hormonal triggers
  - Sometimes associated with prominent large psammoma body calcifications
  - Can form a cluster of calcifications that appears suspicious by mammography
- Lactational adenoma
  - Presents as palpable circumscribed mass during pregnancy or lactation
  - May wax and wane in size with breastfeeding
  - Consists of normal-appearing lactational tissue
    - More likely a hyperplasia than a neoplasia
- Lactational abscess

ANATOMIC STRUCTURE AND LIFECYCLE CHANGES

- o Lactation is most common period for breast infections
- o Cracks in nipple can lead to infection by skin bacteria
- o *Staphylococcus* species are most common bacterial cause, followed by *Streptococci*
- o Usually adequately treated with antibiotics and expression of milk
- Galactocele
  - o Presents as palpable mass
  - o Rupture of ducts leads to extravasation of milk into stroma
  - o Milk causes chronic inflammatory response
- Infarction of benign lesions
  - o High rate of proliferation during 1st 2 trimesters
    - Benign lesions, such as fibroadenomas, can grow in size and may infarct
  - o Mitoses and necrosis can mimic malignant changes in benign lesions
    - Possibility of pregnancy should always be considered before making diagnosis of malignancy
- Bloody nipple discharge
  - o May occur during pregnancy
  - o Likely related to rapid tissue remodeling and growth
- Carcinoma diagnosed during pregnancy
  - o Very rare: In only 1 of 3,000-10,000 pregnancies is cancer diagnosed during or within 1st year after delivery
  - o Often presents at a higher stage due to delay in diagnosis
  - o Increased risk of cancer persists for a period of time after pregnancy; longer length for older individuals
    - Possibly related to profound stromal changes and remodeling during pregnancy and post-pregnancy involution
    - Similar gene expression pattern as in wound healing
    - May facilitate rapid progression from in situ to invasive carcinoma, growth of invasive carcinoma, &/or metastasis
  - o Over longer period of time, risk of carcinoma decreases
    - Thought to be due to terminal differentiation of milk-producing epithelial cells, reducing potential pool of precursor cells
  - o For young pregnant women (late teens to early 20s), protective effects outweigh increased risk
    - Reduces lifetime risk of ER-positive cancer by about 1/2
    - Additional pregnancies further decrease risk (~ 7%)
  - o For older pregnant women (35 and above), increased risk is greater than benefit

Post-Lactation Changes

- Enlarged lobules developed during pregnancy and lactation undergo involution and regression
  - o Involution usually proceeds unevenly and takes months
  - o Involuting lobules are infiltrated by lymphocytes and plasma cells

- Increase in periductal and perivascular stromal connective tissue
- Lobules do not completely regress and remain increased in size compared to nulliparous women

Menopause-related Changes

- Decreased hormonal stimulation affects epithelium and stroma
  - o Progressive atrophy and involution
    - Myoepithelial cells become more prominent and spindled in shape ("myoepithelial atrophy")
  - o Reduction in size and complexity of TDLU
    - In older women, only ducts may remain
  - o Loss of specialized intralobular stroma
  - o Generalized fatty replacement of breast parenchyma
    - Breast tissue becomes less dense on mammography
- Postmenopausal hormone replacement therapy stimulates breast tissue
  - o May lead to increase in mammographic density

BREAST IMAGING

Nipple-Areolar Complex

- Nipple usually everted
  - o Seen in profile in standard mammographic views
  - o New nipple inversion requires search for subareolar pathology
- Subareolar region is normally hypervascular secondary to ductal and vascular network
  - o May intensely enhance on MR

Breast Parenchyma

- Mammography
  - o Fibrous tissue appears white, adipose tissue black
    - Normal breast tissue is a mixture of both and has a gray textured appearance
    - Majority of breast lesions replace adipose tissue and thus appear white
  - o Calcifications are radiodense and appear white
    - Scattered calcifications are frequent finding in normal breasts
    - Calcifications associated with malignancy are usually numerous, clustered, variable in size and shape, and may increase over time
    - Calcifications that appear to outline ductal system (linear and branching) are often associated with either DCIS or duct ectasia
  - o Normal TDLUs are ordinarily not visible
  - o Dilated ducts may be seen in subareolar region
    - Isolated peripheral dilated ducts merit careful evaluation for possible obstructing mass
  - o Fibrous tissue is replaced by adipose tissue with age in most women
    - Mammography increases in sensitivity with age as it is easier to detect masses and calcifications without obscuring fibrous tissue
    - Breast density on mammography is a risk factor for carcinoma most likely because it is a marker of the number of potential precursor cells in ducts and lobules

ANATOMIC STRUCTURE AND LIFECYCLE CHANGES

Anatomic Structures and Associated Lesions

Anatomic Structure	Function	Inflammatory Lesions	Hyperplasias/Tumors
Nipple/areola	Milk ejection	Squamous metaplasia of lactiferous ducts (SMOLD)	Nipple adenoma, leiomyoma, syringomatous adenoma, Paget disease
Large duct system	Conduit for milk	Duct ectasia	Papilloma, encapsulated papillary carcinoma
Terminal duct lobular unit (TDLU)	Luminal cells: Milk production; myoepithelial cells: Contraction for milk ejection	Cysts (rupture), granulomatous lobular mastitis, lymphocytic mastopathy	Epithelial hyperplasia, sclerosing adenosis, carcinoma
Interlobular stroma	Size and shape of breast	Fat necrosis, bacterial infections	Lipoma, angiolipoma, hemangioma, fibromatosis, nodular fasciitis, fibrous tumors, myofibroblastoma, pseudoangiomatous stromal hyperplasia, sarcoma
Intralobular stroma	Support of TDLU	Granulomatous lobular mastitis, lymphocytic mastopathy	Fibroadenoma, phyllodes tumor

Cell Types of the Breast

Cell Types	Function	Markers	Lesions
Luminal cells	TDLU: Milk production, conduit for milk	Luminal keratins 8, 18, E-cadherin, ER, PR	Epithelial hyperplasia, atypical ductal hyperplasia, majority of carcinomas
Myoepithelial cells	Contraction for milk ejection, support of basement membrane, maintenance of luminal cell polarity	Basal keratins 5/6, 14, 17, P-cadherin, muscle markers, p63, CD10	Myoepitheliomas, possible subset of triple negative carcinomas
Stromal fibroblasts and myofibroblasts	Support of epithelial cells, majority of breast volume	CD34 (majority), muscle markers (subset), ER/PR (subset)	Pseudoangiomatous stromal hyperplasia, fibrous tumors, desmoid fibromatosis, myofibroblastoma, fibroadenoma/phyllodes tumors

- Risk is not associated with breast size; large breasts are often composed predominantly of adipose tissue
- Density is increased with postmenopausal hormone replacement therapy
- Ultrasound
  - Different tissue types have characteristic echogenicity
    - Hyperechoic: Adipose tissue
    - Hypoechoic: Solid masses without adipose tissue
    - Anechoic: Fluid-filled cysts
  - Ducts frequently visible as linear, branching, hypo- to isoechoic channels
  - Dilated ducts may be seen during menopause and pregnancy
  - TDLUs on occasion may be visible
  - Normal heterogeneity of breast can be difficult to distinguish from discrete mass-forming lesions
    - Ultrasound is often most helpful to further characterize lesions detected by mammography, MR, or physical exam
- MR
  - Fibroglandular tissues appear white and adipose tissue black on fat-suppressed sequences
    - Appearance without contrast is insufficiently sensitive to identify malignancies
  - Contrast injection is used to determine rate and degree of enhancement
    - Kinetic enhancement curve is used in conjunction with morphology to improve specificity
    - Normal breast and benign lesions typically enhance slowly
    - Malignant lesions typically enhance rapidly
  - Enhancement varies with age and phase of menstrual cycle

SELECTED REFERENCES

1. Hilson JB et al: Phenotypic alterations in ductal carcinoma in situ-associated myoepithelial cells: biologic and diagnostic implications. Am J Surg Pathol. 33(2):227-32, 2009
2. Pan WR et al: A three-dimensional analysis of the lymphatics of a bilateral breast specimen: a human cadaveric study. Clin Breast Cancer. 9(2):86-91, 2009
3. Russo J et al: Full-term pregnancy induces a specific genomic signature in the human breast. Cancer Epidemiol Biomarkers Prev. 17(1):51-66, 2008
4. Suami H et al: The lymphatic anatomy of the breast and its implications for sentinel lymph node biopsy: a human cadaver study. Ann Surg Oncol. 15(3):863-71, 2008
5. Rusby JE et al: Breast duct anatomy in the human nipple: three-dimensional patterns and clinical implications. Breast Cancer Res Treat. 106(2):171-9, 2007
6. Böcker W et al: Common adult stem cells in the human breast give rise to glandular and myoepithelial cell lineages: a new cell biological concept. Lab Invest. 82(6):737-46, 2002
7. Russo J et al: Pattern of distribution of cells positive for estrogen receptor alpha and progesterone receptor in relation to proliferating cells in the mammary gland. Breast Cancer Res Treat. 53(3):217-27, 1999
8. Longacre TA et al: A correlative morphologic study of human breast and endometrium in the menstrual cycle. Am J Surg Pathol. 10(6):382-93, 1986

ANATOMIC STRUCTURE AND LIFECYCLE CHANGES

Nipple Structure

(Left) The nipple-areolar complex is covered by a pigmented squamous epithelium ➡ and contains sebaceous glands (Montgomery tubercles ➡). During lactation, milk is produced in the lobules ➡ and is transported via ducts ➡ that lead to the nipple orifices ➡. *(Right)* Keratin-producing cells ➡ dip down into the nipple orifice 1-3 mm, and a keratin plug may be present. There is an abrupt transition to the normal 2-cell layer of the large duct system ➡.

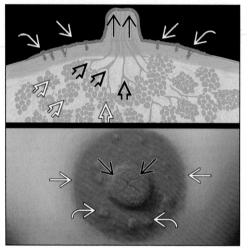

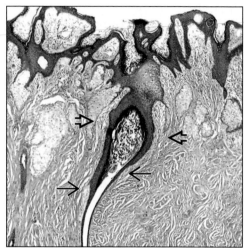

(Left) Toker cells are normal components of nipple skin and are most commonly seen next to duct orifices. The cells have abundant pale cytoplasm ➡ and bland nuclei. Although most commonly present as single cells, clusters and acini may be present. *(Right)* Using IHC, Toker cells are identified in > 80% of nipples. Like luminal cells, they are positive for cytokeratin 7 ➡ as well as other low molecular weight keratins. They are also frequently positive for ER and PR.

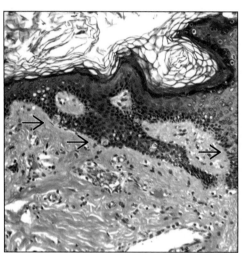

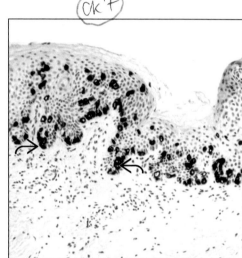

CK 7

(Left) Some of the keratinocytes in nipple skin have cleared out cytoplasm ➡. Spinous processes can be seen ➡. These cells are scattered throughout the thickness of the epidermis. In contrast, Toker cells are preferentially found in the basal portion of the epidermis. *(Right)* The nipple ducts connect with the lactiferous sinuses ➡ at the nipple base. The sinuses serve as reservoirs for milk and are compressed by the suckling infant's mouth, which aids in milk ejection.

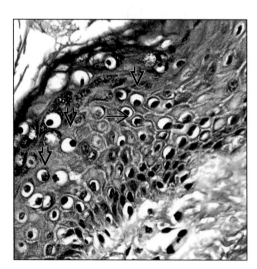

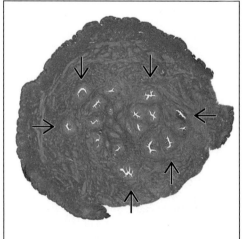

ANATOMIC STRUCTURE AND LIFECYCLE CHANGES

Terminal Duct Lobular Unit (TDLU)

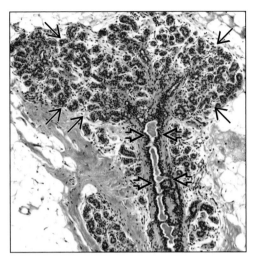

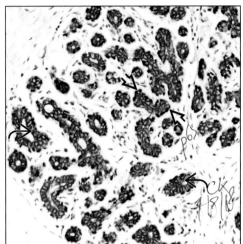

(Left) TDLUs have an architectural organization similar to a tree if the trunk and branches were hollow. The terminal duct ("trunk") ➔ opens into the acini ("branches") ➔ of the lobule. This "lobulocentric" organization is a key microscopic feature in recognizing normal breast structure. *(Right)* There are 2 types of epithelial cells. Luminal cells express keratins 7, 8, and 18 (red cytoplasmic chromogen ➔). Myoepithelial cells express p63 ➔ (brown nuclear chromogen).

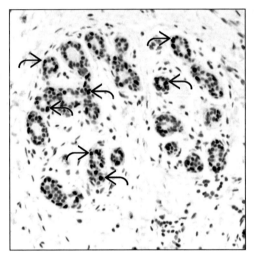

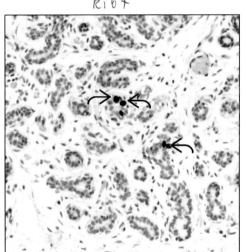

(Left) Not all luminal cells express ER ➔. The content of ER and PR in the normal luminal cells varies with the degree of lobular development, in parallel with cell proliferation. *(Right)* Proliferation is an important part of the growth and development of breast tissue. Scattered Ki-67(+) cells ➔ can be found in the normal TDLU; however, these proliferating cells are negative for ER. Different populations of luminal cells within the breast may interact in a paracrine fashion.

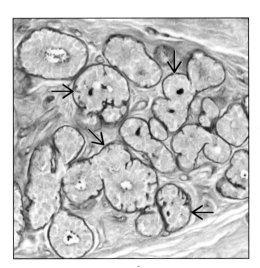

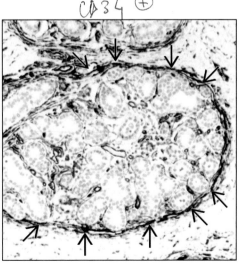

(Left) The basement membrane surrounding the ducts and lobules contains type IV collagen and laminin and appears as a bright pink layer on Alcian blue/PAS staining ➔. This basement membrane is contiguous with that of the large ducts and skin. *(Right)* The TDLU has a specialized intralobular stroma enveloping the acini and consisting of CD34(+) stromal fibroblasts ➔ and capillaries. Lesions arising from this stroma (fibroadenomas and phyllodes tumors) are biphasic.

1

ANATOMIC STRUCTURE AND LIFECYCLE CHANGES

Lifecycle Changes

(Left) During embryologic development, the stroma is the 1st breast tissue to specialize. The overlying epithelium is induced to grow downward and form the large ducts.
(Right) Prior to puberty in females and lifelong in males, the breast consists of large ducts and terminal end buds in a loose cellular stroma. This pattern is characteristic of gynecomastia in men, juvenile hyperplasia in women (diffusely present in both breasts), and gynecomastoid hyperplasia in women (focal mass).

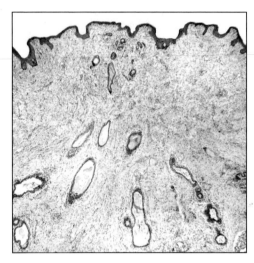 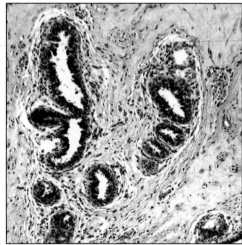

(Left) The breast tissue of most young women is very radiodense (white) due to the predominance of fibrous tissue over adipose tissue. Breast density lowers the sensitivity of mammography as it is difficult to detect calcifications or mass-forming lesions in a background of dense tissue.
(Right) At puberty in women, terminal end buds give rise to acini and form lobules surrounded by specialized stroma. The interlobular stroma also increases in quantity to form the bulk of the breast.

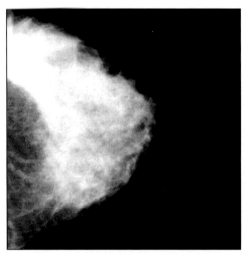 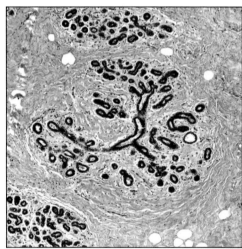

(Left) During lactation, the breasts can appear nodular and dense with a coarse pattern. Mammography should be performed immediately after expression of milk, which will decrease the density.
(Right) During the 1st trimester of pregnancy, epithelial cells proliferate rapidly, and there is a great expansion in both size ⊡ and number of lobules compared to the pre-pregnancy state ➔. The acini dilate and the cells undergo secretory changes in preparation for lactation.

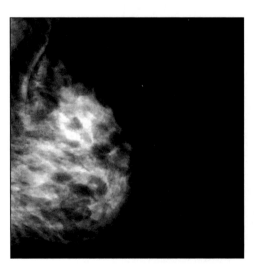 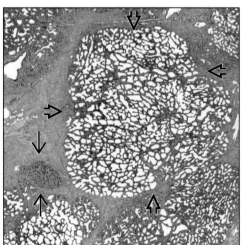

ANATOMIC STRUCTURE AND LIFECYCLE CHANGES

Pregnancy-related Changes

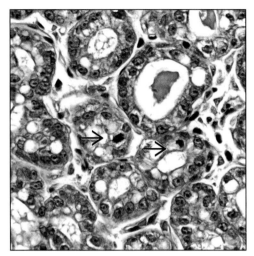

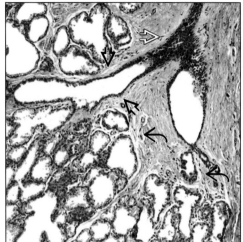

(Left) During pregnancy, the luminal cytoplasm becomes vacuolated and the nuclei enlarge with prominent nucleoli. Mitoses are frequent ➡, particularly in the 1st trimester. Myoepithelial cells become inconspicuous. *(Right)* The large duct system ⇨ can be distinguished from the TDLU ➡ because lactational changes occur in only the luminal cells of the TDLU. There is an abrupt transition ⇨ in the terminal duct.

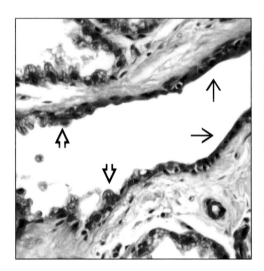

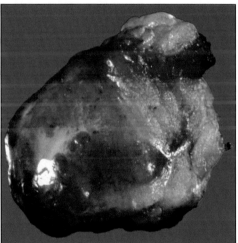

(Left) Only the luminal cells of the TDLU undergo lactational change ⇨ and produce milk. The luminal cells of the large duct system are not milk producing ➡. The biologic reason for this different response to hormones is unknown. *(Right)* Lactational adenomas can form circumscribed masses during pregnancy and lactation. These masses consist of normal-appearing breast tissue and likely represent focal hyperplasias rather than neoplasias.

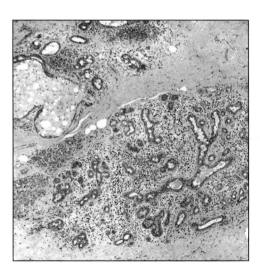

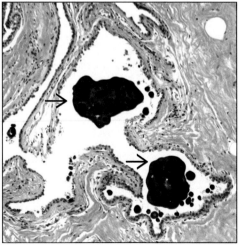

(Left) At the end of lactation, the lobules regress. A prominent lymphocytic infiltrate surrounds the lobules. The lobules do not regress back to the pre-pregnancy state. *(Right)* Lactational changes can occur sporadically in lobules not related to pregnancy or exogenous hormone use. These changes are sometimes associated with multiple psammoma body calcifications ➡ and are detected as clusters of calcifications on mammography.

ANATOMIC STRUCTURE AND LIFECYCLE CHANGES

Involution

(Left) With increasing age, the breast becomes composed of a greater proportion of radiolucent (dark) adipose tissue. This facilitates the detection of radiodense calcifications and masses by mammographic screening. *(Right)* During involution of the breast, the lobules and the specialized lobular stroma begin to disappear. Eventually, only small terminal ducts ➡ are present. The interlobular stroma becomes less fibrous and more fatty, making the breast more radiolucent.

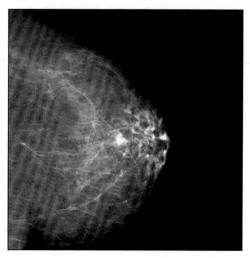 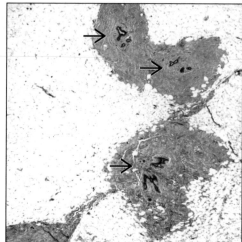

(Left) In an atrophic lobule, the myoepithelial cells and basement membranes become more prominent and the luminal cells regress. The myoepithelial cells sometimes appear spindled in shape. *(Right)* In the aging breast, occluded ducts may recanalize, forming the pattern of "mastitis obliterans." A prior duct is ringed by smaller glandular structures. The appearance resembles recanalization of a thrombus in a blood vessel.

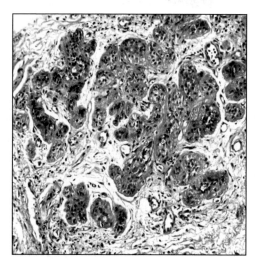 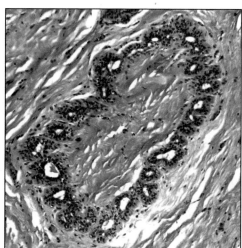

(Left) Large regressing lobules resemble sclerosing adenosis. However, the luminal cells appear small and shrunken, and the basement membranes are prominent. *(Right)* Calcified blood vessels have a characteristic "train track" pattern on mammography and rarely are the source of suspicious clustered calcifications. This finding is common in women over 60 years of age and rare in women younger than 40.

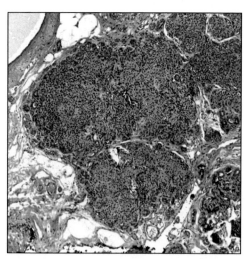 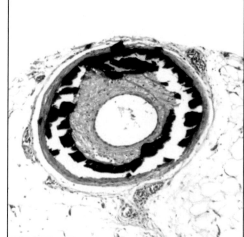

ANATOMIC STRUCTURE AND LIFECYCLE CHANGES

Normal Cells of the Breast

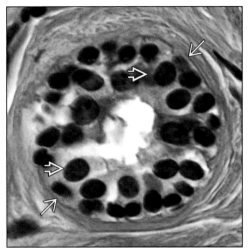

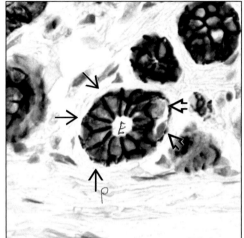

(Left) In normal breast there are 2 cell types. The innermost luminal cells produce milk in the lobules and provide a conduit for milk in the ducts ➡. The outer myoepithelial cells support the basement membrane, maintain polarity of the luminal cells, and contract for milk ejection ➡. (Right) Luminal cells express the cell adhesion protein E-cadherin in a membrane pattern ➡. In contrast, myoepithelial cells are negative ➡ as they express a related protein, P-cadherin.

D2-40 +

SMA

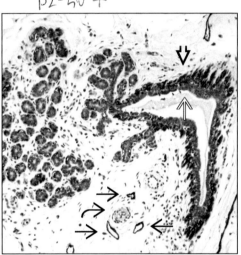

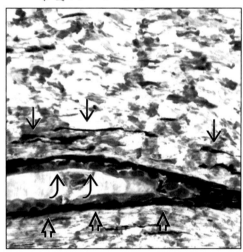

(Left) Lymphatics are positive for podoplanin (D2-40) and are seen here in a characteristic arrangement ➡ surrounding a small arteriole ➡. Myoepithelial cells are often positive for this marker ➡, whereas luminal cells are not ➡. (Right) Myofibroblasts are stromal spindle cells that are often positive for muscle markers such as smooth muscle actin ➡. Myoepithelial cells are also contractile and positive for the same markers ➡. Luminal cells are negative ➡.

CD 34

ER - PR

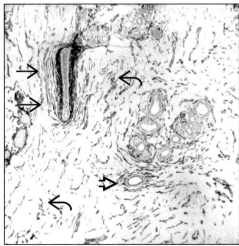

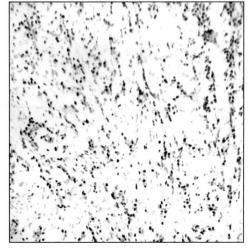

(Left) Many stromal fibroblasts are positive for CD34 ➡, and their numbers may be increased around epithelial structures ➡ or in benign lesions such as sclerosing adenosis. Endothelial cells are also positive for this marker ➡. (Right) Some stromal myofibroblasts are positive for ER &/or PR, as is the smooth muscle of the areola. The tumors arising from these cells, myofibroblastoma and leiomyomas, are also hormone receptor positive.

Breast Specimens, Processing

Checklists for the Examination of Breast Cancer Specimens

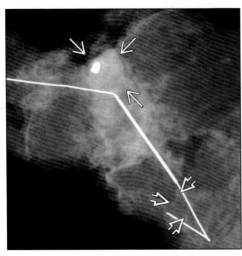

The specimen radiograph is an important guide for specimen processing. In this case, targeted calcifications ⇥ are near the wire tip. An incidental calcified fibroadenoma ➜ is also present.

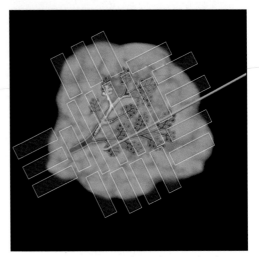

Specimen processing is directed toward adequate sampling to identify the lesion that prompted the biopsy, to find incidental carcinomas, and to evaluate the margins, when appropriate.

COMMUNICATION BETWEEN SURGEONS AND PATHOLOGISTS

Requisition Forms
- Should include information important for optimal processing and interpretation of specimen

Specimen Labeling
- Type of specimen must be clearly indicated

Orientation
- Specimens must have adequate orientation in order to identify sites of possible margin involvement

Specimen Radiography
- Excisions of radiographic lesions must be imaged before transfer to pathology department

INTRAOPERATIVE CONSULTATIONS

Primary Diagnosis
- Frozen sections are > 95% accurate for diagnosis of invasive carcinoma
  - There is a small possibility of error, particularly for small carcinomas and carcinoma in situ
- Frozen sections should not be performed for primary diagnosis except in rare circumstances
  - Technique is limited: Able to freeze only small amount of tissue, ice crystal artifact, loss of nuclear detail, uneven sectioning, and possible tissue loss
  - Should never be performed if entire lesion is frozen; risk to patient of not having an accurate diagnosis outweighs any value of intraoperative diagnosis
  - Should not be performed unless patient has consented to additional surgery based on findings

Margins
- Radiologic margins

  - If patient has prior history of cancer associated with a radiologic finding, specimen radiograph can be used as guide to margin or margins closest to cancer
  - However, DCIS at margins is rarely visualized by radiography
- Gross evaluation
  - Gross distance of palpable cancers to margins can be determined
  - DCIS is rarely grossly apparent and may be present at margins in grossly normal-appearing tissue
- Microscopic evaluation by frozen section
  - Very difficult to evaluate breast specimen margins by frozen section
  - Negative results do not preclude positive margins found by additional sampling for permanent sections
- Microscopic evaluation by touch preparations
  - Margins can be evaluated by scraping specimen surfaces
  - Only evaluate surface for positive margins; close margins are not identified
  - May be of value at centers where only positive margins undergo reexcision

Lymph Node Evaluation: Frozen Section
- Sentinel nodes may undergo intraoperative evaluation if surgeon will complete an axillary dissection if results are positive
- Nodes are carefully dissected away from each other and counted
  - Number of nodes is very important for prognosis and for determining likelihood of additional nodal involvement
  - Each node is thinly sliced and completely frozen
    - Most common source of false-negative results is failure to freeze all slices
  - All macrometastases can be identified by this method

- Additional micrometastases and isolated tumor cells may be seen in additional levels evaluated by permanent section

Lymph Node Evaluation: Touch Preparations

- Nodes are identified as described above and thinly sectioned
- Cut surfaces of each node are scraped and used for touch preparations
- Size of metastasis cannot be determined with certainty

SPECIMEN RADIOGRAPHY

Core Needle Biopsies

- Cores should be radiographed to document that representative calcifications have been removed
  - Cores with calcifications are generally identified separately from cores without calcifications

Wire Localized Excisions

- Specimen must be radiographed to ensure that targeted lesion has been removed
  - Radiologist should issue a report stating whether targeted lesion has been removed
- Copy of radiograph and radiologist's report should be available to pathologist
- **Mammographically guided excisions**
  - Lesions are associated with specific types of pathologic diagnoses
  - Irregular mass
    - 97% invasive carcinoma
    - 2% surgical or trauma-related scarring
    - 1% rare lesions, such as radial sclerosing lesion, fibromatosis, granular cell tumor
  - Circumscribed or lobulated mass
    - 65% fibroadenoma
    - 20% cysts or clusters of cysts
    - 9% other benign lesions, such as nodular sclerosing adenosis, myofibroblastoma, hamartoma, angiolipoma
    - 3% DCIS (intracystic DCIS, DCIS involving a fibroadenoma, DCIS with surrounding stromal fibrosis)
    - 3% invasive carcinoma (especially medullary, mucinous, solid lobular, and triple negative types)
  - Ill-defined mass: May have actual ill-defined margins or may have margins obscured by adjacent fibrous tissue
    - 20% fibroadenoma
    - 15% invasive carcinoma
    - 2% DCIS
    - 63% other benign lesions
  - Calcifications
    - Radiologically suspicious calcifications are clustered, linear, or segmental with amorphous or pleomorphic morphology
    - Many additional nonsuspicious calcifications can be seen radiographically
    - Thus it is essential to be certain that the suspicious radiologic calcifications are sampled for microscopic examination

- 75% benign due to apocrine cysts, sclerosing adenosis, hyalinized fibroadenomas
- 20% DCIS
- 5% invasive carcinoma; generally small (< 1 cm)
  - Architectural distortion
    - Change in texture of breast as compared to other areas, contralateral breast, or over time
    - 33% diffusely invasive carcinoma, especially lobular carcinoma
    - 33% DCIS
    - 33% benign changes
- **Ultrasound-guided excisions**
  - Performed for mass-forming lesions
    - Lesion is usually evident on gross examination
  - Often used to evaluate lesions initially detected by clinical palpation, mammography, or MR
  - 25-50% are carcinoma with majority invasive carcinomas
  - Presence of lesion may be confirmed by radiologist using US
    - An image is generally not provided to pathologist
- **MR-guided excisions**
  - Difficult to perform due to need for open coil and special equipment
  - Lesions are visualized due to vascular uptake of a contrast agent
    - Excised specimens cannot be imaged using same method
    - Lesions are typically small and not grossly evident
  - Correlation of appearance with pathologic findings is generally low
    - Irregular mass: 18% invasive carcinoma, 10% DCIS, 16% fibroadenoma, 56% other benign lesions
    - Circumscribed mass: 11% invasive carcinoma, 3% DCIS, 43% fibroadenoma, 43% other benign lesions
    - Linear/clumped enhancement: 5% invasive carcinoma, 19% DCIS, 12% fibroadenoma, 64% other benign lesions
- **Excisions with > 1 wire**
  - Multiple wires may be used to mark multiple lesions or single lesion that extends over large area
    - Extensive calcifications
    - Large area of architectural distortion
  - If multiple separate lesions are present, distance between lesions should be recorded and tissue between lesion sampled
  - If lesion extends over large area, all tissue should be sampled when practical

Mastectomies

- Generally not sent for radiologic examination by surgeon
  - Radiologic examination prior to processing can be very helpful in the following circumstances
    - Suspicious radiologic lesions that have not been previously biopsied
    - Prior core needle biopsy or biopsies for nonpalpable cancers now marked by clip(s)
    - Post neoadjuvant cancers with marked or complete imaging response, now marked by clip(s)

GENERAL CONSIDERATIONS

FIXATION

Transport to Pathology Department
- Should occur as rapidly as possible
- Tissue can be transported without fixation if within 1-2 hours
  - Preferred if frozen sections, flow cytometry, some types of molecular studies, bacterial culture, or tissue banking are planned
- Intact specimens can be placed into formalin if longer time to specimen processing is anticipated
  - Formalin penetrates tissues slowly
  - Outer surfaces of specimens are often cauterized, which creates a barrier to diffusion
  - Inner portions of specimen will not be fixed for many hours
  - In some cases, surgeon may ink specimen and bisect it to allow better fixation, if necessary, for long transport times
- Optimal fixation is required for histologic detail, preservation of antigenic markers (e.g., ER, PR, and HER2), and preservation of other biomarkers

Ischemic Time
- Tissue starts to deteriorate as soon as it is excised
- Ischemic time is defined as length of time from blood supply being cut off to the time sliced tissue is placed into fixative
- Prolonged ischemic time (> 1 hour) can have deleterious effects on studies for DNA, mRNA, and protein
- Ischemic time should be minimized whenever possible
  - It is helpful to document unusually long ischemic times to help with interpretation of molecular studies
  - If results are negative for such specimens, it may be appropriate to use other specimens for analysis
- Ischemic time does not end when intact specimen is placed in fixative
- Ischemic time ends when sliced specimen is placed into fixative

Fixation Time
- Defined as time from tissue being placed into formalin to time processing begins in preparation for paraffin embedding
- 10% neutral buffered (phosphate) formalin is recommended
  - Crosslinking occurs, which inhibits deterioration
  - Optimal fixation time is at least 6 hours to 72 hours or more
    - Shorter fixation times result in suboptimal antigen preservation for IHC
    - Longer fixation times may result in protein alterations and diminished antigenicity, but antigenicity may be maintained for at least a week after start of fixation

Type of Fixatives
- Clinical assays are generally optimized for tissue fixed in 10% neutral buffered (phosphate) formalin
- Other types of fixatives can alter results of assays
- If other types of fixatives are used for clinical assays, results must be validated as being accurate

TISSUE FOR SPECIAL STUDIES

Clinical Assays
- Routine assays for hormone receptors and HER2 are performed on routine formalin-fixed tissue
- Some commercial assays require fresh tissue
  - Tissue should only be taken for these assays after definitive diagnosis of invasive carcinoma has been made
  - Tissue must be taken in such a way that it will not compromise pathologic evaluation
  - In general, carcinomas < 1 cm in size should not have tissue taken

Research Studies
- Only tissue that is not required for pathologic diagnosis can be taken for research
- Tissue from specimens without diagnosis of invasive carcinoma should not be taken for research unless procedure is performed for cosmetic reasons
- Tissue from lymph nodes without gross metastases should not be taken for research studies

ERRORS IN SPECIMEN PROCESSING

Failure to Find Lesion
- Lesions are rarely missed in small biopsy specimens that are entirely examined microscopically
- Lesions may be missed if an entire specimen is not submitted for microscopic examination
- May not find calcifications in biopsies performed to sample calcifications
  - Specimen radiograph should document that targeted calcifications were removed
  - Tissue containing radiologic calcifications must be sampled as this is most likely location of cancer
    - Tissue and blocks can be radiographed to find cluster of calcifications
  - Reasons for not seeing calcifications
    - Tissue with radiologic calcifications not sampled
    - Calcifications are located deeper in block and can be detected with deeper sections
    - Calcium oxalate not seen; consist of flat pale rhomboid or needle-shaped crystals in apocrine cysts; more easily visible under polarized light
    - Subtle stromal calcifications in hyalinized stroma of fibroadenoma are not seen
    - Very prolonged fixation results in dissolution of calcifications
    - Calcifications lost from tissue; this problem can be minimized in core needle biopsies by having radiologist wrap cores in paper
    - Large calcifications chip out from sections; however, large calcifications are generally not the ones targeted
    - "Calcifications" are actually surgical debris or other radiodense material

Clinical History for Breast Specimens

Relevant Information	Important Features
Patient identifiers	Name, date of birth, medical record number
Type of specimen	Core needle biopsy (free hand, ultrasound, stereotactic, MR guided), incisional biopsy, wire localized excision, excision, mastectomy (type), lymph node biopsy, or axillary dissection
Orientation	Sutures (designations), inks (designations)
Prior history of breast cancer	Type, date, location in breast
Treatment for malignancy in past	Radiation therapy, chemotherapy, endocrine therapy
Neoadjuvant treatment for current cancer	Type of treatment, clinical &/or radiologic response
Pregnancy	Recent pregnancy or breastfeeding
Type of lesion	Palpable mass, radiologic lesion (irregular mass, circumscribed mass, ill-defined mass, calcifications, architectural distortion, MR enhancement, clip marking a biopsy/tumor site), nipple discharge, prophylactic procedure
Size or extent of lesion(s)	Clinical &/or radiologic size
Location of lesions	Quadrant, clock position, &/or distance from nipple
Distance between multiple lesions	Helpful to localize lesions in mastectomy specimens and to determine likely biologic relatedness
Skin &/or nipple involvement	Fixation to skin or retraction, ulceration, scaling crust
Chest wall involvement	Fixation or invasion into chest wall
Prior biopsies of current lesions	Type of biopsy (fine needle aspiration, core needle biopsy, incisional biopsy), results
Special studies on prior biopsies of current lesion	Results of ER, PR, HER2, or other studies
Diseases that could involve breast	Compromised immune system &/or known infections, sarcoidosis, Wegener granulomatosis
Drug use that could affect breast	Hormonal therapy, warfarin (Coumadin), longstanding insulin therapy, cyclosporine, gold treatment
Prior breast surgery	Core needle biopsy, excision, reduction mammoplasty, augmentation (type)

Failure to Find Lymph Nodes

- It is important for surgeon to communicate extent of axillary dissection in mastectomy specimens
  - All tissue potentially containing nodes should be sliced thinly and palpated to identify nodes
- If expected number of nodes not found, additional axillary tissue can be submitted for microscopic examination
  - Very small nodes may not be grossly apparent
  - Nodes with extensive fatty replacement can be difficult to identify
  - In mastectomy specimens, problems with orientation of specimen &/or identification of axillary tissue should be considered
- If no nodes or only a very few nodes are found, this should be documented in pathology report
  - Extent of tissue sampling should be described
  - Clinical reasons for lower than expected numbers should be considered (prior treatment, prior axillary surgery)
  - May be an indication for additional surgery to identify more nodes

REPORTING

Reporting Malignant Results

- Guidelines for reporting invasive carcinoma and DCIS have been issued by the College of American Pathologists (www.cap.org)
  - Recommendations for reporting were determined by broad panel of pathologists, medical oncologists, radiation oncologists, and surgeons
- Use of checklists has been shown to improve completeness of pathology reports

Reporting Benign Results

- Important to document the lesion that prompted the biopsy
- In addition, other lesions that increase risk of invasive carcinoma should be reported

SELECTED REFERENCES

1. Austin R et al: Histopathology reporting of breast cancer in Queensland: the impact on the quality of reporting as a result of the introduction of recommendations. Pathology. 41(4):361-5, 2009
2. Young ES et al: Specimen radiographs assist in identifying and assessing resection margins of occult breast carcinomas. Breast J. 15(5):521-3, 2009
3. Apple SK: Variability in gross and microscopic pathology reporting in excisional biopsies of breast cancer tissue. Breast J. 12(2):145-9, 2006
4. Harvey JM et al: Pathology reporting of breast cancer: trends in 1989-1999, following the introduction of mammographic screening in Western Australia. Pathology. 37(5):341-6, 2005
5. Imperato PJ et al: Improvements in breast cancer pathology practices among medicare patients undergoing unilateral extended simple mastectomy. Am J Med Qual. 18(4):164-70, 2003
6. Wilkinson NW et al: Concordance with breast cancer pathology reporting practice guidelines. J Am Coll Surg. 196(1):38-43, 2003
7. Rubio IT et al: Role of specimen radiography in patients treated with skin-sparing mastectomy for ductal carcinoma in situ of the breast. Ann Surg Oncol. 7(7):544-8, 2000
8. Wiley EL et al: Diagnostic discrepancies in breast specimens subjected to gross reexamination. Am J Surg Pathol. 23(8):876-9, 1999

GENERAL CONSIDERATIONS

Imaging Features and Differential Diagnosis

(Left) The great majority of irregular masses are invasive carcinomas. The irregular border is due to infiltration of the tumor cells into the adjacent stroma ➡. Less common lesions associated with this appearance are fibromatosis, radial sclerosing lesions, or true scars. (Right) Radial sclerosing lesions can form irregular masses that closely mimic invasive carcinomas. The radiating arms are often long compared to the size of the lesion ➡. A lucent center may be present ⇨.

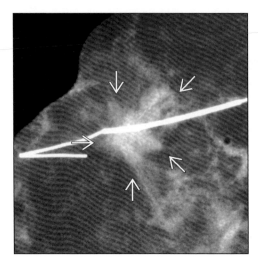 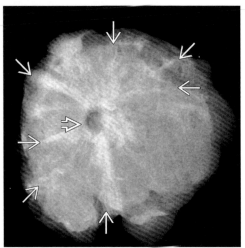

(Left) The majority of circumscribed masses ➡ are benign lesions such as fibroadenomas (65%) or cysts (20%). However, ~ 3% are invasive carcinomas, particularly medullary, solid lobular, mucinous, or triple negative types. DCIS also rarely presents as a circumscribed mass. (Right) Masses that appear to have ill-defined borders ➡ may actually have poorly defined margins or may have discrete borders that are obscured by adjacent breast tissue ⇨.

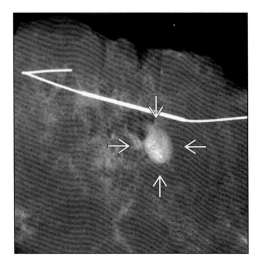 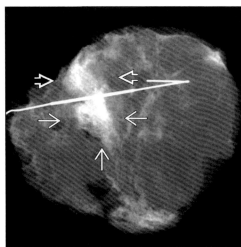

(Left) Excisions for calcification clusters ➡ yield a diagnosis of cancer in 25-30% of cases. The majority of the cancers are DCIS, which is the reason for the apparent increase in this type of cancer with screening mammography. A few cases are due to small invasive carcinomas, usually associated with DCIS. (Right) A linear ➡ and branching ➡ distribution of calcifications is usually associated with comedo DCIS. Less commonly, a similar pattern is seen in secretions in ectatic ducts.

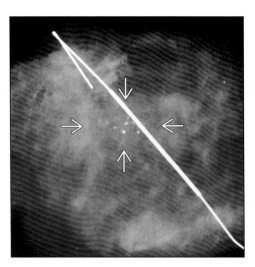 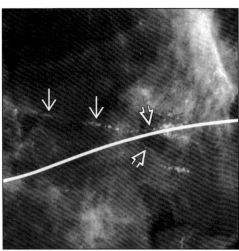

Fixation and Frozen Section Diagnosis

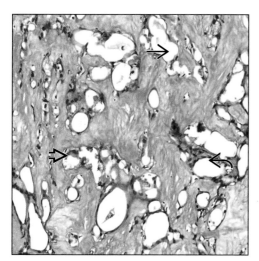 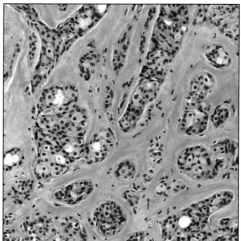

(Left) Delayed or short fixation results in tissue degradation. Histologic changes include artifactual discohesion ⮞, cell loss ➥, and poor nuclear detail ⮥. Antigenicity can also be diminished, and this can cause false-negative results of special studies. (Right) Prompt fixation in formalin for at least 8 hours before processing will result in an optimal histologic appearance and biomarker preservation. However, very prolonged fixation can result in diminished antigenicity.

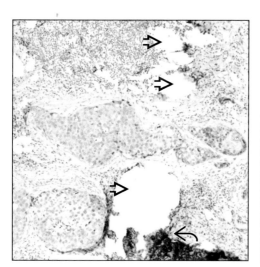 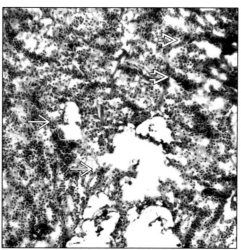

(Left) Prolonged ischemic time can lead to technical problems performing immunohistochemistry and lead to false-negative predictive factor assays, such as HER2. Clues to poor fixation include tissue loss ⮞ and folding ➥ on the slide. (Right) Frozen sections may be limited by poor nuclear detail, ice crystal artifact, tissue tearing ➥, uneven thickness ⮞, and tissue loss. Therefore, this technique should generally not be used for primary diagnosis of breast lesions.

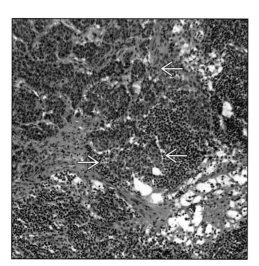 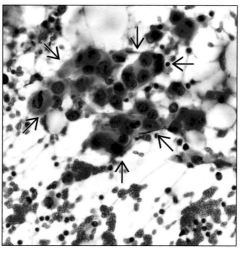

(Left) Frozen sections may be used to examine sentinel lymph nodes intraoperatively if the surgeon will proceed to an axillary dissection based on the finding of a metastasis ➥. The most common reason for missing a macrometastasis is failure to freeze all the slices of the node. (Right) Touch preparations of sentinel lymph nodes can also be used for intraoperative evaluation. Cohesive clusters of large pleomorphic cells ➥ are diagnostic of a metastasis.

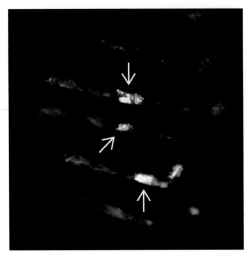

Core needle biopsies for calcifications are radiographed to document that the targeted lesion has been sampled ➡. The cores with calcifications may be separately submitted for more careful processing.

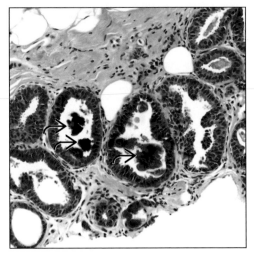

Numerous calcifications ➡ in an area of columnar cell change in a core needle biopsy correlate well with the targeted lesion when found in the cores that harbored the calcifications by radiography.

CORE NEEDLE BIOPSIES

Introduction

- Core needle biopsy (CNB) can be used for initial evaluation of many types of breast lesions
- Patients with benign findings can be spared surgical excision
  - Usually no cosmetic sequelae of breast deformity or skin scarring
  - No tissue scarring that could complicate mammographic interpretation
- Patients with malignant findings also benefit
  - Multiple lesions can be sampled; helpful in determining number of cancers and extent
    - Widely spaced or very extensive cancers may require mastectomy
  - Generally require only 1 subsequent surgical procedure to remove cancer and sample lymph nodes if necessary
  - Information can be used to guide neoadjuvant therapy for eligible patients
- Severe complications after CNB are very rare (< 1% of procedures)
- CNB has advantages and disadvantages in comparison to fine needle aspiration (FNA) biopsy
  - FNA uses smaller needles: 18-, 20-, or 22-gauge
    - Can be performed on palpable masses or under image guidance
    - Slides can be interpreted immediately
    - Single cells rather than tissue are removed
    - Therefore, invasive carcinoma and carcinoma in situ cannot be distinguished with certainty
    - This information is important in deciding whether to sample nodes in subsequent procedure
    - Formalin-fixed, paraffin-embedded tissue sections are preferred specimen to perform special studies for ER, PR, and HER2

- FNA is very useful for sampling palpable or enlarged nodes detected by ultrasound prior to planned neoadjuvant therapy
  - Documents presence of positive node but leaves metastasis in place to be evaluated for treatment response
  - Response in nodal metastases has more prognostic importance than response in breast
- FNA is also useful for distinguishing solid from cystic lesions
  - Masses that can be aspirated to completion and need no further evaluation
  - If fluid is is not bloody, cytologic examination generally not performed

Types of CNB

- Variety of needle sizes are used
  - 16-g: Small size; use generally limited to very dense breast tissue that is difficult to penetrate
  - 14-g: Standard size
  - 11-g: Larger bore needle
- 2 main types of devices
  - Automated, spring-loaded biopsy gun with cutting needle
    - Multiple cores are required to sample lesion; may be obtained through single puncture site using a co-axial needle system
    - May be designated as clock face locations (12:00, 3:00, 6:00, 9:00) and central
    - Used ± imaging guidance
  - Vacuum-assisted devices
    - Employ a vacuum to draw tissue into needle
    - Remove multiple contiguous cores of tissue with 1 insertion
    - Permits use of larger diameter needles yielding larger specimens
    - Can be used under stereotactic, ultrasound, or MR guidance
    - 14-g vacuum-assisted core biopsy is approximately 2x size of 14-g non-vacuum-assisted core

CORE NEEDLE BIOPSIES

- May remove entire lesion if numerous cores are taken
- Clips
  - Generally deployed to mark site of biopsy in case excision is later required
  - Clips marketed by different manufacturers have different shapes
    - If > 1 lesion is biopsied, it is preferable to use clips of different shapes to ensure that each site can be identified
  - Clips are often deployed with gel pledgets
    - Pledgets fill cavity left by needle biopsy
    - Many are small, ovoid, rice-shaped particles; associated with chronic inflammatory reaction with giant cells
    - Larger rectangular gel pledgets are less resorbable and may be surrounded by pseudosynovial lining
    - Pledgets facilitate identification of core site in excisional specimen
    - In ~ 20% of cases, clip is displaced from actual biopsy site; post-procedure radiograph should document location of clip

Identification of Targeted Lesion

- Palpable lesions
  - May be sampled by freehand (Trucut™) core needle biopsies
  - Needle biopsies without imaging tend to push lesions away rather than piercing them
  - If biopsy does not show definite mass-forming lesion (e.g., fibroadenoma or carcinoma), possibility of biopsy not sampling lesion must be considered
- Stereotactic-guided biopsies
  - Can identify masses and calcifications
  - Masses also identified by ultrasound are more easily sampled using this technique
- Ultrasound-guided biopsies
  - Can be used for visible lesions of any size if sufficiently suspicious
  - May be difficult to see masses < 1 cm
- MR-guided biopsies
  - Require open coil and needles compatible with special techniques
  - Only performed for lesions that cannot be identified by other methods

SPECIMEN PROCESSING

Radiologist Handling

- Biopsies for calcifications should be radiographed to ensure that calcifications have been sampled
  - Cores may be separated into those containing and not containing calcifications
  - Cores with calcifications may have more superficial sections taken during slide preparation to ensure they are not missed
  - If calcifications are not seen on initial H&E slides, additional levels can be obtained only on cores with radiologic calcifications
- It is helpful for radiologist to wrap cores in thin paper and submit in tissue cassette in larger container of formalin

- Ensures all tissue fragments are removed from formalin container
  - More likely to keep cores intact
  - More likely to preserve calcifications in tissue
  - As many cassettes as necessary for multiple cores can be used to ensure adequate formalin penetration and fixation
- The time the cores are placed in formalin should be recorded to ensure they are fixed for sufficient amount of time prior to processing
- Radiologist should provide information about targeted lesion(s)
  - Mode of detection (mammography, ultrasound, MR)
  - Type of lesion (mass, calcifications, architectural distortion, type of enhancement on MR)
    - For masses, provide shape (irregular, circumscribed/lobulated, ill defined)
    - Palpable or nonpalpable
  - Size of lesion
  - Distance between lesions if multiple lesions are present
  - Distance from prior excisional sites, if present
- Specialized requisition forms for CNB can be utilized with relevant information in menu form

Pathology Processing

- Cores wrapped in paper can be transferred to labeled cassette for processing
- If there is too much tissue in cassette for adequate fixation, cores can be distributed into more cassettes

Histology Processing

- Multiple levels are usually obtained on each biopsy
  - 3 levels are generally adequate for diagnosis
    - 3rd level should be approximately halfway through thickness of tissue
    - Allows for additional sections should additional studies be necessary
  - For MR biopsies with carcinoma, diagnosis is usually apparent on 1st level
    - Very small cancers are less likely to be detected by MR
- Cores known to have calcifications may have superficial levels taken to make sure calcifications are not missed

REPORTING

General Considerations

- Correlation with imaging findings is essential to ensure lesions are not missed
- Requires adequate information about lesion from radiologist
- Pathologist can document correlation with radiologic finding in some cases
  - Majority of carcinomas will be source of imaging lesion
  - Majority of fibroadenomas will be source of imaging lesion
- In some cases there may be correlation, but pathologist cannot determine this with certainty

CORE NEEDLE BIOPSIES

- ○ Cores for radiologic calcifications with only rare pathologic calcifications seen
- ○ Cores for masses with findings that do not have specific findings on core
  - e.g., lipoma, pseudoangiomatous stromal hyperplasia, hamartoma
- In some cases, there clearly is not a correlation
  - ○ Cores for calcifications without calcifications
    - Radiologic examination of block (direct and lateral views) may be considered to locate them in block
    - Additional deeper levels should be performed
    - Less common reasons for "calcifications" should be considered: Calcium oxalate, metallic debris from prior biopsies, gold from treatment for rheumatoid arthritis
    - Calcium oxalate is best seen using polarized light
  - ○ Cores for mass lesions with only normal tissue identified
- Radiology/pathology correlation conferences are useful for discussing difficult cases

Reporting Cancers

- **Ductal carcinoma in situ (DCIS)**
  - ○ Sometimes difficult to distinguish from atypical ductal hyperplasia (ADH) on CNB
    - Diagnosis may be deferred to excision for borderline lesions
  - ○ Invasive carcinoma will be present on excision in some cases
    - More likely if targeted lesion is a mass
  - ○ Correlation is better for vacuum-assisted biopsies that sample more tissue
    - Reduce number of cases with invasive carcinoma at surgical excision by at least 50%
  - ○ ER may be performed on CNB
    - If results are negative, may be repeated on larger area in excision as there is often marked heterogeneity in DCIS
- **Lobular carcinoma in situ (LCIS)**
  - ○ LCIS may be present as incidental finding
  - ○ If LCIS has atypical features, these should be clearly described
    - High nuclear grade
    - Necrosis
    - Association with calcifications
  - ○ Excision is recommended for LCIS with atypical features due to higher risk of finding invasive carcinoma or DCIS
- **Invasive carcinoma**
  - ○ Useful to report maximum size as seen on CNB
    - Generally smaller than actual size
    - However, size on excision may be smaller than on core for small cancers
    - Helpful to judge reliability of special studies: If only small area of cancer is present on CNB and results are negative, repeat studies on excision may be warranted
    - Clinicians must understand that size on core should not be added to size on excision
  - ○ Histologic type and grade are helpful for counseling patients about likely prognosis and treatment

- Grade may be underscored in ~ 1/3 of cases compared to excisions; rarely overscored
- Special histologic types need to be reevaluated on excisional specimen
- ○ ER, PR, and HER2 may be evaluated
  - CNBs usually have minimal ischemic time and optimal formalin fixation
  - Minimum time for fixation is 6 hours for adequate antigen preservation; shorter times may result in false-negative results
  - However, amount of tumor available may be limited
  - In other cases, tissue disruption and crushing may make evaluation difficult or impossible
  - Repeat of negative results on larger areas of carcinoma on excision should be considered
  - Studies on larger areas of carcinoma may also be better for detecting cases of heterogeneous expression
- ○ For patients undergoing neoadjuvant treatment, results on CNB may be only documentation of their carcinoma
  - Tumor necrosis is predictive of response to therapy
- ○ Most likely lesion to be misinterpreted as invasive carcinoma is sclerosing adenosis
  - It is close mimic when involved by apocrine metaplasia, LCIS, or DCIS
  - Possibility should always be considered and excluded by immunohistochemical studies for myoepithelial cells when warranted
- **Lymph node metastases**
  - ○ Enlarged lymph nodes can be sampled by CNB
    - Fine needle aspiration has advantages as it may be easier to perform in axilla and leaves more of metastasis for evaluation after neoadjuvant therapy
  - ○ If nodal architecture can be identified, this should be specifically stated
    - Breast primary carcinomas occurring in high axilla can be difficult to distinguish from metastases
    - Medullary-type carcinomas can closely resemble lymph node metastasis due to lymphocytic infiltrate
    - Presence of normal breast tissue &/or DCIS supports conclusion that the carcinoma is a primary and not a metastasis
  - ○ Metastases are assumed to be macrometastases if large enough to be sampled by needle biopsy
    - It is helpful to document size of metastasis, particularly if special studies are performed

CLINICAL ISSUES

Accuracy

- Affected by several factors
  - ○ Case selection (palpable vs. screen-detected lesion)
  - ○ Size of needle
  - ○ Number of tissue cores and amount of clinical material obtained
  - ○ Type of lesion: Mass or calcifications

Radiology/Pathologic Correlation: Most Common Lesions

Radiologic Finding	Benign Lesions	Malignant Lesions
Irregular mass	Scars (surgical or trauma), radial sclerosing lesion, fibromatosis, granular cell tumor, abscess	Invasive carcinoma, DCIS (rare), sarcomas, high-grade phyllodes tumors
Circumscribed/lobulated mass	Fibroadenoma, cysts (clusters), papilloma, nodular sclerosing adenosis, pseudoangiomatous stromal hyperplasia, myofibroblastoma, hamartoma, lipoma, angiolipoma, granular cell tumor, fibromatosis	Medullary carcinoma, mucinous carcinoma, triple negative carcinoma, solid lobular carcinoma, encapsulated papillary carcinoma, solid papillary carcinoma, DCIS (rare)
Ill-defined mass	Fibroadenomatoid change, pseudoangiomatous stromal hyperplasia, lymphocytic mastitis, any mass in dense tissue	Any carcinoma in dense tissue
Architectural distortion	Normal breast tissue	Invasive lobular carcinoma, DCIS
Calcifications	Apocrine cysts, sclerosing adenosis, hyalinized fibroadenoma, fat necrosis	DCIS, small invasive carcinoma

- ○ Level of experience of radiologist and pathologist
- Decision as to whether lesion was adequately sampled should be made after close communication between radiologist and pathologist
  - ○ False-negative rate < 1% in most reports
- Factors that can contribute to false-negative CNB
  - ○ Targeting errors due to poor lesion or needle visualization
  - ○ Lesion mobility
  - ○ Deeply located lesions
  - ○ Central lesions in large breast
  - ○ Dense fibrotic tissue resistant to needle penetration
  - ○ Small lesions (≤ 5 mm)
  - ○ Inability of the patient to remain immobile
- Strategies for minimizing false-negative CNB results
  - ○ Adequate sampling may require multiple core samples
  - ○ Always correlate radiographic/imaging findings with pathologic findings
  - ○ If there is discordant result, recommend prompt repeat biopsy or surgical excision

Benign Lesions on CNB That Should Undergo Excision

- Recommendations may be made to excise some benign lesions for 2 reasons
- Benign lesion may be difficult to distinguish from similar malignant lesion
  - ○ Papilloma ± atypia
  - ○ Mucinous (mucocele-like) lesions
  - ○ Radial sclerosing lesions (radial scar)
  - ○ Fibroepithelial lesions with cellular stroma
- Likelihood of carcinoma may be higher in surrounding tissue
  - ○ **ADH**
    - ~ 15-20% will reveal DCIS on excision; < 5% will reveal invasive carcinoma
    - Type of ADH and extent are not sufficiently accurate to predict cases with carcinoma and avoid excision
    - Marked nuclear atypia, micropapillary architecture, and multiple foci are more likely to show adjacent DCIS
    - Larger bore needle biopsies are associated with lower incidence of DCIS
  - ○ **ALH and LCIS**

- Risk of carcinoma is very low if lobular neoplasia is typical in appearance and targeted lesion has been sampled
- ○ **Columnar cell lesions with flat epithelial atypia**
  - 20% likelihood of DCIS on excision
- ○ **Papillary lesions**
  - Risk of carcinoma is very low if papilloma does not show atypical features
- ○ **Radial sclerosing lesions (radial scar)**
  - May be difficult to distinguish from well-differentiated carcinomas on CNB
- Excision may not be necessary in all cases provided there is good radiologic and pathologic correlation

Needle Track Seeding

- Tumor cells can be found in needle track in breast or skin in 20-40% of patients
- Likelihood of finding tumor cells diminishes over time
  - ○ Suggests that artifactually displaced tumor cells may not survive
- Rare patients recur in dermis at core needle site
- Risk is too low to recommend excision of needle site in all patients
  - ○ May be considered in patients not undergoing radiation therapy to core site
- Benign cells, particularly from papillary lesions, can also be pushed into stroma and rarely into lymphatics
  - ○ Should not be overinterpreted as evidence of invasive carcinoma

SELECTED REFERENCES

1. Bilous M: Breast core needle biopsy: issues and controversies. Mod Pathol. 23 Suppl 2:S36-45, 2010
2. Georgian-Smith D et al: Controversies on the management of high-risk lesions at core biopsy from a radiology/pathology perspective. Radiol Clin North Am. 48(5):999-1012, 2010
3. O'Flynn EA et al: Image-guided breast biopsy: state-of-the-art. Clin Radiol. 65(4):259-70, 2010
4. Liebens F et al: Breast cancer seeding associated with core needle biopsies: a systematic review. Maturitas. 62(2):113-23, 2009
5. Kettritz U: Modern concepts of ductal carcinoma in situ (DCIS) and its diagnosis through percutaneous biopsy. Eur Radiol. 18(2):343-50, 2008
6. Schueller G et al: Accuracy of ultrasound-guided, large-core needle breast biopsy. Eur Radiol. 18(9):1761-73, 2008

Benign Findings on CNB

(Left) Many types of masses have specific histologic findings on CNB. For example, the histologic appearance of this lesion is diagnostic of a fibroadenoma and would correlate well with a circumscribed or lobulated mass. *(Right)* Some circumscribed masses do not have specific diagnostic features on CNB. For example, pseudoangiomatous stromal hyperplasia ⊡ can form a mass or be an incidental finding. The diagnosis can only be made if the radiologist confirms that the mass was sampled.

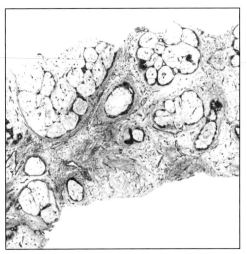
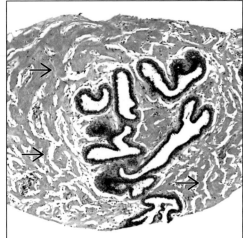

(Left) Irregular masses are almost always invasive carcinomas. In rare cases, benign findings such as biopsy site changes ⊡, radial sclerosing lesions, or fibromatosis can be the cause. *(Right)* Architectural distortion is a change in breast texture without formation of a mass. Although it can be associated with carcinoma, in some cases only normal-appearing breast tissue ⊡ is seen. Radiologic correlation is necessary to ensure that the targeted lesion has been sampled.

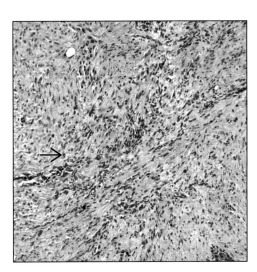
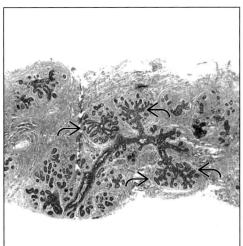

(Left) The most common type of calcification is calcium phosphate, which is seen as refractile dark purple aggregates ⊡. Clusters of calcifications are often associated with sclerosing adenosis ⊡, cysts, and fibroadenomas. *(Right)* Calcium oxalate crystals may be difficult to see because they are usually translucent or pale yellow. They are located in apocrine cysts but may be extruded into the surrounding stroma. These crystals are easily detected using polarized light ⊡.

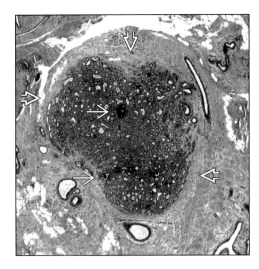
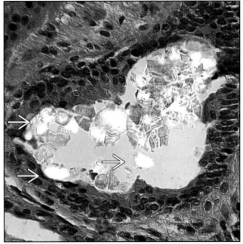

CORE NEEDLE BIOPSIES

CNBs Requiring Excision for Final Diagnosis

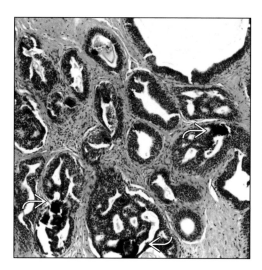

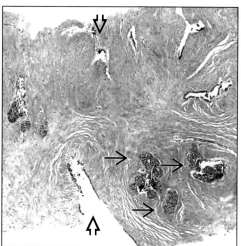

(Left) ADH is often detected due to the association with calcifications ➡. Excision for all cases diagnosed on CNB is recommended; it has not been possible to predict with certainty the subset associated with adjacent DCIS based on extent, histologic appearance, or type of radiologic lesion. (Right) ALH or LCIS ➡ may be seen on CNB as incidental findings. If the targeted lesion such as this fibroadenoma ➡ is identified, the likelihood of cancer on excision is very small.

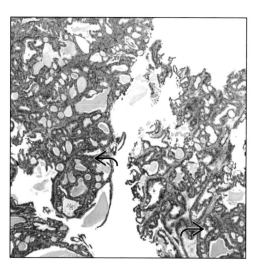

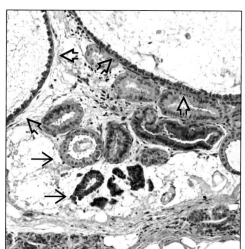

(Left) Papillary lesions can be difficult to classify on CNB. Many are fragmented, and the relationship to the surrounding stroma may not be possible to evaluate. This lesion is involved by an atypical epithelial proliferation ➡ and should be excised for definitive diagnosis. (Right) Mucinous lesions ➡ can be difficult to evaluate on CNB as mucin and epithelium may be displaced into stroma ➡ and simulate invasive carcinoma. These lesions may be evaluated best by excision.

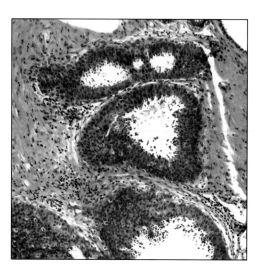

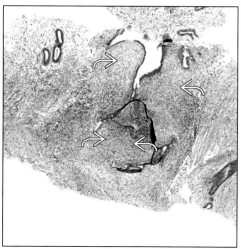

(Left) Columnar cell change with flat epithelial atypia is often seen on CNB due to the association with calcifications. Excision is generally recommended due to a small possibility of finding adjacent DCIS. (Right) Fibroepithelial lesions range from fibroadenomas to high-grade phyllodes tumors. A specific diagnosis cannot always be made due to the limited sampling. The increased cellularity and stromal overgrowth ➡ of this lesion raises the possibility of a phyllodes tumor.

Carcinomas on CNB

(Left) The majority of irregular masses are due to invasive carcinomas ⊟. The presence of tumor necrosis ⊟ is predictive of a good response to chemotherapy. *(Right)* The most common carcinoma associated with the finding of architectural distortion is invasive lobular carcinoma ⊟. These carcinomas have a diffusely infiltrative pattern and can have a minimal desmoplastic response. The presence of fibrous tissue and fat in the carcinoma may not result in formation of a mammographic density.

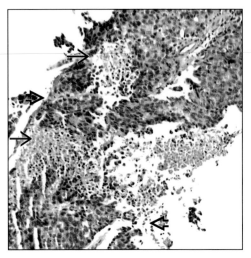
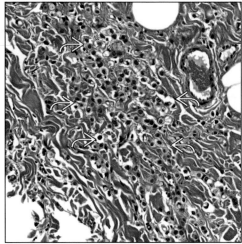

(Left) Although the majority of circumscribed masses are benign, invasive carcinomas of certain histologic types can also present as circumscribed lesions. Mucinous carcinomas ⊟, medullary carcinomas, solid lobular carcinomas, and triple negative carcinomas are the most likely to have rounded or lobulated borders. *(Right)* Spindle cell or fibromatosis-like carcinomas can be very difficult to diagnosis on CNB because they can mimic reactive stroma. IHC for basal-like keratins can identify the tumor cells ⊟.

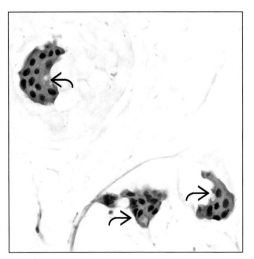
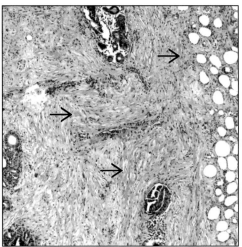

(Left) DCIS most commonly presents as calcifications detected on screening mammography. The calcifications ⊟ are frequently seen in low-grade DCIS with a cribriform pattern ⊟ and with secretions in lumina. *(Right)* Classic LCIS should only be present as an incidental finding as it is not associated with calcifications or masses. However, variant types of LCIS can be associated with necrosis and calcifications ⊟. Excision is recommended for these rare lesions.

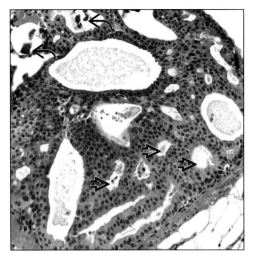
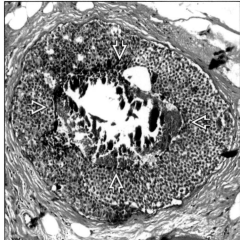

CORE NEEDLE BIOPSIES

Sequelae of CNBs

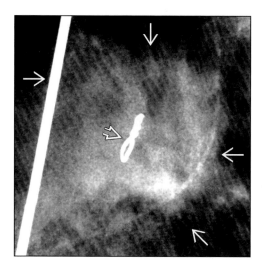
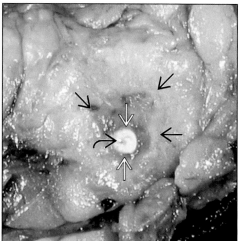

(Left) In most cases, a clip ⊡ is left to mark the site of a CNB, as in this irregular invasive carcinoma ➡. The manufacturer can be recognized by the shape of the clip. This type of clip should be distinguished from surgical clips that may be present on the surface of the specimen. *(Right)* Gel pledgets ➡ and a clip ➡ identify this gross finding as the site of a prior CNB of this invasive carcinoma ➡. The gel pledgets help identify the location of the biopsy.

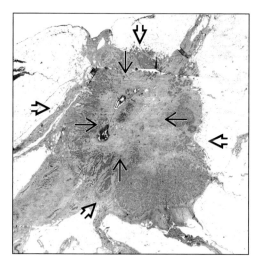
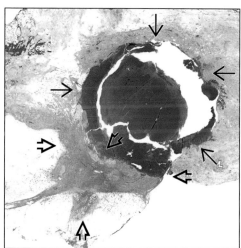

(Left) Ideally, the CNB site ➡ is in the center of an invasive carcinoma ⊡. The size of the carcinoma can be determined, and the adjacent breast tissue can be evaluated for lymphvascular invasion. *(Right)* If a cancer ⊡ is present adjacent to a CNB site ➡, then the size of the cancer cannot be determined with certainty. The size of the cancer on the CNB and the imaging size prior to biopsy should be considered when determining the best AJCC T classification.

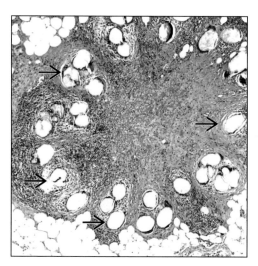
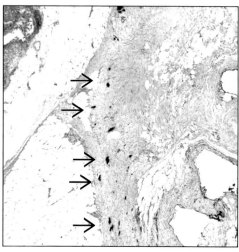

(Left) The gel pledgets left after a CNB fill the resulting holes and should not interfere with diagnosis ➡. The gel will eventually be resorbed by giant cells. *(Right)* CNB can result in epithelial displacement of either benign or malignant cells into the core track. In this case, keratin positive cells are seen strewn along a CNB track ➡. This finding should not be overinterpreted as invasive carcinoma. Myoepithelial cells are sometimes present if the cells are benign.

2

15

EXCISIONS

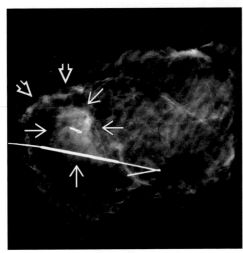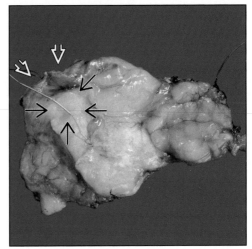

The specimen radiograph is an important guide to the specimen. In this case, there is an invasive carcinoma ➡ close to one margin ⯮ and marked by a prior biopsy clip and the localization wire.

The specimen is sectioned along the plane of the wire, and the findings in the radiograph are clearly seen. The invasive carcinoma ➡ next to the wire is closest to the yellow inked margin ⯮.

INTRODUCTION

Indications for Procedure
- Breast excisions include all procedures with intent to remove entire lesion, but not entire breast
  - Excision is general term for any procedure that does not involve removal of entire breast
  - Biopsy: Used in similar fashion as excision but also includes special types of biopsies such as core needle biopsies or incisional biopsies
  - Lumpectomy: Procedure to remove a palpable mass; also used to generally refer to removal of nonpalpable lesions
  - Quadrantectomy: Removes an entire quadrant of breast
  - Partial mastectomy: Used synonymously with excisions
- Incisional biopsies are less common procedures used to sample, but not completely remove, large lesions
  - In majority of cases, core needle biopsies are used in place of incisional biopsies
- Excisions often result in better cosmetic results than mastectomy
- Performed for initial diagnosis of lesions, treatment of symptoms, and treatment of carcinomas

Initial Investigation of a Lesion
- Breast lesions suspicious for carcinoma require biopsy for evaluation
- Many lesions can be evaluated using core needle biopsy
- Some lesions are not amenable to needle biopsy
  - Location near nipple or deep in breast
  - Patient unable to remain immobile during procedure
  - Lesion difficult to visualize using digital mammography

Treatment of a Symptom
- Some patients have symptoms that may be treated with excision
  - Palpable masses causing cosmetic changes or pain
  - Nipple discharge
  - Inflammatory lesions causing pain ± fistula tracts
    - If due to infectious organisms, incision and drainage may be necessary for cure

Breast-Conserving Therapy (BCT) for Cancer
- Patients with cancer can generally be treated with BCT
  - Eligibility depends on size and location of cancer
  - Survival outcomes of BCT with radiation therapy are similar to those of mastectomy
  - Must be able to maintain acceptable cosmesis
  - Patients must be candidates for radiation therapy
  - Patient preference is also important consideration
- Initial diagnosis of cancer by core needle biopsy aids in patient management
  - Subsequent excision is often larger and more likely to achieve negative margins
  - If clear margins cannot be achieved, mastectomy may be better option
  - For invasive carcinomas, lymph node sampling can be performed in same procedure
- Standard of care is also to treat patients with radiation therapy to reduce risk of local recurrence

SPECIMEN PROCESSING

Requisition Form
- In addition to information that should be provided with all breast specimens, the following information is necessary for gross examination of specimen
  - Type of lesion(s) targeted for removal
    - Palpable mass
    - Imaging finding (mammographic, ultrasound, or MR)
    - Duct excision for nipple discharge

- Orientation of specimen
  - Designations of sutures or clips used to mark specific margins (all 6 margins should be identifiable)
- If adequate information is not provided, additional information should be requested from surgeon

Specimen Radiograph

- If specimen was excised for radiologic lesion, a specimen radiograph should be received with specimen
- Radiologist's interpretation should be available to pathologist
  - States whether or not lesion is present
  - Identifies type of lesion (e.g., mass or calcifications)
  - Often helpful for radiologist to circle or otherwise indicate location of lesion
- Radiograph should be oriented with respect to specimen
  - 4 margins can be identified on radiograph
  - Often provides useful information about closest margin to targeted lesion
  - Surgeons may use radiologic distance to margins to perform a reexcision if diagnosis of carcinoma has been made previously by core needle biopsy or fine needle aspiration
    - However, DCIS at margins is not usually evident by radiography
  - Radiograph can be annotated to designate margins and sites of tissue sampling
- Likely location of targeted lesion in specimen can be approximated using shape of specimen and location of wire
  - Commercial specimen holders with grids are available; these help localize lesions in specimens
- If specimen is transected along plane of the wire, gross appearance is similar to that of specimen radiograph
  - Usually helpful in identifying location of lesion, particularly when lesion is small or difficult to see grossly
  - If cancer is present, it is present at or within 1 cm of radiologic lesion in > 95% of cases
    - Cancers incidental to radiologic lesion are generally LCIS or small low-grade DCIS
- Radiographs of sliced specimen help identify lesions
  - Easier to locate lesions within slices
  - May be more difficult to interpret if lesions are in > 1 slice (e.g., calcification clusters) or if clips are dislodged from specimen
  - Radiographs of blocks with paraffin-embedded tissue can identify calcifications or clips
- Lesions not seen by mammography but present by ultrasound may be localized using same technique
  - Specimens may be imaged by US to document removal of targeted lesion
    - Radiologist's report stating that lesion is present should be provided
    - Sonograph generally not useful to locate lesion in specimen and not provided to pathologist
    - Lesions generally > 1 cm and should be grossly evident
- Specimens cannot be imaged by MR in absence of vascular flow

- Specimen radiograph may be performed but rarely shows targeted lesion
- Unrelated calcifications should not be misinterpreted as the targeted lesion
- Most MR lesions are 1st sampled by core needle biopsy; the clip can be identified by radiography

Gross Description

- Description of intact specimen includes
  - Labeling of specimen as provided by surgeon
  - Size of specimen in 3 dimensions
    - If oriented, dimensions should be designated as superior to inferior, medial to lateral, and anterior to posterior
    - If there are multiple fragments, the number and size of each
  - Presence of a localization wire
    - Present within specimen or dislodged
  - Presence of skin (color, size, presence of scars)
  - Presence of muscle (size and location)
  - Sutures or other means of orientation
    - If specimen has been inked, orientation should be checked
  - Presence of any lesions visible on surface of specimen
  - Presence of defects in surface that could lead to ink leaking into specimen
- Description of sliced specimen should include
  - Appearance of any gross lesions: Size (3 dimensions), shape (irregular, circumscribed, ill defined), color, and consistency (rubbery, firm, hard, mucinous)
  - Distance from each margin
  - If 2 lesions present, distance between lesions
  - Biopsy sites
    - Clips &/or gel pledgets indicating prior core needle biopsy
    - Relationship to other gross lesions
    - Proximity to margins
  - If there is a specimen radiograph, relationship of gross lesion to radiologic lesion
- Extent to which specimen is sampled should be recorded
  - Entire specimen
  - All fibrous tissue
  - % of specimen sampled
- Cassette key
  - Type of tissue in each cassette should be annotated
    - Sections of lesions
    - Margin sections, including designations; ink can run so separate gross identification can help identify sections with > 1 ink color microscopically
    - Sections of tissue between lesions
    - Sections with skin or muscle

Inking Specimen Margins

- Ink adheres better if outer surface of specimen is blotted free of liquid and blood
- 6 margins can generally be identified (anterior, posterior, superior, inferior, medial, and lateral)
- Different colors of ink can be used to identify specific margins

EXCISIONS

○ Helpful to establish system of specific colors for each margin for an institution
• If < 6 ink colors are used, sections should be taken and annotated as to locations of each margin
• Outer surface should be blotted dry before sectioning to avoid smearing ink onto interior surfaces
○ Helpful to change gloves and clean any ink from workspace before proceeding

Sectioning
• Specimen is thinly sectioned into 2-5 mm thick parallel slices, usually perpendicular to its long axis

Sampling
• Lesions are identified, and distances to margins are determined
• Lesions should be sampled in their entirety when practical
○ Very large lesions should be sampled with at least 1 section per cm of greatest dimension
• If multiple lesions present, tissue between lesions is sampled
• Margins generally taken as perpendicular sections
○ En face margins must be specified in description, as interpretation is different than for perpendicular margins
• If a specific gross lesion is not identified, it is preferable to submit all fibrous tissue if practical

DIFFICULT CASES

Excisions for Known DCIS
• It is preferable to completely sample excisions for a known case of DCIS for several reasons
○ Important to determine if there are any areas of invasion
○ Margin status important because cure is possible with complete excision
○ Extent can be determined if completely sampled in systematic fashion
  ▪ For example, sampling can be carried out from medial to lateral
  ▪ Location of sections on specimen radiograph or thickness of slices can be used to estimate extent

Excisions for Nipple Discharge
• Lesion responsible for nipple discharge may be difficult to locate
• Lesions are often small and nonpalpable
• Involved duct may be marked with a suture
○ Ends of duct can be taken as en face margins
○ Remainder of duct may be opened with fine scissors
○ If papilloma is present, it may be seen as polypoid mass on a stalk in the wall

Excisions for MR-Detected Lesions
• Lesions evident by other modalities will be localized using those methods
• ~ 1/4 will have carcinoma
○ 1/2 DCIS (typically high grade)
○ 1/2 invasive carcinoma (usually small, < 1 cm)
• Specimen cannot be imaged using MR in absence of blood flow

• Specimen radiograph may be performed
○ Reveals findings associated with carcinoma in only 20-30% of cases
○ Incidental radiologic findings may be present (calcifications); not associated with targeted lesion
• Carcinomas grossly evident in only 10-20% of cases
• Entire specimen must be examined microscopically in order to identify all carcinomas
• Currently, most MR lesions will be investigated initially by core needle biopsy
○ Clip is left to mark site of lesion

Excisions After Neoadjuvant Therapy
• A clip should be placed prior to treatment to mark site of cancer
• Gross lesion may not be evident after complete, or near complete, response
• Tumor bed may be an ill-defined fibrous area in vicinity of clip
• At least 1 section of tissue per cm of largest dimension of tumor bed or size of carcinoma prior to treatment should be sampled
• If initial sections do not show residual invasive carcinoma, additional sampling should be considered to document a pathologic complete response

SELECTED REFERENCES

1. Kaufmann M et al: Locoregional treatment of primary breast cancer: consensus recommendations from an International Expert Panel. Cancer. 116(5):1184-91, 2010
2. Jones HA et al: Impact of pathological characteristics on local relapse after breast-conserving therapy: a subgroup analysis of the EORTC boost versus no boost trial. J Clin Oncol. 27(30):4939-47, 2009
3. Morrow M: Breast conservation and negative margins: how much is enough? Breast. 18 Suppl 3:S84-6, 2009
4. Carlson JW et al: MRI-directed, wire-localized breast excisions: incidence of malignancy and recommendations for pathologic evaluation. Hum Pathol. 38(12):1754-9, 2007
5. Rosenfeld I et al: The significance of malignancies incidental to microcalcifications in breast spot localization biopsy specimens. Am J Surg. 182(1):1-5, 2001
6. Vicini FA et al: Pathologic and technical considerations in the treatment of ductal carcinoma in situ of the breast with lumpectomy and radiation therapy. Ann Oncol. 10(8):883-90, 1999
7. Nakhleh RE et al: Mammographically directed breast biopsies: a College of American Pathologists Q-Probes study of clinical physician expectations and of specimen handling and reporting characteristics in 434 institutions. Arch Pathol Lab Med. 121(1):11-8, 1997
8. Owings DV et al: How thoroughly should needle localization breast biopsies be sampled for microscopic examination? A prospective mammographic/pathologic correlative study. Am J Surg Pathol. 14(6):578-83, 1990
9. Schnitt SJ et al: Histologic sampling of grossly benign breast biopsies. How much is enough? Am J Surg Pathol. 13(6):505-12, 1989

Processing Excision Specimens

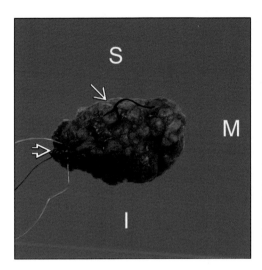

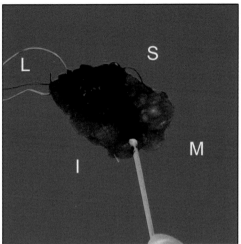

(Left) This excision is oriented with a short suture on the superior margin ➡ and a long suture on the lateral margin ➡. Using these 2 reference points, the remaining 4 margins can be identified. (Right) The outer surface of the specimen is inked to mark the tissue present at the margin. Each margin can be inked a different color, &/or margin sections can be designated as to their location in a cassette code. Both methods are helpful as sometimes ink can become smeared.

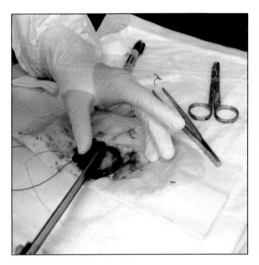

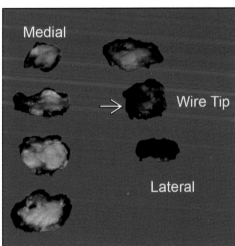

(Left) After inking, the outer surface is blotted dry to prevent ink from being introduced into the interior of the specimen. The workspace and gloves are cleaned of any spilled ink. The specimen is then cut into 2-5 mm slices. If there is a radiograph, a section along the plane of the wire is helpful for correlation. (Right) This specimen has been sectioned from medial to lateral into 7 slices. The location of the wire tip ➡ marks the site of the radiologically targeted lesion.

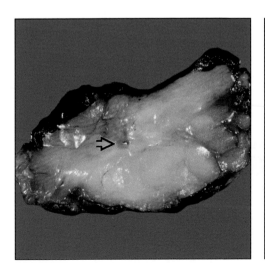

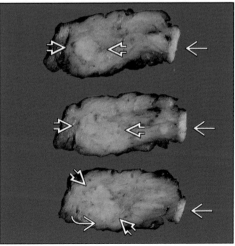

(Left) This is a wire localized excision for a clip marking an area of calcifications shown to be DCIS on a prior needle biopsy. The clip can be seen ➡ associated with normal-appearing fibroadipose tissue. (Right) This specimen contains a white-tan invasive carcinoma ➡ that is clearly separate from the skin ➡. The largest dimension is used for AJCC T classification. The margins are grossly negative for invasive carcinoma with the closest being the red-inked margin ➡.

MARGINS AND REEXCISIONS

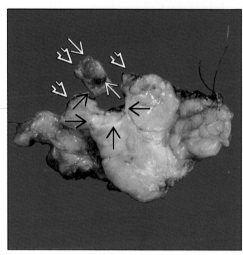

This invasive ductal carcinoma ➡ is closest to the yellow inked margin ➡. A perpendicular margin has been taken. The distance of the invasive carcinoma from the margin can be determined ➡.

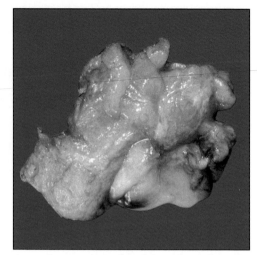

An en face margin is shaved from the surface of a specimen, such as this section of the yellow margin. Although more tissue is sampled, the distance of carcinoma from the margin cannot be measured.

INTRODUCTION

Margins and Local Recurrence Rates

- Carcinoma present at inked margin ("positive" margin) correlates with higher likelihood of residual disease in the breast
  - Carcinoma close to margins also increases likelihood of residual disease, but magnitude of risk is dependent on type of cancer (invasive or in situ), distance from margin, and extent
- Residual carcinoma in the breast is associated with increased risk of local recurrence
- Minimizing risk of local recurrence is important goal
  - Can improve survival for patients whose initial carcinoma is likely curable (carcinoma in situ and small node-negative invasive carcinomas)
  - Reduces need for additional surgery and treatment
  - Reduces possibility of uncontrolled local disease in skin and chest wall ("carcinoma en cuirasse")
  - Recurrence is often very psychologically difficult for patients
    - Often mastectomy is required for treatment as radiation cannot be delivered to chest 2nd time
- Margins for palpable invasive carcinomas are generally negative
  - Surgeon palpates the cancer and excises rim of grossly normal tissue
  - Apparently positive margin on microscopic examination may be due to ink leakage or inadvertent incision into carcinoma
  - Generally several mm of cauterized tissue within biopsy cavity
    - Residual carcinoma at edge of biopsy site will not be viable
  - Therefore, focally positive margin for invasive cancer usually does not correlate with residual invasive carcinoma in the patient

- Margins for nonpalpable invasive carcinomas (due to small size or diffusely invasive pattern) may be positive
  - Surgeon cannot palpate the cancer and, therefore, must make educated guess as to how much tissue to remove
  - If carcinoma is transected, it will be present at margin over broad front
    - Cautery artifact on carcinoma supports that margin is a true surgical margin
    - Extensive residual carcinoma may be present in breast
- Margins are often positive or close for DCIS
  - DCIS is rarely grossly evident
  - Extent of DCIS cannot be determined with certainty by clinical examination or imaging
  - Surgeon cannot definitively know how much tissue to remove
  - Margins can only be evaluated with certainty microscopically on permanent sections

Prediction of Residual Carcinoma

- Even under best conditions, likelihood of residual carcinoma in breast can only be estimated
- Presence of cancer at margins does not predict residual cancer with certainty
  - There may not be breast tissue beyond edge of specimen
    - Particularly relevant for margins adjacent to skin and pectoralis muscle
  - Often several mm of cauterized tissue in biopsy cavity in patient
    - Cautery may destroy small amounts of residual invasive carcinoma
  - Margins may be falsely positive due to ink leakage into cracks or specimen fragmentation
  - Can be gaps between areas of involvement by DCIS
    - Duct at margin can appear free of DCIS, but DCIS can be present further along in duct

○ Margins can be falsely negative if areas of involvement are not sampled or if areas are too small to be present within the width of the section

Risk Factors for Local Recurrence

- Approximately 10% of patients will have local recurrence at 10 years
- Risk factors for recurrence include
  ○ Young patient age
  ○ Poorly differentiated carcinomas
  ○ Positive margins
  ○ Extensive intraductal component (EIC) with DCIS located away from invasive carcinoma
  ○ Extensive lymph-vascular invasion
- Subtypes of breast cancer have different local recurrence rates at 5 years
  ○ Luminal A (ER or PR positive, HER2 negative): 0.8%
  ○ Luminal B (ER or PR positive, HER2 positive): 1.5%
  ○ HER2 (ER and PR negative, HER2 positive): 8.4%
  ○ Triple negative (basal-like) (ER, PR, and HER2 negative): 7.1%
- Growth rate of hormone-positive carcinomas can be inhibited by hormonal therapy over many years
- Patients with HER2-positive carcinomas are now being treated with HER2-targeted therapy over many years
  ○ Treatment reduces likelihood of local recurrence
- Targeted therapy for triple negative carcinomas is not yet available

TYPES OF MARGINS

En Face (Shave)

- Thin (2-4 mm) slice of tissue is taken from surface of specimen; similar to removing section of orange peel
  ○ Any cancer seen in tissue section on glass slide is, by definition, at margin
    ▪ Actual distance from margin cannot be determined
  ○ Larger area can be examined than is seen in perpendicular sections
    ▪ Useful to examine some types of structures such as base of the nipple

Perpendicular (Radial)

- Section of tissue extending from lesion to margin is taken
  ○ Distance to margin can be measured
    ▪ Ink leakage into tissue cracks can be difficult to evaluate
    ▪ Cautery artifact on carcinoma is additional evidence of true margin involvement
  ○ Examines less tissue than is seen in en face margins
  ○ Multiple sections are required to thoroughly examine all margins

Cavity Biopsies

- After removal of main specimen, surgeon takes biopsies of designated margins
  ○ Generally small and not oriented
  ○ Removes problems with ink leakage and orientation
  ○ May not be possible to determine distance to margin

○ Crush and cautery artifact can complicate interpretation of small specimens

Separate Shave Margins

- Taken by surgeon either at time of main excision or in later procedure
  ○ Usually oriented with suture to identify new margin
    ▪ Best inked in 2 colors to show old margin and new margin
- Generally thick enough to take perpendicular margins
  ○ 1 section per cm of longest dimension is suggested for initial sampling

RADIOLOGIC EVALUATION OF MARGINS

Oriented Specimen Radiographs

- 4 margins can be identified on specimen radiograph
  ○ 2nd radiograph may be performed to show remaining 2 margins
- Distance of radiologically evident lesions to margins can be determined
  ○ Some carcinomas (especially DCIS) are not evident radiographically
  ○ All margins need to be evaluated microscopically
- Radiographs can change shape of specimen
  ○ Breast tissue normally "slumps" after excision, resulting in "pancake" shape
  ○ Compression for specimen radiography can also flatten specimens
  ○ May change relationship to margins

SAMPLING MARGINS

Margins of Initial Excisions

- At least 1 perpendicular section of each of the 6 margins should be examined
- Additional sampling should be considered for cases with extensive DCIS or diffusely infiltrating carcinomas
- En face margins are not generally recommended
  ○ If en face margin is submitted, this must be stated in gross description
  ○ Technique combining both en face and perpendicular margins can be used
- Margins should be sampled in area most likely to show involvement by carcinoma
  ○ Areas grossly suspicious for carcinoma
  ○ Fibrous tissue
  ○ Areas with radiologic findings suspicious for carcinoma (e.g., calcifications)

Separate Margin Excisions

- Should be inked in 2 colors designating new margin and old margin
- 1-2 sections per cm of greatest dimension may be taken

MARGINS AND REEXCISIONS

ORIENTATION OF MARGINS

Designation

- Breast specimens have 6 margins
  - Anterior, posterior, superior, inferior, medial, and lateral
- If other names are used, then it may not be possible to orient remaining margins
  - For example, designations such as "next to nipple" should also include name of specific margin
- Posterior margin may be next to muscle fascia
  - Breast tissue is almost never found deep to muscle fascia as identified by surgeon
  - Close posterior margins are unlikely to correlate with residual disease
  - Carcinoma invading into skeletal muscle is most important finding at this margin and could be indication of residual disease in chest wall
- 1 margin may be below skin
  - Often correlates with anterior margin but may be other designated margins
  - Breast tissue is usually not present in dermis
    - In rare cases, particularly close to nipple, ducts and lobules are present in dermis
  - Significance of close or positive margins below skin is often unclear
  - Additional surgery would need to remove skin and subcutaneous tissue

Methods

- Sutures
  - 2 perpendicular sutures can identify all 6 margins
    - Short suture for superior margin and long suture for lateral margin is easy to remember
    - Additional sutures can be used to mark other margins if more specific identification is desirable (e.g., whipstitch marking deep margin)
  - If sutures are placed at opposing margins (e.g., medial and lateral), remaining margins cannot be identified
  - If sutures are placed at edges (e.g., inferior/posterior margin), location of remaining margins is more difficult to identify
- Inks
  - Surgeons can ink margins using colored inks
  - Surgeon has advantage of seeing specimen in situ before changes in shape due to specimen handling
  - Especially helpful for specimens of unusual shape
  - Using both sutures and colored inks is helpful
    - When specimen is inked by surgeon, prosector should double check orientation for accuracy

REPORTING MARGINS

En Face Margins

- Any carcinoma in tissue section on glass slide is reported as positive
- Invasive carcinoma is reported separately from DCIS
- Extent of involvement can be conveyed by size, number of foci, &/or number of blocks

Perpendicular Margins

- Distance to designated margins is reported in mm
- Invasive carcinoma is reported separately from DCIS

Determining Need for Reexcision

- Often a complex decision based on many factors
- Intent of surgery: Cure vs. reduction in local recurrence risk
  - Patients with DCIS and small node-negative carcinomas may benefit most from more extensive surgery
  - Minimizes risk of developing subsequent cancer at higher stage
  - Survival of patients with node-positive or larger carcinomas is unlikely to be diminished by local recurrence
- Status of margins
  - Positive margins are generally an indication for additional surgery
  - Definitions of need to reexcise margins based on proximity of cancer to margin varies widely
    - Invasive carcinoma focally at or close to margin does not correlate well with residual disease; there is usually additional margin of cauterized tissue in patient
    - DCIS close to margins can be used to make educated guess as to likelihood of residual disease
    - Larger margins may be recommended for patients who decline radiation therapy
- Patient preference
  - Some patients' highest priority will be to diminish risk of recurrence as much as possible
  - Some patients may accept slightly higher risk of recurrence to achieve more favorable cosmetic result

SELECTED REFERENCES

1. Hodi Z et al: Comparison of margin assessment by radial and shave sections in wide local excision specimens for invasive carcinoma of the breast. Histopathology. 56(5):573-80, 2010
2. Rizzo M et al: The effects of additional tumor cavity sampling at the time of breast-conserving surgery on final margin status, volume of resection, and pathologist workload. Ann Surg Oncol. 17(1):228-34, 2010
3. Caughran JL et al: Optimal use of re-excision in patients diagnosed with early-stage breast cancer by excisional biopsy treated with breast-conserving therapy. Ann Surg Oncol. 16(11):3020-7, 2009
4. Molina MA et al: Breast specimen orientation. Ann Surg Oncol. 16(2):285-8, 2009
5. Wright MJ et al: Perpendicular inked versus tangential shaved margins in breast-conserving surgery: does the method matter? J Am Coll Surg. 204(4):541-9, 2007
6. Dooley WC et al: Understanding the mechanisms creating false positive lumpectomy margins. Am J Surg. 190(4):606-8, 2005
7. Cellini C et al: Factors associated with residual breast cancer after re-excision for close or positive margins. Ann Surg Oncol. 11(10):915-20, 2004
8. Guidi AJ et al: The relationship between shaved margin and inked margin status in breast excision specimens. Cancer. 79(8):1568-73, 1997

MARGINS AND REEXCISIONS

Microscopic Features

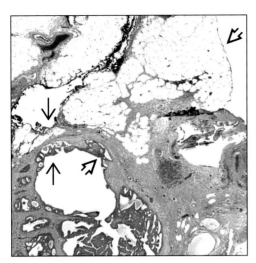

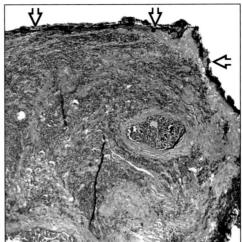

(Left) The distance of a carcinoma to the margin can be measured in perpendicular sections ⬇. However, ink leakage into tissue cracks ➡ can make this evaluation difficult. *(Right)* Surgeons rarely transect palpable invasive carcinomas. Margin involvement is unusual and, if present, is generally focal. However, small or diffusely infiltrative cancers can be difficult to identify grossly. Extensive margin involvement ⬇ may be found for these types of carcinomas.

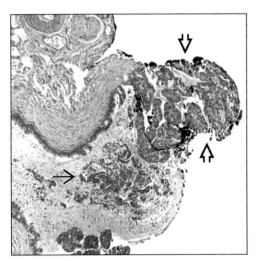

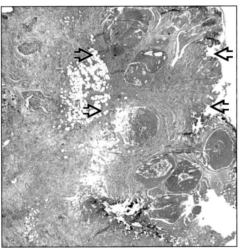

(Left) The presence of ink on tumor cells is the definition of a positive margin ⬇. The presence of cautery artifact in the tissue ➡ is a helpful finding to confirm that the ink indicates a true margin and is not artifactual leakage. *(Right)* Several mm of cauterized nonvital tissue is typically present within the biopsy cavity in the patient's breast ⬇. Thus, carcinoma present at the margin in the excisional specimen may not correlate with residual viable carcinoma in the patient.

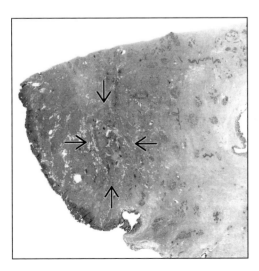

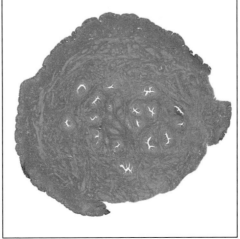

(Left) In an en face margin, any carcinoma in the tissue section indicates a positive margin. Therefore, this margin is positive for DCIS ➡. The actual distance to the margin cannot be determined and could be from 1-4 mm. *(Right)* The base of the nipple is an en face margin for nipple-sparing mastectomies. This section shows all major ducts. In order to see all the major ducts using perpendicular sections, multiple tissue sections and levels would be necessary.

MASTECTOMIES

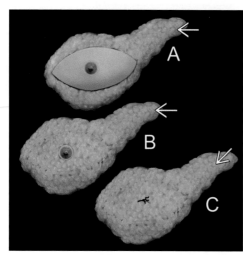

Mastectomies remove all breast tissue in addition to a skin ellipse with nipple (A) and frequently the axillary tail ➡. Skin-sparing (B) and nipple-sparing (C) mastectomies may also be performed.

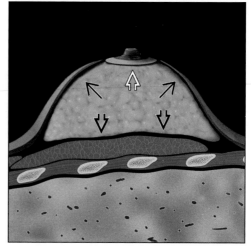

The deep margin of a mastectomy is the pectoralis muscle fascia ⮞. The anterior "margins" are below the skin flaps ➡. The base of the nipple ⮞ is a margin for nipple-sparing mastectomies.

INTRODUCTION

Surgical Procedure

- Mastectomy is intended removal of all breast tissue
- In some women, breast epithelium is present in subcutaneous tissue or axillary tissue beyond the typical extent of the breast
- Therefore, all breast epithelial cells may not be removed by mastectomy
  - Prophylactic mastectomies reduce risk of breast cancer by 90%
  - Rarely, breast cancers arise in residual breast tissue

Indications

- Majority of women can be successfully treated with breast-conserving therapy (BCT) and radiation therapy
  - Rate of local recurrence is higher with BCT, but survival is similar
  - Women with potentially surgically curable disease (DCIS, small node-negative invasive carcinomas) may have a greater benefit from mastectomy as cancer may recur at a higher stage
- Mastectomy may be preferred procedure in some cases
  - Extensive carcinoma or multiple carcinomas that cannot be removed with cosmetically acceptable results
  - Centrally located carcinomas
  - Skin or chest wall involvement; many patients will be treated 1st with neoadjuvant chemotherapy
  - Patients with high risk of subsequent carcinoma (e.g., *BRCA* germline mutation carriers)
  - Patients not eligible for radiation due to previous treatment or collagen vascular disease
  - Patient choice

Types of Mastectomy

- Simple
  - Removes breast tissue and skin ellipse including nipple

- Small amount of muscle may be removed if carcinoma is close to deep margin
- Axillary dissection is not performed
  - However, some lower lymph nodes may be present; lateral tissue should always be examined for nodes
- Radical
  - Removes breast tissue, skin ellipse (including nipple, pectoralis major, and minor muscles), and axillary lymph nodes
  - Currently performed rarely except for carcinomas that invade into chest wall
  - Modified radical mastectomy is a simple mastectomy (without removal of muscle) and axillary dissection
- Skin-sparing
  - Removes breast tissue and nipple with small amount of surrounding skin
- Nipple-sparing
  - Removes breast tissue
  - Does not remove nipple or skin
  - May be appropriate for carcinomas at least 2 cm from nipple with limited amounts of DCIS
  - Base of nipple is a margin that must be sampled separately and submitted by the surgeon
- Subcutaneous
  - Removes 85-90% of breast tissue
  - Does not remove nipple or skin; flaps are usually thick
  - Similar to nipple-sparing mastectomy but removes less breast tissue
    - Most common indication is gynecomastia in men
- Prophylactic
  - Removes breast tissue and skin ellipse including nipple
  - Performed for risk reduction; no known carcinoma is present in the breast at time of surgery
  - Occult invasive carcinomas are found in 3-15% of cases; generally < 1 cm

MASTECTOMIES

Lymph Node Sampling with Mastectomy
- Sentinel node biopsy
  - Sentinel nodes are identified by dye or radioactive tracer
  - Average number of nodes is 2, but more may be identified in some patients
  - Metastases are most often found at the pole of the node stained with blue dye
- Axillary dissection
  - Extent of dissection may include levels I, II, or III
  - Surgeon should indicate extent of dissection
  - Ideally, at least 10 nodes should be found
    - If fewer nodes are present, additional examination of specimen &/or submission of tissue should be considered
- Intramammary nodes
  - Nodes may be present within the breast and are usually located in upper outer quadrant
  - Typically not the sentinel node

SPECIMEN PROCESSING

Requisition Form
- In addition to information germane to all types of breast specimens, additional information is required for mastectomies
  - Number and type of lesions (masses, calcifications, clips, etc.) present
    - Often multiple, thus requiring mastectomy for removal
    - Known or suspected involvement of skin or muscle
  - Distance between lesions and distance from nipple
  - Presence and extent of axillary dissection
    - Specimens should always be examined for lymph nodes even if axillary dissection was not performed
    - Amount of additional gross examination and tissue sampling if lymph nodes are not found is influenced by the number of nodes expected in specimen

Specimen Radiograph
- Mastectomies are generally not sent for radiologic examination by surgeon as this information is not necessary for surgical procedure
- Radiographs can be very helpful prior to sectioning to identify small lesions or lesions that are not apparent on gross examination (e.g., calcifications)
  - Lesions may be lost (e.g., clips) after sectioning or more difficult to identify if transected

Gross Description
- Size of breast tissue in 3 dimensions
  - Size of attached axillary tail
- Size of skin ellipse
  - Size of nipple and areola (note if retracted or if skin lesions are present)
    - Ulceration &/or satellite skin lesions change AJCC T classification
    - Enlargement and erythema of inflammatory carcinoma are not seen in excised specimen

- Scaling crust of Paget disease is usually removed during preparation for surgery
  - Note any lesions on remainder of skin including scars (may be difficult to see if circumareolar)
- Sutures or other markings for orientation
- All lesions should be described
  - Location (quadrant, distance from nipple)
  - Size, color, borders, texture (soft, rubbery, hard)
  - Distance &/or involvement of skin or muscle
  - Distance between lesions
- Cassette key
  - Type of tissue in each cassette should be noted
    - Lesions
    - Skin, nipple, and deep margin
    - Lymph nodes (number &/or ink designations)

Inking Specimen Margins
- Deep margin is smooth fascial plane of pectoralis muscle
  - Usually inked black
  - Note if any skeletal muscle or defects in fascia are present; if so, these are potential areas of tumor invasion and should be specifically sampled
- Anterior breast tissue is adjacent to skin flaps
  - Not a true margin as breast tissue is usually not present in skin flaps
    - However, this will depend on thickness of flap and ductal anatomy of patient
  - Clinical significance of close or positive tissue edges is unclear
  - If inked and evaluated, should be clearly distinguished from deep margin
- Skin is usually not involved by cancer, and margins need not be evaluated
  - If skin is involved (by direct invasion or Paget disease), then skin margins should be evaluated grossly
  - In the absence of gross involvement, microscopic carcinoma is very unlikely
  - Grossly abnormal skin edges should be evaluated
- Base of nipple is a margin for nipple-sparing mastectomies
  - Surgeon should remove base of nipple as an en face section and submit this as a separate specimen
    - Major ducts retract after the nipple is removed, making it difficult to identify this margin
  - Location of nipple base should be marked with suture

Sectioning
- Breast is serially sectioned from posterior aspect
  - Sections are not quite complete at anterior aspect in order to keep the specimen intact
- Axillary tail is thinly sliced and palpated to identify all nodes
  - Most lateral portion of the breast should also be carefully examined for nodes
    - Lymph nodes can be present in mastectomies without formal node dissection ("simple" mastectomies)
  - If fewer than 10 nodes are found, additional examination and sampling should be considered

MASTECTOMIES

Sampling

- Lesions
  - Sample all lesions with at least 1 section per cm
  - Smaller lesions are sampled in their entirety
- Margins
  - Perpendicular section of deep margin closest to carcinomas
  - Base of nipple margin for nipple-sparing mastectomies
- Skin and nipple
  - 1 representative perpendicular section
  - More extensive sampling if gross lesions are present or there is history of inflammatory carcinoma
  - If nipple involvement is suspected, base of nipple may be taken en face and superficial nipple as perpendicular sections
- Lymph nodes
  - All nodes are thinly sliced (2-3 mm) and completely submitted for microscopic examination
  - Each node must be separately identified
    - Ink nodes placed in same cassette different colors

Difficult Cases

- **Mastectomy after core needle biopsy**
  - Lesions are usually small and may not be grossly evident
  - Biopsy sites can heal after 1 month, making it difficult to locate lesion
  - Specimen radiograph prior to sectioning is very helpful to identify the site of core needle biopsy and any radiologic findings (mass, calcifications, or clip)
    - Clips can be dislodged during sectioning
  - If specimen is sliced and core site/lesion is not found, slices can be radiographed
- **Mastectomy after neoadjuvant chemotherapy**
  - Site of carcinoma should be marked with clip before treatment
    - If there is marked or complete response, clip may be the only means of identifying the tumor bed
  - Size and location of carcinoma prior to treatment should be available
    - Tumor bed can be very difficult to identify grossly; may be ill-defined fibrotic area difficult to distinguish from normal breast tissue
  - Initial sampling of tumor bed should be at least 1 section per cm of greatest dimension of the carcinoma prior to treatment
    - If no residual carcinoma is seen in tumor bed or lymph nodes, additional sampling should be considered to document a pathologic complete response
  - Tumor bed should be evident after microscopic examination
  - If tumor bed is not identified after evaluation of initial slides, additional sampling is necessary
    - If tumor bed is not found, pathologic complete response cannot be determined with certainty
- **Mastectomy for women with positive axillary lymph node and no primary carcinoma by imaging**
  - Rarely, women present with palpable axillary node with metastatic breast carcinoma

- Prognosis is similar to women with same extent of nodal involvement
- Prognosis is not changed by presence or absence of primary carcinoma documented in breast
  - Majority of carcinomas are found with mammography, ultrasound, &/or MR
    - If no lesions are detected by these modalities, it is unlikely the primary will be found by gross examination
  - Gross examination is best performed shortly after removal of the breast and before fixation
    - Normal tissue is softer, making detection of small invasive carcinomas easier
    - Extensive sampling is unnecessary as finding the cancer will not alter stage or treatment of patient
  - Primary carcinomas may not be evident for several possible reasons
    - Carcinoma is very small
    - Carcinoma regressed (no evidence for this phenomenon but theoretically possible)
    - Metastasis in "lymph node" is actually primary carcinoma; some medullary-like carcinomas can closely resemble nodes due to circumscribed borders and dense lymphocytic infiltrate
    - Carcinoma arose in benign inclusion in lymph node (theoretically possible)
- **Mastectomy with extensive DCIS**
  - DCIS can extensively involve all 4 quadrants of breast
  - May be impractical to microscopically examine all involved tissue to look for invasion
  - All grossly firm to hard areas that could harbor invasive carcinoma should be sampled
- **Mastectomy for inflammatory carcinoma**
  - Clinical signs of enlarged erythematous breast are due to plugging of dermal lymphatics by tumor cells
    - These findings are not apparent in excised breast due to absence of blood flow
  - Patients typically do not have easily definable mass by palpation or imaging
  - Majority of patients will undergo neoadjuvant chemotherapy prior to surgery
    - Skin findings are often the 1st to respond to treatment
  - It may be difficult to determine site of tumor bed
    - If mass was present before treatment, this area should be sampled
    - If biopsy was performed and a clip deployed, clip must be identified
    - In addition to nipple skin, other areas of skin should be sampled to look for skin involvement

SELECTED REFERENCES

1. Skytte AB et al: Breast cancer after bilateral risk-reducing mastectomy. Clin Genet. 79(5):431-7, 2011
2. Brachtel EF et al: Occult nipple involvement in breast cancer: clinicopathologic findings in 316 consecutive mastectomy specimens. J Clin Oncol. 27(30):4948-54, 2009
3. Yi M et al: Predictors of contralateral breast cancer in patients with unilateral breast cancer undergoing contralateral prophylactic mastectomy. Cancer. 115(5):962-71, 2009

MASTECTOMIES

Gross and Imaging Features

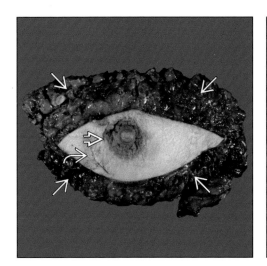

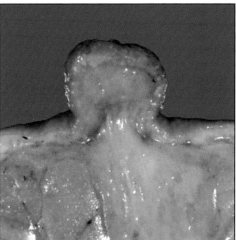

(Left) The most common type of mastectomy consists of skin, nipple and areola ⇒, and breast tissue. A cicatrix is present ➡, marking the site of a prior biopsy. The anterior breast tissue ➡ corresponds to the skin flap "margins." (Right) A single cross section of the nipple shows a few of the major ducts and lactiferous sinuses. If carcinoma involving the nipple is suspected, an en face margin of the nipple base and perpendicular sections of the nipple should be examined.

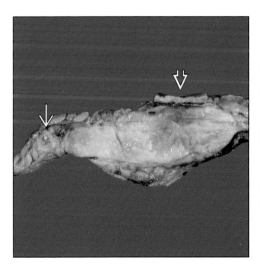

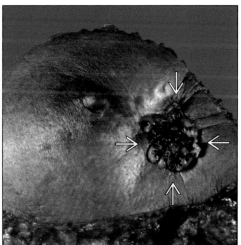

(Left) Blue dye can be injected in the skin near the nipple ⇒ for sentinel node identification. The dye is water soluble and is not seen in histologic sections. There is a far lateral invasive carcinoma containing a gel pledget ➡ from a prior core needle biopsy. (Right) Large, locally advanced carcinomas may ulcerate ➡ through the skin. Ulceration &/or satellite skin nodules are important findings to document, as these carcinomas are classified as AJCC T4b.

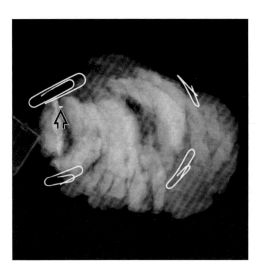

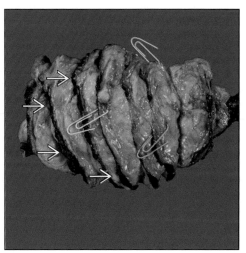

(Left) Mastectomies are often necessary if multiple lesions are present. In this case, a specimen radiograph was helpful to find the clip ⇒ identifying a biopsy site, as well as 3 other areas of suspicious calcifications by the other paperclips. (Right) The deep margin of this mastectomy was inked black ➡, and it has been sectioned starting at the posterior surface from medial to lateral. Three paperclips have been used to mark the sites of 3 different small carcinomas.

REDUCTION MAMMOPLASTIES

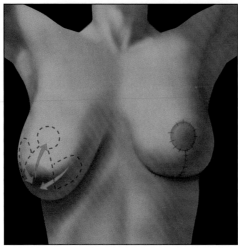

To reduce the size of the breasts, multiple portions of breast tissue and skin are resected. The nipple is preserved and repositioned. Tissue from each breast should be separately identified.

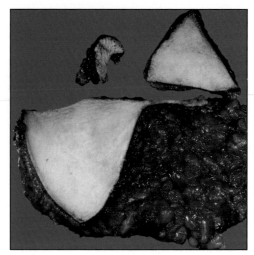

The specimen consists of multiple fragments of breast tissue with or without skin and is generally not oriented. Any suspicious areas identified grossly are submitted for microscopic examination.

TERMINOLOGY

Abbreviations
- Reduction mammoplasty (RM)

Synonyms
- Breast reduction surgery

Definitions
- Surgical procedure to reduce size of breast; skin and breast tissue (but not nipple) are removed

INTRODUCTION

Breast Reduction Surgery
- Indications
  - Congenital breast asymmetry
  - Symptomatic macromastia
  - Asymmetry following breast cancer surgery
- Insurance plans may only reimburse RM for physical symptoms and not for cosmetic reasons
  - May require that only minimal amount of breast tissue is removed (typically 300 g)
- RM has proven to be safe and relieves symptoms due to macromastia
  - Associated with overall excellent patient satisfaction
- Follow-up studies after breast reduction surgery
  - Significantly better quality of life
  - Fewer breast-associated symptoms
  - Less depression and anxiety; better self-esteem when compared with preoperative evaluation

Macromastia
- Benign condition of breast hypertrophy
- Defined as disproportionately heavy breasts on an otherwise average-sized woman
  - Women may seek consultation for RM because of psychological reasons, physical reasons, or both
  - Obesity may be contraindication for surgery
    - May increase post-op complication rates

- Symptomatic macromastia has multiple presentations
  - Back and shoulder pain
  - Kyphosis
  - Excoriation from bra straps
  - Chronic intertrigo in breast skin folds
- Severe breast hypertrophy can severely limit normal activity of daily living
  - May limit exercise ability
  - May cause difficulty sleeping
- Conservative measures such as weight loss, physical therapy, and special brassieres may provide some relief of symptoms
- Some patients may suffer from low self-esteem or depression due to unhappiness with body image
  - Counseling and psychological assessment may be appropriate in some cases

Occult Cancers in RM Specimens
- Occult malignant and premalignant lesions are rarely found in RM
  - Incidence of invasive carcinoma is 0.06-0.4% in population-based studies
    - Single-center studies suggest a slightly higher incidence of invasive cancers (0.3-1.4%)
  - ≤ 1% have occult DCIS or LCIS
  - ≤ 4% have atypical ductal or lobular hyperplasia
  - Younger patients (< 40) are less likely to have occult cancers compared with older women
- Women with history of breast cancer are more likely to have cancer found in contralateral RM
  - Invasive carcinomas are unlikely as most of these women will have had recent breast imaging
  - ~ 1/3 will have either DCIS or LCIS in contralateral breast

Breast Imaging After RM
- RM can produce mammographic and histologic changes
  - Skin thickening, retroareolar fibrosis may develop

REDUCTION MAMMOPLASTIES

- ○ Fat necrosis, formation of oil cysts, fibrosis, calcifications
- Postoperative breast changes following RM do not significantly hinder assessment of screening mammography
  - ○ Recall rates for further imaging assessment are similar between patients who are status post RM compared with no surgery

Screen-Detected Cancer After RM
- Lower age adjusted breast cancer rates have been reported for women who have undergone RM
  - ○ Relative risk 0.2-0.7
  - ○ Associated with removal of > 800 g of tissue
  - ○ Reason for decreased cancer risk hypothesized to be due to removal of potential epithelial precursor cells

MACROSCOPIC FINDINGS

Specimen Handling
- Breast tissue from reduction mammoplasties should be sent for pathologic examination
  - ○ Right and left breast tissue should be received as separate specimens
  - ○ In most cases, specimens are received as multiple fragments of breast tissue ± skin and are not oriented
  - ○ Tissue is weighed and measured in aggregate for each breast
    - ■ Tissue is usually weighed in operating room because a minimal weight may be required for insurance reimbursement
    - ■ Operating room weight and pathology weight are usually concordant; differences may be due to fluid loss
  - ○ Tissue segments are thinly sectioned and grossly examined
    - ■ All suspicious areas should be sampled
    - ■ If no discrete lesions are identified grossly, 2-4 samples of representative breast tissue and 1 sample of skin from each breast can be submitted for microscopic examination

- ○ More extensive histologic evaluation should be considered in patients > 40 years of age or with prior history of breast cancer
  - ■ In patients < 30 years, careful gross examination ± minimal microscopic study is most likely adequate
- If carcinoma is found on initial slides, additional examination is indicated
  - ○ Specimen may be reexamined grossly
  - ○ Specimen radiography can be considered if patient has not undergone recent screening mammography
    - ■ May reveal suspicious calcifications or small densities; helps guide sampling of specimen
    - ■ Preferable that women > 40 undergoing RM have screening mammogram prior to procedure
    - ■ If screening mammography did not show lesions, it is unlikely that radiography of specimen will show significant findings

SELECTED REFERENCES

1. Saariniemi KM et al: The outcome of reduction mammaplasty remains stable at 2-5 years' follow-up: a prospective study. J Plast Reconstr Aesthet Surg. 64(5):573-6, 2011
2. Campbell MJ et al: The role of preoperative mammography in women considering reduction mammoplasty: a single institution review of 207 patients. Am J Surg. 199(5):636-40, 2010
3. Hernanz F et al: Reduction mammaplasty: an advantageous option for breast conserving surgery in large-breasted patients. Surg Oncol. 19(4):e95-e102, 2010
4. Muir TM et al: Screening for breast cancer post reduction mammoplasty. Clin Radiol. 2010 Mar;65(3):198-205. Epub 2010 Jan 22. Erratum in: Clin Radiol. 65(6):498, 2010
5. Clark CJ et al: Incidence of precancerous lesions in breast reduction tissue: a pathologic review of 562 consecutive patients. Plast Reconstr Surg. 124(4):1033-9, 2009
6. Dotto J et al: Frequency of clinically occult intraepithelial and invasive neoplasia in reduction mammoplasty specimens: a study of 516 cases. Int J Surg Pathol. 16(1):25-30, 2008
7. Golshan M et al: Sentinel lymph node biopsy for occult breast cancer detected during breast reduction surgery. Am Surg. 72(5):397-400, 2006
8. Colwell AS et al: Occult breast carcinoma in reduction mammaplasty specimens: 14-year experience. Plast Reconstr Surg. 113(7):1984-8, 2004

IMAGE GALLERY

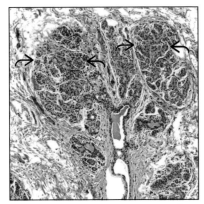 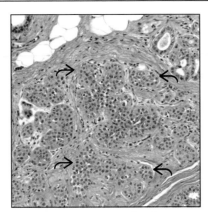 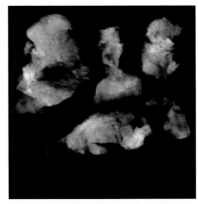

(Left) Reduction mammoplasty specimens from younger women (< 40 years of age) most commonly have normal fibroglandular breast tissue ➘. *(Center)* Clinically significant lesions such as atypical lobular hyperplasia ➘, LCIS, or DCIS are more commonly found in older patients. Occult invasive carcinomas are very rare. *(Right)* If carcinoma is found in the initial samples, tissue may be radiographed to determine if calcifications that would guide further sampling are present.

CHECKLIST FOR THE REPORTING OF INVASIVE BREAST CARCINOMA

Invasive Carcinoma of the Breast: Complete Excision (Less Than Total Mastectomy, Including Specimens Designated Biopsy, Lumpectomy, Quadrantectomy, and Partial Mastectomy ± Axillary Contents) and Mastectomy (Total, Modified Radical, Radical ± Axillary Contents)

Surgical Pathology Cancer Case Summary (Checklist)

Specimen

____ Partial breast

____ Total breast (including nipple and skin)

____ Other (specify): _____

____ Not specified

Procedure

____ Excision without wire-guided localization

____ Excision with wire-guided localization

____ Total mastectomy (including nipple and skin)

____ Other (specify): _____

____ Not specified

Lymph Node Sampling (select all that apply) (required only if lymph nodes are present in specimen)

____ No lymph nodes present

____ Sentinel lymph node(s)

____ Axillary dissection (partial or complete dissection)

____ Lymph nodes present within breast specimen (i.e., intramammary lymph nodes)

____ Other lymph nodes (e.g., supraclavicular or location not identified)

Specify location, if provided: _____

*Specimen Integrity

*____ Single intact specimen (margins to be evaluated)

*____ Multiple designated specimens (e.g., main excision and identified margins)

*____ Fragmented (margins cannot be evaluated with certainty)

*____ Other (specify): _____

Specimen Size (for excisions less than total mastectomy)

Greatest dimension: _____ cm

*Additional dimensions: _____ x _____ cm

____ Cannot be determined

Note: Specimen size is required but may be reported in the gross description.

Specimen Laterality

____ Right

____ Left

____ Not specified

*Tumor Site: Invasive Carcinoma (select all that apply)

*____ Upper outer quadrant

*____ Lower outer quadrant

*____ Upper inner quadrant

*____ Lower inner quadrant

*____ Central

*____ Nipple

Position: _____ o'clock

*____ Other (specify): _____

*____ Not specified

Tumor Size: Size of Largest Invasive Carcinoma

____ Microinvasion only (≤ 0.1 cm)

Greatest dimension of largest focus of invasion > 0.1 cm: _____ cm

CHECKLIST FOR THE REPORTING OF INVASIVE BREAST CARCINOMA

____ *Additional dimensions: _____ x _____ cm

____ No residual invasive carcinoma after presurgical (neoadjuvant) therapy

____ Cannot be determined

> Note: The size of the invasive carcinoma should take into consideration the gross findings correlated with the microscopic examination. In some cases, it may be helpful to use information about tumor size from imaging studies. If multiple foci of invasion are present, the size listed is the size of the largest contiguous area of invasion. The size of multiple invasive carcinomas should not be added together. The size does not include adjacent DCIS. If there has been a prior core needle biopsy or incisional biopsy showing a larger area of invasion than in the excisional specimen, the largest dimension of the invasive carcinoma in the prior specimen should be used for T classification, if known. If there has been prior treatment and no invasive carcinoma is present, the cancer is classified as Tis if there is residual DCIS and T0 if there is no remaining carcinoma.

Tumor Focality (required only if > 1 focus of invasive carcinoma is present)

____ Single focus of invasive carcinoma

____ Multiple foci of invasive carcinoma

____ *Number of foci: _____

____ *Sizes of individual foci: _____

____ No residual invasive carcinoma after presurgical (neoadjuvant) therapy

____ Indeterminate

> Note: If there are multiple invasive carcinomas, size, grade, histologic type, and the results of studies for estrogen receptor (ER), progesterone receptor (PR), and HER2/neu should pertain to the largest invasive carcinoma.

Macroscopic and Microscopic Extent of Tumor (required only if involved structures are present) (select all that apply)

Skin

____ Skin is not present

____ Invasive carcinoma does not invade into dermis or epidermis

____ Invasive carcinoma directly invades into dermis or epidermis without skin ulceration

____ Invasive carcinoma directly invades into dermis or epidermis with skin ulceration (classified as T4b)

____ Satellite microscopically evident skin foci of invasive carcinoma are present (i.e., not contiguous with invasive carcinoma in breast) (classified as T4b)

____ Satellite microscopic skin foci of invasive carcinoma are present (i.e., not contiguous with invasive carcinoma in breast) (does not change T classification)

> Note: Dermal lymph-vascular invasion is reported separately.

Nipple

____ DCIS does not involve nipple epidermis

____ DCIS involves nipple epidermis (Paget disease of nipple)

> Note: This finding does not change the T classification of invasive carcinomas.

Skeletal muscle

____ No skeletal muscle present

____ Skeletal muscle is present and is free of carcinoma

____ Carcinoma invades skeletal muscle

____ Carcinoma invades skeletal muscle and into chest wall (classified as T4a)

> Note: Invasion into pectoralis muscle is not considered chest wall invasion, and cancers are not classified as T4a unless there is invasion deeper than this muscle.

Ductal Carcinoma In Situ (DCIS) (select all that apply)

____ No DCIS present

____ DCIS is present

*____ Extensive intraductal component (EIC) negative

*____ EIC positive

*____ Only DCIS is present after presurgical (neoadjuvant) therapy

Size (extent) of DCIS

____ *Estimated size (extent) of DCIS (greatest dimension using gross and microscopic evaluation) is at least _____ cm

____ *Additional dimensions: _____ x _____ cm

____ *Number of blocks with DCIS: _____

____ *Number of blocks examined: _____

> Note: The size (extent) of DCIS is an estimation of the volume of breast tissue occupied by DCIS. This information may be helpful for cases with a predominant component of DCIS (e.g., DCIS with microinvasion) but may not be necessary for cases of EIC negative invasive carcinomas.

**Architectural patterns (select all that apply)

CHECKLIST FOR THE REPORTING OF INVASIVE BREAST CARCINOMA

*____ Comedo

*____ Paget disease (DCIS involving nipple skin)

*____ Cribriform

*____ Micropapillary

*____ Papillary

*____ Solid

*____ Other (specify): _____

*Nuclear grade

*____ Grade I (low)

*____ Grade II (intermediate)

*____ Grade III (high)

*Necrosis

*____ Not identified

*____ Present, focal (small foci or single cell necrosis)

*____ Present, central (expansive "comedo" necrosis)

Lobular Carcinoma In Situ (LCIS)

*____Not identified

*____Present

Histologic Type of Invasive Carcinoma

____ Ductal carcinoma in situ with microinvasion

____ Lobular carcinoma in situ with microinvasion

____ Ductal carcinoma in situ involving nipple skin (Paget disease) with microinvasion

____ Invasive ductal carcinoma (no special type or not otherwise specified)

____ Invasive lobular carcinoma

____ Invasive carcinoma with ductal and lobular features ("mixed-type carcinoma")

____ Invasive mucinous carcinoma

____ Invasive medullary carcinoma

____ Invasive papillary carcinoma

____ Invasive micropapillary carcinoma

____ Invasive tubular carcinoma

____ Invasive cribriform carcinoma

____ Invasive carcinoma; type cannot be determined

____ No residual invasive carcinoma after presurgical (neoadjuvant) therapy

____ Other(s) (specify): _____

> Note: Histologic type corresponds to the largest carcinoma. If there are smaller carcinomas of a different type, this information should be included under "Additional Pathologic Findings." Inflammatory carcinoma requires the presence of clinical findings of erythema and edema involving at least 1/3 of skin of breast.

Histologic Grade: Nottingham Score

Glandular (acinar)/tubular differentiation

____ Score 1: > 75% of tumor area forming glandular/tubular structures

____ Score 2: 10-75% of tumor area forming glandular/tubular structures

____ Score 3: < 10% of tumor area forming glandular/tubular structures

____ Only microinvasion present (not graded)

____ No residual invasive carcinoma after presurgical (neoadjuvant) therapy

____ Score cannot be determined

Nuclear pleomorphism

____ Score 1: Nuclei small with little increase in size in comparison with normal breast epithelial cells, regular outlines, uniform chromatin, little variation in size

____ Score 2: Cells larger than normal with open vesicular nuclei, visible nucleoli, and moderate variability in both size and shape

____ Score 3: Vesicular nuclei, often with prominent nucleoli, exhibiting marked variation in size and shape, occasionally with very large and bizarre forms

____ Only microinvasion present (not graded)

____ No residual invasive carcinoma after presurgical (neoadjuvant) therapy

____ Score cannot be determined

Mitotic count

CHECKLIST FOR THE REPORTING OF INVASIVE BREAST CARCINOMA

____ Score 1 (≤ 3 mitoses per mm²)

____ Score 2 (4-7 mitoses per mm²)

____ Score 3 (≥ 8 mitoses per mm²)

____ Only microinvasion present (not graded)

____ No residual invasive carcinoma after presurgical (neoadjuvant) therapy

____ Score cannot be determined

    *Number of mitoses per 10 high-power fields: _____

    *Diameter of microscope field: _____ mm

Overall grade

____ Grade 1: Scores of 3, 4, or 5

____ Grade 2: Scores of 6 or 7

____ Grade 3: Scores of 8 or 9

____ Only microinvasion present (not graded)

____ No residual invasive carcinoma after presurgical (neoadjuvant) therapy

____ Score cannot be determined

    Note: Grade corresponds to largest area of invasion. If there are smaller foci of invasion of a different grade, this information should be included under "Additional Pathologic Findings."

Margins (select all that apply)

____ Margins cannot be assessed

____ Margins uninvolved by invasive carcinoma

    Distance from closest margin: _____ mm

      *Specify margins:

        *Distance from superior margin: _____ mm

        *Distance from inferior margin: _____ mm

        *Distance from anterior margin: _____ mm

        *Distance from posterior margin: _____ mm

        *Distance from medial margin: _____ mm

        *Distance from lateral margin: _____ mm

        *Distance from other specified margin: _____ mm

          *Designation of margin: _____

____ Margins uninvolved by DCIS (if present)

    Distance from closest margin: _____ mm

      *Specify margins

        *Distance from superior margin: _____ mm

        *Distance from inferior margin: _____ mm

        *Distance from anterior margin: _____ mm

        *Distance from posterior margin: _____ mm

        *Distance from medial margin: _____ mm

        *Distance from lateral margin: _____ mm

        *Distance from other specified margin: _____ mm

          *Designation of margin: _____

____ Margin(s) positive for invasive carcinoma

      *Specify margin(s): _____

      *Specify margin(s) and extent of involvement

        *____ Superior margin

          *____ Focal

          *____ Minimal/moderate

          *____ Extensive

        *____ Inferior margin

          *____ Focal

          *____ Minimal/moderate

          *____ Extensive

        *____ Anterior margin

          *____ Focal

CHECKLIST FOR THE REPORTING OF INVASIVE BREAST CARCINOMA

    *____ Minimal/invasive

    *____ Extensive

  *____ Posterior margin

    *____ Focal

    *____ Minimal/moderate

    *____ Extensive

  *____ Medial margin

    *____ Focal

    *____ Minimal/moderate

    *____ Extensive

  *____ Lateral margin

    *____ Focal

    *____ Minimal/moderate

    *____ Extensive

____ Margin(s) positive for DCIS

  *Specify margin(s): _____

  *Specify margin(s) and extent of involvement

    *____ Superior margin

      *____ Focal

      *____ Minimal/moderate

      *____ Extensive

    *____ Inferior margin

      *____ Focal

      *____ Minimal/moderate

      *____ Extensive

    *____ Anterior margin

      *____ Focal

      *____ Minimal/moderate

      *____ Extensive

    *____ Posterior margin

      *____ Focal

      *____ Minimal/moderate

      *____ Extensive

    *____ Medial margin

      *____ Focal

      *____ Minimal/moderate

      *____ Extensive

    *____ Lateral margin

      *____ Focal

      *____ Minimal/moderate

      *____ Extensive

*Treatment Effect: Response to Presurgical (Neoadjuvant) Therapy

*In breast

  *____ No known presurgical therapy

  *____ No definite response to presurgical therapy in invasive carcinoma

  *____ Probable or definite response to presurgical therapy in invasive carcinoma

  *____ No residual invasive carcinoma is present in breast after presurgical therapy

*In lymph nodes

  *____ No known presurgical therapy

  *____ No lymph nodes removed

  *____ No definite response to presurgical therapy in metastatic carcinoma

  *____ Probable or definite response to presurgical therapy in metastatic carcinoma

  *____ No lymph node metastases; fibrous scarring, possibly related to prior lymph node metastases with pathologic complete response

  *____ No lymph node metastases and no prominent fibrous scarring in nodes

CHECKLIST FOR THE REPORTING OF INVASIVE BREAST CARCINOMA

*Lymph-Vascular Invasion

*____ Not identified

*____ Present

*____ Indeterminate

*Dermal lymph-vascular invasion

   *____ No skin present

   *____ Not identified

   *____ Present

   *____ Indeterminate

Lymph Nodes (required only if lymph nodes are present in specimen)

Number of sentinel lymph nodes examined: _____

Total number of lymph nodes examined (sentinel and nonsentinel): _____

Number of lymph nodes with macrometastases (> 0.2 cm): _____

Number of lymph nodes with micrometastases (> 0.2 mm to 2.0 cm &/or > 200 cells): _____

Number of lymph nodes with isolated tumor cells (≤ 0.2 mm and ≤ 200 cells): _____

Size of largest metastatic deposit (if present): _____

   Note: Sentinal node is usually the first involved lymph node. In the unusual situation in which a sentinel node is not involved by metastatic carcinoma but a nonsentinel node is involved, this information should be included in a note.

*Extranodal extension

   *____ Present

   *____ Not identified

   *____ Indeterminate

*Method of evaluation of sentinel lymph nodes (select all that apply)

   *____ Hematoxylin and eosin (H&E), 1 level

   *____ H&E, multiple levels

   *____ Immunohistochemistry

   *____ Sentinel lymph node biopsy not performed

   *____ Other (specify): _____

Pathologic Staging (based on information available to the pathologist) (pTNM)

TNM descriptors (required only if applicable) (select all that apply)

   ____ m (multiple foci of invasive carcinoma)

   ____ r (recurrent)

   ____ y (post-treatment)

Primary tumor (invasive carcinoma) (pT)

   ____ pTX: Primary tumor cannot be assessed

   ____ pT0: No evidence of primary tumor#

   ____ pTis (DCIS): Ductal carcinoma in situ#

   ____ pTis (LCIS): Lobular carcinoma in situ#

   ____ pTis (Paget): Paget disease of nipple **not** associated with invasive carcinoma &/or carcinoma in situ (DCIS &/or LCIS) in underlying breast parenchyma#

      pT1: Tumor ≤ 20 mm in greatest dimension

         ____ pT1mi: Tumor ≤ 1 mm in greatest dimension (microinvasion)

         ____ pT1a: Tumor > 1 mm but ≤ 5 mm in greatest dimension

         ____ pT1b: Tumor > 5 mm but ≤ 10 mm in greatest dimension

         ____ pT1c: Tumor > 10 mm but ≤ 20 mm in greatest dimension

      ____ pT2: Tumor > 20 mm but ≤ 50 mm in greatest dimension

      ____ pT3: Tumor > 50 mm in greatest dimension

      pT4: Tumor of any size with direct extension to chest wall &/or to skin (ulceration or skin nodules)

         Note: Invasion of dermis alone does not qualify as pT4.

         ____ pT4a: Extension to chest wall, not including only pectoralis muscle adherence/invasion

         ____ pT4b: Ulceration &/or ipsilateral satellite nodules &/or edema (including peau d'orange) of skin, which does not meet criteria for inflammatory carcinoma

         ____ pT4c: Both T4a and T4b

         ____ pT4d: Inflammatory carcinoma##

CHECKLIST FOR THE REPORTING OF INVASIVE BREAST CARCINOMA

#For the purposes of this checklist, these categories should only be used in the setting of preoperative (neoadjuvant) therapy for which a previously diagnosed invasive carcinoma is no longer present after treatment.

##Inflammatory carcinoma is a clinical-pathologic entity characterized by diffuse erythema and edema (peau d'orange) involving 1/3 or more of the skin of the breast. The skin changes are due to lymphedema caused by tumor emboli within dermal lymphatics, which may or may not be obvious in a small skin biopsy. However, a tissue diagnosis is still necessary to demonstrate an invasive carcinoma in the underlying breast parenchyma or at least in the dermal lymphatics, as well as to determine biological markers such as ER, PR, and HER2 status. Tumor emboli in dermal lymphatics without the clinical skin changes described above do not qualify as inflammatory carcinoma. Locally advanced breast cancers directly invading the dermis or ulcerating the skin without the clinical skin changes also do not qualify as inflammatory carcinoma. Thus the term "inflammatory carcinoma" should not be applied to neglected locally advanced cancer of the breast presenting late in the course of a patient's disease. The rare case that exhibits all the features of inflammatory carcinoma but in which skin changes involve less than 1/3 of the skin should be classified by the size and extent of the underlying carcinoma.

Regional lymph nodes (pN) (choose a category based on lymph nodes received with specimen; immunohistochemistry &/or molecular studies are not required)

If internal mammary lymph nodes, infraclavicular nodes (level III axillary), or supraclavicular lymph nodes are included in specimen, consult the AJCC Cancer Staging Manual for additional lymph node categories.

Modifier (required only if applicable)

____ (sn): Only sentinel node(s) evaluated; if ≥ 6 sentinel nodes &/or supraclavicular lymph nodes are removed, this modifier should not be used

Category (pN)

____ pNX: Regional lymph nodes cannot be assessed (e.g., previously removed or not removed for pathologic study)

____ pN0: No regional lymph node metastasis is identified histologically

Note: Isolated tumor cell clusters (ITC) are defined as small clusters of cells ≤ 0.2 mm or single tumor cells, or < 200 cells in a single histologic cross section.# ITCs may be detected by routine histology or by immunohistochemical (IHC) methods. Nodes containing only ITCs are excluded from the total positive node count for purposes of N classification but should be included in the total number of nodes evaluated.

____ pN0(i-): No regional lymph node metastases histologically, negative IHC

____ pN0(i+): Malignant cells in regional lymph node(s) ≤ 0.2 mm and < 200 cells (detected by H&E or IHC including ITC)

____ pN0(mol-): No regional lymph node metastases histologically, negative molecular findings (reverse transcriptase polymerase chain reaction [RT-PCR])

____ pN0(mol+): Positive molecular findings (RT-PCR), but no regional lymph node metastases detected by histology or IHC

____ pN1mi: Micrometastases (> 0.2 mm &/or > 200 cells, but none > 2.0 mm)

____ pN1a: Metastases in 1-3 axillary lymph nodes (at least 1 metastasis > 2.0 mm)

____ pN2a: Metastases in 4-9 axillary lymph nodes (at least 1 tumor deposit > 2.0 mm)

____ pN3a: Metastases in 10 or more axillary lymph nodes (at least 1 tumor deposit > 2.0 mm)

#Approximately 1,000 tumor cells are contained in a 3-dimensional 0.2 mm cluster. Thus, if > 200 individual tumor cells are identified as single dispersed tumor cells or as a nearly confluent elliptical or spherical focus in a single histologic section of a lymph node, there is a high probability that > 1,000 cells are present in the lymph node. In these situations, the node should be classified as containing a micrometastasis (pN1mi). Cells in different lymph node cross sections or longitudinal sections or levels of the block are not added together; the 200 cells must be in a single node profile even if the node has been thinly sectioned into multiple slices. It is recognized that there is substantial overlap between the upper limit of the ITC and the lower limit of the micrometastasis categories due to inherent limitations in pathologic nodal evaluation and detection of minimal tumor burden in lymph nodes. Thus, the threshold of 200 cells in a single cross section is a guideline to help pathologists distinguish between these 2 categories. The pathologist should use judgment regarding whether it is likely that the cluster of cells represents a true micrometastasis or is simply a small group of isolated tumor cells.

*Distant metastasis (M)

*____ Not applicable

*____ cM0(i+): No clinical or radiographic evidence of distant metastasis, but deposits of molecularly or microscopically detected tumor cells in circulating blood, bone marrow, or other nonregional nodal tissue that are no larger than 0.2 mm in a patient without symptoms or signs of metastasis

*____ pM1: Distant detectable metastasis as determined by classic clinical and radiographic means &/or histologically proven larger than 0.2 mm

Note: The MX designation has been eliminated from the AJCC/UICC TNM system.

Only the applicable T, N, or M category is required for reporting; the definitions need not be included in the final report.

*Additional Pathologic Findings

*Specify: _____

Ancillary Studies

(These elements are required only in the primary report of the results)

Estrogen receptor

Specimen used for this assay (required only if results were obtained on a specimen other than the one currently being reported)

____ Performed on this specimen

____ Performed on another specimen

CHECKLIST FOR THE REPORTING OF INVASIVE BREAST CARCINOMA

____ *Specify specimen (accession number): _____

____ Pending

____ Not performed

____ No residual invasive carcinoma after presurgical (neoadjuvant) therapy

____ Other (specify): _____

Results and interpretation

____ Positive (_____ % of tumor cells with nuclear positivity)

____ Negative (< 1% of tumor cells with nuclear positivity)

____ Negative (no tumor cells with nuclear positivity)

____ Results unknown

____ Other (specify): _____

Average intensity of tumor cell nuclei staining

____ Absent

____ Weak

____ Moderate

____ Strong

____ Unknown

____ Other (specify): _____

Progesterone receptor

Specimen used for this assay (required only if results were obtained on a specimen other than the one currently being reported)

____ Performed on this specimen

____ Performed on another specimen

____ *Specify specimen (accession number): _____

____ Pending

____ Not performed

____ No residual invasive carcinoma after presurgical (neoadjuvant) therapy

____ Other (specify): _____

Results and interpretation

____ Positive (_____ % of tumor cells with nuclear positivity)

____ Negative (< 1% of tumor cells with nuclear positivity)

____ Negative (no tumor cells with nuclear positivity)

____ Results unknown

____ Other (specify): _____

Average intensity of tumor cell nuclei staining

____ Absent

____ Weak

____ Moderate

____ Strong

____ Unknown

____ Other (specify): _____

Note: It is optional to provide additional information using other scoring systems.

HER2 (results for invasive carcinoma performed on this specimen or a prior core needle biopsy or incisional biopsy)

Immunoperoxidase studies

Specimen used for this assay (required only if results were obtained on a specimen other than the one currently being reported)

____ Performed on this specimen

____ Performed on another specimen

____ *Specify specimen (accession number): _____

____ Pending

____ Not performed

____ No residual invasive carcinoma after presurgical (neoadjuvant) therapy

____ Other (specify): _____

Results

____ Negative (score 0)

____ Negative (score 1+)

CHECKLIST FOR THE REPORTING OF INVASIVE BREAST CARCINOMA

____ Equivocal (score 2+)

____ Positive (score 3+)

____ Other

Specify: _____

____ Results unknown

Fluorescence in situ hybridization (FISH) for HER2

Specimen used for this assay (only required if results were obtained on a specimen other than the one currently being reported)

____ Performed on this specimen

____ Performed on another specimen

*Specify specimen (accession number): _____

____ Pending

____ Not performed

____ No residual invasive carcinoma after presurgical (neoadjuvant) therapy

____ Other (specify): _____

Results

____ Not amplified (HER2 gene copy < 4.0 or ratio < 1.8)

____ Equivocal (HER2 gene copy 4.0-6.0 or ratio 1.8-2.2)

____ Amplified (HER2) gene copy > 6.0 or ratio > 2.2

*Average number of HER2 gene copies per cell: _____

*Average number of CEP17 per cell: _____

*Ratio: _____

____ Results unknown

____ Other (specify): _____

*Other ancillary studies (results for invasive carcinoma performed on this specimen or a prior core needle biopsy or incisional biopsy)

*____ Performed on this specimen

*____ Performed on another specimen

*Specify specimen (accession number): _____

*Name of test: _____

Results: _____

*Microcalcifications (select all that apply)

*____Not identified

*____Present in DCIS

*____Present in invasive carcinoma

*____Present in nonneoplastic tissue

*____Present in both carcinoma and nonneoplastic tissue

*Clinical History (select all that apply)

*Current clinical/radiologic breast findings for which this surgery is performed include

*____ Palpable mass

*____ Radiologic finding

*____ Mass or architectural distortion

*____ Calcifications

*____ Other (specify): _____

*____ Nipple discharge

*____ Prior history of breast cancer

*Specify site, diagnosis, and prior treatment: _____

*____ Prior presurgical (neoadjuvant) therapy for this diagnosis of invasive carcinoma

*Specify type: _____

*Data elements with asterisks are not required. However, these elements may be clinically important but are not yet validated or regularly used in patient management. Adapted with permission from College of American Pathologists, "Protocol for the Examination of Specimens from Patients with Invasive Carcinoma of the Breast." Web posting date: October 2009, www.cap.org.

CHECKLIST FOR THE REPORTING OF DUCTAL CARCINOMA IN SITU

DCIS of Breast: Complete Excision (Less Than Total Mastectomy, Including Specimens Designated Biopsy, Lumpectomy, Quadrantectomy, and Partial Mastectomy; With or Without Axillary Contents) and Mastectomy (Total, Modified Radical, Radical; With or Without Axillary Contents)

Surgical Pathology Cancer Case Summary (Checklist)

Specimen

____ Partial breast

____ Total breast (including nipple and skin)

____ Other (specify): _____

____ Not specified

Procedure

____ Excision without wire-guided localization

____ Excision with wire-guided localization

____ Total mastectomy (including nipple and skin)

____ Other (specify): _____

____ Not specified

Lymph Node Sampling (select all that apply)

____ No lymph nodes present

____ Sentinel lymph node(s)

____ Axillary dissection (partial or complete dissection)

____ Lymph nodes present within breast specimen (i.e., intramammary lymph nodes)

____ Other lymph nodes (e.g., supraclavicular or location not identified)

Specify location, if provided: _____

Specimen Integrity

____ Single intact specimen (margins can be evaluated)

____ Multiple designated specimens (e.g., main excisions and identified margins)

____ Fragmented (margins cannot be evaluated with certainty)

____ Other (specify): _____

Specimen Size (for excisions less than total mastectomy)

Greatest dimension: _____ cm

*Additional dimensions: _____ x _____ cm

____ Cannot be determined

Specimen Laterality

____ Right

____ Left

____ Not specified

Tumor Site (select all that apply)

*____ Upper outer quadrant

*____ Lower outer quadrant

*____ Upper inner quadrant

*____ Lower inner quadrant

*____ Central

*____ Nipple

*Position: _____ o'clock

*____ Other (specify): _____

*____ Not specified

Size (Extent) of DCIS

Estimated size (extent) of DCIS (greatest dimension using gross and microscopic evaluation): At least _____ cm

*Additional dimensions _____ x _____ cm

*Number of blocks with DCIS: _____

CHECKLIST FOR THE REPORTING OF DUCTAL CARCINOMA IN SITU

*Number of blocks examined: _____

Note: Size (extent) of DCIS is an estimation of volume of breast tissue occupied by DCIS

Histologic Type

____ Ductal carcinoma in situ; classified as Tis (DCIS) or Tis (Paget)

*Architectural Patterns (select all that apply)

*____ Comedo

*____ Paget disease (DCIS involving nipple skin)

*____ Cribriform

*____ Micropapillary

*____ Papillary

*____ Solid

*____ Other (specify): _____

Nuclear Grade

____ Grade I (low)

____ Grade II (intermediate)

____ Grade III (high)

Necrosis

____ Not identified

____ Present, focal (small foci or single cell necrosis)

____ Present, central (expansive "comedo" necrosis)

Margins (select all that apply)

____ Margins cannot be assessed

____ Margin(s) uninvolved by DCIS

Distance from closest margin: _____ mm

*Specify margins:

*Distance from superior margin: _____ mm

*Distance from inferior margin: _____ mm

*Distance from medial margin: _____ mm

*Distance from lateral margin: _____ mm

*Distance from anterior margin: _____ mm

*Distance from posterior margin: _____ mm

*Distance from other specified margin: _____ mm

*Designation of margin: _____

____ Margin(s) positive for DCIS

*Specify which margin(s) and extent of involvement

*____ Superior margin

*____ Focal

*____ Minimal/moderate

*____ Extensive

*____ Inferior margin

*____ Focal

*____ Minimal/moderate

*____ Extensive

*____ Anterior margin

*____ Focal

*____ Minimal/moderate

*____ Extensive

*____ Posterior margin

*____ Focal

*____ Minimal/moderate

*____ Extensive

*____ Medial margin

*____ Focal

CHECKLIST FOR THE REPORTING OF DUCTAL CARCINOMA IN SITU

    *____ Minimal/moderate

    *____ Extensive

   *____ Lateral margin

    *____ Focal

    *____ Minimal/moderate

    *____ Extensive

Treatment Effect: Response to Presurgical (Neoadjuvant) Therapy

 *____ No known presurgical therapy

 *____ No definite response to presurgical therapy

 *____ Probable or definite response to presurgical therapy

Lymph Nodes (required only if lymph nodes are present in specimen)

Number of sentinel nodes examined: _____

Total number of nodes examined (sentinel and nonsentinel): _____

Number of lymph nodes with macrometastases (> 0.2 cm): _____

Number of lymph nodes with micrometastases (> 0.2 mm to 0.2 cm &/or > 200 cells): _____

Number of lymph nodes with isolated tumor cells (≤ 0.2 mm and ≤ 200 cells): _____

Size of largest metastatic deposit (if present): _____

*Extranodal extension

 *____ Present

 *____ Not identified

 *____ Indeterminate

*Method of evaluation of sentinel lymph nodes (select all that apply)

 *____ Hematoxylin and eosin (H&E), 1 level

 *____ H&E, multiple levels

 *____ Immunohistochemistry

 *____ Sentinel lymph node biopsy not performed

 *____ Other (specify): _____

  Note: Sentinel node is usually the first involved lymph node. In the unusual situation in which a sentinel node is not involved by metastatic carcinoma but a nonsentinel node is involved, this information should be included in a note

Pathologic Staging (pTNM)

TNM descriptors (required only if applicable) (select all that apply)

 ____ r (recurrent)

 ____ y (post-treatment)

Primary tumor (pT)

 ____ pTis (DCIS): Ductal carcinoma in situ

 ____ pTis (Paget): Paget disease of nipple **not** associated with invasive carcinoma &/or carcinoma in situ (DCIS & or LCIS) in underlying breast parenchyma

  Note: If there has been a prior core needle biopsy, the pathologic findings from the core, if available, should be incorporated in the T classification. If invasive carcinoma or microinvasion were present on core, protocol for invasive carcinomas of breast should be used and should incorporate this information

Regional lymph nodes (pN) (choose a category based on lymph nodes received with specimen; immunohistochemistry &/or molecular studies are not required)

Note: If internal mammary lymph nodes, infraclavicular nodes, or supraclavicular lymph nodes are included in the specimen, consult the AJCC Staging Manual for additional lymph node categories.

Modifier (required only if applicable)

____ (sn) Only sentinel node(s) evaluated; if ≥ 6 sentinel nodes &/or nonsentinel nodes are removed, this modifier should not be used

Category (pN)

____ pNX: Regional lymph nodes cannot be assessed (e.g., previously removed, or not removed for pathologic study)

____ pN0: No regional lymph node metastasis identified histologically

  Note: Isolated tumor cell clusters (ITC) are defined as small clusters of cells ≤ 0.2 mm or single tumor cells, or a cluster of < 200 cells in a single histologic cross-section.† ITCs may be detected by routine histology or by immunohistochemical (IHC) methods. Nodes containing only ITCs are excluded from total positive node count for purposes of N classification but should be included in total number of nodes evaluated.

____ pN0(i-): No regional lymph node metastases histologically, negative IHC

____ pN0(i+): Malignant cells in regional lymph node(s) ≤ 0.2 mm and ≤ 200 cells (detected by H&E or IHC including ITC)

CHECKLIST FOR THE REPORTING OF DUCTAL CARCINOMA IN SITU

____ pN0(mol-): No regional lymph node metastases histologically, negative molecular findings (reverse transcriptase polymerase chain reaction [RT-PCR])

____ pN0(mol+): Positive molecular findings (RT-PCR), but no regional lymph node metastases detected by histology or IHC

____ pN1mi: Micrometastases (> 0.2 mm &/or > 200 cells, but none > 2.0 mm)

____ pN1a: Metastasis in 1-3 axillary lymph nodes, at least 1 metastasis > 2.0 mm

____ pN2a: Metastases in 4-9 axillary lymph nodes (at least 1 tumor deposit > 2.0 mm)

____ pN3a: Metastases in 10 or more axillary lymph nodes (at least 1 tumor deposit > 2.0 mm)

Distant metastasis (M)

____ Not applicable

____ cM0(i+): No clinical or radiographic evidence of distant metastasis, but deposits of molecularly or microscopically detected tumor cells in circulating blood, bone marrow, or other nonregional nodal tissue that are no larger than 0.2 mm in a patient without symptoms or signs of metastasis

____ pM1: Distant detectable metastasis as determined by classic clinical and radiographic means &/or histologically proven larger than 0.2 mm

Note: Presence of distant metastases in a case of DCIS would be very unusual. Additional sampling to identify invasive carcinoma in breast or additional history to document prior or synchronous invasive carcinoma is advised in evaluation of such cases

*Additional Pathologic Findings

*Specify: _____

*Ancillary Studies

*Estrogen receptor (results of special studies performed on this specimen or a prior core needle biopsy)

*____ Immunoreactive tumor cells present

*____ No immunoreactive tumor cells present

*____ Pending

*____ Not performed

*____ Other (specify): _____

     *Name of antibody: _____

     *Name of vendor: _____

     *Type of fixative: _____

*Progesterone receptor (results of special studies performed on this specimen or a prior core biopsy)

*____ Immunoreactive tumor cells present

*____ No immunoreactive tumor cells present

*____ Pending

*____ Not performed

*____ Other (specify): _____

     *Name of antibody: _____

     *Name of vendor: _____

     *Type of fixative: _____

*Microcalcifications (select all that apply)

*____ Not identified

*____ Present in DCIS

*____ Present in nonneoplastic tissue

*____ Present in both DCIS and nonneoplastic tissue

CHECKLIST FOR THE REPORTING OF DUCTAL CARCINOMA IN SITU

*Clinical History (select all that apply)

Current clinical/radiologic breast findings for which this surgery is performed include

*____ Palpable mass

*____ Radiologic finding

    *____ Mass or architectural distortion

    *____ Calcifications

    *____ Other (specify): _____

*____ Nipple discharge

*____ Other (specify): _____

*____ Prior history of beast cancer

    *Specify site, diagnosis, and prior treatment: _____

*____ Prior neoadjuvant treatment for this diagnosis of DCIS

    *Specify type: _____

*Data elements with asterisks are not required. However, these elements may be clinically important but are not yet validated or regularly used in patient management. †Approximately 1,000 tumor cells are contained in a 3-dimensional 0.2 mm cluster. Thus, if > 200 individual tumor cells are identified as single dispersed tumor cells or as a nearly confluent elliptical or spherical focus in a single histologic section of a lymph node, there is a high probability that > 1,000 cells are present in the lymph node. In these situations, the node should be classified as containing a micrometastasis (pN1mi). Cells in different lymph node cross-sections or longitudinal sections or levels of the block are not added together; the 200 cells must be in a single node profile even if the node has been thinly sectioned into multiple slices. It is recognized that there is substantial overlap between the upper limit of the ITC and the lower limit of the micrometastasis categories due to inherent limitations in pathologic nodal evaluation and detection of minimal tumor burden in lymph nodes. Thus, the threshold of 200 cells in a single cross-section is a guideline to help pathologists distinguish between these 2 categories. The pathologist should use judgment regarding whether it is likely that the cluster of cells represents a true micrometastasis or is simply a small group of isolated tumor cells. Adapted with permission from College of American Pathologists, "Protocol for the Examination of Specimens from Patients with Ductal Carcinoma In Situ (DCIS) of the Breast." Web posting date October 2009, www.cap.org.

Disorders of Development

JUVENILE PAPILLOMATOSIS

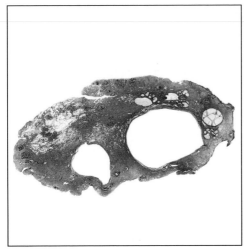

Juvenile papillomatosis is also termed "Swiss cheese" disease due to its appearance on gross and microscopic examination as multiple cysts of varying sizes within a discrete mass-forming lesion.

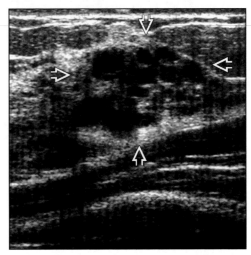

Young women and men with juvenile papillomatosis generally present with a firm, palpable, circumscribed, mobile mass. The presence of multiple cysts ⬌ is clearly seen on ultrasound examination.

TERMINOLOGY

Abbreviations
- Juvenile papillomatosis (JP)

Synonyms
- "Swiss cheese" disease

Definitions
- Rare mass-forming lesion of breast, composed of cysts and epithelial proliferation, occurring in young patients

ETIOLOGY/PATHOGENESIS

Etiology
- 1/3-2/3 of women with JP report family history of breast cancer
  - Affected relatives are usually mothers and maternal aunts
- 1/2 of male infants with JP have neurofibromatosis 1
- Suggests genetic basis for at least some cases

CLINICAL ISSUES

Epidemiology
- Incidence
  - Rare: < 1% of all excised breast masses
- Age
  - Mean age: 23 (range: 12-48 years)
    - 70% are under age 26
  - May occur in infants
- Gender
  - Occurs in both females and males

Presentation
- Presents as palpable, circumscribed, mobile mass
  - Often pre-biopsy diagnosis is fibroadenoma
- Not associated with nipple discharge

Natural History
- Can recur if not completely excised
  - ~ 10-15% of patients have concurrent cancer, and ~ 10% may subsequently develop cancer
- Subgroup of patients is at higher risk for subsequent cancer if any of the following features are present
  - Family history
  - Epithelial atypia
  - Bilateral lesions
  - Multiple lesions
  - Recurrent lesions
  - Diagnosis at an older age (> 25 years)

Prognosis
- Patients should be followed clinically due to increased risk of subsequent carcinoma in some patients

IMAGE FINDINGS

Mammographic Findings
- May be negative or shows asymmetric density

Ultrasonographic Findings
- Ill-defined mass with cysts

MR Findings
- Focal enhancement with internal cystic areas

MACROSCOPIC FEATURES

General Features
- Firm discrete mass
  - Borders are not well defined
- Multiple small (1-2 mm) cysts
  - Cysts confer "Swiss cheese" appearance on gross examination

Size
- 1-8 cm (average: 4 cm)

JUVENILE PAPILLOMATOSIS

Key Facts

Terminology
- Rare mass-forming lesion of breast, composed of cysts and epithelial proliferation, occurring in young patients
- Also termed "Swiss cheese" disease

Etiology/Pathogenesis
- 1/3-2/3 of women with JP report family history of breast cancer
- 1/2 of male infants with JP have neurofibromatosis 1

Clinical Issues
- Rare: < 1% of all excised breast masses
- Mean age: 23 (range: 12-48 years)
- Occurs in both females and males
- Presents as palpable, circumscribed, mobile mass
- Can recur if not completely excised
  - ~ 10-15% of patients have concurrent cancer, and ~ 10% may subsequently develop cancer

MICROSCOPIC PATHOLOGY

Histologic Features
- Several different histologic lesions are generally present
  - Cysts
    - Often with inspissated secretions and foamy histiocytes
  - Epithelial hyperplasia
    - Usually florid
    - Necrosis present in ~ 15%
  - Apocrine metaplasia
  - Papillomas
- Atypical architectural patterns (cribriform or micropapillary) are present in ~ 40%
- Fibroadenomas are often present as separate lesions
- Concurrent carcinoma is present in 10-15% of patients; several types are reported
  - Invasive lobular carcinoma
  - Invasive secretory carcinoma
  - Invasive carcinoma of no special type
  - Lobular carcinoma in situ

DIFFERENTIAL DIAGNOSIS

Fibrocystic Changes
- Any of the findings associated with JP can be present as multiple small lesions in the breast

  - However, essential diagnostic criterion for JP is presence of changes within a grossly defined palpable mass in young person

Papillomas
- Papillomas are often 1 of the changes associated with JP
- JP is not synonymous with finding of 1 or multiple papillomas in young patient
  - Discrete palpable mass with cysts must be present

SELECTED REFERENCES

1. Chung EM et al: From the archives of the AFIP: breast masses in children and adolescents: radiologic-pathologic correlation. Radiographics. 29(3):907-31, 2009
2. Gill J et al: Juvenile papillomatosis and breast cancer. J Surg Educ. 64(4):234-6, 2007
3. Tan TY et al: Juvenile papillomatosis of the breast associated with neurofibromatosis 1. Pediatr Blood Cancer. 49(3):363-4, 2007
4. Pacilli M et al: Juvenile papillomatosis of the breast in a male infant with Noonan syndrome, café au lait spots, and family history of breast carcinoma. Pediatr Blood Cancer. 45(7):991-3, 2005
5. Rice HE et al: Juvenile papillomatosis of the breast in male infants: two case reports. Pediatr Surg Int. 16(1-2):104-6, 2000
6. Rosen PP et al: Juvenile papillomatosis of the breast. A follow-up study of 41 patients having biopsies before 1979. Am J Clin Pathol. 93(5):599-603, 1990
7. Rosen PP et al: Juvenile papillomatosis and breast carcinoma. Cancer. 55(6):1345-52, 1985

IMAGE GALLERY

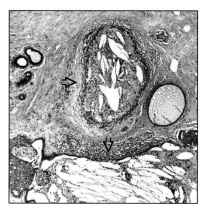 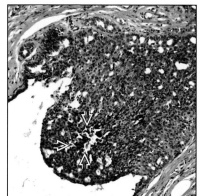 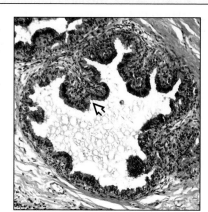

(Left) The cysts in juvenile papillomatosis are often filled with inspissated secretions and foamy histiocytes ➡. *(Center)* Florid epithelial hyperplasia is usually present. In almost 1/2 of patients, the hyperplasia has atypical features. Necrosis ➡ is reported in about 15%. *(Right)* Papillomas ➡ are another type of epithelial proliferation typical of juvenile papillomatosis; however, papillomas alone are insufficient to make this diagnosis in the absence of other criteria.

GYNECOMASTIA

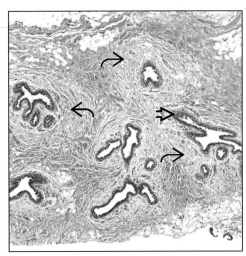

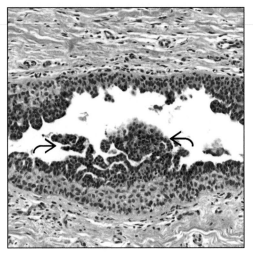

Gynecomastia results from a hormonal imbalance (estrogen/androgens) that stimulates proliferation of periductal stroma ⊿ and ductal epithelium ⊅. The stroma typically has a myxoid appearance.

The early phase of gynecomastia exhibits varying degrees of epithelial hyperplasia, which can be quite florid. The hyperplasia may form finger-like papillary projections extending into the lumen ⊿.

TERMINOLOGY

Definitions
- Nonneoplastic enlargement of the male breast due to hyperplasia of both epithelium and stroma

ETIOLOGY/PATHOGENESIS

Endocrine Alterations and Pathogenesis
- Gynecomastia develops because of alterations in ratio of free androgen to estrogen
  - Affected by serum levels of sex hormone-binding globulin
- Many causes are recognized
  - Obesity resulting in enhanced peripheral aromatization of androgen to estrogen
    - Due to displacement of estrogen from sex hormone-binding globulin or decreased metabolism
  - Declining androgen synthesis with age
  - Medications
    - Digitalis, tricyclic antidepressants, amiodarone, simvastatin, atorvastatin, omeprazole, marijuana, topical agents, spironolactone, many anti-hypertensive medications
    - Anabolic steroid use in body builders
    - Nonsteroidal antiandrogen monotherapy treatment in patients with prostate cancer
  - Liver disease (cirrhosis, liver transplantation)
  - Renal disease (chronic renal failure, dialysis, kidney transplantation)
  - Hormone deficiency (hypogonadism, pituitary adenoma) and prostate cancer
  - Gonadal failure: Decreased testosterone
    - Primary gonadal failure includes Klinefelter syndrome (47,XXY; 50% of affected men develop gynecomastia), mumps orchitis, castration
    - Secondary gonadal failure includes hypothalamic and pituitary disease
  - Hormone-producing tumors
    - Leydig cell tumor
    - Sertoli cell tumor
    - Granulosa cell tumor
- In at least 25% of cases, no cause is identified

CLINICAL ISSUES

Epidemiology
- Incidence
  - Gynecomastia is common finding
    - Palpable breast tissue can be detected in 36% of healthy young adult males
    - 57% of healthy older men and 70% of hospitalized elderly males show evidence of gynecomastia
  - 3 distinct peaks of gynecomastia occur during male life span
    - Infancy: 60-90% of male infants show transient gynecomastia due to maternal estrogens; may produce milk ("witch's milk")
    - Puberty: 48-64% of males develop gynecomastia (peak incidence: 13-14 years); over 1/2 have family history of gynecomastia
    - Older age: Highest prevalence seen in males between 50-80 years of age
  - Incidence of symptomatic gynecomastia is markedly lower

Site
- Subareolar and just superior to nipple

Presentation
- Most often presents as a palpable, tender, firm, mobile, disc-shaped mound of tissue
- May be painful; most common in 1st 6 months; possibly associated with stromal edema
- May be unilateral or bilateral
- Can be localized or diffuse

GYNECOMASTIA

Key Facts

Terminology
- Nonneoplastic enlargement of male breast due to hyperplasia of epithelium and stroma

Etiology/Pathogenesis
- Gynecomastia develops due to imbalance in ratio of free androgen to estrogen (variety of etiologies)

Clinical Issues
- 3 distinct peaks in occurrence of gynecomastia
  - Male infants (60-90%), transient
  - Males at puberty (48-64%, peak age: 13-14)
  - Highest prevalence in older males (50-80 years)
- Gynecomastia is benign, usually self-limited
  - For persistent or symptomatic lesions, pharmacological and surgical options are available

Microscopic Pathology
- Hormonal imbalance stimulates stromal and glandular tissue in gynecomastia
- Early changes (active florid phase)
  - Proliferation of periductal connective tissue, edema, inflammation
  - Mammary ductular epithelial hyperplasia
- Later changes (inactive fibrous phase)
  - Flattening of ductal epithelium
  - Progressive fibrosis of adjacent stroma
- Histological appearance of gynecomastia is same regardless of underlying cause

Top Differential Diagnoses
- Male breast cancer
- Myofibroblastoma

Natural History
- Benign condition and is usually self-limited
  - Over time, fibrotic tissue gradually replaces symptomatic proliferation of glandular tissue, and tenderness resolves
    - If regression occurs, no therapeutic intervention is necessary
  - When work-up is negative for other underlying pathology, reassurance and periodic follow-up are recommended
- If gynecomastia persists and is associated with pain, pharmacological and surgical options are available
- Gynecomastia associated with specific drug use can be treated by withdrawing causative agent
  - May result in regression of gynecomastia and decrease pain

Treatment
- Surgical approaches
  - Simple surgical excision may be indicated for symptomatic lesions that are persistent
    - Most commonly used technique is subcutaneous mastectomy
    - Surgical treatment typically produces good cosmesis and is well tolerated
- Adjuvant therapy
  - Symptomatic gynecomastia of recent onset may respond to antiestrogen therapy
    - Short course of estrogen receptor modifiers (tamoxifen or raloxifene)
    - Reported to lead to reductions in pain and nodule size without long-term adverse effects

Prognosis
- Benign condition: Only necessary to treat due to concerns with pain &/or cosmetic appearance

IMAGE FINDINGS

Mammographic Findings
- 3 patterns depending on duration and cause
  - Early (< 1 year)
    - Discrete subareolar mass extending posteriorly in fan-shaped pattern
  - Late (> 1 year)
    - Flame-shaped central mass with linear projections into peripheral tissue
  - Diffuse (related to exogenous estrogen treatment, e.g., patients with prostate cancer or transsexual patients)
    - Dense nodular parenchyma resembling female breast
    - Lacks Cooper ligaments

MACROSCOPIC FEATURES

General Features
- Usually ill-defined area of fibrous breast tissue

Size
- 2-6 cm

MICROSCOPIC PATHOLOGY

Histologic Features
- Normal adult breast tissue consists of nipple and rudimentary large ducts
- In gynecomastia, there is increase in glandular elements, fibrous stroma, and adipose tissue
  - Epithelial component consists primarily of branching ducts and terminal ductules
    - Absent or minimal lobule formation
    - Receptors for androgens and estrogens are present
- Histologic appearance changes over time
- Early changes (active florid phase)
  - Increase in proliferation of periductal connective tissue, edema, and inflammation
    - Myxoid stroma contains fibroblasts, myofibroblasts, lymphocytes, and plasma cells
    - Pseudoangiomatous stromal hyperplasia often present
  - Epithelial hyperplasia common

GYNECOMASTIA

- Hyperplasia can be florid with papillary tufts
- Papillae have broad base and narrow "pinched" apex
- Surrounding epithelium is also hyperplastic
- Narrow-based papillae with bulging tips &/or complex architecture are not seen
- Atypical ductal hyperplasia, atypical lobular hyperplasia, DCIS, and LCIS are uncommon and should be diagnosed with caution
- Later changes (inactive fibrous phase)
  - Gradual resolution of inflammatory reaction
    - Flattening of ductal epithelium
    - Squamous metaplasia may be present
    - Progressive fibrosis of adjacent stromal elements
    - Hyalinized periductal stroma
  - Lesions may regress completely, or there may be residual fibrous nodule
- Histologic appearance of gynecomastia is same regardless of underlying cause
- Incidental carcinoma in subcutaneous mastectomies for gynecomastia is very unusual
  - < 1% of males under 21 years
  - ~ 6% of all patients have atypical ductal hyperplasia
    - Significance of this finding for risk of later development of breast cancer is unknown

ANCILLARY TESTS

Immunohistochemistry
- Hormone receptors
  - Estrogen, progesterone, and androgen receptor expression is seen in virtually all cases of gynecomastia
  - Patients with Klinefelter syndrome and gynecomastia exhibit markedly elevated expression of ER and PR in ductal epithelium
    - Cases of gynecomastia due to other causes do not demonstrate such a significant elevation of these receptors
- Prostate specific antigen (PSA)
  - Gynecomastia induced by antiandrogen therapy may show strong focal PSA reactivity in ductal epithelium
    - This finding should not be misinterpreted as evidence of metastasis to breast from underlying prostate cancer
    - Prostatic acid phosphatase is negative

DIFFERENTIAL DIAGNOSIS

Pseudogynecomastia
- Accumulation of subareolar fat without proliferation of glandular tissue
- Physical examination reveals diffuse breast enlargement without subareolar palpable nodule
- Usually older obese males

Male Breast Cancer
- Only 0.5-1% of breast cancers occur in men
- Risk factors

- *BRCA2* carriers (4-30% of men with breast cancer, 6% lifetime risk), Cowden syndrome, *CHEK2* mutation carriers
- Klinefelter syndrome (4-20% of men with breast cancer)
- Increasing age
- Infertility, undescended testis, orchiectomy, orchitis
- Estrogen therapy
- Chest radiation
- Gynecomastia is **not** thought to be a risk factor
- Invasive carcinoma presents as palpable mass
  - Often found at larger size and with more frequent skin and muscle involvement than cancers in females
  - Papillary carcinomas are more common in men than in women
  - Majority positive for ER and PR
  - Must be distinguished from metastatic prostate carcinomas
    - Prostate cancers are negative for cytokeratin 7, may be positive for ER-α, and are positive for prostate specific antigen and prostatic acid phosphatase
    - Breast cancers are positive for cytokeratin 7, ER, and PR, may be positive for prostate specific antigen, and are negative for prostatic acid phosphatase
- DCIS is rare (5% of male breast cancers); may present as nipple discharge
  - Papillary pattern involving large nipple ducts is common
  - Micropapillary DCIS must be distinguished from gynecomastia
    - Papillae have narrow bases and bulbous ends ("drumstick" or "light bulb" morphology)
    - Other complex architectural patterns may be present
    - Intervening epithelium is generally flat
    - Cells are monomorphic in appearance
    - Associated calcifications are common
    - Necrosis may be present

Myofibroblastoma
- Clinical presentation (elderly man, palpable nodule) may overlap with gynecomastia
  - Usually discrete circumscribed mass rather than diffuse enlargement
- Only tumor to occur with equal frequency in male and female breasts
- Solid proliferation of spindle-shaped myofibroblasts
  - Epithelial elements are not present within mass

SELECTED REFERENCES

1. Johnson RE et al: Gynecomastia: pathophysiology, evaluation, and management. Mayo Clin Proc. 84(11):1010-5, 2009
2. Niewoehner CB et al: Gynaecomastia and breast cancer in men. BMJ. 336(7646):709-13, 2008

GYNECOMASTIA

Microscopic Features

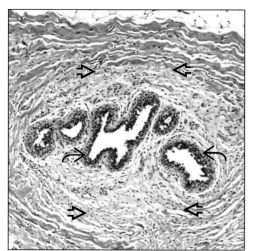

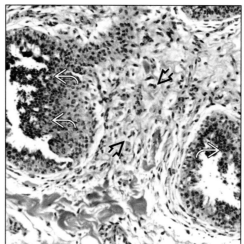

(Left) Gynecomastia is a benign proliferation of mammary ductal elements ⮕ and stroma ⮕ in male breast tissue. Small ducts are present, but lobule formation is very uncommon. *(Right)* The early (active or florid) phase of gynecomastia is characterized by loose hypercellular, myxoid, and edematous stroma ⮕. The edema may contribute to the pain associated with some cases. Scattered lymphocytes may be present. Epithelial hyperplasia is a common feature ⮕.

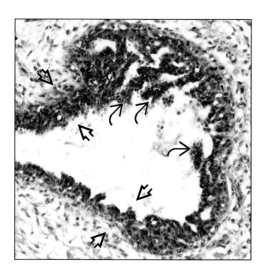

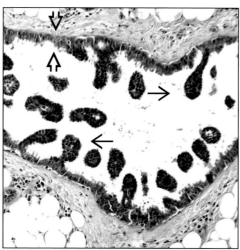

(Left) Hyperplastic ductal epithelium commonly forms papillary tufts that tend to be broad-based & taper near the tips ⮕. Intervening epithelium is also hyperplastic ⮕. *(Right)* Papillary hyperplasia associated with gynecomastia must be distinguished from micropapillary DCIS, which is characterized by papillae with narrow necks & bulbous ends ⮕. Intervening epithelium is generally flat ⮕. Calcifications are common, and necrosis is sometimes present.

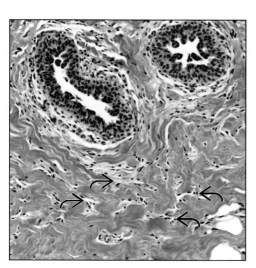

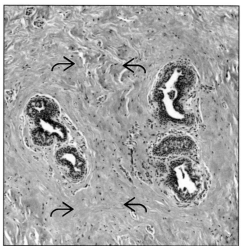

(Left) In later stages of gynecomastia, there is gradual resolution of inflammatory reaction with progressive fibrosis of the periductal stroma. Not uncommonly, pseudoangiomatous stromal hyperplasia ⮕ is present in adjacent fibrotic stroma. *(Right)* Later changes in gynecomastia have been referred to as inactive or fibrotic phase. As seen here, there is dense fibrosis and hyalinization of the periductal stroma ⮕. In some cases, the lesion resolves.

HAMARTOMA (FIBROADENOLIPOMA)

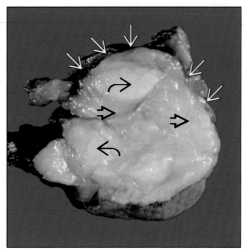

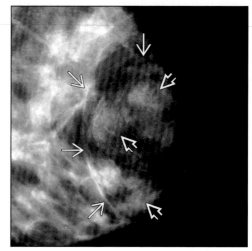

Hamartomas form circumscribed ➡ or lobulated masses consisting of an admixture of adipose tissue ⇨ and normal-appearing breast tissue with fibrous stroma ➡.

Mammogram shows an 8 cm encapsulated mass ➡ containing fat (black areas) and parenchymal densities ⇨ compatible with hamartoma in this 39 year old. Despite its size, the mass was not palpable.

TERMINOLOGY

Abbreviations
- Mammary hamartoma (MH)

Synonyms
- Fibroadenolipoma, adenolipofibroma

Definitions
- Hamartomas, distinct subtype of benign tumors
  - Proliferation of cells that show normal differentiation but are disorganized with respect to architecture
- MHs are well-circumscribed lesions composed of a disorganized overgrowth of benign mammary tissues
  - Variously composed of ductal and lobular epithelium and stromal mesenchymal elements
  - Typical MH shows considerable overlap with other benign breast lesions

ETIOLOGY/PATHOGENESIS

PTEN Hamartoma Tumor Syndromes
- MHs are more commonly observed in patients with dysgenetic disorders such as Cowden syndrome
  - Cowden syndrome is autosomal dominant disorder associated with increased risk of developing benign and malignant tumors
    - Breast, thyroid, skin, central nervous system, and GI tract are most frequently affected
    - Solitary MHs are associated with Cowden syndrome
  - Cowden syndrome is caused by germline mutation in tumor suppressor gene *PTEN*
    - Loss of *PTEN* increases activation and signaling of PI3K/Akt/mTOR pathway
    - MHs probably result from dysgenesis of mesenchymal cells leading to abnormal growth resulting from this altered cellular signaling

CLINICAL ISSUES

Epidemiology
- Incidence
  - MH has a reported incidence of 0.1-0.7%
    - Many authors consider this entity underdiagnosed
    - Findings in some MHs may be misinterpreted as other benign lesions
- Age
  - Range is wide (20-80 years)
    - Mean age: 45 years
- Gender
  - Almost exclusively seen in female patients

Presentation
- Typical patient will present with painless, soft to firm, palpable breast mass
  - Clinical impression is often that of fibroadenoma
- May be detected on screening mammogram
  - MHs may be solitary or multiple
    - May occur in ectopic breast tissue in axillary or inguinal areas

Treatment
- No treatment is necessary for most patients
  - Consider surgical excision for lesion with atypical appearance on imaging
    - Suspicious calcifications or intrinsic mass lesion would be unusual for typical MH
  - Consider surgical excision for large symptomatic lesions
    - Extremely large lesions may require mammoplasty or reconstruction

Prognosis
- MH is benign lesion
  - Most patients can be followed
  - Consider surgical excision for symptomatic cases or atypical clinical presentation

HAMARTOMA (FIBROADENOLIPOMA)

Key Facts

Terminology
- Mammary hamartoma (MH)
- Synonyms: Fibroadenolipoma, adenolipofibroma
  - Well-circumscribed mass, disorganized overgrowth of mature benign mammary tissues
  - Variously composed of ductal and lobular epithelium and stromal mesenchymal elements

Clinical Issues
- Reported incidence of 0.1-0.7%
- Benign lesion
- Consider surgical excision for symptomatic cases or atypical appearance

Image Findings
- Classic appearance has been described as "breast within a breast" on mammogram

Macroscopic Features
- Cut surface shows variable fat and fibrotic stroma

Microscopic Pathology
- Stroma of MH can consist of a variety of different mesenchymal tissues
  - Different stromal elements can coexist in single lesion
  - Adipose tissue is typically seen in variable amounts
  - Cases with prominent myoid changes are referred to as myoid hamartomas
- Typical lesions will show glands that resemble normal terminal ductal lobular units

Top Differential Diagnoses
- Fibroadenoma
- Benign phyllodes tumor

IMAGE FINDINGS

General Features
- Best diagnostic clue
  - Classic appearance has been described as "breast within a breast" on mammogram
- Location
  - May occur anywhere within breast
- Size
  - Extremely variable size range for MH has been reported
    - Lesion sizes may be from 1.2 cm to > 14 cm
    - Typically MH is 3-6 cm at diagnosis

Mammographic Findings
- MH presents as ovoid to round or lobulated, well-circumscribed mass lesion
  - Mixed heterogeneous density with mottled center
  - Degree of mammographic density will depend upon fat component of lesion
  - Other benign mass-forming breast lesions typically do not include fat
- Thin smooth "pseudocapsule" with peripheral radiolucent zones is common finding
- MH will displace adjacent normal breast tissue mammographically
- Benign-appearing calcifications may be present within lesion

Ultrasonographic Findings
- Well-encapsulated mass lesion with variably echogenic rim
  - Heterogeneous internal echogenicity
    - Mixture of sonolucent fat and echogenic glandular elements
    - May be uniformly hyperechoic if minimal fat component

MR Findings
- Well-encapsulated mass with dark, smooth, thin rim
  - Ovoid in shape with internal heterogenicity
  - Heterogeneous gadolinium enhancement

- Internal fat intensity is demonstrated in most lesions

MACROSCOPIC FEATURES

General Features
- Gross examination shows nodular masses that are rounded and possess smooth pushing contours
  - Some lesions will have been "shelled out" or marginally excised at time of surgery because of encapsulated nature of MHs
  - Lesions are soft to firm on palpation
  - Cut surface shows variable fatty areas within fibrotic stroma, tan-white to yellow in color
  - Clefts and fronds within lesion are typically not present
- Macroscopic nodules are well demarcated from adjacent breast tissue

MICROSCOPIC PATHOLOGY

Histologic Features
- MHs are composed of mixture of glandular structures and different stromal elements
  - Disproportionate growth of these tissue components will show disorganization of mature mammary tissues
  - Stromal component may spread around and through lobular structures
- Stromal components
  - Stroma of MH can consist of a variety of different mesenchymal tissues
    - Often several different types can coexist in single lesion
  - Varying degrees of dense hyalinized stroma is seen between individual lobules in most cases
    - Fibrotic stroma may show areas of pseudoangiomatous changes
    - Some lesions will show predominance of dense fibrotic stroma
  - Adipose tissue is typically noted within stroma in variable amounts

HAMARTOMA (FIBROADENOLIPOMA)

- ▪ Adipose tissue can account for 5-90% of stromal area
  - ○ Less common stromal changes in MH
    - ▪ Smooth muscle differentiation or myoid changes
    - ▪ Cases with prominent myoid changes have been referred to as myoid hamartomas
    - ▪ Bizarre stromal giant cells
    - ▪ Foci of cartilaginous or osseous metaplasia
- **Epithelial components**
  - ○ Glandular tissue of MH can exhibit a range of different appearances
    - ▪ Typical lesions will show glands that resemble normal terminal ductal lobular units
    - ▪ Will contain normal luminal and myoepithelial layers
  - ○ Mild epithelial hyperplasia without atypia may be seen but is uncommon
    - ▪ Rare lesions have been reported to contain foci of ADH or DCIS
  - ○ Some lesions can show cystic changes, apocrine metaplasia, and adenosis

Cytologic Features

- Glandular and stromal components of MH should show normal differentiation and lack atypia

ANCILLARY TESTS

Immunohistochemistry

- Hormone receptors
  - ○ ER and PR expression in MH resembles what is seen in normal breast tissues
    - ▪ Positive in 10-20% of luminal epithelial cells
- Growth factor receptors and tumor suppressor genes
  - ○ HER2 and p53 expression should be uniformly negative in all cases
- Mesenchymal and myoepithelial cell markers
  - ○ Muscle-specific actin will highlight stromal smooth muscle in myoid MH
  - ○ S100 protein will highlight adipose tissue and areas of cartilaginous metaplasia
  - ○ Myoepithelium surrounding luminal cells will stain with p63, CK5/6, calponin, muscle specific actin
- Pattern of protein expression seen in MH is reflective of nonneoplastic, "hamartomatous" nature of these lesions

Cytogenetics

- Chromosome 12 translocation breakpoints have been described in MH that map within multiple aberration region (MAR)
  - ○ MAR is known to be a major cluster region of chromosome 12 breakpoints
  - ○ Chromosome 12 breakpoints are frequent in a number of benign tumors
    - ▪ e.g., uterine leiomyomas, lipomas, and pleomorphic salivary gland adenomas

DIFFERENTIAL DIAGNOSIS

Fibroadenoma

- Morphologic appearance of MH can overlap with other fibroepithelial breast lesions that have glandular and stromal components
  - ○ MH can be misinterpreted as fibroadenoma, particularly in limited sample (needle biopsy)
- Fibroadenoma will have more orderly epithelial/ stromal organization compared to MH
  - ○ Epithelial component will be more disorganized and irregularly dispersed in fibroadipose stroma in MH
- MH may be softer than fibroadenoma depending on amount of adipose tissue
- Significant adipose tissue component would not typically be seen in fibroadenoma

Benign Phyllodes Tumor

- Another fibroepithelial breast lesion with admixed glands and stromal elements
  - ○ Phyllodes tumor may contain neoplastic adipose tissue (e.g., well-differentiated liposarcoma)
  - ○ Phyllodes tumors may also invade into surrounding normal adipose tissue
  - ○ Stromal adipose tissue component of MH will appear mature and benign
- Stroma of MH is less cellular than that of phyllodes tumor
  - ○ Stromal atypia and pleomorphism is not seen in MH and would suggest phyllodes tumor
- Cleft-like epithelial-lined spaces due to stromal overgrowth are typically present in phyllodes tumor and not seen in MH

DIAGNOSTIC CHECKLIST

Pathologic Interpretation Pearls

- Core needle biopsy usually shows nonspecific mixture of benign breast tissue elements
  - ○ Findings may be insufficient for specific histopathologic diagnosis
  - ○ Presence of fibrous tissue within lobules, or admixed fibrous tissue, muscle, and fat in stroma, should raise possibility of hamartoma
- Correlation with imaging findings and clinical impression may be necessary for definitive diagnosis

SELECTED REFERENCES

1. Blumenthal GM et al: PTEN hamartoma tumor syndromes. Eur J Hum Genet. 16(11):1289-300, 2008
2. Georgian-Smith D et al: The mammary hamartoma: appreciation of additional imaging characteristics. J Ultrasound Med. 23(10):1267-73, 2004
3. Herbert M et al: Breast hamartomas: clinicopathological and immunohistochemical studies of 24 cases. Histopathology. 41(1):30-4, 2002
4. Tse GM et al: Hamartoma of the breast: a clinicopathological review. J Clin Pathol. 55(12):951-4, 2002

HAMARTOMA (FIBROADENOLIPOMA)

Microscopic Features

PB

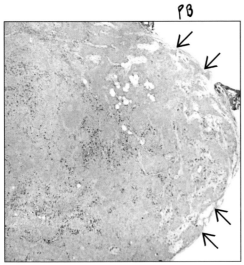

AT

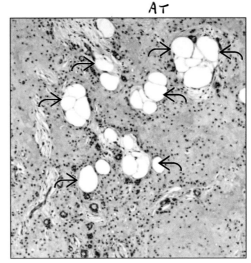

(Left) MH is a benign fibroepithelial lesion that classically presents as a well-defined mobile mass with sharply "geographic," pushing borders ➡. Some lesions will have been shelled out at the time of surgery due to this circumscribed growth pattern. (Right) Adipose tissue ➡ is frequently seen as a component of the stroma and can vary from 5-90% of a MH. The fat cells in the stroma of MH are well differentiated and mature and lack cytologic atypia.

gs

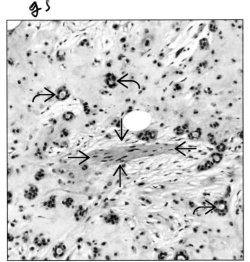

M

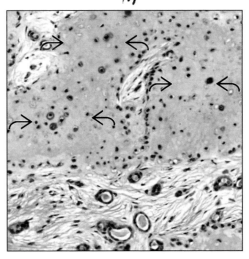

M

(Left) MH consists of benign glandular structures ➡ and mature stromal mesenchymal elements. Areas showing muscle differentiation can be seen ➡ and, when prominent, the designation of myoid hamartoma may be used. (Right) Different mature stromal mesenchymal elements can coexist in the stroma of MH. Although rare, areas of cartilaginous stromal metaplasia ➡ have been reported. The mature features and lack of atypia are important considerations for a correct diagnosis.

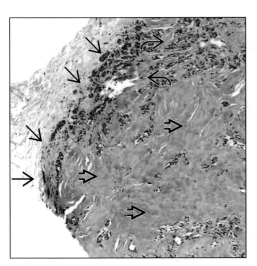

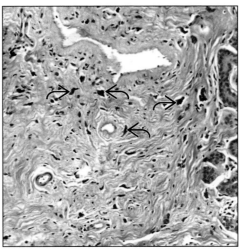

(Left) The stromal portion of MH is often densely hyalinized ➡ and can spread around and through lobular structures ➡. MHs are well circumscribed ➡ like fibroadenomas but lack an orderly epithelial stromal relationship. (Right) Occasionally, MHs may contain bizarre stromal giant cells ➡ within a fibrotic stroma. These cells are dispersed and contain enlarged irregular hyperchromatic nuclei. This finding should not be overinterpreted as indicating malignancy.

Benign Epithelial Lesions

EPIDEMIOLOGY: LESIONS CONFERRING INCREASED RISK OF BREAST CARCINOMA

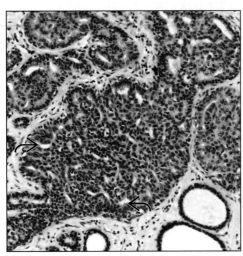

Epithelial hyperplasia ⇗ is associated with an increased bilateral risk of invasive cancer. Genetic studies suggest that this lesion is not a direct precursor but rather an indicator of risk.

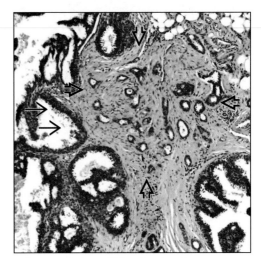

Columnar cell change ⇲ is often found in proximity to tubular carcinomas ⇲, and both share similar genetic changes. Therefore, columnar cell change is thought to be a predictor of risk and a potential precursor.

TERMINOLOGY

Abbreviations
- Benign breast disease (BBD)

Definitions
- BBD can be classified according to subsequent risk of developing invasive breast cancer

INTRODUCTION

Study of Benign Breast Lesions
- Widespread use of mammographic screening has led to increased detection of BBD
- Studies have identified 2 main classes of benign lesions
  - Risk indicators for development of invasive breast cancer
    - Predict generalized increased risk to both breasts
    - May be associated with other risk factors such as those related to hormone exposure
  - Precursor lesions for invasive carcinoma
    - Cells or lesions that may accumulate additional changes to eventually evolve into carcinoma
    - Lesions are nonobligate precursors; majority do not progress during patient's lifetime
- Some lesions are both risk indicators and precursors
  - For example, 60% of cancers developing after atypical hyperplasia (AH) are ipsilateral, and 40% are contralateral
    - Suggests that AH not only is an indicator of bilateral risk but can also act as a precursor in same breast

Morphologic Studies
- BBD was originally classified according to histologic appearance
- Association with carcinoma was postulated based on appearance and location

- Some BBD resembles carcinoma
  - Hyperplasia resembles atypical ductal hyperplasia (ADH), which resembles DCIS
  - Atypical lobular hyperplasia (ALH) and LCIS are cytologically identical to invasive lobular carcinoma
  - Radial sclerosing lesions are similar in appearance to tubular carcinoma
- BBD is frequently seen adjacent to invasive carcinomas
  - ALH and LCIS near invasive lobular carcinoma
  - ADH and DCIS near invasive ductal carcinoma
  - Columnar cell change (± flat epithelial atypia), ALH/LCIS, and tubular carcinoma ("Rosen triad")

Epidemiologic Studies
- In 3 large studies, BBD in breast biopsies from women without cancer were categorized
  - Nashville Study
  - Nurses' Health Study
  - Mayo Clinic Study
- Women were followed over time to determine groups most likely to develop invasive carcinoma
- Each study confirmed importance of classification of BBD to predict risk of subsequent carcinoma
- Estimates of risk associated with each group of lesions were similar

Biologic Studies
- Attempt to separate markers of risk from true precursors of invasive carcinoma
  - Loss of heterozygosity (LOH) for selected markers
  - Gene expression profiling
  - Comparative genomic hybridization
- Most common recognized precursors are similar to ER-positive cancers
  - "Low-grade neoplasia" family includes columnar cell lesions, flat epithelial atypia, ADH, ALH, LCIS, and low-grade DCIS
    - Show strong diffuse positivity for ER

EPIDEMIOLOGY: LESIONS CONFERRING INCREASED RISK OF BREAST CARCINOMA

- In normal breast, only ER-negative cells undergo division
- Therefore, there must be a change in regulation of cell proliferation
  - Often associated with invasive tubular carcinoma, invasive cribriform carcinoma, grade 1 and 2 lobular carcinomas, and grade 1 invasive ductal carcinomas
    - All share deletions of 16q and gains of 1p
  - Radial sclerosing lesions are sometimes associated with tubular carcinomas or lobular carcinomas
    - Some are associated with loss of 16q
    - In some cases, it may be difficult to distinguish radial sclerosing lesion from low-grade invasive carcinoma
  - High-grade ER-positive cancers also show 16q deletions and are likely etiologically related to low-grade ER-positive cancers
- Precursors for ER-negative cancer have not been established
  - Carcinomas are heterogeneous and include triple negative (basal-like), HER2 positive, apocrine, and other types
  - Characterized by aneuploidy and numerous genetic changes
    - Most frequent changes are losses at 1p, 8p, and 17p and gains at 1q and 8q
    - Amplifications are common and include 1q, 8q, 17q (site of HER2), and 20q
    - Minority have deletion of 16q, characteristic of low-grade carcinomas
- Several possible precursor lesions have been proposed
  - Myoepithelial precursor lesion
    - Normally ER negative
    - Some carcinomas have features very similar to myoepithelial cells
    - Histologically recognizable neoplastic myoepithelial lesions are quite rare
    - Myoepithelial precursor lesion might progress rapidly to invasive carcinoma as a 2nd normal population of cells supporting basement membrane would not be present
    - Very short in situ phase could explain why ER-negative carcinomas are rarely associated with extensive ER-negative DCIS
  - ER-positive ADH
    - ER-negative carcinomas may arise from ER-positive ADH that loses ER expression
    - Some cases of DCIS show markedly heterogeneous expression of ER (less common in ADH)
    - Could explain reduction of subsequent cancers due to tamoxifen treatment or oophorectomy for women with cancer who have *BRCA1* germline mutations
    - However, genetic changes in ER precursors differ from ER-negative carcinomas; loss of 16q is very unusual
    - In addition, ER-negative carcinomas are almost never associated with ER-positive precursors in adjacent tissue
  - Apocrine metaplasia
    - Shares morphologic features with cases of apocrine DCIS and invasive carcinoma

- Normally ER negative and androgen receptor positive
- Increased immunoreactivity for HER2 is present in ~ 50% of cases but is not associated with gene amplification; ~ 1/2 of apocrine carcinomas show gene amplification and HER2 overexpression
- Myoepithelial cells may be diminished in number
- At least some lesions are clonal; may share genetic gains and losses with adjacent DCIS and invasive carcinoma
- Apocrine metaplasia without atypia associated with cysts; not associated with increased risk of breast cancer
- Possible that there are apocrine precursors with nuclear or architectural (complex papillary hyperplasia) atypia that can act as precursor lesions
  - Microglandular adenosis (MGA)
    - Very rare infiltrative lesion of breast
    - Normally ER negative
    - Although the name "adenosis" suggests an in situ lesion, this is an invasive tumor that lacks myoepithelial cells
    - Better classified as a type of nonmetastasizing invasive carcinoma rather than a benign precursor lesion

EPIDEMIOLOGY

Incidence
- BBD in breast biopsies without cancer
  - Nonproliferative changes: 40-70%
  - Proliferative breast disease without atypia: 30-60%
  - Atypical hyperplasia: 10-15%
    - ADH is more common than ALH due to the association with mammographic calcifications

CLINICAL IMPLICATIONS

Clinical Significance of Lesions of Risk
- Lesions conferring an increased risk of breast cancer are useful in counseling patients
  - Family history in addition to BBD may slightly elevate risk
- Models of risk incorporate types of BBD
  - AH is used to calculate risk using Gail model
  - Proliferative disease and AH are used in Rosner and Colditz model
- Women at very high risk can consider options for risk reduction
  - Risk of ≥ 1.66% within next 5 years using Gail model is used for eligibility for chemoprevention with tamoxifen
    - Also reduces BBD and likelihood of undergoing breast biopsy
  - Increased surveillance at shorter intervals or using additional modalities (e.g., MR) may detect cancers earlier
  - Bilateral mastectomy reduces risk by > 90%

EPIDEMIOLOGY: LESIONS CONFERRING INCREASED RISK OF BREAST CARCINOMA

Potential Precursor Lesions for Carcinoma

Type of Lesion	ER	Clonality	Genetic Changes	Comment
Suggested Precursors for ER-positive Carcinomas				
Epithelial hyperplasia	Positive/negative	Rarely clonal; mixture of cell types	Rare, not consistent, not similar to cancers	Unlikely to be a precursor
Columnar cell change/ flat epithelial atypia	Positive	Clonal	Gains at 16p, 15q, 17q, 19q; losses at 16q, X	Likely precursor; often found in association with ADH, ALH, LCIS, and low-grade carcinomas
ALH/LCIS	Positive	Clonal	Gains at 1q 6q; losses at 16q, 16p, 17p; E-cadherin mutations	Nonobligate precursor for lobular carcinomas
ADH	Positive	Clonal	Gains at 1q; losses at 1q, 16q, 17p	Nonobligate precursor for carcinomas
Radial sclerosing lesion	Positive/negative	May be clonal	May have loss at 16q	May be associated with tubular and lobular carcinomas
Suggested Precursors for ER-negative Carcinomas				
Apocrine metaplasia	Negative	May be clonal	Gains at 2q, 13q, 1p; losses at 1p, 10q, 11q, 13q, 16q, others	Atypical lesions may be precursors for some apocrine carcinomas
Myoepithelial cells	Negative	Unknown	Unknown	Some carcinomas have expression profiles similar to myoepithelial cells; histologic lesions are rare
Microglandular adenosis	Negative	Clonal	Gains at 2q, 8q; losses at 5q, 14q	Better classified as a nonmetastasizing carcinoma
ER-positive precursors	Positive	May be clonal	Losses at 16q	Some lesions show heterogeneity with loss of ER; however, not genetically related to ER-negative carcinoma

- Weight reduction, exercise, and dietary changes may have small effect, but primary benefit is reduced risk of cardiovascular disease

Core Needle Biopsies
- BBD is often detected on core needle biopsies due to association with mammographic lesions
- Excision is indicated when sufficient risk of adjacent DCIS or invasive carcinoma
  - ADH is often present adjacent to DCIS; excisions yield DCIS in ~ 15% of cases
  - Columnar cell change with flat epithelial atypia: Excisions yield DCIS in ~ 15% of cases
  - Papillomas with atypia: Associated with carcinoma on excision in 20-60% of cases
- Routine excision of other types of BBD on core needle biopsy is debated
  - With good pathologic and radiologic correlation, likelihood of a missed carcinoma is small (< 5%)

MICROSCOPIC FINDINGS

Classification of BBD
- **Nonproliferative changes: No increased risk** (~ 4% lifetime risk of invasive carcinoma)
  - Fibroadenoma (lacking complex features)
  - Gross or microscopic cysts
  - Apocrine metaplasia
  - Duct ectasia
  - Mild hyperplasia: 3-4 cell layers
- **Proliferative disease without atypia: 1.5-2x increased risk** (5-7% lifetime risk of invasive carcinoma)
  - Sclerosing adenosis
  - Papilloma
  - Radial sclerosing lesion
  - Fibroadenoma with complex features (sclerosing adenosis, apocrine cysts)
  - Moderate to florid epithelial hyperplasia
  - Columnar cell change ± flat epithelial atypia
- **Proliferative disease with atypia: 4-5x increased risk** (13-17% lifetime risk of invasive carcinoma)
  - Atypical ductal hyperplasia: Multifocality may increase risk
  - Atypical lobular hyperplasia: Risk is higher in premenopausal women or if pagetoid spread is present

SELECTED REFERENCES

1. Aroner SA et al: Columnar cell lesions and subsequent breast cancer risk: a nested case-control study. Breast Cancer Res. 12(4):R61, 2010
2. Lopez-Garcia MA et al: Breast cancer precursors revisited: molecular features and progression pathways. Histopathology. 57(2):171-92, 2010
3. Manfrin E et al: Benign breast lesions at risk of developing cancer--a challenging problem in breast cancer screening programs: five years' experience of the Breast Cancer Screening Program in Verona (1999-2004). Cancer. 115(3):499-507, 2009
4. Brandt SM et al: The "Rosen Triad": tubular carcinoma, lobular carcinoma in situ, and columnar cell lesions. Adv Anat Pathol. 15(3):140-6, 2008
5. Allred DC et al: The origins of estrogen receptor alpha-positive and estrogen receptor alpha-negative human breast cancer. Breast Cancer Res. 6(6):240-5, 2004

EPIDEMIOLOGY: LESIONS CONFERRING INCREASED RISK OF BREAST CARCINOMA

Predictors of Increased Risk of Breast Cancer

Apocrine met

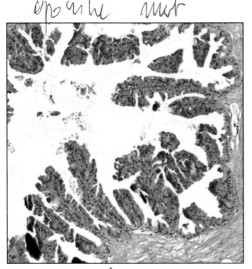

Scler adenosis

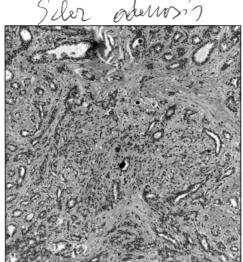

(Left) Typical apocrine metaplasia is commonly found in cysts and does not increase the risk of cancer. However, biologic and genetic changes shared with apocrine carcinomas suggest that at least some atypical apocrine lesions may act as precursors. (Right) Sclerosing adenosis is associated with a slightly increased cancer risk. Although it closely mimics the appearance of invasive carcinoma, it is considered a marker of risk and not a true precursor of invasive carcinoma.

Intraductal papilloma

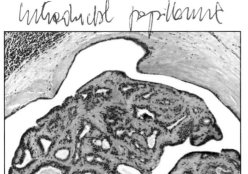

RSL

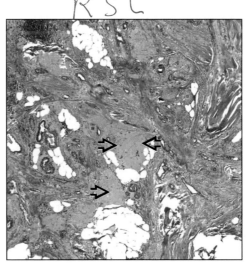

(Left) Intraductal papillomas slightly increase the risk of breast cancer. Some are associated with atypia and may be involved by carcinoma. A relationship to papillary carcinoma has not been established. (Right) Radial sclerosing lesions morphologically resemble invasive carcinomas ⊡, and some may be clonal proliferations with loss of 16q. They may be associated with tubular or lobular carcinomas.

ADH

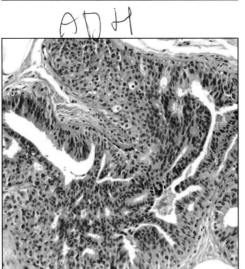

ALH

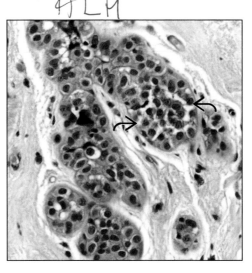

(Left) ADH shares morphologic and molecular features with low-grade DCIS; 60% of subsequent cancers are ipsilateral, supporting that ADH is a predictor of risk as well as a nonobligate precursor. (Right) ALH ➜, LCIS, and invasive lobular carcinomas share similar genetic changes and loss of E-cadherin. ALH and LCIS are associated with a slightly greater risk in the ipsilateral breast and, like ADH, are likely nonobligate precursor lesions as well as predictors of bilateral risk.

NONPROLIFERATIVE CHANGES

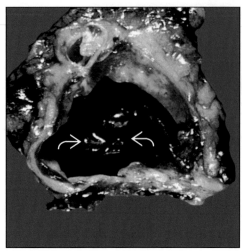

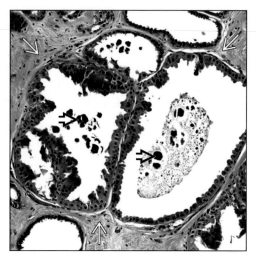

Simple cysts are often aspirated to completion and do not need further evaluation. Cysts containing debris or blood ➡ may appear solid and require biopsy to exclude the possibility of carcinoma.

Calcifications ▣ are often found within clusters of apocrine cysts ➡. When detected on mammographic screening, biopsy is warranted as DCIS is also frequently associated with multiple calcifications.

TERMINOLOGY

Abbreviations
- Benign breast disease (BBD) with nonproliferative changes

Synonyms
- Fibrocystic breast disease
- Fibrocystic changes

Definitions
- Commonly encountered constellation of benign breast changes including cysts, apocrine metaplasia, stromal fibrosis, and adenosis

ETIOLOGY/PATHOGENESIS

Hormonal Effects
- Responsiveness of breast tissues to monthly changes of estrogen and progesterone levels plays an important role in pathogenesis of BBD
  - May be related to excess hormonal stimulation &/or hypersensitivity of breast tissue
- Clinical factors associated with increased risk of BBD
  - Late age at menopause, estrogen replacement therapy, nulliparity, low body mass index, and family history of breast cancer
- Clinical factors associated with decreased risk of BBD
  - High parity, oral contraceptives, physical activity
  - Tamoxifen, when used for breast cancer prevention, is associated with 28% reduction in prevalence of BBD (relative risk 0.72)

CLINICAL ISSUES

Epidemiology
- Incidence
  - Very common

- Some elements of BBD are evident in up to 50-60% of women of reproductive age
  - Increased incidence of BBD seen in postmenopausal women receiving estrogens ± progestins for > 8 years (relative risk increased by 1.70)

Presentation
- Mammographic screening
  - May present with densities or calcifications
- Palpable lumps
  - Diffuse symmetrical lumpiness is commonly found on physical examination
  - Size and symptoms may fluctuate over course of menstrual cycle
- Cyclic breast pain may occur during late luteal phase of menstrual cycle

Natural History
- BBD with nonproliferative changes does not increase risk of breast cancer

IMAGE FINDINGS

Mammographic Findings
- Masses: May be circumscribed or ill defined
- Calcifications: Usually clustered

MR Findings
- BBD has wide spectrum of morphologic and kinetic features on MR
- MR should preferably be performed in 1st 1/2 of menstrual cycle to minimize false-positive findings

MACROSCOPIC FEATURES

General Features
- Cut surface has whitish, firm, rubbery appearance
- Unopened larger "blue-dome" cysts contain turbid fluid that is brown or blue in color

4

NONPROLIFERATIVE CHANGES

Key Facts

Terminology

- Benign breast disease (BBD) with nonproliferative changes includes a commonly encountered constellation of pathologic findings
  - Stromal fibrosis
  - Cysts
  - Apocrine metaplasia
  - Calcifications
  - Adenosis

Clinical Issues

- Frequent findings: Evident in up to 50-60% of women of reproductive age
- Nonproliferative changes do not increase risk of breast cancer
- Often presents as palpable masses (cysts) or mammographic lesions (densities or calcifications)

Top Differential Diagnoses

- BBD with proliferative changes &/or atypia
  - These changes increase subsequent risk of developing breast carcinoma

Reporting Considerations

- "Fibrocystic changes" or "fibrocystic disease" can include a number of different pathologic processes
  - Can be useful descriptive terms but not as diagnostic terms for pathologic diagnosis
- Clinically more relevant to list specific types of benign lesions present including
  - Lesion conferring highest risk of subsequent carcinoma (if present)
  - Lesion that correlates with symptom or radiologic finding that prompted biopsy

MICROSCOPIC PATHOLOGY

Histologic Features

- Most common features of BBD encountered in histologic sections include cysts, apocrine metaplasia, fibrosis, and adenosis
  - Changes are usually bilateral and multifocal
- **Fibrosis**
  - Stromal fibrosis contributes to palpable densities on breast exam and increased density on imaging
  - Attributed to repeated cyst rupture, inflammation, and scarring
  - Must be distinguished from normal dense breast tissue in young women not associated with cysts and inflammation
- **Apocrine metaplasia**
  - Cells have abundant granular eosinophilic cytoplasm; may be vacuolated
    - Resembles normal apocrine epithelium of sweat glands
  - Nuclei are enlarged and round and contain prominent nucleoli
    - Some cells are tetraploid
    - Moderate degrees of nuclear variation may be present but not true cytologic atypia
  - Apocrine cells are ER/PR negative and positive for androgen receptor and GCDFP-15
    - May show membrane enhancement for HER2
  - Architecture can be flat or papillary
  - Apocrine changes can be seen in both benign and malignant breast lesions
    - Lesions with apocrine change are difficult to evaluate as cells are monomorphic due to metaplasia rather than neoplasia
    - Focal apocrine metaplasia is more common in benign lesions
    - Cytologic atypia, necrosis, mitoses, or complex architecture raises possibility of an apocrine neoplasm
- **Cysts**
  - Common finding
    - May be due to unfolding of lobules
  - May be microscopic or grossly visible
    - May present clinically as large, firm, palpable mass
    - Clusters of cysts can form masses
  - Typically lined by single layer of luminal epithelial cells
    - Apocrine (type I cysts)
    - Flattened luminal cells (type II cysts)
    - Mild epithelial hyperplasia may be present
  - Contents vary
    - Clear fluid
    - Blood and fibrin: May appear as solid mass on imaging
    - Secretory debris: Often associated with calcifications
    - Mucin: Associated with mucocele formation
  - Cysts may rupture, spilling contents into surrounding stroma
    - Incites chronic inflammatory reaction
    - Ochrocytes are histiocytes with brown granular cytoplasm due to phagocytosis of lipids
    - May be associated with fat necrosis
    - Resulting fibrosis can form irregular mass by palpation or imaging
    - Calcifications may be found in surrounding stroma associated with a giant cell response
- **Calcifications**
  - Numerous calcifications are detected microscopically
    - Mammography can only detect calcifications approximately 100 microns in size or multiple clustered overlapping calcifications
    - Only calcifications with suspicious features as determined by imaging (i.e., numerous, clustered, irregular, or linear and branching) are associated with malignancy
    - Therefore, it is imperative that the pathologist examine the tissue harboring radiologic calcifications
  - Often difficult to correlate calcifications seen microscopically with those seen by imaging according to number or size

NONPROLIFERATIVE CHANGES

- Imaging visualizes calcifications in 3 dimensions; tissue sections on slides are essentially 2 dimensional
- Thus it is essential to be certain that the tissue harboring radiologic calcifications has been examined
  - "Milk of calcium" is a radiology term used to describe calcifications that change in relative position in the 2 different mammographic views
    - On horizontal-cranial-caudal view, cysts are flattened and calcifications are not influenced by gravity
    - On upright medial-lateral-oblique view, calcifications appear to line bottom of cysts under influence of gravity in "tea cup" pattern
    - Correlates with calcifications in large cysts that can layer out on bottom of cyst
  - Calcifications may be calcium phosphate or calcium oxalate
  - Calcium phosphate appears as granular dark purple crystals
    - May be associated with secretory debris, necrotic debris, mucin, or dense collagenized stroma in fibroadenomas
    - Do not polarize
  - Calcium oxalate crystals are flat rhomboid or needle-shaped crystals
    - More easily seen under polarized light
    - Only found in association with cysts with apocrine metaplasia; if there has been cyst rupture, crystals may be present in surrounding stroma
    - Never associated with malignancy
  - Special stains can be used to identify calcium deposits
    - If calcifications are not evident by light microscopy, they are very small and unlikely to correlate with mammographic calcifications
    - Therefore, special stains are rarely useful in practice
  - If calcifications cannot be identified, the following should be considered
    - Calcifications not biopsied: All specimens removed to evaluate calcifications should be radiographed to ensure calcifications are present
    - Tissue with calcifications not sampled: Tissue and paraffin blocks can be radiographed to identify location of calcifications
    - Calcifications dissolved: Can occur if tissue is left in formalin for multiple days
    - Calcifications lost from small specimens, particularly core needle biopsies: Helpful for radiologists to wrap cores in paper and place them in a cassette prior to placing in formalin
    - "Calcifications" not present: Radiodense metallic debris from prior surgery, trauma, or gold treatments for rheumatoid arthritis can mimic radiographic calcifications
- **Adenosis**
  - Increased number of acini per terminal ductal lobular unit

- Acini are often enlarged or dilated but not distorted, as is seen in sclerosing adenosis
- Often associated with columnar cell change ± flat epithelial atypia
- **Mastitis**
  - Scattering of lymphocytes is normal finding
  - Chronic inflammation is increased at end of each menstrual cycle and after pregnancy or lactation
  - Inflammatory response after cyst rupture and spillage of secretory material into stroma may contribute to fibrosis

DIFFERENTIAL DIAGNOSIS

BBD with Proliferative Changes &/or Atypia
- Some benign changes increase subsequent risk of developing breast carcinoma
  - Include sclerosing adenosis, radial sclerosing lesions, papillomas, moderate to florid epithelial hyperplasia, columnar cell change, complex fibroadenomas, atypical ductal hyperplasia, and atypical lobular hyperplasia
- These changes should be specifically reported when present

REPORTING CRITERIA

Terminology
- "Fibrocystic changes" or "fibrocystic disease" can include a large number of different pathologic processes
  - Useful for describing a group of lesions but not as diagnostic terms in pathology reports
- Clinically more relevant to list specific types of benign lesions present
- Most important benign lesions are
  - Those that confer highest risk of subsequent cancer
  - Those that correlate with finding that prompted biopsy

SELECTED REFERENCES

1. Wells CA et al: Non-operative breast pathology: apocrine lesions. J Clin Pathol. 60(12):1313-20, 2007
2. Santen RJ et al: Benign breast disorders. N Engl J Med. 353(3):275-85, 2005
3. van den Bosch MA et al: Magnetic resonance imaging characteristics of fibrocystic change of the breast. Invest Radiol. 40(7):436-41, 2005

NONPROLIFERATIVE CHANGES

Imaging and Microscopic Features

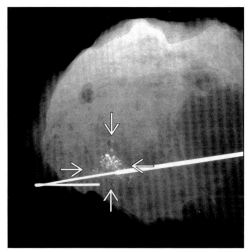

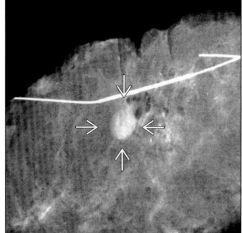

(Left) Cysts are often seen as clustered calcifications ➡ on mammography. The calcifications form on membranes in secretions that provide a regular repeating structure allowing for crystallization. (Right) Cysts present as circumscribed masses ➡ when filled with secretory debris or hemorrhage. A cluster of small cysts can also appear to be a dense circumscribed or lobulated mass. The mass sometimes disappears if a core needle biopsy causes the cyst to collapse.

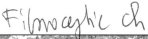

Fibrocystic ch

Ca++ oxalate

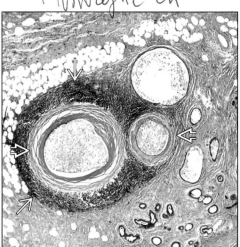

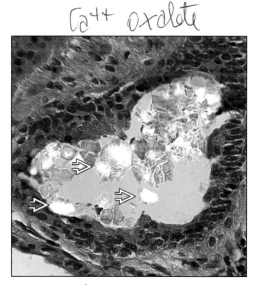

(Left) The "fibro-" of fibrocystic changes is due to cyst rupture followed by a chronic inflammatory response ➡ and periductal scarring fibrosis ➡. This type of dense breast tissue must be distinguished from the normal breast stroma in young women. (Right) Calcium oxalate crystals only occur in association with apocrine cysts or adjacent to ruptured cysts. The crystals can be difficult to see on H&E as they are colorless or pale yellow. However, polarized light makes them readily apparent ➡.

Apocr. Met

Adenosis?

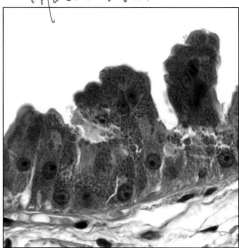

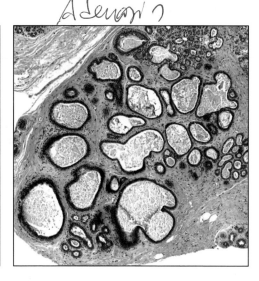

(Left) Apocrine metaplasia closely resembles apocrine sweat glands. The nuclei are enlarged and round and have prominent nucleoli. The cytoplasm is abundant and eosinophilic and may have bright red granules. (Right) Adenosis refers to increased acini per lobule. This lobule would not be classified as sclerosing adenosis as the lumens are not compressed by a prominent stromal component. Columnar cell change is often seen associated with this type of lobule.

COLUMNAR CELL CHANGE WITH OR WITHOUT FLAT EPITHELIAL ATYPIA

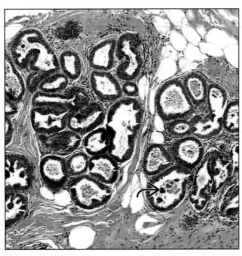

The terminal ductal lobular units in columnar cell change demonstrate prominent distension and cystic dilatation. The luminal spaces contain secretions with granular punctate calcifications ➯.

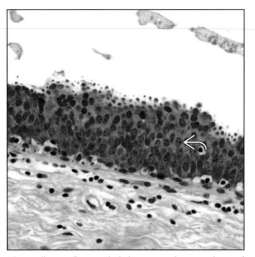

The cells in flat epithelial atypia show a loss of nuclear polarity and appear stratified here. There is monomorphous low-grade cytologic atypia with chromatin changes and punctate nucleoli ➯.

TERMINOLOGY

Abbreviations
- Columnar cell change (CCC)
- Flat epithelial atypia (FEA)

Synonyms
- Columnar cell hyperplasia
- Columnar alteration with prominent apical snouts and secretions
- Atypical cystic lobules
- Unfolding breast lobules
- Term CCC is preferred
  - Encompasses spectrum of lesions with characteristic cytoarchitectural features

Definitions
- CCC characterized by presence of columnar epithelial cells
  - Cells line dilated terminal ductal lobular units (TDLUs)
- Cystic spaces frequently contain luminal secretions and flocculent material
  - Frequently associated with microcalcifications
- Encountered with increasing frequency in breast needle core biopsies
  - Most frequently seen in biopsies performed for mammographic microcalcifications

ETIOLOGY/PATHOGENESIS

Genetic Changes
- Molecular studies show genetic changes similar to those found in low-grade DCIS and invasive cancer
  - May represent nonobligate precursor lesion
  - Likely early lesion in low-grade breast neoplasia development

CLINICAL ISSUES

Site
- Often a multifocal process that may be bilateral
  - Rarely will produce palpable abnormality
- Reported association and coexistence with other more serious low-grade neoplastic processes
  - Atypical ductal hyperplasia, atypical lobular hyperplasia
  - Low-grade ductal carcinoma in situ, lobular carcinoma in situ
  - Invasive low-grade ductal carcinomas (tubular carcinoma), invasive lobular carcinoma

Presentation
- Microcalcifications on screening mammography
  - Finding will prompt needle core biopsy

Treatment
- Surgical approaches
  - FEA found on needle core biopsy
    - Surgical excision is recommended
    - Diagnosis is upgraded to more serious lesion in 20-30% of cases
  - CCC found on needle core biopsy (without atypia)
    - Most likely incidental finding as result of microcalcifications
    - Can be followed as long as there are no other worrisome clinical or mammographic findings

Prognosis
- Follow-up studies suggest low risk of progression to invasive cancer
- Need to exclude association with more serious lesion, such as low-grade DCIS or tubular carcinoma

IMAGE FINDINGS

Mammographic Findings
- Presence of microcalcifications frequent finding

COLUMNAR CELL CHANGE WITH OR WITHOUT FLAT EPITHELIAL ATYPIA

Key Facts

Terminology
- Columnar cell change (CCC)
- Flat epithelial atypia (FEA)
- Encountered with increasing frequency in breast biopsies performed for mammographic microcalcifications

Microscopic Pathology
- CCC
  - TDLUs with variably dilated acini lined by 1 or 2 layers of columnar epithelial cells
  - Cells are uniform with ovoid to elongated nuclei oriented perpendicular to basement membrane
  - Cystic spaces contain luminal secretions, flocculent material, and frequent microcalcifications
- FEA: Similar architectural features to CCC and columnar cell hyperplasia (CCH)

- Epithelial cells demonstrate low-grade, monomorphic-type cytologic atypia
- Cells show nuclear enlargement, stratification, and variable nucleoli
- May coexist with areas that fulfill diagnostic criteria for ADH or low-grade DCIS

Diagnostic Checklist
- FEA may show genetic changes similar to those seen in low-grade DCIS and invasive carcinomas
- Risk of FEA progressing to invasive cancer appears to be low when present as isolated finding
- Presence of FEA should alert pathologist to search for other frequently associated lesions
  - ADH, DCIS, lobular neoplasia, and invasive carcinoma

MACROSCOPIC FEATURES

General Features
- Typically no gross findings in absence of other associated lesions

MICROSCOPIC PATHOLOGY

Histologic Features
- CCC
  - TDLUs with variably dilated acini lined by 1 or 2 layers of columnar epithelial cells
    - Enlargement and cystic dilatation of TDLUs
    - Flat growth pattern by lining epithelial cells, may show some stratification
  - Cells are uniform with ovoid to elongated nuclei
    - Nuclei show polarity, oriented in regular fashion
    - Typically perpendicular to basement membrane
  - Evenly dispersed chromatin without conspicuous nucleoli or atypia
    - Mitotic figures rarely encountered
  - Apical cytoplasmic blebs or snouts often present at luminal surface of epithelial cells
  - Flocculent secretions typically present in lumina of involved acini
  - Luminal calcifications frequently present and may be prominent
- Columnar cell hyperplasia (CCH)
  - Features similar to CCC
  - Epithelial lining cells show varying cellular stratification, > 2 cell layers
  - Nuclei ovoid to elongated and, for the most part, oriented perpendicular to basement membrane
    - Lack conspicuous nucleoli or atypia
  - Proliferating columnar cells form small mounds, tufts, or abortive micropapillations
    - Cellular tufts and mounds are broader at base than at tips
- FEA
  - Similar architectural features as seen in CCC and CCH

- Morphologic spectrum based on presence and degree of epithelial atypia
- FEA represents columnar cell lesion with varying degrees of cytologic atypia
  - Epithelial cells demonstrate low-grade, monomorphic-type cytologic atypia
  - Typically show relatively round or ovoid enlarged nuclei
  - Increased nuclear to cytoplasmic ratio
  - Nuclei can show stratification
    - Loss of polarity
    - Loss of perpendicular orientation to basement membrane
  - Nuclear chromatin may be evenly dispersed or slightly marginated
    - Nucleoli may be present and variably prominent
  - Cytologic features similar to those seen in low-grade DCIS, lesions lack architectural changes
  - FEA may coexist with areas that fulfill diagnostic criteria for ADH or low-grade DCIS
  - Finding of FEA should prompt diligent search for such areas
    - May require careful examination of deeper levels &/or additional sections

ANCILLARY TESTS

Immunohistochemistry
- Cells are strongly ER(+) throughout lesion
- Luminal low molecular weight keratin 8/18 positive
- High molecular weight keratin 5/6 negative

Array CGH
- FEA is clonal proliferation
- Genetic changes have been described, including losses of 16q
- Changes similar to those seen in low-grade DCIS and invasive carcinoma

4

COLUMNAR CELL CHANGE WITH OR WITHOUT FLAT EPITHELIAL ATYPIA

Flat Epithelial Atypia, Differential Diagnosis

	Flat Epithelial Atypia	ADH/DCIS	Apocrine Metaplasia
Cytology	Low-grade, monomorphic cytologic atypia	Low-grade, monomorphic cytologic atypia	Cells lack atypia, low nuclear to cytoplasmic ratio with eosinophilic cytoplasm
Architecture	Flat growth pattern	Complex architectural growth	Flat or micropapillary growth pattern
Calcifications	Frequent	Frequent	May be present

DIFFERENTIAL DIAGNOSIS

Apocrine Metaplasia
- May show cystically dilated spaces and calcifications similar to CCC
- Apocrine metaplasia shows low nuclear to cytoplasmic ratio, eosinophilic granular cytoplasm, and round nuclei with nucleoli
- Flat growth pattern or micropapillary growth pattern

Atypical Ductal Hyperplasia/Low-Grade Ductal Carcinoma In Situ
- Complex architectural patterns
  - Well-developed micropapillations
  - Rigid cellular bridges, bars, and arcades
  - "Punched-out" fenestrations
- Complex architectural patterns should be considered either ADH or DCIS
- FEA may coexist with ADH and DCIS

High-Grade Ductal Carcinoma In Situ, Flat or "Clinging" Pattern
- High-grade cytologic atypia with marked nuclear pleomorphism is not a feature of FEA
- High-grade nuclear features merit designation of high-grade DCIS
  - Classified as DCIS even when neoplastic cells comprise only single cell layer (flat or clinging pattern)
- Such lesions are rarely seen in absence of high-grade DCIS exhibiting other architectural patterns

DIAGNOSTIC CHECKLIST

Clinically Relevant Pathologic Features
- Encountered with increasing frequency in breast biopsies for mammographic calcifications
- FEA may show genetic changes similar to those seen in low-grade DCIS and invasive carcinomas
  - May represent precursor lesion or early stage of low-grade DCIS in some cases
- Risk of FEA progressing to invasive cancer appears to be low when present as isolated finding
  - Data are limited, and further studies will be required to help define relationship between CCC, FEA, and breast neoplasia
- Presence of FEA should alert pathologist to search for other frequently associated lesions
  - ADH and DCIS
  - Lobular neoplasia
  - Invasive carcinoma

Pathologic Interpretation Pearls
- Look for dilated TDLUs with flat growth pattern of lining epithelium, luminal secretions, and microcalcifications
- Look for cytologic atypia (nuclear enlargement, loss of polarization, nuclear stratification, chromatin changes, mitotic figures)
- Look for other more serious associated neoplastic epithelial lesions
- If FEA is encountered on excision
  - Perform multiple levels to look for architectural changes of ADH or low-grade DCIS
  - Submit all tissue for microscopic examination

SELECTED REFERENCES

1. Jara-Lazaro AR et al: Columnar cell lesions of the breast: an update and significance on core biopsy. Pathology. 41(1):18-27, 2009
2. Abdel-Fatah TM et al: Morphologic and molecular evolutionary pathways of low nuclear grade invasive breast cancers and their putative precursor lesions: further evidence to support the concept of low nuclear grade breast neoplasia family. Am J Surg Pathol. 32(4):513-23, 2008
3. Boulos FI et al: Histologic associations and long-term cancer risk in columnar cell lesions of the breast: a retrospective cohort and a nested case-control study. Cancer. 113(9):2415-21, 2008
4. Lerwill MF: Flat epithelial atypia of the breast. Arch Pathol Lab Med. 132(4):615-21, 2008
5. Abdel-Fatah TM et al: High frequency of coexistence of columnar cell lesions, lobular neoplasia, and low grade ductal carcinoma in situ with invasive tubular carcinoma and invasive lobular carcinoma. Am J Surg Pathol. 31(3):417-26, 2007
6. Collins LC et al: Clinical and pathologic features of ductal carcinoma in situ associated with the presence of flat epithelial atypia: an analysis of 543 patients. Mod Pathol. 20(11):1149-55, 2007
7. Datrice N et al: Do breast columnar cell lesions with atypia need to be excised? Am Surg. 73(10):984-6, 2007
8. Pinder SE et al: Lobular in situ neoplasia and columnar cell lesions: diagnosis in breast core biopsies and implications for management. Pathology. 39(2):208-16, 2007
9. Dabbs DJ et al: Molecular alterations in columnar cell lesions of the breast. Mod Pathol. 19(3):344-9, 2006
10. O'Malley FP et al: Interobserver reproducibility in the diagnosis of flat epithelial atypia of the breast. Mod Pathol. 19(2):172-9, 2006
11. Schnitt SJ et al: Columnar cell lesions of the breast. Adv Anat Pathol. 10(3):113-24, 2003
12. Rosen PP: Columnar cell hyperplasia is associated with lobular carcinoma in situ and tubular carcinoma. Am J Surg Pathol. 23(12):1561, 1999

4

COLUMNAR CELL CHANGE WITH OR WITHOUT FLAT EPITHELIAL ATYPIA

Microscopic Features

Cytt / lumi secr.

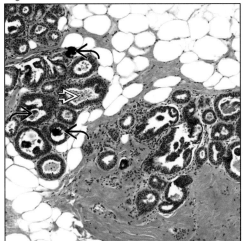

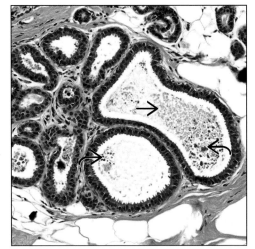

(Left) This low-power view shows a TDLU with cystically dilated acini with luminal secretions ⊟. While CCC is typically a microscopic finding without a mass lesion, patients frequently come to clinical attention due to associated calcifications ⊟. (Right) These dilated spaces contain abundant luminal secretions ⊟, which may show calcifications ⊟ and are lined by 2 cell layers of luminal cells and myoepithelial cells. The luminal cells are orderly and uniform.

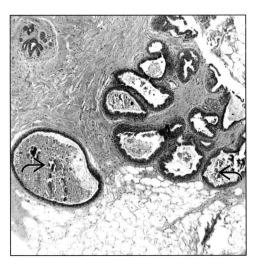

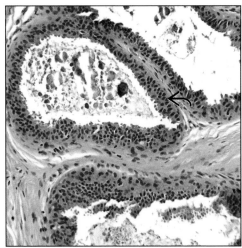

(Left) CCC on needle core biopsy is being seen with increasing frequency, associated with the work-up of mammographic calcifications ⊟. The lesion is usually easily identified at low power due to cystic dilation of the TDLU. Microcalcifications are frequently associated with luminal secretions. (Right) On higher power examination, the lining epithelium of this case of CCC consists of 2 layers of relatively uniform and orderly columnar epithelial cells ⊟.

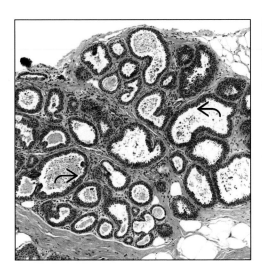

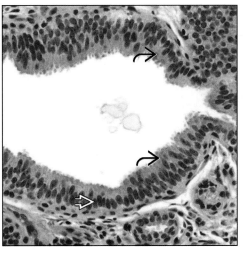

(Left) An important diagnostic feature for CCC is the lack of any evidence of architectural complexity with a simple "flat" epithelial lining ⊟. (Right) The cells lining the cystic spaces in CCC are uniform, oval to elongated, and oriented perpendicular to the underlying basement membrane ⊟. The cells seen here demonstrate dispersed nuclear chromatin and lack atypia. The cells show nuclear polarity with nuclei located toward the basement membrane side of the cells ⊟.

COLUMNAR CELL CHANGE WITH OR WITHOUT FLAT EPITHELIAL ATYPIA

Microscopic Features

(Left) The epithelial lining in some cases of CCC can show varying degrees of stratification of nuclei ➡. Such cases may show cytologic atypia, and a careful evaluation of the cytologic features is warranted. *(Right)* Proliferating columnar cells can form small mounds, tufts, or abortive micropapillations broader at base than tips ➡. This epithelial proliferation appears disorganized with varying nuclear sizes consistent with flat epithelial atypia (FEA).

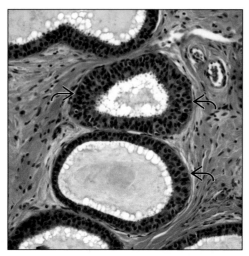
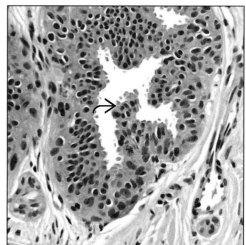

(Left) Low-power view of CCC shows a characteristic cystically dilated TDLU ➡ with flocculent luminal secretions. This characteristic appearance is usually readily apparent on low-power examination. *(Right)* Higher magnification shows some evidence of nuclear stratification in this case of CCC ➡, which should be followed by a careful evaluation of the epithelial lining for evidence of monomorphic low-grade cytologic atypia.

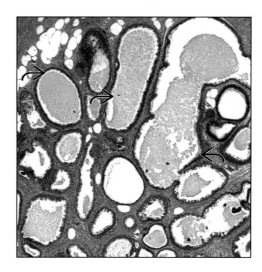
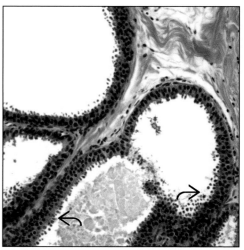

(Left) CCC with marked cytologic atypia (FEA) is shown. Atypical features are nuclear stratification, loss of polarity, and loss of perpendicular orientation to the basement membrane, resulting in a disorganized appearance ➡. *(Right)* On higher power examination, this lesion shows evidence of nuclear enlargement, stratification, vesicular chromatin with nucleoli and mitotic figures ➡. These findings should prompt a careful search for more serious low-grade neoplastic processes.

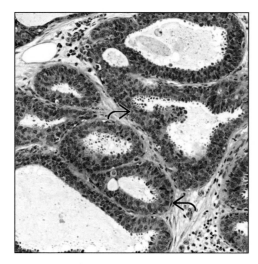
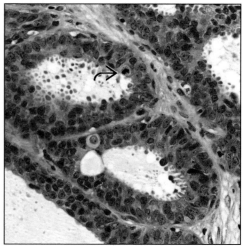

COLUMNAR CELL CHANGE WITH OR WITHOUT FLAT EPITHELIAL ATYPIA

Differential Diagnosis

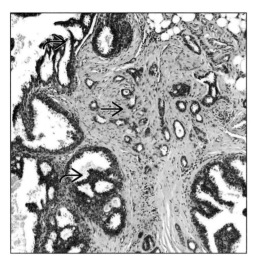

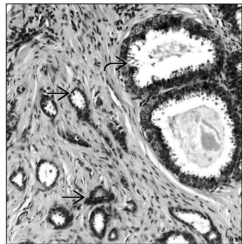

(Left) CCC & FEA can be associated with atypical ductal hyperplasia ➡ and tubular carcinoma ➡. The reported association between CCC and tubular carcinoma has led some authors to suggest that some columnar cell lesions may represent a neoplastic precursor to low-grade mammary neoplasia. *(Right)* Higher magnification shows infiltrating tumor cells in a desmoplastic stroma ➡ adjacent to the cystically dilated spaces of CCC ➡.

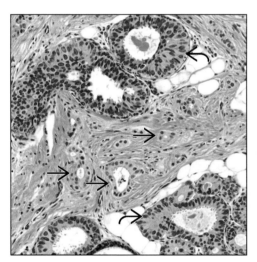

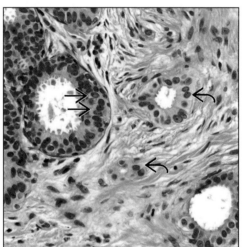

(Left) FEA associated with tubular carcinoma is shown. The FEA ➡ shows characteristic cystically dilated spaces lined by atypical epithelial cells with stratification. The infiltrating carcinoma ➡ shows angulated glandular spaces, which lack surrounding myoepithelial cells. *(Right)* On higher power examination, the cells within the FEA ➡ have a similar cytologic appearance to the tubular carcinoma ➡, further supporting the idea that FEA may represent a precursor lesion.

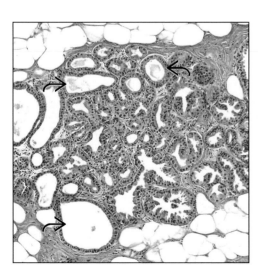

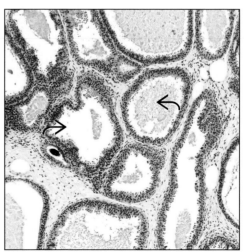

(Left) Apocrine metaplasia can demonstrate cystic dilatation of spaces ➡ with secretions and calcifications similar to CCC. The cells of apocrine metaplasia show granular eosinophilic cytoplasm and characteristic round nuclei, often with prominent nucleoli. *(Right)* CCC has a characteristic low-power appearance including cystically dilated spaces with luminal secretions ➡. The cytology of the lining epithelium is different allowing for diagnostic distinction from other cystic lesions.

MUCOCELE-LIKE LESIONS

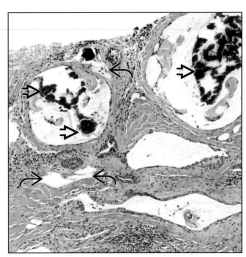

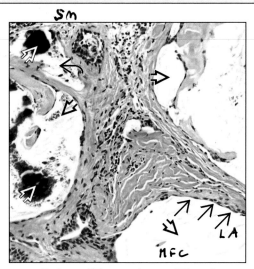

Mucocele-like lesions typically consist of multiple dilated mucinous cysts that may rupture with discharge of mucin into the surrounding stroma ➔. Coarse calcifications are commonly seen ➔.

Mucin-filled cysts ➔, stromal mucin ➔, and coarse calcifications ➔ are readily identified. The epithelial lining consists of a single layer of uniform attenuated cells ➔ that lack atypia.

TERMINOLOGY

Abbreviations
- Mucocele-like lesion (MLL)

Synonyms
- Mucocele-like tumor

Definitions
- Uncommon breast lesion, composed of mucin-containing cysts that may rupture
  o Analogous to mucocele of minor salivary glands
- MLL of breast was initially described as benign lesion
  o However, MLL may be associated with atypical ductal hyperplasia (ADH), ductal carcinoma in situ (DCIS), &/or invasive carcinoma
    ▪ Associated DCIS and invasive carcinoma are usually mucin producing
- MLL may represent spectrum of lesions ranging from benign to neoplastic

ETIOLOGY/PATHOGENESIS

Relationship with Mucinous Carcinoma
- Several lines of evidence suggest that at least some MLLs may be related to mucinous carcinoma
  o ADH reported in up to 50% of patients with MLL
    ▪ Some may later develop mucinous carcinoma
  o Some MLLs contain areas of DCIS and invasive mucinous carcinoma at initial diagnosis
  o Mucin found in MLL is identical to that found in mucinous carcinoma

CLINICAL ISSUES

Epidemiology
- Age
  o Wide range at presentation
    ▪ 27-79 years (mean: 48 years)

Presentation
- MLL is usually asymptomatic
  o Screening mammograms may show mass or calcifications
- Less commonly, MLL is detected as palpable mass

Treatment
- Diagnosis of MLL on needle core biopsy warrants excision for further evaluation
  o Careful evaluation of excised tissue sample for atypia or carcinoma is required
  o Multiple H&E levels on tissue with mucin in stroma may be helpful to exclude invasive mucinous carcinoma
- If no carcinoma is found after complete excision, no additional treatment is necessary

Prognosis
- MLL without associated carcinoma is benign lesion

IMAGE FINDINGS

Mammographic Findings
- Pleomorphic &/or amorphous coarse calcifications are most common finding
- Less common is lobulated and circumscribed dense mass
  o Indistinct margins may be due to rupture and extravasation of mucin into stroma

Ultrasonographic Findings
- Multiple cysts with calcified or noncalcified solid components, often multiple, may suggest diagnosis of MLL
  o Hypoechoic round, oval, or lobulated solid masses may be present
  o Intracystic mural nodules correlate with mucin within cysts

MUCOCELE-LIKE LESIONS

Key Facts

Terminology
- Mucocele-like lesion (MLL)
  - Uncommon lesion involving breast, composed of mucin-containing cysts that may rupture
  - Analogous to mucocele of minor salivary glands

Clinical Issues
- MLL is usually asymptomatic
- Screening mammograms may show mass or calcifications
- Less commonly, MLL is detected as palpable mass
- MLL without associated carcinoma is benign lesion

Microscopic Pathology
- Cystically dilated ducts contain luminal mucin
  - Spaces lined by cuboidal to attenuated epithelium

- Epithelium may show spectrum of proliferative changes including hyperplasia, ADH, or DCIS
- May include associated ruptured ducts with extravasated mucin within surrounding stroma
- Histocytes and inflammatory cells may be present
- Strips or clusters of epithelial cells may become detached from wall, floating free in mucin
  - Multiple H&E levels may be necessary to exclude invasive mucinous carcinoma

Top Differential Diagnoses
- MLL with ADH/DCIS
  - ADH is reported in 50% of cases
- Mucinous carcinoma
- Mucinous cystadenocarcinoma
- Nodular mucinosis
- Cystic hypersecretory breast lesions

MICROSCOPIC PATHOLOGY

Histologic Features
- Cystically dilated ducts contain luminal mucin
  - Spaces are lined by cuboidal to attenuated (flattened) epithelium
  - Epithelium may show spectrum of proliferative changes including hyperplasia, ADH, or DCIS
- Ruptured ducts may be associated with extravasated mucin within surrounding stroma
  - Histologic picture resembles mucocele of minor salivary glands found in oral cavity
  - Histocytes and inflammatory cells may be seen in extravasated mucin
  - Distinctive large granular calcifications may be seen within mucin
  - Strips or clusters of epithelial cells may become detached from wall and float free in mucin
    - It is important not to overinterpret detached free-floating lining epithelium as mucinous carcinoma
    - Multiple levels of areas of mucin extravasation may be helpful to look for possible areas of invasion
  - Features favoring MLL with epithelial detachment
    - Linear configuration of epithelial cells (resembling lining)
    - Associated myoepithelial cells; in some cases, immunohistochemical studies for myoepithelial markers may be helpful
    - Associated findings that suggest presence of core needle biopsy track
- Distinction between MLL and mucinous carcinoma is often not possible on needle core biopsy when there is extravasated mucin

Cytologic Features
- Epithelial lining consists of uniform flattened to low cuboidal cells
  - Uniform oval nuclei
  - Absence of cytologic atypia
  - Associated with underlying myoepithelial cell layer

- Low columnar epithelium and minor papillary elements may be present in some lesions
- Atypical epithelial alterations have been reported in association with MLL
  - Columnar cell change ± atypia
  - Atypical ductal hyperplasia
  - DCIS (micropapillary and cribriform patterns)
  - Awareness of association with atypia should prompt close histological scrutiny of any epithelial proliferative changes accompanying MLL
- In background of MLL, diagnosis of ADH and DCIS relies on conventionally described cytoarchitectural criteria

MLL: Neutral and Nonsulfated Acid Mucin
- Mucin in cysts and stroma of MLL is largely composed of neutral and nonsulfated acid mucin
- Identical results are obtained when the mucin from MLL and mucinous carcinoma are compared with ancillary testing

ANCILLARY TESTS

Histochemistry
- Alcian blue at pH 2.7
  - Reactivity: Positive
  - Staining pattern
    - Diffuse strong staining of mucin
- PAS-diastase
  - Reactivity: Positive
  - Staining pattern
    - Diffuse strong staining of mucin
- Mucicarmine
  - Reactivity: Positive
  - Staining pattern
    - Diffuse strong staining of mucin
- Alcian blue at pH 0.9
  - Reactivity: Equivocal
  - Staining pattern
    - Weak to negative staining of mucin

4

Immunohistochemistry
- MUC2 and MUC6 are predominant mucins demonstrated by IHC in both MLL and mucinous carcinoma

DIFFERENTIAL DIAGNOSIS

MLL with ADH/DCIS
- Up to 50% of MLLs will show areas of ADH &/or DCIS
  - Morphologic features of MLL are readily apparent in all cases showing atypia and DCIS
  - Associated DCIS is low grade and often demonstrates cribriform or micropapillary patterns
- It is important to exclude the possibility of DCIS by examining adequate tissue samples when MLL is found on biopsy
  - Look for architectural complexity and low-grade cytonuclear atypia in epithelium
- No appreciable differences in age, tumor size, or laterality between patients with MLL vs. MLL with atypia/DCIS/carcinoma

Mucinous Carcinoma
- Can be paucicellular with large quantities of stromal mucin and a few floating nests of neoplastic epithelium
  - Clumps and nests of tumor cells are usually grade 1 and sometimes grade 2
    - Nuclear atypia favors diagnosis of mucinous carcinoma
- Myoepithelial cells should not be seen in association with epithelial nests of mucinous carcinoma
  - Demonstration of associated myoepithelial cells supports a diagnosis of MLL with detached epithelium
  - Changes of previous core or needle biopsy in the vicinity (e.g., granulation tissue, fat necrosis, or hemorrhage) increases the likelihood of epithelial displacement
- MLL lesions with areas diagnostic of mucinous carcinoma have been described

Mucinous Cystadenocarcinoma
- Very rare breast neoplasm
- Histologically reminiscent of mucinous cystadenocarcinomas in pancreas and ovary
  - Multilocular cystic appearance can mimic MLL
  - Lining epithelial cells are tall and columnar with cytoplasmic mucin and basally oriented nuclei, differing from MLL
- Mucin extravasation has also been described in mucinous cystadenocarcinoma

Nodular Mucinosis
- Lesions typically located under or near nipple
  - Poorly circumscribed and unencapsulated
  - Soft and gelatinous consistency
- Mucinous tissue consists of acid mucopolysaccharides
  - Will stain positive with Alcian blue and Hale colloidal iron
  - Mucicarmine stain may be faintly positive
  - Periodic acid-Schiff (PAS) negative
- Can be distinguished from MLL by location and staining properties of mucous substances

Cystic Hypersecretory Breast Lesions
- Includes both cystic hypersecretory hyperplasia and cystic hypersecretory carcinoma
  - May bear superficial similarity to MLL due to presence of cystically dilated duct spaces
  - Luminal contents from cystic hypersecretory lesion differ from MLL
    - Contain gelatinous eosinophilic material resembling colloid of thyroid

DIAGNOSTIC CHECKLIST

Pathologic Interpretation Pearls
- MLL is typically benign, although can be associated with atypia &/or malignancy
- Differentiating MLL from mucinous carcinoma can be difficult on core needle biopsy
  - Surgical excision is recommended for women of all age groups to exclude possibility of ADH, DCIS, or mucinous carcinoma
  - Examination of entire pathologic specimen is necessary to exclude more worrisome lesion
- MLL may represent 1 end of pathologic spectrum of low-grade mucinous breast neoplasia
- Patients diagnosed with MLL warrant close follow-up because of association with ADH and malignancy

SELECTED REFERENCES

1. Tan PH et al: Mucinous breast lesions: diagnostic challenges. J Clin Pathol. 61(1):11-9, 2008
2. Kim JY et al: Benign and malignant mucocele-like tumors of the breast: mammographic and sonographic appearances. AJR Am J Roentgenol. 185(5):1310-6, 2005
3. Carder PJ et al: Surgical excision is warranted following a core biopsy diagnosis of mucocoele-like lesion of the breast. Histopathology. 45(2):148-54, 2004
4. Glazebrook K et al: Original report. Mucocele-like tumors of the breast: mammographic and sonographic appearances. AJR Am J Roentgenol. 180(4):949-54, 2003
5. Michal M et al: Nodular mucinosis of the breast: report of three cases. Pathol Int. 48(7):542-4, 1998
6. Hamele-Bena D et al: Mammary mucocele-like lesions. Benign and malignant. Am J Surg Pathol. 20(9):1081-5, 1996
7. Weaver MG et al: Mucinous lesions of the breast. A pathological continuum. Pathol Res Pract. 189(8):873-6, 1993
8. Rosen PP: Mucocele-like tumors of the breast. Am J Surg Pathol. 10(7):464-9, 1986

MUCOCELE-LIKE LESIONS

Microscopic Features and Differential Diagnosis

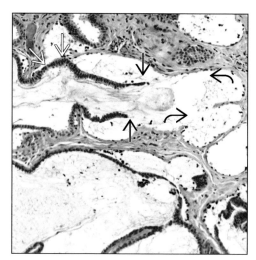
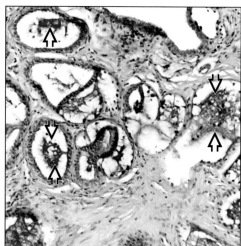

(Left) The dilated mucin-filled ducts show evidence of rupture ➡ with extravasated mucinous material spilling into the surrounding stroma ➡. The epithelial lining in this case consists of uniform cuboidal cells ➡ that lack atypia. The epithelial cells remain attached to the wall of the cyst. *(Right)* The mucin in the cysts and stroma of MLL is largely composed of neutral and nonsulfated acid mucins, which show strong diffuse mucicarmine staining ➡.

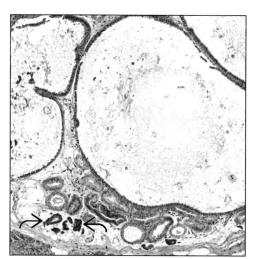
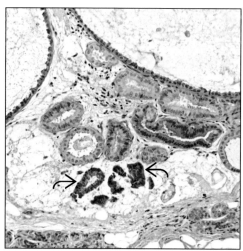

(Left) A diagnosis of benign MLL can be rendered after careful examination to exclude evidence of carcinoma. Epithelial cells may become detached from the wall of the cysts ➡ and float freely in the extravasated mucin and thus mimic a mucinous cancer. *(Right)* It is important not to overinterpret detached free-floating epithelium as malignancy. Features that favor MLL with epithelial displacement include a linear configuration of epithelial cells ➡ and associated myoepithelial cells.

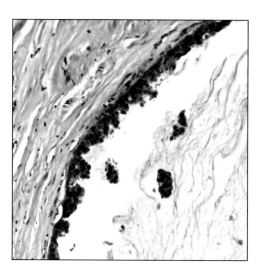
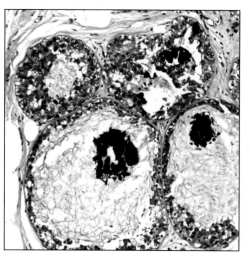

(Left) Atypical hyperplasia is often found in MLLs. In this case, severely atypical cells line the wall of the cyst, and detached papillary tufts are present within the mucin. Invasive mucinous carcinoma was present elsewhere in the specimen. *(Right)* In this case of DCIS associated with mucin production, coarse calcifications have formed in the mucin. Unlike MLLs, the malignant cells show marked nuclear atypia and are piled up in multiple layers in an abnormal architectural pattern.

COLLAGENOUS SPHERULOSIS

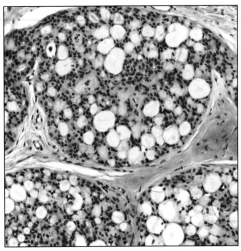

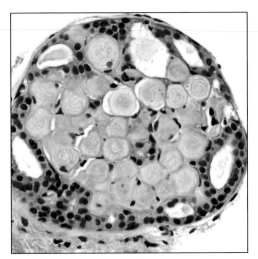

Collagenous spherulosis of the breast is shown. This lesion is characterized by aggregates of eosinophilic fibrillar or hyaline spherules surrounded by an inner layer of myoepithelial cells and luminal cells.

A higher power view shows dense spherules of eosinophilic basement membrane-like material surrounded by cells. This arrangement gives the proliferation a fenestrated or cribriform appearance.

TERMINOLOGY

Abbreviations
- Collagenous spherulosis (CS)

Synonyms
- Mucinous spherulosis

Definitions
- Incidental microscopic finding in 1-2% of biopsies that contain hyperplastic ductal lesions
  - Important to recognize CS because lesion may superficially resemble cribriform DCIS
  - CS may also superficially resemble low-grade adenoid cystic carcinoma

CLINICAL ISSUES

Presentation
- Incidental finding
  - Typically seen in breast tissue containing other sclerosing benign proliferative lesions
    - Includes sclerosing adenosis, papillomas, ductal hyperplasia, and atypical ductal hyperplasia
  - Calcification of CS can lead to mammographic detection and diagnosis by needle core biopsy

Treatment
- CS may be seen associated with atypical ductal hyperplasia, LCIS, or DCIS
- Appropriate treatment is related to other lesions present

Prognosis
- Benign process
- No evidence that CS is directly associated with precancerous lesions or predisposes to future development of breast cancer

IMAGE FINDINGS

Mammographic Findings
- CS may be detected mammographically for those lesions with calcifications

MICROSCOPIC PATHOLOGY

Histologic Features
- CS characterized by lobulocentric aggregates of eosinophilic fibrillar &/or hyaline spherules of extracellular material
- Spherules composed of varying amounts of basement membrane-like material, including polysaccharides, laminin, and type IV collagen
  - Positive staining for PAS and Alcian blue by histochemistry
  - In some cases, spherules contain mucoid-like material ("mucinous spherulosis")
- Spherules surrounded by inner myoepithelial layer and outer luminal layer of cells
  - Myoepithelial cells may become attenuated and difficult to appreciate in H&E sections
  - Immunohistochemical stains for myoepithelial cells (calponin, p63, myosin heavy chain) to highlight myoepithelial cells may be helpful
- Spherules and cellular arrangement give rise to appearance of cribriform or fenestrated proliferation when viewed at low power

DIFFERENTIAL DIAGNOSIS

Low-Grade Cribriform DCIS
- Microlumens formed and surrounded by single monotonous population of neoplastic epithelial cells
- Nuclei of cells tend to stand apart and appear polarized around microlumens

COLLAGENOUS SPHERULOSIS

Key Facts

Terminology

- Collagenous (mucinous) spherulosis (CS)
- Incidental microscopic finding in 1-2% of biopsies that contain hyperplastic ductal lesions
- Important to recognize CS because lesion may superficially resemble cribriform DCIS

Clinical Issues

- Typically seen in breast tissue containing sclerosing lesions
- Calcification of CS can lead to mammographic detection and diagnosis by needle core biopsy
- Benign process; no evidence that CS is directly associated with precancerous lesions or is risk factor for breast cancer

Microscopic Pathology

- CS is characterized by eosinophilic fibrillar &/or hyaline spherules consisting of basement membrane-like material (polysaccharides, laminin, and type IV collagen) within areas of epithelial hyperplasia
- In foci of CS, myoepithelial cells are present around periphery and also surround inner spherules
- Immunohistochemical studies to demonstrate presence of myoepithelial cells around cribriform spaces and associated with spherules can be helpful

Top Differential Diagnoses

- Low-grade cribriform DCIS
  - CS involved by LCIS can be difficult to distinguish from cribriform DCIS
- Low-grade adenoid cystic carcinoma

- Gives rise to a rigid or "punched-out" appearance due to microlumens with round or smooth internal contours
  - Microluminal spaces may be empty, contain secretions, necrotic cells, or calcifications
- Stains to highlight myoepithelial component of CS may be helpful in difficult cases

Low-Grade Adenoid Cystic Carcinoma

- Typically demonstrates invasive growth pattern at periphery with tumor infiltrating beyond central gross nodule
- Tumor is composed of 2 different components
  - True glandular component (formed by luminal-type cells)
  - "Pseudoglandular" component consisting of basement membrane deposition surrounded by myoepithelial-like cells
  - Different components typically show heterogeneity in distribution throughout tumor
- Higher grade lesions typically show areas with solid growth pattern
- Adenoid cystic carcinomas may have luminal cells positive for C-Kit (CD117) whereas cells of CS are negative for this marker

DIAGNOSTIC CHECKLIST

Clinically Relevant Pathologic Features

- Tissue distribution
  - Ductal or lobular process only
  - May involve intraductal papillomas
  - Most often seen in association with sclerosing adenosis, ductal hyperplasia, and papillomas
- Usually incidental finding
  - Important to recognize because it can mimic other more serious processes
- Rarely CS can be involved by lobular neoplasia
  - Neoplastic lobular cells displace indigenous luminal cells, leaving myoepithelium and spherules in place
  - May be difficult to distinguish from cribriform DCIS

- Presence of basement membrane material and dyshesive quality of lobular cells may be helpful
- Immunostains for E-cadherin and myoepithelial cells can identify 2 cell types

Pathologic Interpretation Pearls

- Cribriform or fenestrated proliferation
  - Luminal spaces tend to have irregular or angulated shapes
  - Look for acellular spherules of basement membrane-like material within luminal spaces
  - Look for attenuated myoepithelial cells surrounding luminal spaces admixed with luminal cells
    - Immunostains can help to highlight different cell types
- CS typically associated with other sclerosing and benign proliferative lesions

SELECTED REFERENCES

1. Hill P et al: Collagenous spherulosis with lobular carcinoma in situ: a potential diagnostic pitfall. Pathology. 39(3):361-3, 2007
2. Rabban JT et al: Immunophenotypic overlap between adenoid cystic carcinoma and collagenous spherulosis of the breast: potential diagnostic pitfalls using myoepithelial markers. Mod Pathol. 19(10):1351-7, 2006
3. Resetkova E et al: Collagenous spherulosis of breast: morphologic study of 59 cases and review of the literature. Am J Surg Pathol. 30(1):20-7, 2006
4. Mooney EE et al: Spherulosis of the breast. A spectrum of municous and collagenous lesions. Arch Pathol Lab Med. 123(7):626-30, 1999
5. Sgroi D et al: Involvement of collagenous spherulosis by lobular carcinoma in situ. Potential confusion with cribriform ductal carcinoma in situ. Am J Surg Pathol. 19(12):1366-70, 1995
6. Stephenson TJ et al: Nodular basement membrane deposits in breast carcinoma and atypical ductal hyperplasia: mimics of collagenous spherulosis. Pathologica. 86(3):234-9, 1994
7. Clement PB et al: Collagenous spherulosis of the breast. Am J Surg Pathol. 11(6):411-7, 1987

COLLAGENOUS SPHERULOSIS

Microscopic Features

(Left) Collagenous spherulosis is a benign sclerosing process, typically seen with other benign sclerosing lesions. This example is associated with florid sclerosing adenosis. The lesion gives the appearance of an intraductal proliferation; however, studies of the earliest phases suggest that the process usually affects lobules. **(Right)** A higher power view shows the typical fenestrated or cribriform appearance of the epithelium surrounding eosinophilic hyaline material.

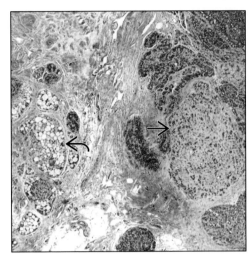
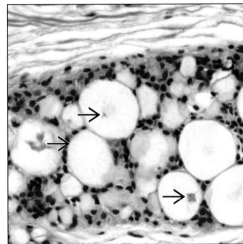

(Left) This example shows an intraductal papilloma with a fibrovascular core, associated with CS. Surrounding areas show the typical fenestrated pattern with hyaline basement membrane material within the spaces associated with a fibrous stroma. **(Right)** A higher power image of 1 of these areas shows that, despite the architectural complexity, there is variability to the cells within the proliferation and flattened myoepithelial cells surrounding the pseudoluminal spaces.

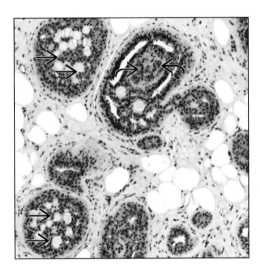
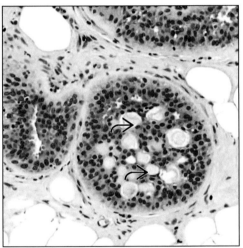

(Left) The internal aspects of the pseudolumens in CS can appear somewhat angulated and irregular in contour. The cells are not uniformly distributed, and parts of these spaces are lined by thin eosinophilic septae. **(Right)** At higher power, attenuated myoepithelial cells in CS are seen between pseudolumens. Thickened and fibrillar eosinophilic basement membrane material is readily seen within and surrounding these spaces.

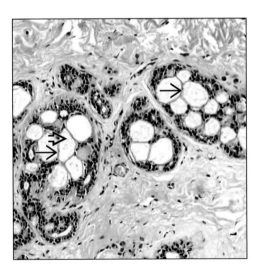
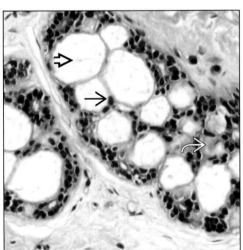

4

COLLAGENOUS SPHERULOSIS

Microscopic Features

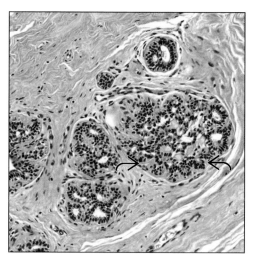

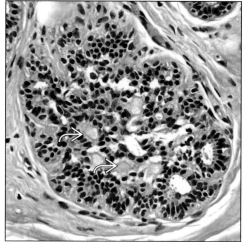

(Left) In CS, the cribriform or fenestrated proliferation often appears to arise within larger ducts; however, the study of early stage lesions supports that this process begins within the TDLUs ➔. The epithelial proliferation may unfold the TDLU and create the appearance of a duct. (Right) When seen at higher magnification, the characteristic fibrillar eosinophilic deposits of basement membrane-like material ➔ appear to originate in the TDLU for this case of early CS.

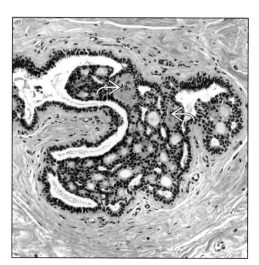

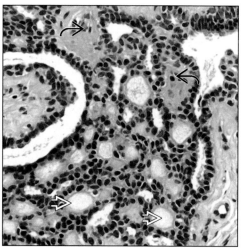

(Left) The fenestrated cribriform proliferation seen here appears to be arising within a mammary duct in association with an intraductal papilloma. Note the fibrovascular cores ➔. (Right) When viewed at higher power the pseudolumens seen here contain the eosinophilic deposits that are characteristic of CS ➔. The fibrovascular cores ➔ are more clearly seen, consistent with CS arising in an intraductal papilloma.

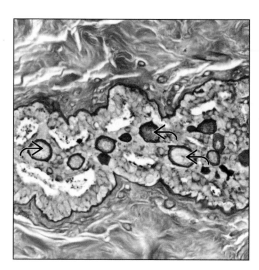

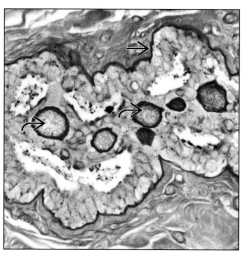

(Left) The fibrillar deposits seen in CS are composed of varying amounts of basement membrane-like material, including polysaccharides, laminin, and type IV collagen, which show positive staining with an Alcian blue/PAS stain ➔. (Right) When viewed under higher magnification, the fibrillar depositions in CS ➔ show similar staining features to those of the basement membrane seen at the periphery of this mammary duct ➔.

Differential Diagnosis

(Left) Both CS and low-grade cribriform DCIS appear fenestrated. CS demonstrates basement membrane material ➡ within pseudolumens, which are surrounded by myoepithelial cells ➡.
(Right) Low-grade cribriform DCIS forms microlumens with rigid "punched-out" spaces ➡ surrounded by a monomorphous population of cells that appear polarized to the lumens. The luminal spaces are either empty or contain secretions or necrotic cells ➡.

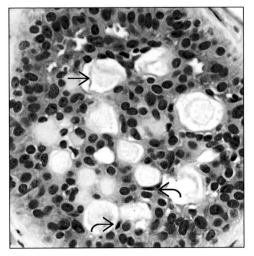
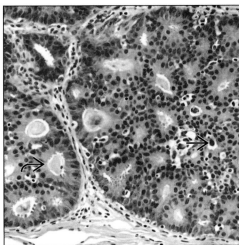

(Left) Cribriform DCIS retains myoepithelial cells at the periphery next to the basement membrane, as shown by nuclear p63 staining ➡. Myoepithelial cells do not line the cribriform spaces ➡. The tumor cells are uniformly positive for cytokeratin AE1/AE3 (red cytoplasmic immunoreactivity) and negative for p63. *(Right)* The cribriform spaces in CS are lined by myoepithelial cells, reacting here with p63 ➡. Luminal epithelial cells show red cytokeratin staining ➡.

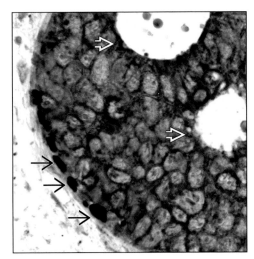
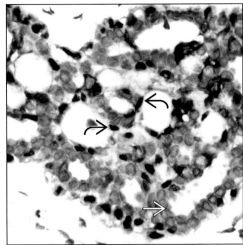

(Left) CS with basement membrane material ➡ can at times be confused with a low-grade adenoid cystic carcinoma (LGACC). *(Right)* Similar to CS, LGACC also demonstrates deposition of basement membrane material ➡ giving rise to a pseudoglandular appearance. LGACC tends to be heterogeneous and typically demonstrates an invasive growth pattern at the periphery with tumor infiltrating beyond a central gross nodule ➡. In contrast, CS is typically a localized lesion.

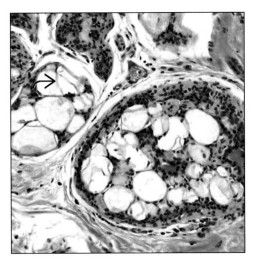
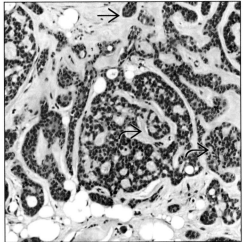

COLLAGENOUS SPHERULOSIS

Differential Diagnosis

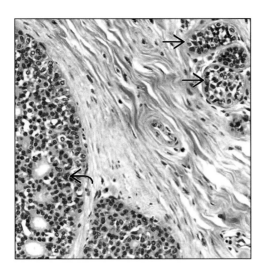
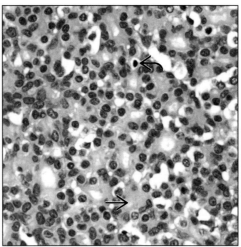

(Left) On occasion, lobular neoplasia ➔ can involve areas of CS creating a monotonous and monomorphic appearance and a resemblance to cribriform DCIS ➔. (Right) At higher power, the presence of attenuated myoepithelial cells ➔, basement membrane-like material in pseudolumens ➔, and a dyshesive quality to the lobular cells are clues to the correct diagnosis. Immunostains for E-cadherin and myoepithelial cells may be helpful in problematic cases.

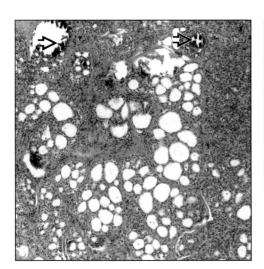
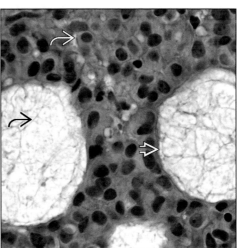

(Left) This core needle biopsy for calcifications shows LCIS involving collagenous spherulosis. The calcifications ➔ are associated with CS. (Right) The spaces are filled by fibrillary material ➔ and lined by a densely eosinophilic cuticle ➔. The cells of LCIS between the spaces are monomorphic and rounded with small gaps between the cells ➔.

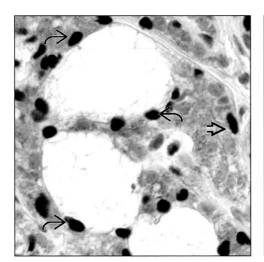
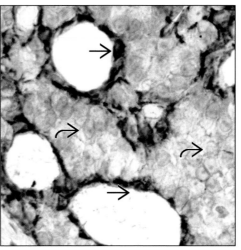

(Left) An immunoperoxidase study for p63 demonstrates myoepithelial cells lining the internal cribriform spaces ➔ and the basement membrane around the periphery of the space ➔. (Right) Two populations of cells are evident. LCIS surrounds the cribriform spaces, and the cells are negative for E-cadherin ➔. The myoepithelial cells lining the spaces show weak E-cadherin positivity ➔. In contrast, DCIS would have strong membrane reactivity for E-cadherin throughout.

GYNECOMASTOID HYPERPLASIA

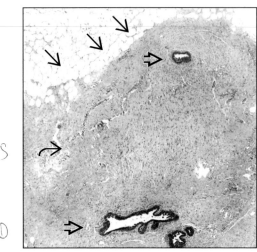

GH is characterized by end ducts without lobule formation ⊡ in an area of abundant fibrous stroma ⇗ in a female, associated with a mass. The borders may be circumscribed ⊡ or poorly defined.

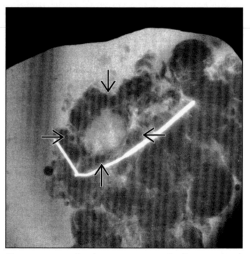

On mammography, the most common finding associated with GH is an asymmetric density. Less commonly, GH forms a circumscribed mass ⊡.

TERMINOLOGY

Abbreviations
• Gynecomastoid hyperplasia (GH)

Synonyms
• Gynecomastia-like changes of female breast
• Gynecomastia-like lesion of female breast

Definitions
• Histologic changes in breast identical to those seen in male gynecomastia, usually forming palpable mass or asymmetric density by mammography

ETIOLOGY/PATHOGENESIS

Pathogenesis
• Absence of lobule formation suggests abnormal developmental response
  ○ Alteration in balance between estrogen and androgens may play a role
  ○ Some women have history of infertility or amenorrhea
• Unlike gynecomastia in males, no specific medical disorders or drug therapy are associated with GH in females

CLINICAL ISSUES

Epidemiology
• Incidence
  ○ Rare: ~ 0.15% of all breast biopsies
• Age
  ○ Younger women; range: 19-42 years (mean age: 32 years)

Presentation
• Usual clinical presentation is as palpable mass
• May show asymmetric density on mammography

Prognosis
• Benign process
• No recurrences have been reported

IMAGE FINDINGS

Mammographic Findings
• Asymmetric density or nodular mass

Ultrasonographic Findings
• May not be visible
• May show solid mass with indistinct margins

MACROSCOPIC FEATURES

General Features
• Soft to slightly firm, irregular to ovoid masses of fibroadipose tissue without discrete borders

Size
• Ranges from microscopic involvement to palpable lesions up to 5 cm

MICROSCOPIC PATHOLOGY

Histologic Features
• Identical to gynecomastia of male breast
  ○ Poorly circumscribed microscopically
  ○ Borders may be difficult to define, as fibrous tissue merges with surrounding breast tissue
• Absence of lobule formation is an important diagnostic feature
• Involved ducts often exhibit epithelial hyperplasia with formation of micropapillae
  ○ Papillary projections are thinner at tips and wider at base
  ○ Epithelial cells at tips are smaller and more hyperchromatic compared with cells at base

GYNECOMASTOID HYPERPLASIA

Key Facts

Terminology

- Gynecomastoid hyperplasia (GH)
  - Focal occurrence in a female of histologic changes identical to those seen in male gynecomastia

Clinical Issues

- Usual clinical presentation is as palpable mass
- GH is most commonly seen mammographically as area of asymmetric density but may form nodular mass

Microscopic Pathology

- Ducts without lobule formation surrounded by periductal fibrosis and edema
- Epithelial hyperplasia with formation of micropapillae

Top Differential Diagnoses

- Low-grade micropapillary DCIS
- Mammary hamartoma
- Juvenile hypertrophy

- Papillae arise on background of epithelial hyperplasia
- Complex architecture (cribriform spaces, rigid arches) is absent
- No necrosis or calcifications are associated with hyperplasia
- Stromal proliferative changes are seen adjacent to involved ducts
  - Periductal stromal fibrosis and edema typical
- GH is frequently associated with other benign changes in surrounding breast parenchyma

DIFFERENTIAL DIAGNOSIS

Low-Grade Micropapillary DCIS

- DCIS is a clonal population of cells
  - Cells have uniform monotonous appearance throughout lesion
- Micropapillae typically arise on a flat 2-3-cell layer lining involved ducts
- Micropapillae usually have bulbous expanded tips and narrow tapered base
  - Complex architectural patterns may be present: Rigid arches, cribriform spaces
- Often associated with calcifications
  - Less commonly associated with necrosis
- Micropapillary DCIS is often associated with other architectural types of DCIS such as cribriform

Mammary Hamartoma

- Hamartomas have sharply circumscribed borders

- Borders of GH may be more difficult to define
- Hamartomas consist of both glands and prominent dense stromal component
  - Lobules are typically present
  - Stroma may contain smooth muscle or cartilaginous elements
- Gynecomastia-like changes can be component of mammary hamartoma

Juvenile Hypertrophy

- Occurs at onset of puberty (typically ages 11-14)
  - GH occurs in women over the age of 19
- Characterized by massive bilateral enlargement of both breasts
  - Enlargement may be synchronous or metachronous
  - GH is a focal mass-forming lesion
- Increase in both stroma and epithelium
  - Gynecomastia-like changes may be present

SELECTED REFERENCES

1. Kang Y et al: Gynecomastia-like changes of the female breast. Arch Pathol Lab Med. 125(4):506-9, 2001
2. Selland DL et al: Gynecomastoid hyperplasia: imaging findings in six patients. Radiology. 214(2):553-5, 2000
3. Umlas J: Gynecomastia-like lesions in the female breast. Arch Pathol Lab Med. 124(6):844-7, 2000

IMAGE GALLERY

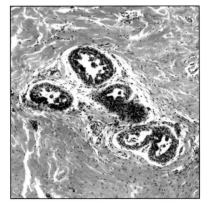 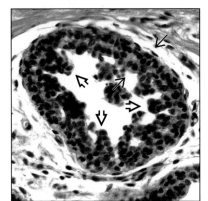 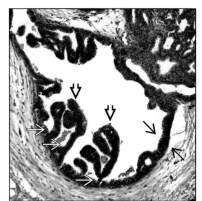

(Left) GH is characterized by the presence of small ducts in the absence of lobule formation in dense surrounding stroma. (Center) Small, abortive, short, and tapering papillae are typical ➡. Hyperplasia is also present lining the remainder of the duct wall ➡. (Right) The papillae of micropapillary DCIS are characterized by a narrow base ➡ supporting a bulging tip, often with complex architecture ➡. The remainder of the duct shows little hyperplasia ➡.

SYRINGOMATOUS ADENOMA OF THE NIPPLE

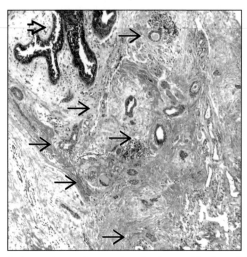

Syringomatous adenoma is a benign proliferation of eccrine-like ductal structures ⇨ in the dermis of the nipple. The adenoma typically surrounds lactiferous ducts ⊳ and areolar smooth muscle.

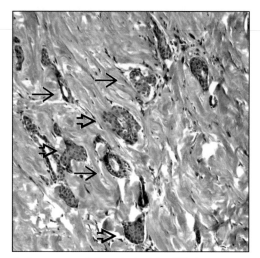

Both squamous ⊳ and glandular ⇨ elements are present. The tumor forms a firm subareolar dermal mass that may be painful. The overlying skin may become irritated and acanthotic.

TERMINOLOGY

Abbreviations
- Syringomatous adenoma of the nipple (SAN)

Synonyms
- Infiltrating syringomatous adenoma
- Syringomatous tumor

Definitions
- Benign, locally invasive neoplasm of probable eccrine duct origin that forms palpable mass in areolar dermis

ETIOLOGY/PATHOGENESIS

Cell of Origin
- Most likely origin is intraepidermal eccrine sweat ducts of nipple
- Morphologically identical to syringomas of skin in other parts of body that arise from eccrine ducts

CLINICAL ISSUES

Epidemiology
- Incidence
  - Very rare
- Age
  - Mean: 40 years (range: 11-76 years)
- Gender
  - Almost all patients have been female
    - Only 1 reported case in a male

Presentation
- Solitary firm mass in subareolar or nipple region
- May be associated with
  - Pain or tenderness
  - Skin crusting or ulceration
  - Nipple discharge
  - Nipple retraction

Treatment
- Surgical approaches
  - Should be completely excised with negative margins

Prognosis
- Benign lesion
  - No reported cases of regional or distant metastasis
  - May recur locally if not completely excised (30% of cases with positive margins)

IMAGE FINDINGS

General Features
- May be indistinguishable from carcinoma on mammography or ultrasonography

Mammographic Findings
- Mass-forming lesion in subareolar region
  - Borders may be irregular
  - Calcifications may be present

Ultrasonographic Findings
- Ill-defined mass with heterogeneous internal echoes

MACROSCOPIC FEATURES

General Features
- Ill-defined, firm, white mass with minute cystic spaces in the dermis of the nipple and areola

Size
- 1-3 cm

MICROSCOPIC PATHOLOGY

Histologic Features
- Small nests with both squamous and glandular features

SYRINGOMATOUS ADENOMA OF THE NIPPLE

Key Facts

Terminology
- Benign neoplasm morphologically similar to dermal syringoma

Clinical Issues
- Presents as palpable, solitary, firm dermal mass in subareolar or nipple region
- Management is complete local excision to achieve negative margins
  - Local recurrences in up to 30% of incompletely excised lesions
  - No risk for local recurrence if completely excised with negative margins
- Does not metastasize

Image Findings
- May be indistinguishable from carcinoma on mammography or ultrasonography

Microscopic Pathology
- Infiltrative proliferation of eccrine duct-like structures
- Squamous cell nests and glandular structures are present
- Infiltration into smooth muscle bundles and nerves simulates malignant neoplasm
- Cells have small uniform nuclei
- Mitotic figures are not usually present
- Overlying epidermis may be acanthotic

Top Differential Diagnoses
- Tubular carcinoma
- Low-grade adenosquamous carcinoma

- Tubules are lined by > 1 cell layer: Luminal and basal cells
  - Basally located cells may be positive for actin
  - Lumens may be empty or contain granular eosinophilic secretions
  - Inner cells are often flattened, and cytoplasm may resemble eosinophilic cuticle
- Squamous nests may be solid or cystic
  - Cysts contain keratin, may have calcifications
  - Cells are positive for p63
- Some nests have both squamous and glandular areas
  - Lined by flattened to cuboidal cells
  - Often comma-shaped
  - May show complex branching patterns
- Nuclei are small and uniform
- Mitoses are absent or rare
- Tumor invades around smooth muscle and lactiferous sinuses of nipple
  - Extent can be difficult to define as portions of tumor can appear to be located at a distance, separated by normal-appearing dermis
- Tumor cells should not invade into epidermis or deeply into subcutaneous adipose tissue
  - Focal involvement of subcutaneous tissue may be present
- Perineural invasion may be present
- Background fibrous stroma shows myxoid or hyaline change
- Overlying epidermis can be acanthotic

ANCILLARY TESTS

Immunohistochemistry
- Hormone receptors
  - Negative for estrogen and progesterone receptors
- p63
  - Positive in areas of squamous differentiation
- Actin
  - May be positive in basal layer

DIFFERENTIAL DIAGNOSIS

Tubular Carcinoma (TC)
- Well-differentiated adenocarcinoma usually present within breast parenchyma, only rarely involving dermis
  - Tubules are often angulated and can resemble comma-shaped tumor nests of SAN
  - Apical snouts are common
  - Tubules have single cell layer
- Frequently associated with micropapillary or cribriform types of low-grade DCIS
- TC is not associated with squamous metaplasia
- IHC can be helpful to distinguish TC from SAN
  - TC is usually strongly positive for ER and PR
    - SAN is negative for hormone receptors
  - TC lacks positivity for myoepithelial markers
    - SAN may show p63 positivity in squamous cells and actin positivity in basal cells

Low-Grade Adenosquamous Carcinoma (LGASC)
- SAN is histologically similar to LGASC
- LGASC can metastasize and cause death in rare cases
- Major distinguishing feature is location within breast
  - LGASC arises within breast parenchyma
  - Rarely involves subareolar tissue or nipple
- May be difficult or impossible to distinguish in small &/or superficial biopsies

SELECTED REFERENCES

1. Oo KZ et al: Infiltrating syringomatous adenoma of the nipple: clinical presentation and literature review. Arch Pathol Lab Med. 133(9):1487-9, 2009
2. Sarma DP et al: Infiltrating syringomatous eccrine adenoma of the nipple: a case report. Cases J. 2:9118, 2009
3. Ku J et al: Syringomatous adenoma of the nipple. Breast. 13(5):412-5, 2004

SYRINGOMATOUS ADENOMA OF THE NIPPLE

Microscopic Features

(Left) The initial diagnosis of SAN is usually made on a small punch biopsy of the skin. In this biopsy, the adenoma ⇨ is present in the dermis, just deep to the nipple duct orifices ⇨. *(Right)* The tumor is composed of small, well-formed glandular structures ⇨ with an infiltrative pattern in the dermis. The tumor cells should not invade into the epidermis or deep into subcutaneous adipose tissue. In such cases, low-grade adenosquamous carcinoma or another type of malignancy should be considered.

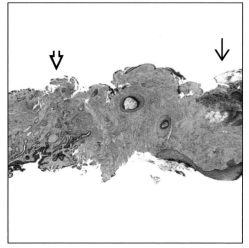
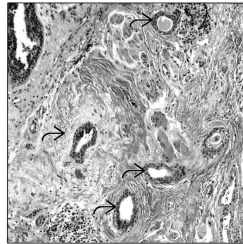

(Left) The tubules have multiple cell layers and are often comma-shaped. A basal cell layer positive for actin can be identified by IHC. The inner cells are often flattened and may show squamous differentiation by histologic appearance or immunoreactivity for p63. *(Right)* The lumens are usually empty but may be filled with eosinophilic secretory material. The nuclei are small and bland with inconspicuous nucleoli. Mitoses are absent or very rare. Necrosis is not a feature.

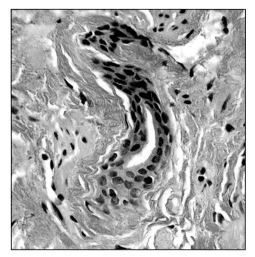
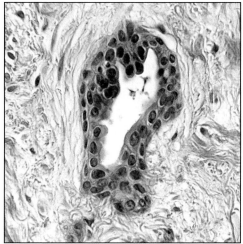

(Left) Perineural invasion ⇨ by tumor cells ⇨ may be present. SAN may recur locally, but neither metastasis to regional lymph nodes nor distant metastasis has been reported. *(Right)* SAN resembles these normal eccrine ducts ⇨ present in the dermis of the nipple, as well as other tumors of sweat duct origin. However, the true cell of origin is unknown.

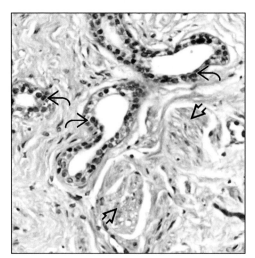
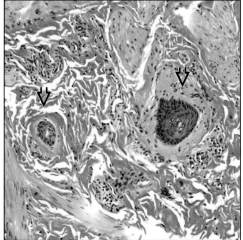

SYRINGOMATOUS ADENOMA OF THE NIPPLE

Differential Diagnosis

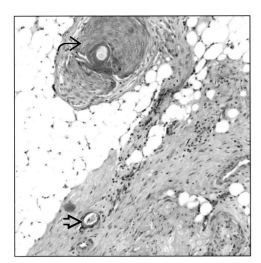
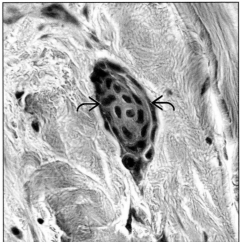

(Left) LGASC closely resembles SAN but occurs deeper in breast parenchyma. Similar squamous elements ➚ and glandular elements ⮕ are present. It may be impossible to distinguish these 2 lesions in small &/or superficial biopsies. (Right) Comma-shaped nests of squamous cells ➚ are characteristic of both SAN and LGASC. Such nests are not a feature of tubular carcinoma and are useful to exclude this diagnosis. In addition, multiple cell layers would not be present.

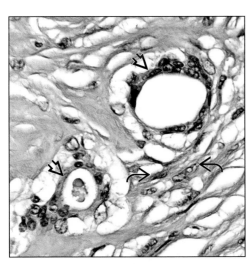
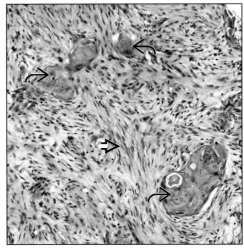

(Left) In LGASC, some of the spindle cells ➚ adjacent to tubules ⮕ have nuclear atypia and are neoplastic keratin-positive cells. These cells would not be seen in SAN. (Right) SAN should not be mistaken for squamous cell carcinoma. The squamous cells have pleomorphic nuclei ➚ and form irregular nests. They are associated with malignant spindle cells ⮕. The degree of atypia and the spindle cell background would not be present in SAN.

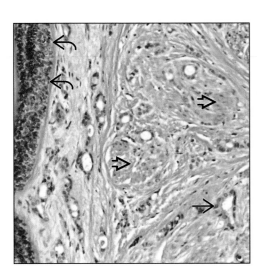
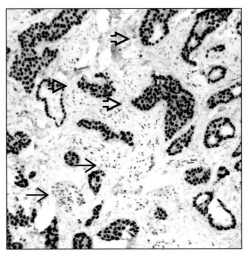

(Left) This tubular carcinoma presented as a subareolar nodule, infiltrating around large mammary ducts ➚ and into smooth muscle bundles ⮕, mimicking SAN. The tubules have a single cell layer ➚ and do not show areas of squamous differentiation. (Right) This well-differentiated invasive carcinoma in the dermis is easily distinguished from SAN by the presence of strong positivity for ER ⮕. The smooth muscle of the areola ➚ is also ER positive.

SCLEROSING ADENOSIS

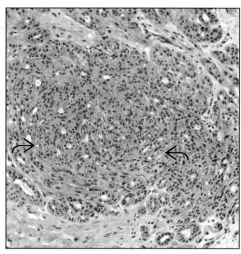

Sclerosing adenosis is an enlarged lobular unit with the acini distorted and compressed by stromal sclerosis, typically with a swirling appearance ➘. Myoepithelial cells surround each acinus.

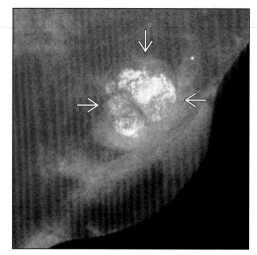

Sclerosing adenosis is often detected as a mammographic nodular density with ➡ or without calcifications. Less common presentations are as architectural distortion or as a palpable mass.

TERMINOLOGY

Abbreviations
- Sclerosing adenosis (SA)

Definitions
- Lobulocentric proliferation of acini around a central duct with stromal sclerosis and compression of lumens

ETIOLOGY/PATHOGENESIS

Dysregulation of Estrogen Receptor
- SA demonstrates increased expression of ER and Ki-67 over normal benign breast elements
  - SA and other proliferative lesions are more common in women receiving hormone replacement therapy
  - Association with obesity (increased endogenous estrogen levels)
- Hormone imbalance and dysregulation of ER may play a role in development of SA
- Risk for developing SA and other proliferative lesions may be increased in women who have > 25% fibroglandular breast tissue density

CLINICAL ISSUES

Epidemiology
- Incidence
  - Frequent incidental finding in breast biopsies
    - Present in 12% of breast biopsies without cancer
- Age
  - Most common in perimenopausal women

Presentation
- Most common: Finding during screening mammography
- Less commonly presents as a palpable mass
  - Termed nodular SA or adenosis tumor
  - May be associated with pain and tenderness

- Can also be a frequent incidental finding in breast specimens removed for other indications

Prognosis
- Benign proliferative lesion
- Classified as proliferative disease without atypia
  - 1.5-2x increased relative risk for development of invasive carcinoma or 5-7% actual lifetime risk
  - Increased risk is for both breasts

Core Needle Biopsy
- Most common benign lesion mistaken for invasive carcinoma
  - Closely mimics carcinoma when involved by apocrine metaplasia, LCIS, or DCIS
  - More difficult to diagnose on core needle biopsy when borders and lobulocentric pattern may not be evaluable
- Should always be considered in the differential diagnosis of invasive carcinomas
  - IHC for myoepithelial markers can be used to make the correct diagnosis

IMAGE FINDINGS

Mammographic Findings
- Microcalcifications most common finding
  - Clustered amorphous calcifications typical
  - Pleomorphic and punctate calcifications may also be seen
- Mass-forming lesions are generally circumscribed or lobulated
  - Less commonly, borders are ill defined or irregular
  - May be associated with calcifications
- Rare cases present as architectural distortion

Ultrasonographic Findings
- Circumscribed, hypoechoic, solid mass

SCLEROSING ADENOSIS

Key Facts

Clinical Issues
- Can present as a lesion on mammography, as a palpable mass, or as an incidental finding
- Classified as proliferative disease without atypia
  - 1.5-2x increased risk for development of invasive carcinoma in either breast
- Most common benign lesion misdiagnosed as invasive carcinoma
  - Can be difficult to diagnose on core needle biopsies

Image Findings
- Microcalcifications (clustered amorphous) most common finding
- Can also form rounded or lobulated masses

Microscopic Pathology
- Circumscribed lobulocentric architecture

- Lumens variably distorted and compressed by background collagen
- Can closely mimic invasive carcinoma if involved by apocrine metaplasia, DCIS, or LCIS
- Frequently associated with papillomas, complex sclerosing lesions, and fibroadenomas

Ancillary Tests
- Immunohistochemistry to detect myoepithelial cells may be helpful to distinguish SA from invasive carcinoma
- Expression of some markers is reduced

Top Differential Diagnoses
- Normal breast
- Invasive ductal carcinoma
- Microglandular adenosis

MR Findings
- Typical lesions are indistinguishable from breast parenchyma
  - May show enhancement in up to 30% of cases

MACROSCOPIC FEATURES

General Features
- SA presenting as a mass by palpation or imaging may be grossly evident
  - Rubbery circumscribed nodule
- Majority are small and not grossly apparent

MICROSCOPIC PATHOLOGY

Histologic Features
- Arises within terminal duct lobular unit
  - Must be at least 2x larger than average lobule
  - However, lobules can vary greatly in size in same breast, making this requirement difficult to assess
- Lobulocentric pattern is an important diagnostic feature
  - Refers to a cluster of tubules or acini
  - Often a central larger duct or ducts
  - Lobulocentric growth pattern is best appreciated at lower magnification
- Acini appear to swirl around central duct
  - Acini are formed by luminal cells and myoepithelial cells
  - Acini conform in shape to one another and are tightly clustered
    - In less typical cases, acini on periphery can be located farther apart and appear to "wander" through surrounding breast tissue
  - Myoepithelial cells may be spindled in shape and can be prominent
  - 2 cell layers may be best appreciated at periphery
    - May be difficult to see if center of lesion is sampled in a core needle biopsy

- Sclerosis refers to stromal hyalinization that compresses and distorts acini
  - Luminal spaces may be completely obliterated
  - Acini may have appearance of solid cords in swirling pattern
  - Glandular compression and distortion may be most marked in center of lesions
- Microcalcifications are present in > 50% of cases and may be prominent
- Multiple confluent areas of SA are sometimes seen
  - When large, can form a mammographic density or palpable mass
- Pseudoperineural invasion may be seen
  - Tubules are present within nerves
  - Not an indication of malignancy
- Luminal cells lack atypia and may appear cuboidal or flattened
- SA is frequently associated with other proliferative lesions
  - e.g., sclerosing papilloma, complex sclerosing lesion, fibroadenoma
- SA can be involved by apocrine metaplasia
  - Term "apocrine adenosis" is used for these lesions
  - May be mistaken for carcinoma due to monomorphic appearance of cells with enlarged nuclei
- SA can be involved by LCIS and DCIS
  - Such involvement may be mistaken for invasive carcinoma, particularly on needle biopsy
  - Features supporting SA include
    - Myoepithelial cells on H&E or by IHC
    - Lobulocentric architecture
    - Dense rather than desmoplastic stroma
    - Swirling back-to-back glands in concentric arrays

ANCILLARY TESTS

Immunohistochemistry
- Myoepithelial markers
  - SA is always associated with a prominent myoepithelial layer

SCLEROSING ADENOSIS

Differential Diagnosis

Features	Sclerosing Adenosis	Microglandular Adenosis	Tubular Carcinoma
Configuration/growth pattern	Circumscribed and lobulocentric, swirling and back-to-back	Scattered around normal breast ducts and lobules	Haphazard and infiltrative
Luminal epithelium	Cuboidal or flattened	Cuboidal (may be clear cell)	Cuboidal (may have apical snouts)
Luminal spaces	Flattened or obliterated	Round open lumens	Angulated open lumens
Myoepithelial cells	Present	Absent	Absent
Stromal response	Sclerotic or fibrotic	Absent or minimal	Hypercellular, desmoplastic
Estrogen receptor	Positive	Negative	Positive
S100 protein	Luminal cells negative (may stain myoepithelial cells)	Uniform strong reactivity	Negative

- o Most useful markers are p63 and smooth muscle myosin heavy chain
- o Use of more than 1 myoepithelial marker or a "cocktail" of markers can be helpful
- o Expression of some markers is reduced in sclerosing lesions
  - ▪ Expression of CK5/6 is reduced to greatest extent; absent in about 1/3
  - ▪ Calponin and p63 are least affected; reduced in < 10%

DIFFERENTIAL DIAGNOSIS

Normal Breast
- Adenosis is defined as an increase in number of tubules or acini
- Breast lobules normally enlarge during pregnancy; this is an example of normal adenosis
- Lobules partially regress after pregnancy and end of lactation
- Lobules also undergo involution with age
- Large involuting lobules may be difficult to distinguish from SA
  - o Myoepithelial cells are prominent and basement membranes are thickened
  - o Luminal cells diminish in size and appear atrophic
  - o Thus, involuting lobules appear more eosinophilic than SA, which is dominated by luminal cells with plump blue nuclei

Invasive Ductal Carcinoma (IDC)
- SA can mimic low-grade IDC such as tubular carcinoma
  - o Distinction is particularly difficult when SA is involved by DCIS, LCIS, or apocrine metaplasia
- IDC shows haphazard infiltrating growth pattern
  - o Does not conform to lobulocentric architecture
  - o Tubules are more widely spaced and are not in parallel arrays
  - o Borders are irregular rather than circumscribed or lobulated
- IDC shows angulated glands with open lumens
  - o Tubules lack surrounding myoepithelial cells
  - o IHC can be helpful to confirm absence of myoepithelial cells

- o Myofibroblasts adjacent to malignant tubules are positive for muscle markers and should not be mistaken for myoepithelial cells
- IDC is associated with a more cellular desmoplastic stromal reaction

Microglandular Adenosis
- Composed of small round tubules scattered around normal breast structures
  - o Luminal spaces are open with round contours and contain eosinophilic secretions
  - o Little or no stromal response
- Distinguished from SA by IHC
  - o Lacks myoepithelial cells
  - o ER(-)
  - o Strongly S100(+)
- Can recur and is often associated with frankly invasive carcinoma

SELECTED REFERENCES
1. Taskin F et al: Sclerosing adenosis of the breast: radiologic appearance and efficiency of core needle biopsy. Diagn Interv Radiol. 2011 Feb 15. doi: 10.4261/1305-3825. DIR. Epub ahead of print, 3785
2. Hilson JB et al: Phenotypic alterations in myoepithelial cells associated with benign sclerosing lesions of the breast. Am J Surg Pathol. 34(6):896-900, 2010
3. Pavlakis K et al: Myoepithelial cell cocktail (p63+SMA) for the evaluation of sclerosing breast lesions. Breast. 15(6):705-12, 2006
4. Gill HK et al: When is a diagnosis of sclerosing adenosis acceptable at core biopsy? Radiology. 228(1):50-7, 2003
5. Shoker BS et al: Abnormal regulation of the oestrogen receptor in benign breast lesions. J Clin Pathol. 53(10):778-83, 2000
6. Oberman HA et al: Noninvasive carcinoma of the breast presenting in adenosis. Mod Pathol. 4(1):31-5, 1991
7. Jensen RA et al: Invasive breast cancer risk in women with sclerosing adenosis. Cancer. 64(10):1977-83, 1989
8. Taylor HB et al: Epithelial invasion of nerves in benign diseases of the breast. Cancer. 20(12):2245-9, 1967

SCLEROSING ADENOSIS

Microscopic Features

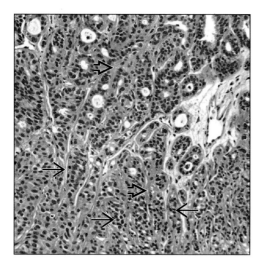
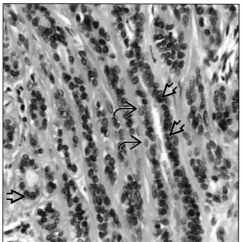

(Left) In SA, stromal fibrosis ➡ usually compresses and causes collapse of acinar lumens ➡. The resulting cords of cells are arranged in closely approximated parallel arrays, often in a swirling pattern. (Right) The luminal cells in SA may appear cuboidal ➡ or flattened and lack cytologic atypia. Myoepithelial cells ➡ usually are seen in H&E sections but may be spindled in shape and difficult to identify. IHC will identify a myoepithelial cell layer in difficult cases.

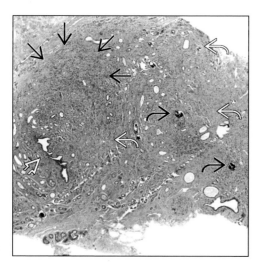
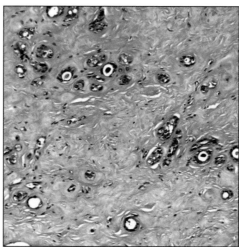

(Left) The lobulocentric pattern of SA consists of numerous small back-to-back tubules ➡ surrounding a larger central duct ➡. Calcifications ➡ are often present. Multiple confluent areas of SA can form lobulated masses ➡. (Right) Some of the peripheral acini of SA can have a "wandering" pattern into stroma and appear to invade around normal ducts and lobules. These small tubules can closely mimic invasive well-differentiated carcinoma or microglandular adenosis.

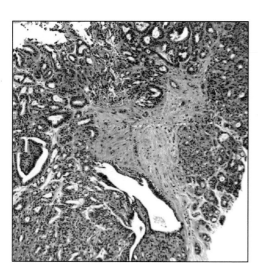
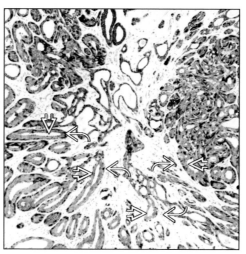

(Left) SA is the lesion most commonly misdiagnosed as invasive carcinoma. The diagnosis can be particularly difficult in needle biopsies where the lobulocentric pattern and circumscribed borders may be difficult to appreciate. (Right) IHC is very helpful to confirm the presence of luminal cells (CK18, red) ➡ and myoepithelial cells (p63 and CK5/6, brown) ➡ in SA. SA should always be considered when diagnosing a well- or moderately differentiated invasive ductal carcinoma.

Difficult Cases

(Left) When DCIS ⊟ involves SA ⊞, the pattern can closely resemble invasive carcinoma. The involved spaces are generally closer together than typical for carcinomas, and the stroma is usually sclerotic rather than desmoplastic. *(Right)* IHC for myoepithelial markers such as smooth muscle actin can be used to identify myoepithelial cells in areas of DCIS ⊟ as well as in the areas of DCIS involving SA in a complex pattern ⊞. The back-to-back pattern is easily appreciated.

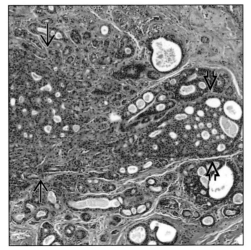
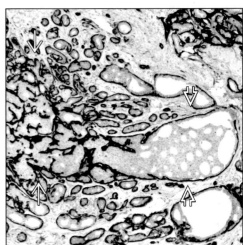

(Left) This core needle biopsy of a 1.5 cm irregular mass was misdiagnosed as invasive carcinoma. Although a monomorphic neoplastic cell population is present ⊞, the circumscribed border ⊟ and flattened peripheral tubules suggestive of a swirling pattern ⊞ would be unusual. *(Right)* IHC for myoepithelial cells identified this lesion as SA. The neoplastic cell population partially involving the SA was confirmed as LCIS by the absence of E-cadherin positivity ⊞.

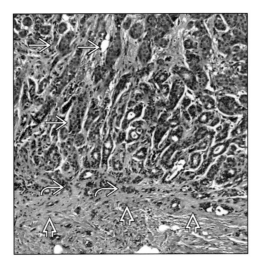
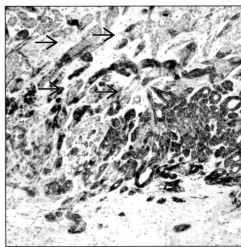

(Left) Apocrine metaplasia can be present in SA. The luminal cells are monomorphic in appearance with large nuclei and prominent nucleoli. The compressed tubules and sometimes inconspicuous myoepithelial cells make distinction from invasive carcinoma difficult. *(Right)* SA can involve nerves in a pattern that closely mimics malignant perineural invasion. However, the benign nature of the tubules is shown by the presence of a p63(+) layer of myoepithelial cells ⊞.

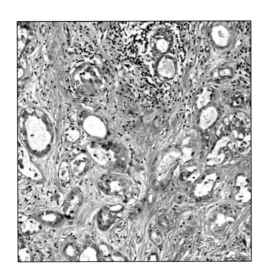
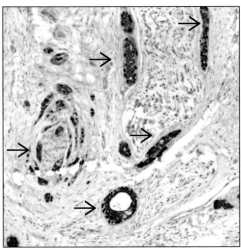

SCLEROSING ADENOSIS

Differential Diagnosis

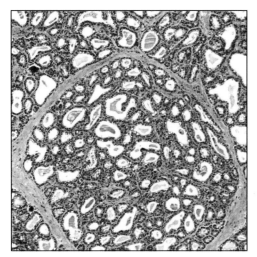

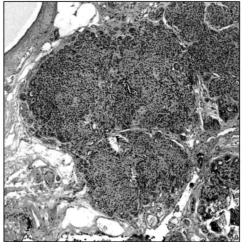

(Left) Lobules normally enlarge during pregnancy and lactation due an increase in the number and size of the acini. However, unlike SA, in normal breast tissues, the acini remain round in shape with open lumens and the stroma is not sclerotic. (Right) After lactation ceases and with age, lobules regress until only the large duct system remains. A large regressing lobule can resemble SA. However, the myoepithelial cells are more prominent, and the epithelial cells become small and atrophic.

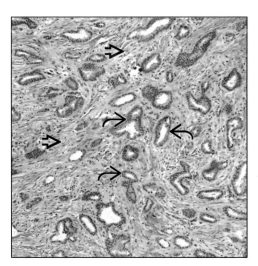

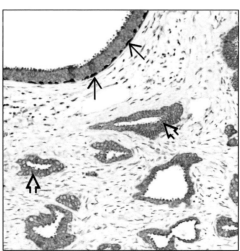

(Left) Compared to SA, tubular carcinoma has a haphazard infiltrating pattern ⇨ and lacks a lobulocentric architecture. The tubules are widely separated by a cellular reactive desmoplastic stroma ⇨. (Right) Carcinomas are positive for cytokeratin (CK18, cytoplasmic red) ⇨ but lack myoepithelial cells. SA is composed of cytokeratin(+) luminal cells and myoepithelial cells (p63, nuclear brown), as is this adjacent normal duct ⇨.

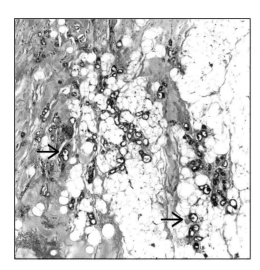

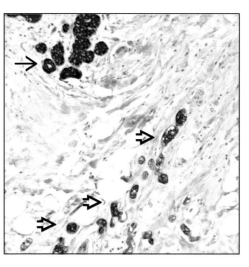

(Left) Like SA, microglandular adenosis consists of small tubules. However, the tubules are rounded and contain characteristic eosinophilic secretions ⇨ and are not closely approximated in a lobulocentric pattern. There is little or no stromal reaction. (Right) Unlike SA, microglandular adenosis ⇨ lacks myoepithelial cells, which would be detected by p63 ⇨ in sclerosing adenosis. Microglandular adenosis also differs in being negative for ER and strongly positive for S100.

EPITHELIAL HYPERPLASIA

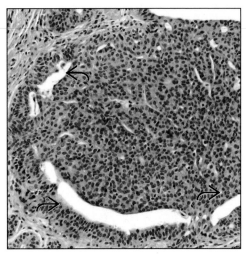

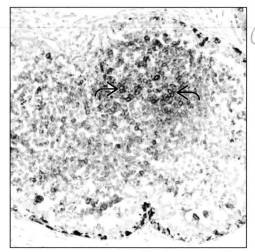

Usual epithelial hyperplasia in an involved duct space distended by a heterogeneous proliferation with a haphazard arrangement of overlapping cells. The fenestrated spaces are slit-like ⊿.

The cellular proliferation shows a mosaic pattern of staining with the HMW cytokeratin CK5/6 ⊿*. This finding supports the heterogeneous nature of UDH, which is composed of a mixture of cell types.*

TERMINOLOGY

Abbreviations
- Usual type ductal epithelial hyperplasia (UDH)

Synonyms
- Ductal epithelial hyperplasia

Definitions
- UDH: Benign intraductal epithelial proliferation
  - Proliferation tends to fill and bridge across involved spaces
  - Considerable variability in degree of proliferation
    - Mild proliferation: 2-4 cell layers
    - Florid proliferation: > 4 cell layers filling and distending duct spaces
    - Florid UDH may show solid, fenestrated, or micropapillary-type architecture
  - Florid UDH must be distinguished from atypical ductal epithelial hyperplasia (ADH) and low-grade ductal carcinoma in situ (LGDCIS)

ETIOLOGY/PATHOGENESIS

Molecular Changes in UDH
- Molecular studies have shown loss of heterozygosity in subsets of UDH
  - No consistent molecular alterations have been reported
  - Fewer genetic abnormalities compared with ADH, LGDCIS, and invasive cancer from same patients
- Molecular data support the concept that UDH does not represent a direct cancer precursor
- Current concept: Moderate to florid UDH is a marker of generalized increased cancer risk

CLINICAL ISSUES

Epidemiology
- Incidence
  - UDH can be found in up to 25% of benign breast biopsies
- Age
  - Majority of women with UDH are 35-60 years of age
    - UDH is less frequent in patients > 60 years of age

Presentation
- Microscopic finding and is not clinically apparent
- UDH is frequent constituent of benign epithelial changes
  - Can include any of the following
    - Apocrine cysts
    - Sclerosing adenosis
    - Papillary apocrine metaplasia
    - Stromal hyperplasia and fibrosis
- Benign epithelial changes may present as indeterminate mammographic calcifications
  - Calcifications are usually associated with cysts or sclerosing adenosis
  - UDH is not typically associated with calcifications
- These changes may also present as palpable abnormality
  - Most often, mass is ill-defined palpable area of breast thickening

Treatment
- UDH is benign process requiring no further treatment
  - Patients should be encouraged to participate in regular clinical follow-up
    - Follow-up programs should include physician examinations and imaging
    - Follow-up is important due to slight increased risk of developing carcinoma associated with florid UDH

EPITHELIAL HYPERPLASIA

Key Facts

Terminology
- Usual type ductal epithelial hyperplasia (UDH)

Clinical Issues
- UDH found in up to 25% of breast biopsies
- UDH is frequent constituent of benign epithelial changes
- Florid UDH associated with 1.5-2x increased relative risk of developing subsequent carcinoma

Microscopic Pathology
- Solid pattern
  ○ Heterogeneity in cell size, shape, and placement
  ○ Haphazard arrangement of cells
- Fenestrated pattern
  ○ Luminal spaces irregular and variable in size and shape (slit-like)

○ Peripherally located luminal spaces
- Cellular proliferation may have syncytial appearance
  ○ Individual cell borders are inconspicuous
  ○ Cellular proliferation has benign cytologic features
- Some cases may show spindle-shaped cells with prominent streaming or swirling pattern

Ancillary Tests
- UDH shows diffuse or mosaic pattern of staining with high molecular weight cytokeratin
- Cells of UDH show variable expression of ER and PR
- Stains for CK5/6 or 34BE12 may be helpful for distinguishing UDH from ADH

Top Differential Diagnoses
- Atypical ductal hyperplasia
- Low-grade ductal carcinoma in situ

■ Intervals for follow-up should be based on comprehensive assessment of risk for individual patient

Prognosis
- UDH is associated with a 1.5-2x increased relative risk of developing subsequent carcinoma
  ○ This means that 5-7% of women with UDH are expected to develop breast cancer during their lifetimes
  ○ Subsequent risk is higher with diagnosis of ADH (5x increase in relative risk)
  ○ Subsequent cancer risk applies to both breasts
  ○ Subsequent cancer risk will be higher in women with UDH and positive family history of breast cancer

IMAGE FINDINGS

Mammographic Findings
- Manifestations of benign epithelial changes associated with UDH are variable
  ○ UDH is rarely associated with calcifications or mammographic densities
  ○ Cysts may be associated with calcifications
  ○ Sclerosing adenosis or papillomas may be associated with calcifications or circumscribed or lobulated density
  ○ Findings may require biopsy to exclude malignancy

MICROSCOPIC PATHOLOGY

Histologic Features
- Architectural patterns of UDH
  ○ Solid pattern
    ■ Heterogeneity in cell size, shape, and placement
    ■ May demonstrate peripheral slit-like luminal spaces
    ■ Myoepithelial layer maintained
  ○ Fenestrated pattern

■ Luminal spaces irregular and variable in size and shape
■ Frequently slit-like and located peripherally
  ○ Micropapillary pattern
    ■ Tuft-like papillary projections tapered at tips
    ■ Resembles pattern of hyperplasia seen in gynecomastia

Cytologic Features
- Cellular proliferation may have syncytial appearance
  ○ Individual cell borders are inconspicuous
- Cellular proliferation shows benign cytologic features
  ○ Cells vary in size, shape, and nuclear orientation
  ○ Cells do not show polarization around luminal spaces
  ○ Cells arranged in haphazard pattern and appear to be overlapping
  ○ Some cases may show spindle-shaped cells with prominent streaming or swirling pattern

ANCILLARY TESTS

Immunohistochemistry
- Cells of UDH show variable expression of ER and PR
  ○ Some lesions show marked diffuse ER expression in most cells
    ■ Most commonly seen in florid UDH cases
    ■ Up to 60% of florid UDH cases demonstrate diffuse expression of ER
    ■ ER may play role in driving cellular proliferation of lesion
- Heterogeneous nature of intraductal cellular proliferation can be highlighted by IHC
  ○ UDH shows diffuse or mosaic pattern of staining with high molecular weight cytokeratin
  ○ Stains for CK5/6 or 34BE12 may be helpful for distinguishing UDH from ADH
    ■ UDH: Diffuse or mosaic staining pattern
    ■ ADH: Absence of staining indicating homogeneous (clonal) proliferation
    ■ Surrounding myoepithelial layer will be highlighted by these markers

EPITHELIAL HYPERPLASIA

Differential Diagnosis: Intraductal Epithelial Proliferation

Feature	Usual Epithelial Hyperplasia	Atypical Ductal Hyperplasia	Low-Grade Ductal Carcinoma In Situ
Cell population	Heterogeneous	Variable (partially heterogeneous)	Monotonous
Cytologic features	Variation in size, shape, orientation	Admixed monotonous and heterogeneous	Monotonous, uniform, small, round nuclei
Cell borders	Overlapping cells; borders poorly defined	2 populations; overlapping and well-defined borders	Not overlapping, evenly spaced; well-defined borders
Nuclei	Variable; round and spindle-shaped	2 populations, variable and monotonous	Monotonous, uniform, round nuclei
Growth pattern	Solid, fenestrated, micropapillary	Solid, fenestrated, micropapillary	Solid, fenestrated, micropapillary
Luminal spaces	Irregular, variable size (slit-like)	Admixture of luminal space patterns	Rigid, round, "punched-out" spaces
Polarization of cells around luminal spaces	Absent	May be present	Almost always present
Bridges	Stretched, central attenuation	Variable pattern	Bridges and arcades have uniform thickness
LOH studies	~ 10%, usually only 1 or few loci	~ 50% LOH, pattern similar to DCIS	50-80%, numerous loci, similar pattern seen in invasive cancer
Clonality	Polyclonal proliferation (97%)	Monoclonal proliferation (51%)	Monoclonal proliferation (100%)
HMWCK (CK5/6, 14, 34βE12)	Diffuse &/or mosaic staining pattern	Usually negative (may be variable)	Negative
ER/PR	Variable	Usually diffusely positive	Diffusely positive
High-grade cytologic features	Absent	Absent	Absent

ADH is a proliferative ductal lesion that demonstrates some but not all features of low-grade ductal carcinoma in situ.

- Ki-67 proliferative index should be very low
  - Usually < 5% of cells

- UDH does not have a uniform appearance and does not have well-formed architectural features

DIFFERENTIAL DIAGNOSIS

Atypical Ductal Hyperplasia
- ADH has appearance of small monoclonal population of cells but insufficient for diagnosis of DCIS
  - Uniform population of monotonous cells typically only partially fills duct spaces
  - Architectural features (e.g., cribriform spaces and papillae) are not as well formed as in DCIS
  - UDH consists of multiple cell types and does not appear clonal
- IHC for high molecular weight cytokeratin can be helpful in problematic cases
  - Clonal-appearing areas of ADH are typically negative for high molecular weight cytokeratin
  - Mixed cell population in UDH usually shows partial positivity for high molecular weight cytokeratin
- If a lesion is difficult to classify as ADH or UDH, UDH should be favored

Low-Grade Ductal Carcinoma In Situ
- Involved ductal spaces dilated and filled with a monotonous clonal population of cells
  - Complex architectural patterns are well formed (cribriform, solid, micropapillary)
  - Uniform involvement of duct spaces
  - Typically involves multiple adjacent duct spaces
- Monotonous uniform cells that stand apart
  - Cells do not overlap; frequent sharp cellular boundaries

SELECTED REFERENCES

1. Johnson NB et al: Update on percutaneous needle biopsy of nonmalignant breast lesions. Adv Anat Pathol. 16(4):183-95, 2009
2. Yu Q et al: Analysis of the progression of intraductal proliferative lesions in the breast by PCR-based clonal assay. Breast Cancer Res Treat. 114(3):433-40, 2009
3. MacGrogan G et al: Impact of immunohistochemical markers, CK5/6 and E-cadherin on diagnostic agreement in non-invasive proliferative breast lesions. Histopathology. 52(6):689-97, 2008
4. Nofech-Mozes S et al: The role of cytokeratin 5/6 as an adjunct diagnostic tool in breast core needle biopsies. Int J Surg Pathol. 16(4):399-406, 2008
5. Ashbeck EL et al: Benign breast biopsy diagnosis and subsequent risk of breast cancer. Cancer Epidemiol Biomarkers Prev. 16(3):467-72, 2007
6. Page DL et al: Anatomic markers of human premalignancy and risk of breast cancer. Cancer. 66(6 Suppl):1326-35, 1990
7. Page DL et al: Premalignant conditions and markers of elevated risk in the breast and their management. Surg Clin North Am. 70(4):831-51, 1990
8. Page DL et al: Atypical hyperplastic lesions of the female breast. A long-term follow-up study. Cancer. 55(11):2698-708, 1985
9. Page DL et al: Relation between component parts of fibrocystic disease complex and breast cancer. J Natl Cancer Inst. 61(4):1055-63, 1978

EPITHELIAL HYPERPLASIA

Microscopic Features

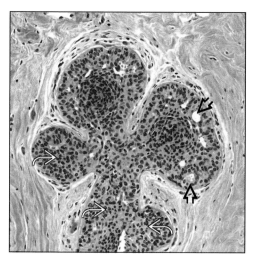
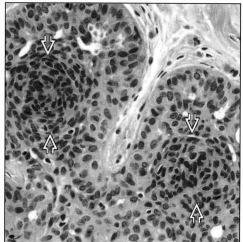

(Left) UDH represents a benign intraductal proliferation of epithelial cells that can show considerable variability in the extent of involvement of duct spaces. The architectural patterns can be solid ➤ or fenestrated, with peripheral luminal spaces ➤. *(Right)* On higher magnification, the haphazard nature of the cellular proliferation is readily apparent. The cells show variability in their size and shapes and can demonstrate a flowing or swirling appearance ➤.

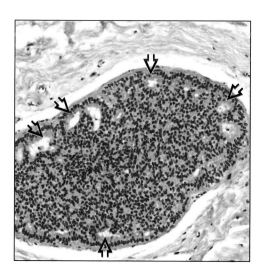
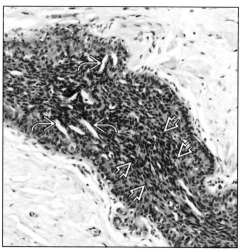

(Left) Florid UDH shows a proliferation of multiple cells that will begin to fill and distend duct spaces. The proliferation may form luminal spaces that are variable in size and frequently peripherally located ➤. *(Right)* The proliferating cells of UDH are variable in size, frequently overlap, and appear disorganized in general. In some cases, spindle-shaped cells will be oriented in parallel, imparting a streaming appearance ➤. Typical slit-like spaces ➤ can be seen.

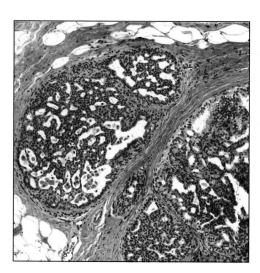
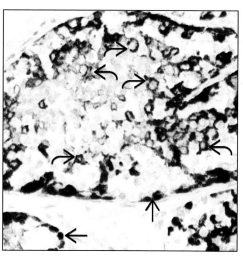

(Left) Florid UDH represents a heterogeneous proliferation of different cell types. Some cases of florid UDH can be challenging and must be distinguished from ADH. *(Right)* The heterogeneous nature of the intraductal cellular proliferation can be highlighted by immunohistochemistry for high molecular weight cytokeratins. CK5/6 expression can be seen in myoepithelial cells ➤ and also shows a mosaic pattern of staining ➤ within the intraductal proliferation in UDH.

RADIAL SCLEROSING LESION/RADIAL SCAR

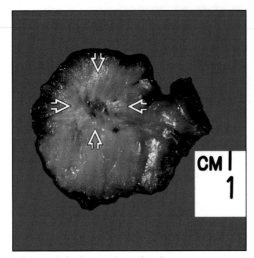

A large radial sclerosing lesion has the gross appearance of an irregularly shaped mass ⊳. Generally, only the central nidus is firm or hard and not the entire lesion (as are invasive carcinomas).

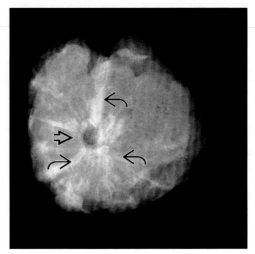
The radiographic appearance of a radial sclerosing lesion is a stellate-shaped radiodense mass with long radially arranged fibrous septae ⊳ and a central lucent region ⊳.

TERMINOLOGY

Abbreviations
- Radial sclerosing lesion (RSL)

Synonyms
- Radial scar
- Complex sclerosing lesion (CSL)

Definitions
- RSL shows variable combinations of the following elements
  o Epithelial proliferation, which may be florid
  o Stromal fibrosis and dense sclerosis
  o As a result, RSL shows irregular contours
- Clinically, mammographically, and pathologically, this lesion closely resembles invasive carcinoma
- "Radial scar" is term used for same lesion; "scar" does not imply prior surgery or trauma
- CSL is less specific term
  o Sometimes defined as a RSL > 1 cm in size
  o CSL may also include lesions consisting of confluent sclerosing adenosis, sclerosing papillomas, &/or multiple RSLs

CLINICAL ISSUES

Presentation
- Most RSLs are microscopic findings
- Larger RSLs may present as mammographic density or even palpable mass
- Both in situ and invasive carcinomas have been reported in association with RSL

Treatment
- Surgical approaches
  o Most authors recommend surgical excision for RSL diagnosed by needle core biopsy
    ▪ Some RSLs are reported to coexist with malignancy

  ▪ RSL on core needle biopsy may be difficult to distinguish from invasive carcinomas

Prognosis
- RSL is histologic risk factor for subsequent development of breast carcinoma
- Presence of epithelial atypia, increased size, and multiple lesions are likely associated with increased risk for development of malignancy
- However, additional risk after adjusting for proliferative disease and atypical hyperplasia is small

IMAGE FINDINGS

Mammographic Findings
- RSL presents as irregular mass
  o Length of radiating arms is long in relation to size of mass, as compared to carcinomas
  o Center of mass may be lucent
- Microcalcifications are present in some lesions
  o Typically seen in association with accompanying sclerosing adenosis or ADH
- Most mammographically detected lesions are < 2 cm
  o Average size: < 1 cm
  o Associated carcinomas more common with RSL > 2 cm

Ultrasonographic Findings
- RSL most commonly seen as hypoechoic area/mass
- Parenchymal distortion without hypoechoic mass may be seen

MR Findings
- Irregular enhancing lesion by MR
  o RSLs tend to show less enhancement by MR, as compared with invasive carcinoma

RADIAL SCLEROSING LESION/RADIAL SCAR

Key Facts

Terminology
- Radial sclerosing lesion (RSL)
  - Radially organized combination of epithelial proliferation, central stromal fibrosis, and sclerosis resulting in mass-like lesion
- Clinically, mammographically, and pathologically RSL may mimic invasive carcinoma

Clinical Issues
- Most RSLs are microscopic findings
- Larger RSL may present as mammographic or palpable mass
  - Risk factor for subsequent development of breast carcinoma
- Surgical excision recommended for RSL diagnosed by core needle biopsy

- Both in situ and invasive carcinomas have been reported in association with RSL

Image Findings
- Irregular appearance on mammography

Microscopic Pathology
- Central nidus, varying degrees of fibrosis and fibroelastosis in stellate or radial configuration
  - Associated proliferative epithelial component
  - Varying degrees of proliferative epithelial changes
  - Smaller ducts can become entrapped in dense fibrous stroma within central fibrotic region

Top Differential Diagnoses
- Tubular carcinoma

MACROSCOPIC FEATURES

General Features
- Irregular firm mass
  - Yellow-white color, indurated with central retraction
  - Lesions are usually firm but not as hard as invasive carcinomas
  - However, lesions may grossly be indistinguishable from invasive carcinoma

Size
- Most lesions are < 2 cm

MICROSCOPIC PATHOLOGY

Histologic Features
- Central nidus, sclerotic zone composed of varying degrees of fibrosis and fibroelastosis in stellate or radial configuration
  - Dense granular eosinophilic stroma, sometimes showing weakly basophilic quality
  - Elastic component of stroma may be highlighted by van Gieson stain, which shows dense curvilinear elastic fibrils
  - Stroma usually hypocellular
- Associated proliferative epithelial component
  - Ducts and lobular elements radiate from central fibroelastotic zone
  - Demonstrates varying degrees of benign alteration and proliferative changes
  - Florid ductal epithelial hyperplasia, sclerosing adenosis, and epithelial cyst formation
  - Radiating epithelial components appear to expand or enlarge moving away from central fibroelastotic region
  - ADH, ALH, in situ and invasive carcinoma can occur in association with RSL
  - Atypical hyperplasias and carcinomas more common in larger lesions
  - Atypical hyperplasias and associated carcinomas more common in women > 50 years

- Entrapped ducts
  - Smaller ducts can be seen entrapped in dense fibrous stroma within central region of lesion
  - Ducts may become distorted and appear angulated giving rise to a pseudoinfiltrative appearance
  - Appearance may mimic tubular carcinoma, especially on core needle biopsy
  - Entrapped ducts retain myoepithelial layer of cells
  - Surrounding stroma typically paucicellular, absence of loose desmoplastic reaction
  - Immunohistochemistry for myoepithelial cells may be helpful to exclude invasive carcinoma

ANCILLARY TESTS

Immunohistochemistry
- Studies to identify myoepithelial cells may be helpful in difficult cases
  - However, results of myoepithelial cell studies to rule out malignancy must be interpreted with caution
    - Myoepithelial cells may only be identified around some of entrapped glands
    - Myoepithelial cells may not be present in plane of section used for the study
  - Use of more than 1 myoepithelial cell marker is recommended to improve likelihood of detection
    - p63, calponin, and smooth muscle myosin heavy chain have good sensitivity and specificity
    - Cocktails of > 1 myoepithelial marker may be helpful
    - p63 is nuclear marker; nuclei may not be present on all levels
    - Cytoplasmic myoepithelial markers are more likely to detect cell body of myoepithelial cells

DIFFERENTIAL DIAGNOSIS

Tubular Carcinoma (TC)
- May be significant mammographic, macroscopic, and histologic overlap between large RSLs and TC

RADIAL SCLEROSING LESION/RADIAL SCAR

Differential Diagnosis

Feature	Tubular Carcinoma	Radial Sclerosing Lesion
Mammographic appearance	Stellate irregular mass; spicules are shorter than size of the mass	Stellate irregular mass (may show radiolucent central area); spicules are longer than size of the mass
Microscopic appearance	Haphazard distribution of neoplastic ducts, central and peripheral	Stellate "centrifugal" pattern; radiating proliferation increases in size away from central region
Stromal appearance	Desmoplastic stroma, more cellular, present throughout	"Hyalinized," fibroelastotic stroma, less cellular, confined to center of lesion
Entrapped glands	Neoplastic ducts distributed in desmoplastic stroma throughout lesion	Confined to central portion of lesion, entrapped and distorted by fibroelastotic stroma
Myoepithelial cells	Absent around malignant tubules	Present, surrounding entrapped ducts (may be focal or patchy); multiple myoepithelial markers may be needed to demonstrate
Associated in situ proliferation	Atypical ductal hyperplasia, flat epithelial atypia, and low-grade DCIS frequent findings; admixed with malignant tubules	ADH and low-grade DCIS may be present but uncommon; typically seen at periphery of lesion

- o Proliferating neoplastic ducts of TC are associated with desmoplastic stroma (increased cellularity)
  - Entrapped ducts of RSL are surrounded by hyalinized fibroelastotic stroma (low cellularity)
- o Proliferating neoplastic ducts of TC show haphazard arrangement, usually throughout lesion
  - Entrapped ducts of RSL limited to central fibroelastotic region of lesion
- o Proliferating neoplastic ducts of TC show single cell layer and lack surrounding myoepithelial cells
  - Entrapped ducts of RSL demonstrate surrounding myoepithelial cells
- Immunohistochemistry for myoepithelial cells may be helpful in difficult cases
  - o Infiltrating neoplastic ducts of TC lack surrounding myoepithelial cells by IHC
- TC typically demonstrates low-grade monomorphous atypia, which can be subtle in some cases
- TC is more commonly associated with adjacent DCIS or ADH

DIAGNOSTIC CHECKLIST

Clinically Relevant Pathologic Features

- Gross appearance
  - o RSLs are most often incidental microscopic finding
  - o Larger RSLs can clinically, mammographically, and histologically be mistaken for invasive carcinoma
- RSL is histologic risk factor for subsequent development of breast carcinoma
  - o 2x increased risk of subsequent breast cancer, independent of other benign histologic features
  - o Risk may be further increased in women with larger lesions or multiple lesions, > 50 years of age

Pathologic Interpretation Pearls

- Look for central fibroelastotic region with entrapped ducts
  - o Central area typically paucicellular-cellular and densely hyalinized
  - o Entrapped ducts contain surrounding myoepithelial layer

- Look for circumferential radial arrangement of peripheral ducts and lobules with associated varying degrees of adenosis and hyperplasia
  - o Epithelial proliferation may be florid in some cases and demonstrate atypia
    - Atypia is more common in larger lesions

SELECTED REFERENCES

1. Berg JC et al: Breast cancer risk in women with radial scars in benign breast biopsies. Breast Cancer Res Treat. 108(2):167-74, 2008
2. Manfrin E et al: Risk of neoplastic transformation in asymptomatic radial scar. Analysis of 117 cases. Breast Cancer Res Treat. 107(3):371-7, 2008
3. Douglas-Jones AG et al: Radial scar lesions of the breast diagnosed by needle core biopsy: analysis of cases containing occult malignancy. J Clin Pathol. 60(3):295-8, 2007
4. Doyle EM et al: Radial scars/complex sclerosing lesions and malignancy in a screening programme: incidence and histological features revisited. Histopathology. 50(5):607-14, 2007
5. de Moraes Schenka NG et al: p63 and CD10: reliable markers in discriminating benign sclerosing lesions from tubular carcinoma of the breast?. Appl Immunohistochem Mol Morphol. 14(1):71-7, 2006
6. Sanders ME et al: Interdependence of radial scar and proliferative disease with respect to invasive breast carcinoma risk in patients with benign breast biopsies. Cancer. 106(7):1453-61, 2006
7. Fasih T et al: All radial scars/complex sclerosing lesions seen on breast screening mammograms should be excised. Eur J Surg Oncol. 31(10):1125-8, 2005
8. Farshid G et al: Assessment of 142 stellate lesions with imaging features suggestive of radial scar discovered during population-based screening for breast cancer. Am J Surg Pathol. 28(12):1626-31, 2004
9. Iqbal M et al: Molecular and genetic abnormalities in radial scar. Hum Pathol. 33(7):715-22, 2002
10. Alvarado-Cabrero I et al: Neoplastic and malignant lesions involving or arising in a radial scar: A clinicopathologic analysis of 17 cases. Breast J. 6(2):96-102, 2000
11. Jacobs TW et al: Radial scars in benign breast-biopsy specimens and the risk of breast cancer. N Engl J Med. 340(6):430-6, 1999

RADIAL SCLEROSING LESION/RADIAL SCAR

Imaging, Gross, and Microscopic Features

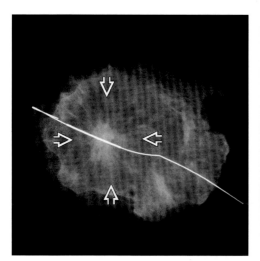

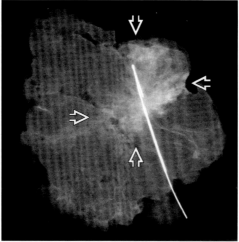

(Left) RSLs typically have spiculations ⊳ (or radiating arms) longer than the central portion of the mass, as seen in this case. In contrast, invasive carcinomas generally have a relatively large central mass with short spicules. (Right) This RSL presented radiographically as an ill-defined mass ⊳. The margins cannot be seen clearly due to the surrounding dense tissue. RSLs are often surrounded by lesions that can also cause mammographic densities (e.g., sclerosing adenosis).

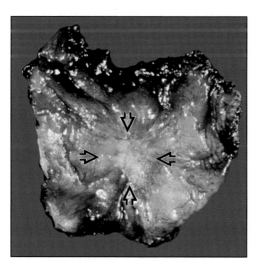

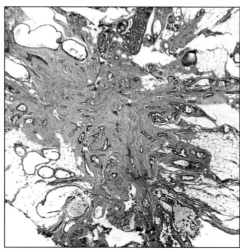

(Left) This RSL had the gross appearance of an invasive carcinoma with irregular margins ⊳. However, by palpation the lesion had a hard central nidus but was less firm around the periphery. Invasive carcinomas are typically hard throughout the lesion and have a distinct edge at the junction with the surrounding normal tissue. (Right) The irregular margins of this RSL can be clearly seen in contrast to the adjacent tissue. The compressed glands in the fibrotic center are typical.

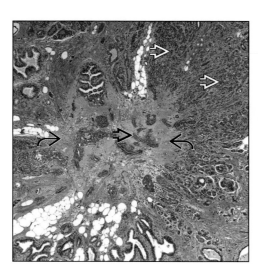

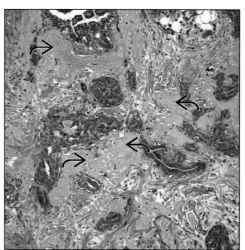

(Left) This RSL forms a stellate-shaped mass with a central area of stromal sclerosis ⊡ that contains entrapped and distorted glands and epithelial cell nests ⊳. The periphery of RSL is frequently associated with adenosis ⊳ and epithelial hyperplasia. (Right) On higher magnification, the central fibroelastotic zone of a typical RSL demonstrates a dense sclerotic stroma ⊡, which is paucicellular and at times can have a blue-gray color due to elastosis.

4

Ancillary Techniques

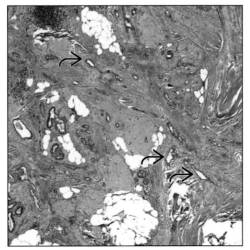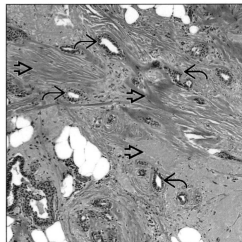

(Left) The central sclerotic zone of a RSL entraps and distorts small ducts ➤ giving rise to a pseudoinfiltrative appearance, which could be confused with a tubular carcinoma. An important diagnostic feature is that the ducts are confined to the center of the RSL. *(Right)* The entrapped glands ➤ are surrounded and distorted by dense hyalinized paucicellular stroma ➤ that lacks the typical desmoplastic appearance of stroma associated with invasive carcinomas.

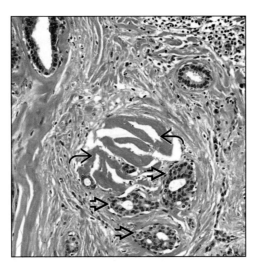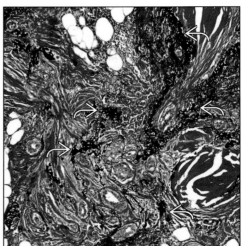

(Left) The central fibrotic region may show dense, keloid-like hyalinized stroma ➤. The entrapped glands have a myoepithelial layer, which can be seen by H&E ➤ or with stains for myoepithelial cells. *(Right)* The central sclerotic zone is composed of varying degrees of fibrosis and fibroelastosis in a stellate or radial configuration. The elastic component of the stroma shows a weakly basophilic appearance on H&E and is highlighted by a van Gieson elastic stain ➤.

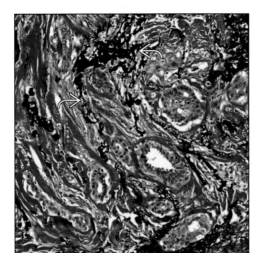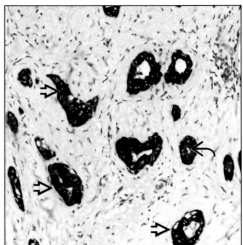

(Left) On higher magnification, an elastic stain shows dense curvilinear elastic fibrils ➤ admixed with dense collagen. *(Right)* A RSL will be composed of luminal cells positive for keratin (red cytoplasmic signal) ➤ and myoepithelial cells positive for nuclear p63 (brown nuclear signal) ➤. In some cases, IHC may be helpful to distinguish entrapped glands of an RSL from an invasive carcinoma.

RADIAL SCLEROSING LESION/RADIAL SCAR

Differential Diagnosis

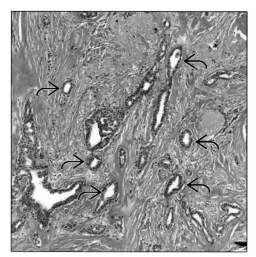

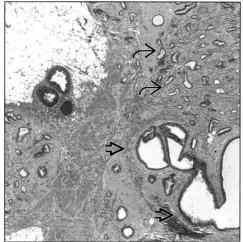

(Left) The entrapped glandular elements of a RSL can be numerous ➡, and myoepithelial cells can become attenuated and difficult to appreciate on routine H&E stained sections. The distinction between a RSL and an invasive carcinoma may be difficult, especially in limited biopsy samples. *(Right)* In this tubular carcinoma, the neoplastic tubules show a haphazard infiltrative pattern ➡ and surround adjacent ducts and lobules ➡. The desmoplastic stroma is very cellular.

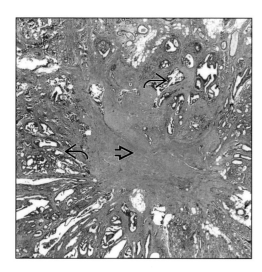

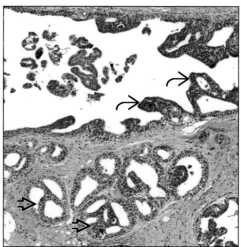

(Left) This large RSL has a characteristic central hyalinized fibroelastotic region ➡. A florid epithelial proliferation with a radial configuration is present and appears to expand away from the central sclerotic zone ➡. *(Right)* On higher magnification, the epithelial proliferation in this case demonstrates architectural complexity with cribriform ➡ and micropapillary ➡ areas and atypia. These architectural and cytologic features are diagnostic of ADH.

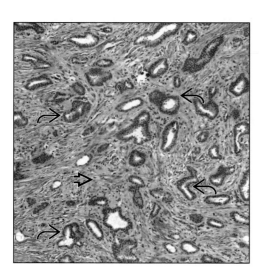

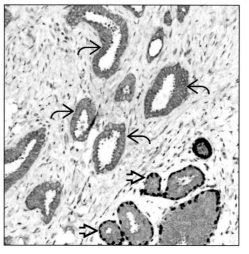

(Left) This case shows a tubular carcinoma (TC) with an infiltrative arrangement of angulated neoplastic glands ➡. The adjacent stroma is more cellular, showing a typical desmoplastic reaction ➡ to the tumor. *(Right)* The malignant tubules of TC are positive for cytokeratin (red cytoplasmic signal) and lack a surrounding myoepithelial cell layer ➡. In contrast, adjacent normal ducts have a layer of peripheral myoepithelial cells ➡, positive for p63 (brown nuclear signal).

PAPILLOMA, LARGE DUCT AND SMALL DUCT

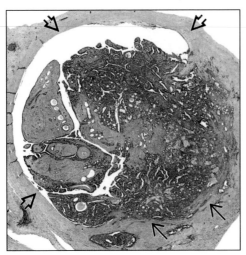

Large duct papillomas arise in the lactiferous sinuses ⇨ below the nipple and are attached to the wall by a stalk ⇥. The presenting symptom is often clear or hemorrhagic nipple discharge.

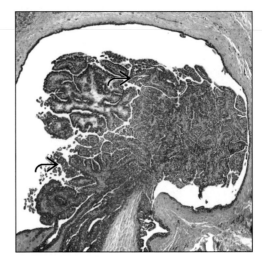

Small duct papillomas are usually peripherally located and are frequently multiple. The luminal epithelial cells of these papillomas are more likely to show hyperplasia ⇨ or atypia.

TERMINOLOGY

Abbreviations
- Large duct papilloma (LDP)
- Small duct papilloma (SDP)

Synonyms
- Central papilloma
- Peripheral papilloma
- Intraductal papilloma

Definitions
- Benign epithelial proliferative lesions characterized by papillary ingrowths into major ducts (LDP) or smaller ducts (SDP)

CLINICAL ISSUES

Epidemiology
- Age
  - LDP: Most frequent in women 35–50 years old
  - SDP: Usually younger

Site
- LDP: Centrally located in subareolar lactiferous ducts; usually solitary
- SDP: Peripherally located; often multiple ("papillomatosis")

Presentation
- LDP
  - Nipple discharge present in 80% of cases
    - In women < 60, 7% of cases with discharge are associated with malignancy
    - In women > 60, 30% of cases with discharge are associated with malignancy
  - Nipple discharge associated with pathologic lesions is unilateral and spontaneous
    - Sanguinous or serosanguinous: 70%
    - Bloody (less common): May be due to papilloma twisting on stalk and infarction
    - Other causes: Duct ectasia, mastitis, cysts, carcinoma (especially papillary and micropapillary DCIS)
  - Palpable subareolar mass
    - May form a lobulated mass on mammography
- SDP
  - Finding on screening mammography
  - Incidental finding in a biopsy for another lesion
  - Usually does not cause discharge or a palpable mass

Treatment
- Surgical approaches
  - Symptomatic papillomas are excised for diagnosis and treatment of nipple discharge
  - For benign lesions on excision, no further surgical treatment is necessary

Prognosis
- Papillomas are benign
- Mild increased risk of subsequent carcinoma: 1.5-2.0x relative risk or ~ 5-7% lifetime risk
  - Risk similar to that for moderate or florid ductal epithelial hyperplasia
  - Classified as proliferative disease without atypia
  - Breast cancer risk is slightly higher for women with multiple peripheral SDP (papillomatosis)
  - Can occur in either breast and at any site

Core Needle Biopsies
- Usually fragmented and can be difficult to evaluate
- IHC can be helpful in difficult cases
  - Confirm the presence of myoepithelial cells at periphery and in fibrovascular cores
  - Cytokeratin 5/6 is generally positive in benign papillomas and absent in papillary carcinomas
- Excision may be warranted in the following situations
  - Large (~ 2 cm) &/or palpable lesions
  - Papillomas with nuclear atypia

PAPILLOMA, LARGE DUCT AND SMALL DUCT

Key Facts

Terminology
- **Large duct papilloma (LDP)**
  - Usually centrally located; often solitary
  - Originates in lactiferous sinus or large mammary ducts
- **Small duct papilloma (SDP)**
  - Usually peripherally located; smaller lesions involving terminal ductal lobular units
  - Often multiple (papillomatosis)
  - Epithelium more likely to show foci of ADH or DCIS compared with LDP

Clinical Issues
- LDP may present with pathologic nipple discharge
  - Larger lesions may be palpable
- Standard treatment for LDP is complete excision

- Benign lesions on excision need no further surgical treatment
- Solitary LDPs have an increased relative risk of developing breast carcinoma (1.5–2.0x)
  - Risk is slightly higher for women with multiple peripheral SDP (papillomatosis)

Microscopic Pathology
- Arborizing fronds of tissue with well-developed central fibrovascular core
  - Lined by epithelial cells, myoepithelial cell layer

Top Differential Diagnoses
- Papillary DCIS
- Encapsulated (intracystic) carcinoma
- Solid papillary carcinoma
- Nipple adenoma

- Papillomas partially involved by proliferations that would be diagnostic of ADH or DCIS if outside of the papilloma
- Management of lesions diagnosed as benign papillomas on core needle biopsy is controversial
  - Risk of carcinoma on excision of benign papillomas is very low
    - When cases are carefully selected and there is good radiologic/pathologic correlation, carcinomas on excision are absent or rare (< 5%)
  - However, distinction between benign papillomas and atypical papillomas can be difficult, and some authorities recommend excision of all papillary lesions on core needle biopsy
  - Papillomas with atypia should be excised as 20-60% of cases will reveal carcinoma on excision

IMAGE FINDINGS

Mammographic Findings
- LDP may not be visible by mammography
- SDP can present as lobulated mass or cluster of calcifications

Ultrasonographic Findings
- LDP: Intraductal, well-defined, hypoechoic mass near nipple
  - May have both solid and cystic components
  - Adjacent ducts often dilated
- SDP: Small circumscribed or lobulated masses

Ductography
- LDP associated with nipple discharge may be diagnosed by ductography
  - Involved ductal orifice is often dilated
    - Very difficult to cannulate a duct in the absence of discharge
  - Contrast agent can show 1 or multiple filling defects with smooth contours in the duct
    - Papilloma interrupts flow of contrast
- Ductography may help localize lesion for excision

MACROSCOPIC FEATURES

General Features
- Excisions for nipple discharge require special processing
  - May lack a mass detectable by palpation or imaging
  - Surgeon excises subareolar tissue beneath duct orifice with discharge
  - Dilated duct should be marked with a suture
  - Involved duct is opened longitudinally and examined for gross lesions
- LDP may be visible macroscopically
  - Appears as tan-pink, circumscribed nodule protruding into a dilated duct or cystically dilated space
    - Cystic spaces may be filled with serosanguinous fluid and hemorrhage
  - Verrucous, bosselated, or frankly papillary appearance
- Many papillomas, including the majority of SDPs, are not evident on gross exam
- Excisions for palpable masses or mammographically detected lesions do not require special processing

Size
- LDP is usually < 2 cm but can be as large as 4-5 cm
- SDP is usually < 1 cm

MICROSCOPIC PATHOLOGY

Histologic Features
- **LDP**
  - Originates in lactiferous sinus or large mammary ducts
  - Arborizing finger-like fronds of fibrovascular stromal digitations
  - Covered by luminal epithelial cells with associated myoepithelial cells
  - Presence of myoepithelial cells and their distribution in lesion is helpful diagnostic feature

- May require use of myoepithelial markers to aid in the diagnostic evaluation in problematic cases
  o Apocrine metaplasia may be present and is supportive of benign diagnosis
  o Epithelial hyperplasia can be present and may be florid
  o "Sclerosing papilloma" refers to LDP with extensive fibrosis of fibrovascular cores &/or lesions with associated sclerosing adenosis
  o Squamous metaplasia may be present
    - Rarely, spindle or squamous cell carcinomas can arise in association with papillomas
  o Infarction, necrosis, and hemorrhage can occur if the LDP twists on its stalk
- **SDP**
  o Usually peripherally located small lesions involving terminal ductal lobular units
  o Often multiple (papillomatosis)
  o Fibrovascular cores are usually well defined
    - May show varying degrees of fibrosis and sclerosis
    - Demonstration of myoepithelium by IHC may be helpful for problematic cases
    - Fibrosis may entrap benign glands and solid epithelial nests
    - Entrapped glands may mimic infiltrating carcinoma
- **Papilloma with atypia**
  o 2 types
    - Entire papilloma appears atypical
    - Focal areas within papilloma fulfill criteria for ADH or DCIS
  o Atypical features in an entire papilloma include
    - Monomorphic-appearing epithelial cells
    - Complex architectural patterns (e.g., cribriform, micropapillary, or solid)
    - Thin, delicate fibrovascular cores
    - Absence of apocrine metaplasia or squamous metaplasia
    - IHC to demonstrate a myoepithelial cell layer is helpful to exclude papillary carcinoma
    - Surrounding tissue should be examined to find areas of carcinoma away from the papilloma
  o Papillomas with focal atypical areas are also seen
    - Criteria for diagnosing DCIS within a papilloma vary
    - It has been suggested that DCIS should not be diagnosed if area is < 0.3 cm or < 30% of papilloma
    - However, others favor diagnosing DCIS if criteria for diagnosis would be fulfilled if outside of the papilloma
    - Presence of DCIS in surrounding breast tissue is helpful to support diagnosis of DCIS and is more significant for determining patient's risk of subsequent breast cancer
    - Clinical significance of DCIS limited to a papilloma and completely excised is unclear; risk of subsequent breast cancer is at least equivalent to a diagnosis of ADH; multiple lesions may also increase risk
    - IHC for high molecular weight cytokeratins (CK5/6) can be helpful to distinguish hyperplasia

(patchy positivity) from ADH (negative) or DCIS (negative)
- **Spindle cell carcinoma arising in papilloma**
  o Squamous metaplasia may occur in papillomas, especially if associated with trauma or infarction
  o Spindle cell carcinomas can arise adjacent to these areas
  o Spindle cells may be difficult to distinguish from reactive fibroblasts in fibrous capsule of papilloma
    - Nuclear atypia and mitoses may be present
  o IHC for keratin (particularly basal types) and p63 is helpful to establish epithelial origin of spindle cells
- **Infarction**
  o Extensive coagulative necrosis can be seen in papillomas
    - May be focal or involve entire lesion
  o Can be associated with prior needle biopsies or twisting of stalk
  o Can result in a clinical bloody discharge
  o Completely necrotic papillary lesions can be difficult to classify
- **Epithelial displacement**
  o Entrapment of benign epithelium in core needle biopsy sites, surgical sites, or other areas of stromal disturbance occurs most frequently with papillary lesions
  o Benign cells can be pushed into lymphatics and be seen in sentinel node
    - Usually, a few cells are present and would be classified as isolated tumor cells
  o IHC can be helpful in many cases to demonstrate presence of both myoepithelial and epithelial cells
  o If myoepithelial cells are absent, diagnosis of invasive carcinoma &/or metastatic carcinoma should be made with great caution if artifactual displacement is a possibility

ANCILLARY TESTS

Immunohistochemistry
- Myoepithelial markers
  o Benign papillomas usually have prominent myoepithelial cell layer
  o IHC for myoepithelial cells can be helpful to document their presence
    - Papillary carcinomas lack myoepithelial cells
  o p63 is most helpful for evaluation of fibrovascular cores
    - Both myoepithelial cells and endothelial cells are positive for muscle markers
    - Blood vessels can be closely opposed to basal portion of epithelial cells and can be misidentified as myoepithelial cells
- Cytokeratin 5/6
  o Florid hyperplasia in papillomas can be difficult to distinguish from ADH or DCIS
  o Hyperplasia usually shows patchy positivity for cytokeratin 5/6, whereas ADH and DCIS are generally negative

PAPILLOMA, LARGE DUCT AND SMALL DUCT

Differential Diagnosis of Papillary Lesions

Diagnosis	Most Common Presentation	Papillae	Myoepithelial Cells: Periphery	Myoepithelial Cells: Papillae	Focal Apocrine Metaplasia	CK5/6
Large duct papilloma	Nipple discharge, circumscribed subareolar mass	Thick, may be infarcted	Present	Present, often prominent	Frequent	Usually positive
Small duct papilloma	Mammographic lobulated mass or calcifications	Thick	Present	Present	May be present	Usually positive
Papilloma with atypia	Mammographic lobulated mass or calcifications	Thick or thin	Present	Usually present except in areas of atypia/DCIS	May be present	Absent in areas of atypia
Papillary DCIS	Mammographic calcifications, nipple discharge	Thin	Present	Absent but may be present if papilloma is involved	Absent	Usually negative
Encapsulated papillary carcinoma	Circumscribed deep subareolar mass, nipple discharge	Thin	Absent	Absent	Absent	Usually negative
Solid papillary carcinoma	Multinodular mass	Solid growth pattern	May be absent, very focal, or present	Absent	Absent; may have mucinous features	Usually negative
Invasive papillary carcinoma	Irregular mass by palpation or mammography	Thin	Absent	Absent	Absent	Usually negative

DIFFERENTIAL DIAGNOSIS

Papillary DCIS

- Epithelial cells are monomorphic in appearance and may be hyperchromatic
  - Scattered globoid cells are often present and have more abundant pale cytoplasm than other tumor cells
  - Can mimic myoepithelial cells
  - Often immunoreactive for GCDFP-15
- Architectural complexity such as solid, cribriform, or micropapillary areas may be present
- Fibrovascular cores are usually thin and delicate
  - Myoepithelial cells are usually absent or rare
- In some cases, DCIS involves preexisting papillomas
  - Residual fibrovascular cores from papillomas have myoepithelial cells
- Myoepithelial cells are present at periphery of involved duct spaces
- May present as nipple discharge

Encapsulated (Intracystic) Carcinoma

- Usually presents as central circumscribed mass but located deeper in breast than LDP
- May be associated with nipple discharge
- Fibrovascular cores are usually thin and delicate
- Myoepithelial cells are absent within fibrovascular cores and around periphery
- If completely excised, clinical behavior is similar to DCIS

Solid Papillary Carcinoma

- Presents as multiple solid nodules consisting of monomorphic cells
  - Fibrovascular cores are present within cell nests
- Often difficult to distinguish invasive solid papillary carcinoma from solid papillary DCIS

  - IHC is helpful to determine presence and distribution of myoepithelial cells

Nipple Adenoma (NA)

- May be considered variant of papilloma
- Usually involves multiple nodular spaces directly under and often involving epidermis
- NA often consists of complex pattern of papillary areas, solid areas, and sclerosing adenosis
- Typically presents as palpable dermal mass or focal erosion of nipple skin

SELECTED REFERENCES

1. Chang JM et al: Papillary lesions initially diagnosed at ultrasound-guided vacuum-assisted breast biopsy: rate of malignancy based on subsequent surgical excision. Ann Surg Oncol. Epub ahead of print, 2011
2. Reisenbichler ES et al: Luminal cytokeratin expression profiles of breast papillomas and papillary carcinomas and the utility of a cytokeratin 5/p63/cytokeratin 8/18 antibody cocktail in their distinction. Mod Pathol. 24(2):185-93, 2011
3. Hardie M et al: Transported papillary lesions of the breast in axillary lymph nodes: a report of two cases. Pathology. 42(7):686-8, 2010
4. Pathmanathan N et al: Diagnostic evaluation of papillary lesions of the breast on core biopsy. Mod Pathol. 23(7):1021-8, 2010
5. Ahmadiyeh N et al: Management of intraductal papillomas of the breast: an analysis of 129 cases and their outcome. Ann Surg Oncol. 16(8):2264-9, 2009
6. Nagi C et al: Epithelial displacement in breast lesions: a papillary phenomenon. Arch Pathol Lab Med. 129(11):1465-9, 2005
7. Gobbi H et al: Metaplastic spindle cell breast tumors arising within papillomas, complex sclerosing lesions, and nipple adenomas. Mod Pathol. 16(9):893-901, 2003

PAPILLOMA, LARGE DUCT AND SMALL DUCT

Microscopic Features

(Left) Fibrovascular cores of papillomas are lined by luminal cells ⇥ and myoepithelial cells ⇥. Apocrine metaplasia ⇥ is a helpful finding as it is common in benign papillomas and would be unusual in papillary carcinomas. (Right) A well-developed myoepithelial cell layer is highlighted by nuclear positivity for p63 within the fibrovascular cores ⇥ and around the periphery ⇥. The cores in benign papillomas are typically thick ⇥ but can be very thin ⇥.

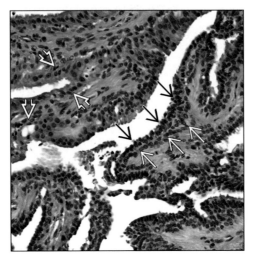 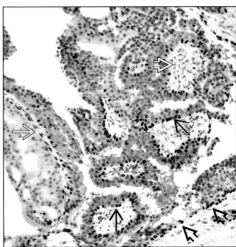

(Left) Large papillomas can show areas of florid epithelial hyperplasia that appear architecturally complex ⇥ and may be difficult to distinguish from atypia. (Right) IHC can be helpful to confirm areas of usual hyperplasia in papillomas. CK5/6 and p63 (brown in cytoplasm and nuclei) are positive in myoepithelial cells ⇥, and CK18 (red cytoplasm) is positive in luminal cells ⇥. The cells in the hyperplasia have a mixed pattern ⇥, supporting a diagnosis of florid hyperplasia.

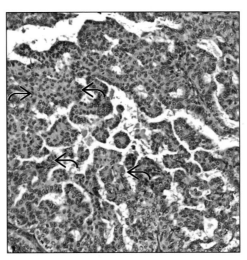 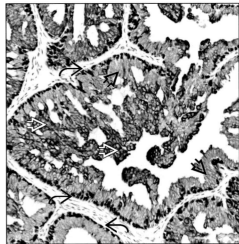

(Left) Large duct papillomas can twist on their stalk, resulting in infarction, necrosis, and bloody nipple discharge. Areas of granulation tissue and squamous metaplasia ⇥ are often present in these areas of trauma. (Right) Spindle cell carcinomas ⇥ can rarely arise from foci of squamous metaplasia in papillomas. Areas of cellular stroma should be carefully examined for nuclear atypia. IHC for basal-type keratins and p63 are helpful to identify the cells as carcinoma.

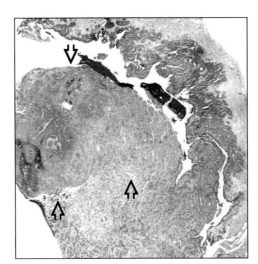 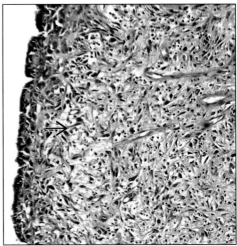

PAPILLOMA, LARGE DUCT AND SMALL DUCT

Papillomas with Atypia

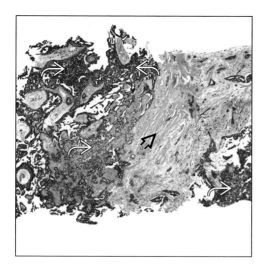
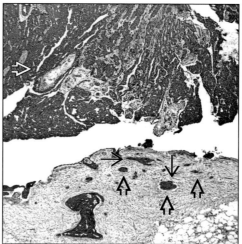

(Left) Papillomas can be difficult to evaluate on needle core biopsies as the lesions are often fragmented. This palpable lesion has papillary areas with marked epithelial proliferation ➡ and dense sclerosis ➡. (Right) This large papilloma ➡ had undergone core needle biopsy. Multiple epithelial nests are present in adjacent fibrous tissue ➡. Myoepithelial cells are identified by positivity for p63 ➡, demonstrating that this is epithelial displacement.

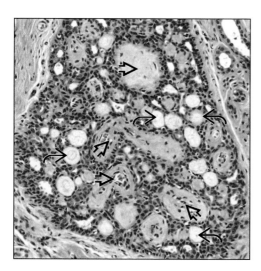
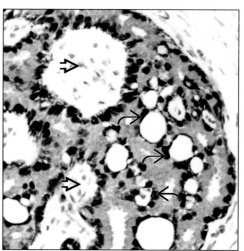

(Left) Collagenous spherulosis can involve papillomas, giving rise to a fenestrated architectural appearance ➡ that mimics DCIS. Identification of basement membrane material may be helpful ➡. (Right) IHC for myoepithelial cells is helpful to identify collagenous spherulosis. IHC for CK5/6 and p63 highlights myoepithelial cells around fibrovascular cores ➡ and the pseudoluminal spaces ➡, supporting the diagnosis of collagenous spherulosis involving an intraductal papilloma.

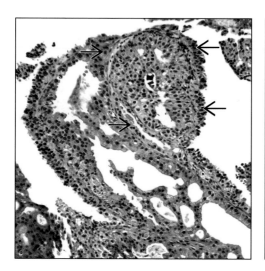
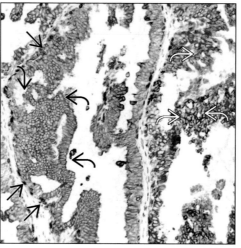

(Left) Papillomas can be focally involved by monomorphic cell proliferations ➡ that would be classified as ADH or DCIS if present in breast tissue outside of a papilloma. (Right) The combination of CK18 (red) and p63 and CK5/6 (brown) is helpful diagnostically. Myoepithelial cells are readily apparent ➡ due to nuclear positivity for p63. Areas of florid hyperplasia ➡ are CK5/6 positive. A cribriform proliferation that is only positive for CK18 ➡ is consistent with ADH.

PAPILLOMA, LARGE DUCT AND SMALL DUCT

Papillomas with Atypia

(Left) Some papillomas have a globally atypical appearance. This papilloma is monomorphic throughout with very thin fibrovascular cores. Hyalinized cores and apocrine metaplasia are not present. *(Right)* The cells of this atypical papilloma have nuclear atypia, and mitotic figures are present ⏩. The fibrovascular cores are very thin ➡. Globoid cells ➔ have more abundant pale cytoplasm and can mimic myoepithelial cells. These cells are often positive for GCDFP-15.

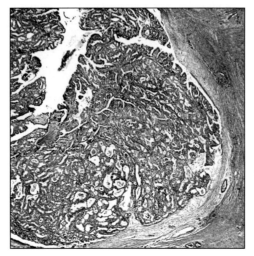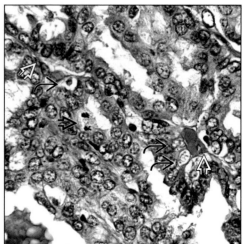

(Left) This atypical papilloma has a very well-developed myoepithelial cell layer throughout, as shown by this IHC study for smooth muscle actin. Therefore, despite the monomorphic appearance, it would not be classified as a papillary carcinoma but rather as a papilloma with atypia. *(Right)* Benign papillomas can be involved by ADH and DCIS. This papilloma has thick fibrovascular cores ⏩ and focal apocrine metaplasia ➔. In other areas, the papilloma is involved by DCIS ⏩.

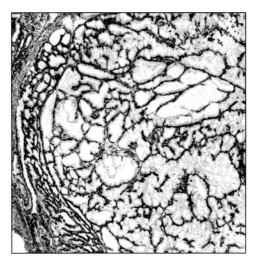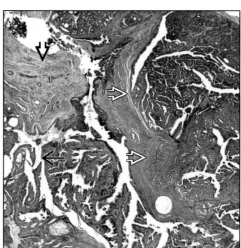

(Left) This sclerosing papilloma is involved by extensive epithelial hyperplasia that has a somewhat monomorphic appearance. An IHC study for high molecular weight keratin showed patchy positivity. This finding supports classification as hyperplasia rather than as carcinoma. *(Right)* A p63 study in this sclerosing papilloma showed normal myoepithelial cells in the central portion ⏩. However, at the periphery, the myoepithelial cells were scant or in abnormal locations ➔.

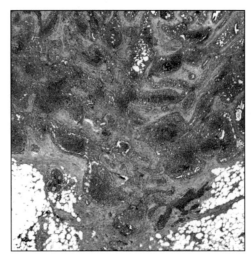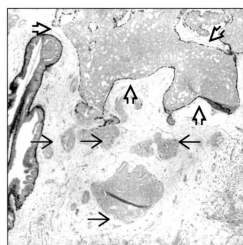

PAPILLOMA, LARGE DUCT AND SMALL DUCT

Differential Diagnosis

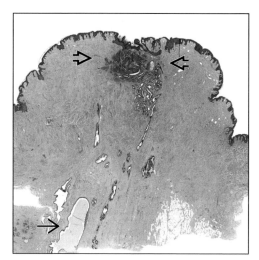
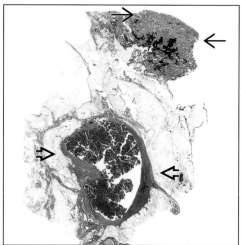

(Left) Nipple adenomas ⇗ arise in the large ducts directly below the nipple skin and usually have a complex multinodular architecture. Large duct papillomas are typically found in the deeper lactiferous sinuses and involve a single duct ➡. (Right) Like large duct papillomas, encapsulated papillary carcinomas involve a single ductal space ⇗ and may be associated with nipple discharge. However, they are generally located deeper in the breast relative to the skin surface ➡.

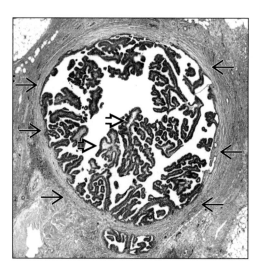
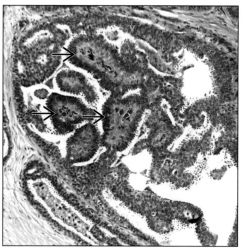

(Left) Papillary DCIS can involve large duct spaces. Myoepithelial cells are absent from the thin delicate fibrovascular cores ⇗ but are present around the periphery of the duct spaces ➡. (Right) DCIS often has a mixed pattern of papillary and micropapillary areas. The fibrovascular cores may have many myoepithelial cells ➡, possibly due to involvement of a preexisting benign papilloma. The pattern is often complex and may be difficult to classify.

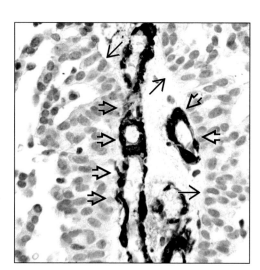
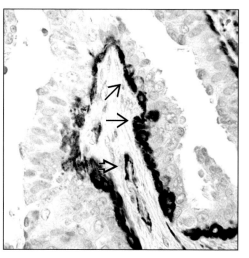

(Left) Papillary carcinomas lack myoepithelial cells as shown by IHC for smooth muscle actin ➡. However, blood vessels are also positive for muscle markers and may be apposed to the basal aspect of the tumor cells ⇗ in the thin fibrovascular cores. IHC for p63 is often easier to evaluate. (Right) IHC for muscle markers will demonstrate a myoepithelial cell layer lying above the basement membrane in benign papillomas ➡. Blood vessels are also positive for these makers ⇗.

SUB ARBOLAIR DUCTS **NIPPLE ADENOMA**

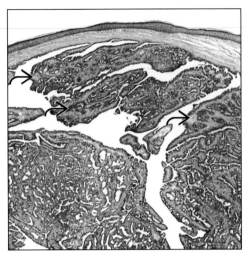

Nipple adenomas are benign epithelial proliferations arising from subareolar ducts. There are several histologic patterns. This lesion is an example of the papillomatosis pattern ➔.

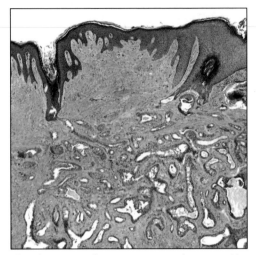

The sclerosing papillomatosis pattern is characterized by a prominent dense stromal component. Patients present with a palpable mass without changes in the overlying skin.

TERMINOLOGY

Abbreviations
- Nipple adenoma (NA)

Synonyms
- Florid papillomatosis
- Erosive adenomatosis
- Superficial papillary adenomatosis
- Subareolar duct papillomatosis
- Nipple duct adenoma

Definitions
- Benign lesion characterized by florid epithelial hyperplasia, arising from lactiferous ducts of nipple

CLINICAL ISSUES

Epidemiology
- Incidence
  - ~ 1-2% of breasts
- Age
  - Wide age range at presentation
  - Most often seen in 4th or 5th decade
- Gender
  - Occurs in males and females

Presentation
- Bloody nipple discharge
  - Unilateral and spontaneous
- Skin changes
  - Crusting, nodularity, tenderness, swelling, erosion, and erythema
  - Can mimic Paget disease
- Ill-defined palpable subcutaneous or protruding mass
  - Usually < 1 cm

Treatment
- Surgical approaches

- Local excision is necessary for diagnosis and treatment

Prognosis
- Benign lesion but can recur locally if not completely excised
- Association with carcinoma can occur but is rare

IMAGE FINDINGS

General Features
- Mammographic and ultrasound features may suggest carcinoma

MACROSCOPIC FEATURES

General Features
- Firm mass under nipple epidermis with irregular borders
  - Macroscopic features similar to invasive carcinoma
- Overlying epidermis may be scaly, eroded, or ulcerated

MICROSCOPIC PATHOLOGY

Histologic Features
- NA occurs just below skin of nipple and has multinodular pattern
  - Continuity with overlying squamous epithelium of skin may be seen
- Histologic changes are quite diverse; grouped into 4 major categories by Rosen
  - **Sclerosing papillomatosis pattern**
    - Papillary growth within ducts
    - Prominent stromal proliferation: Typically collagenous bands, myxoid change, or elastosis
    - Overlying skin is intact but thickened
    - Squamous cysts are often present in duct orifices

NIPPLE ADENOMA

Key Facts

Terminology
- Benign proliferative lesion arising in major ducts of nipple

Clinical Issues
- Patients present with nipple discharge (bloody or clear) &/or ill-defined indurated mass
- Skin changes (crusting, erosion) can mimic Paget disease of nipple
- Local excision is necessary for diagnosis and treatment
- Occasional recurrences have been described after incomplete excision
- Rare patients present with carcinomas involving NA

Microscopic Pathology
- Diverse array of possible histologic patterns
  - Sclerosing papillomatosis pattern
  - Papillomatosis pattern
  - Adenosis pattern
  - Mixed patterns
- Some features can be difficult to distinguish from malignancy
  - Florid hyperplasia
  - Focal necrosis
  - Sclerosing adenosis resembling invasive carcinoma
  - Skin erosion

Top Differential Diagnoses
- Invasive ductal carcinoma
- Papillary carcinoma
- DCIS involving large ducts

    - Focal central necrosis can be present in areas of florid hyperplasia
    - Usually presents as mass with serous discharge
  - **Papillomatosis pattern**
    - Papillary growth within large ducts
    - Less prominent stromal proliferation
    - Epidermis replaced by glandular epithelium; creates clinical appearance of erythematous granular surface
    - Focal necrosis can be present
    - Usually presents with skin erosion and bloody discharge in an indurated area of nipple; may be mistaken for Paget disease clinically
  - **Adenosis pattern**
    - Proliferation of small glands similar to sclerosing adenosis
    - Entrapped ducts can have pseudoinfiltrative pattern; may closely mimic invasive carcinoma
    - Myoepithelial hyperplasia is present; IHC can be helpful to demonstrate presence in difficult cases
    - Necrosis is uncommon
    - Usually presents with bloody or serous discharge
  - **Mixed pattern**
    - Any combination of these patterns can be seen
- Florid epithelial hyperplasia is common
  - Nuclei lack significant pleomorphism
  - High molecular weight keratins show patchy pattern of positivity
- Toker cell hyperplasia may be present in overlying epithelium
  - In superficial biopsy, presence of Toker cells in association with clinically evident skin changes can be mistaken for Paget disease
- Invasive carcinoma and DCIS are rarely present within NA
  - Paget disease in overlying epidermis supports diagnosis of DCIS
  - IHC for myoepithelial markers is useful to confirm diagnosis of invasive carcinoma
  - In absence of these findings, diagnosis of malignancy should only be made when clearly present

DIFFERENTIAL DIAGNOSIS

Invasive Ductal Carcinoma
- Invasive carcinomas are rarely present at the periphery of a nipple adenoma
- In difficult cases, IHC can be used to confirm absence of a myoepithelial cell layer

Papillary Carcinoma
- Typically deeper in breast and less likely to be just below epidermis
- Cells are monomorphic in appearance
- IHC can confirm absence of myoepithelial cells

DCIS Involving Large Ducts
- DCIS present below nipple typically involves a single duct
  - Multinodular pattern as seen in NA would be unusual
- Generally high grade and positive for HER2
  - Paget disease of nipple skin may be present
- IHC for high molecular weight keratin may be helpful

SELECTED REFERENCES

1. Da Costa D et al: Common and unusual diseases of the nipple-areolar complex. Radiographics. 27 Suppl 1:S65-77, 2007
2. Jones MW et al: Coexistence of nipple duct adenoma and breast carcinoma: a clinicopathologic study of five cases and review of the literature. Mod Pathol. 8(6):633-6, 1995
3. Myers JL et al: Florid papillomatosis of the nipple: immunohistochemical and flow cytometric analysis of two cases. Mod Pathol. 3(3):288-93, 1990
4. Rosen PP et al: Florid papillomatosis of the nipple. A study of 51 patients, including nine with mammary carcinoma. Am J Surg Pathol. 10(2):87-101, 1986

Histologic Patterns

(Left) The sclerosing papillomatosis pattern is associated with formation of a firm palpable mass due to the presence of dense stroma ➡. This may cause irritation leading to hyperkeratosis ➡ and the white scaly appearance of the overlying skin. The findings can be mistaken for Paget disease. Superficial squamous cysts are often present ➡. *(Right)* The squamous cysts at the orifices of the ducts can be quite prominent. These cysts are filled with keratin.

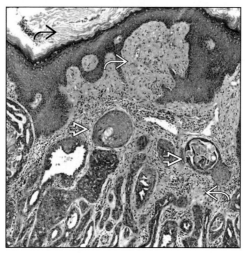
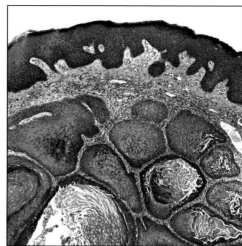

(Left) Foci of necrosis ➡ can be present in the center of hyperplastic nests of cells in NA. This finding should not be interpreted as evidence of malignancy. This is the only benign lesion of the breast frequently associated with necrosis. *(Right)* The squamous cells of the epidermis ➡ and in the squamous cysts ➡ are positive for p63. Deeper in the NA, the myoepithelial cells ➡ are also p63 positive. IHC can be helpful to exclude invasive carcinoma in difficult cases.

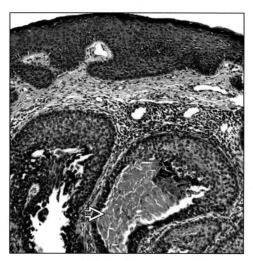
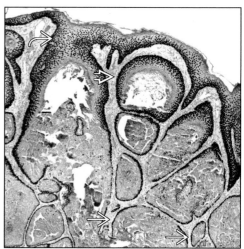

(Left) The adenosis pattern of NA consists of numerous glands ➡ in a back-to-back arrangement. The stromal component is not prominent. Most patients have a palpable nodule, and some have bloody or serous nipple discharge. Changes in the overlying epidermis are uncommon ➡. *(Right)* The presence of myoepithelial cells surrounding the tubules is demonstrated by the positivity for calponin ➡. Myoepithelial cells can be quite prominent in some NAs.

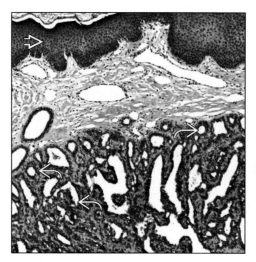
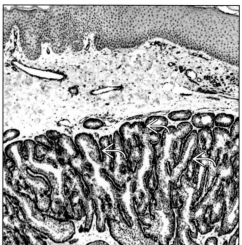

NIPPLE ADENOMA

Histologic Patterns

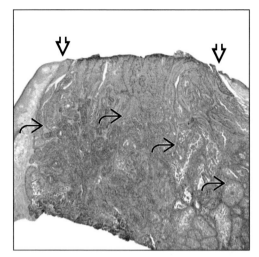

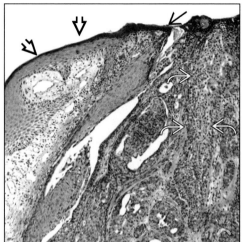

(Left) In the papillomatosis pattern ⇒, the glandular cells can extend to and replace the overlying squamous epithelium ⊋. Clinically, the patient presents with nipple erosion and erythema, often accompanied by bloody nipple discharge. The findings closely mimic those of carcinoma. *(Right)* The papillary and solid areas of proliferating epithelial cells in the ducts ⇒ have replaced the normal squamous epithelium ⊋ of the nipple, producing an area of surface erosion ⇒.

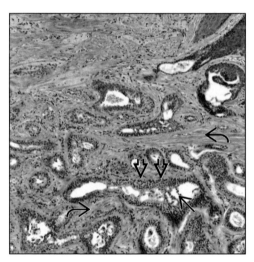

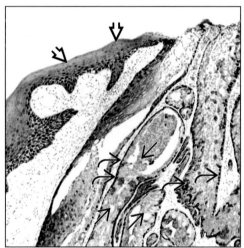

(Left) An adenosis pattern within sclerotic stroma ⇒ with minimal epithelial hyperplasia ⇒ can closely mimic an invasive carcinoma. However, myoepithelial cells are readily identified ⊋ surrounding ductal epithelium. *(Right)* IHC highlights CK5/6 (brown) in the cytoplasm of squamous ⊋ and myoepithelial cells ⇗ and luminal cytokeratins (CK8/18, red) in the luminal cells ⊋ in this NA. IHC can be very helpful to exclude malignancy.

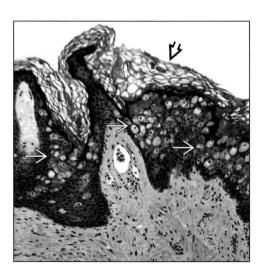

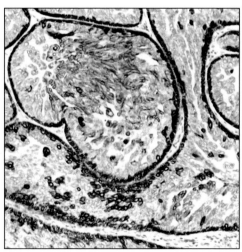

(Left) Toker cell hyperplasia ⇒ and hyperkeratosis ⊋ may be present in the skin overlying NA. In a superficial biopsy, these findings may closely resemble Paget disease; however, the Toker cells typically show minimal nuclear pleomorphism and are negative for HER2. *(Right)* Areas with epithelial proliferation show an admixture of luminal (red) and basal cells (brown) consistent with florid epithelial hyperplasia in NA. IHC studies can be helpful to exclude a diagnosis of DCIS.

MICROGLANDULAR ADENOSIS

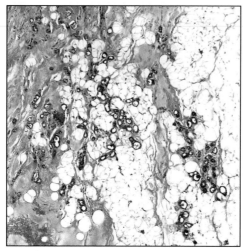

Microglandular adenosis consists of small round tubules infiltrating through fibrous tissue and adipose tissue and around normal ducts and lobules without an associated stromal response.

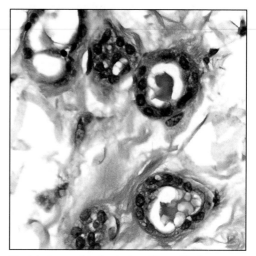

The tubules consist of a single cell layer. The lumens are typically filled with eosinophilic secretory material.

TERMINOLOGY

Abbreviations
- Microglandular adenosis (MGA)

Definitions
- Proliferation of small round tubules with a single cell layer distributed in an infiltrative pattern

ETIOLOGY/PATHOGENESIS

Pathogenesis
- Currently classified as benign lesion
  - Only benign epithelial lesion that lacks myoepithelial cells
- Associated with invasive carcinoma in about 25% of cases (at presentation or after recurrence) and is molecularly related to carcinoma
  - MGA in its classic appearance has never been reported to metastasize

CLINICAL ISSUES

Presentation
- Most commonly presents as palpable mass
- Less commonly, MGA forms mammographic density or is incidental finding
- Women over wide age range, from 20s to 80s, are affected (mean: Mid 50s)

Treatment
- Complete excision with negative margins due to risk of local recurrence

Prognosis
- Carcinomas capable of metastasis may arise in association with MGA at presentation or after local recurrence

MACROSCOPIC FEATURES

General Features
- Not associated with marked desmoplastic response; lesions may be ill-defined mass or not be apparent

MICROSCOPIC PATHOLOGY

Histologic Features
- Consists of haphazard arrangement of small round tubules in and around normal ducts and lobules
  - Little or no stromal reaction
- Tubules are round and consist of single cell layer
  - Tubules contain characteristic eosinophilic (PAS- and mucicarmine-positive) secretory material

Cytologic Features
- Cells are cuboidal and have clear &/or foamy cytoplasm
  - Apocrine snouts are not present
- Nuclei are round with small nucleoli and minimal pleomorphism

ANCILLARY TESTS

Immunohistochemistry
- Immunoperoxidase studies for myoepithelial markers confirm absence of myoepithelial cells
- MGA is negative for estrogen receptor, progesterone receptor, HER2, and epithelial membrane antigen
  - Should be considered if lesion thought to be well-differentiated carcinoma is negative for hormone receptors
- Shows strong cytoplasmic positivity for S100 and is reported to be cathepsin-D positive
- Tubules are surrounded by basement material as demonstrated by collagen IV and laminin

MICROGLANDULAR ADENOSIS

Key Facts

Terminology
- Proliferation of small round tubules with a single cell layer (i.e., without both luminal and myoepithelial cells) in an infiltrative pattern

Etiology/Pathogenesis
- Associated with invasive carcinoma in about 25% of cases (at presentation or after recurrence)
  - MGA is molecularly related to invasive carcinoma
- MGA in its classic appearance has never been reported to metastasize

Clinical Issues
- Treatment: Complete excision with negative margins due to risk of local recurrence

Microscopic Pathology
- Negative for estrogen and progesterone receptors

- MGA should be considered if a lesion thought to be a well-differentiated carcinoma is estrogen receptor negative
- Shows strong cytoplasmic positivity for S100 and is reported to be cathepsin D positive
- Tubules are surrounded by basement material as demonstrated by collagen IV and laminin

Top Differential Diagnoses
- Invasive tubular carcinoma
- Sclerosing adenosis
- MGA with atypia or carcinoma arising in MGA
  - These carcinomas share features with MGA and may be of unusual types (basaloid or metaplastic)

Differential Diagnosis of Breast Lesions Consisting of Small Tubules

Features	Microglandular Adenosis	Invasive Tubular Carcinoma	Sclerosing Adenosis
Distribution of tubules	Haphazard in normal stroma	Radiating with irregular margins	Lobulocentric, swirling, but some glands may "wander"
Shape of tubules	Round	Pointed	Compressed, slit-like
Apical snouts	Absent	Often present	May be present
Luminal contents	Dense, eosinophilic	Calcifications or pink secretory material may be present	Calcifications may be present
Stromal reaction	Absent or minimal	Desmoplastic	Sclerosing
Myoepithelial cell layer	Absent	Absent	Present, prominent
Hormone receptors	Absent	Present	Present
S100	Strongly positive	Usually negative or weak	Usually negative or weak

DIFFERENTIAL DIAGNOSIS

Invasive Tubular Carcinoma
- Tubules are angulated and cells often have apocrine snouts
- Ductal carcinoma in situ, lobular carcinoma in situ, atypical ductal hyperplasia, and atypical lobular hyperplasia are frequently present in adjacent tissue

Sclerosing Adenosis
- Tubules are most commonly arranged in lobulocentric pattern with swirling back-to-back glands
  - In some cases, glands can appear to "wander" around adjacent uninvolved lobules and ducts
- Tubules are compressed and often slit-like in center portion; at periphery, they may be more open

MGA with Atypia or Carcinoma Arising in MGA
- Features not characteristic of MGA include
  - Architectural complexity: Cribriform nests, solid nests, single cells
  - Nuclear atypia: Pleomorphism, large nucleoli, frequent &/or atypical mitoses
  - Increased numbers of cells instead of single cell layer

- Carcinomas arising in association with MGA usually have features in common with MGA
  - Carcinomas are negative for estrogen receptors, progesterone receptors, and HER2, and positive for S100
  - Unusual subtypes with basaloid, metaplastic, or biphasic features have been reported, including squamous cell carcinoma, carcinomas with matrix production, and adenoid cystic carcinomas

SELECTED REFERENCES

1. Geyer FC et al: Microglandular adenosis or microglandular adenoma? A molecular genetic analysis of a case associated with atypia and invasive carcinoma. Histopathology. 55(6):732-43, 2009
2. Shin SJ et al: Molecular evidence for progression of microglandular adenosis (MGA) to invasive carcinoma. Am J Surg Pathol. 33(4):496-504, 2009
3. Khalifeh IM et al: Clinical, histopathologic, and immunohistochemical features of microglandular adenosis and transition into in situ and invasive carcinoma. Am J Surg Pathol. 32(4):544-52, 2008
4. Salarieh A et al: Breast carcinoma arising in microglandular adenosis: a review of the literature. Arch Pathol Lab Med. 131(9):1397-9, 2007

MICROGLANDULAR ADENOSIS

Microscopic Features

(Left) A normal lobule consists of luminal cells with cytoplasmic positivity for cytokeratin (red) and myoepithelial cells with nuclear positivity for p63 (brown) ➡. MGA consists of cytokeratin-positive cells (red) without a separate myoepithelial cell layer ⇨. (Right) The tubules of MGA show strong cytoplasmic immunoreactivity for S100.

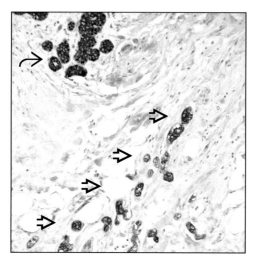
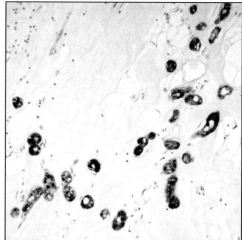

(Left) MGA is negative for estrogen receptor ⇨, progesterone receptor, and HER2. A normal duct shows nuclear positivity for estrogen receptor in the luminal cells ➡. (Right) The tubules of MGA are surrounded by basement membrane material as demonstrated by collagen IV (in this photograph) or laminin immunohistochemical studies.

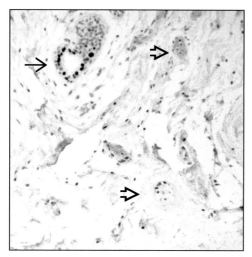
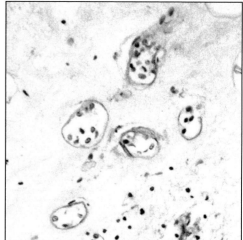

(Left) This case of MGA has atypical features. Although most of the tubules are round, some show more complex architecture. The nuclei show moderate pleomorphism, and a mitotic figure is present ⇨. (Right) This cell nest in a case of MGA with atypia has an increased number of cells (instead of the typical single layer) and shows marked nuclear atypia.

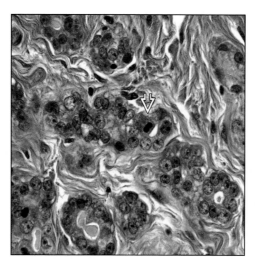
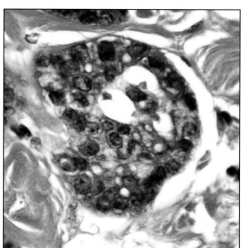

4

MICROGLANDULAR ADENOSIS

Differential Diagnosis

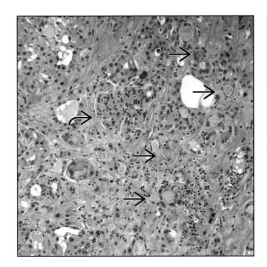
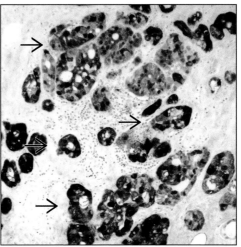

(Left) This invasive carcinoma arose in an area of MGA and infiltrates around a normal lobule ➡. Some of the carcinoma consists of tubules with eosinophilic secretions ➡. In other areas, there are solid nests of cells or single cells. (Right) Carcinomas arising in the context of MGA usually have the same immunohistochemical profile. In this case, the carcinoma shows strong cytoplasmic S100 positivity ➡ and was negative for ER, PR, and HER2.

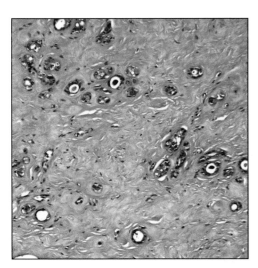
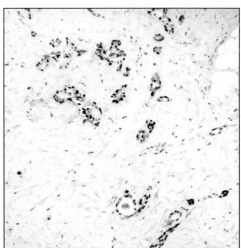

(Left) In most cases of sclerosing adenosis, there is a solid back-to-back arrangement of glands in a swirling pattern that is easily distinguished from MGA. However, in other cases such as the one shown here, the glands are scattered in the stroma ("wandering" adenosis). (Right) An immunohistochemical study for p63 clearly shows the presence of myoepithelial cells associated with the small tubules, supporting a diagnosis of sclerosing adenosis and excluding the possibility of MGA.

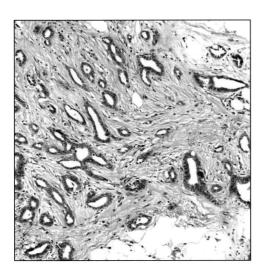
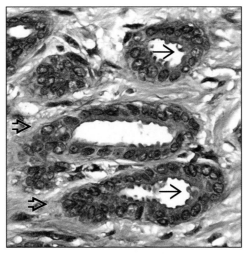

(Left) Like MGA, tubular carcinomas lack myoepithelial cells. Tubular carcinomas can be distinguished from MGA by the presence of irregular, generally empty glands in a reactive cellular desmoplastic stroma. (Right) In tubular carcinomas, the tubules are usually angulated ➡ with compressed lumens, and apocrine snouts ➡ are frequently found. Tubular carcinomas are essentially always positive for ER and PR whereas MGA is negative for these markers.

ATYPICAL DUCTAL HYPERPLASIA = (≈ DCIS)

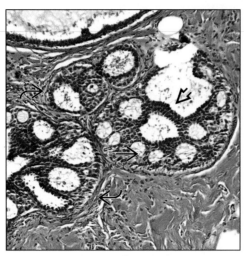

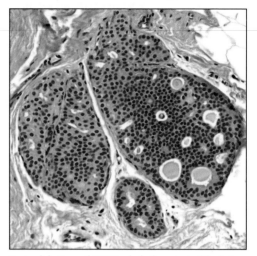

ADH has some, but not all, of the features of DCIS. Although some of the bridges appear rigid ➤, others have a streaming pattern ➡. A 2nd cell population also appears to be present ➱.

Some definitions of ADH include the extent of the lesion. The proliferation may need to involve at least 2 spaces, such as in this case, or be > 2 mm to be sufficient for low-grade DCIS.

TERMINOLOGY

Abbreviations
- Atypical ductal hyperplasia (ADH)

Synonyms
- Ductal intraepithelial neoplasia (DIN) type 1b or 1c, depending on system used

Definitions
- Clonal intraductal proliferation with architectural and cytologic features approaching those seen in low-grade ductal carcinoma in situ (LGDCIS)

ETIOLOGY/PATHOGENESIS

Molecular Pathology
- DNA studies show genetic similarity between ADH and LGDCIS
  - Shared alterations include chromosomal gain of 1q and loss of 16q
    - Also seen in low-grade invasive ductal carcinoma (LGIDC)
- Gene expression profiling data also show similarities shared by low-grade lesions
  - ADH, LGDCIS, and LGIDC have similar gene expression patterns
  - Differences are in quantitative levels of expression
  - No significant qualitative differences in expression patterns
  - Low-grade carcinomas express a unique set of genes rarely seen in high-grade carcinomas
- ADH likely represents an early stage in a low-grade breast neoplasia pathway
- However, majority of ADH does not progress to carcinoma
  - Factors responsible for progression from ADH to DCIS and IDC are poorly understood

CLINICAL ISSUES

Epidemiology
- Incidence
  - Present in 15-20% of breast biopsies performed to evaluate mammographic microcalcifications
- Age
  - Peak: Women in mid 40s

Presentation
- Most commonly detected as clustered calcifications on screening mammography

Treatment
- Risk reduction
  - Interventions to decrease risk of subsequent breast cancer must address both breasts
  - Surgical approach would require bilateral mastectomies
  - Chemoprevention with tamoxifen reduces risk of ER-positive cancers
  - Majority of women opt for careful surveillance

Prognosis
- ADH is a marker of increased risk for developing invasive carcinoma and a nonobligate precursor of carcinoma
  - Associated with a 4-5x increased relative risk or a 13-17% lifetime risk of invasive carcinoma
    - Cancer risk approximately equal in both breasts
    - Some (but not all) studies show increased risk for women with positive family history

Core Needle Biopsy
- ADH on core needle biopsy is an indication for excision
  - DCIS is found in adjacent tissue in ~ 15-20% of cases
    - Likelihood of DCIS is less for larger bore core needle biopsies
  - Invasive carcinoma is present in < 5%

4

ATYPICAL DUCTAL HYPERPLASIA

Key Facts

Terminology
- Atypical ductal hyperplasia (ADH) is an intraductal proliferation with some, but not all, features of low-grade DCIS

Etiology/Pathogenesis
- Molecular studies support that ADH and low-grade DCIS are genetically related
- ADH likely represents an early stage in a low-grade breast neoplasia pathway

Clinical Issues
- ADH is considered a marker of increased risk of carcinoma and a nonobligate precursor of carcinoma
  - Increased relative risk is 4-5x or an actual lifetime risk of 13-17%
  - Both breasts are at increased risk

- ADH on core needle biopsy should be excised due to risk of adjacent DCIS

Image Findings
- ADH is most often detected associated with calcifications on mammographic screening

Microscopic Pathology
- Diagnosis includes both qualitative and quantitative criteria
- Differential diagnosis for ADH should include low-grade DCIS
- Borderline lesions may be described as "ADH bordering on DCIS"

Top Differential Diagnoses
- Usual ductal hyperplasia
- Low-grade ductal carcinoma in situ

- Extent or type of ADH on core does not predict with certainty which patients will or will not have DCIS on excision
- Factors associated with increased likelihood of malignant diagnosis on surgical excision
  - Marked nuclear atypia
  - Multiple foci of ADH
  - Micropapillary architecture

IMAGE FINDINGS

Mammographic Findings
- Amorphous calcifications most common finding
  - Clustered distribution
  - Other calcification morphologies (punctate, pleomorphic, fine linear) favor DCIS
- ADH may be an incidental microscopic finding associated with other benign lesions
  - Papilloma, fibroadenoma, apocrine cysts, radial sclerosing lesion, gynecomastia

MACROSCOPIC FEATURES

Gross Findings
- ADH does not form grossly apparent lesions

MICROSCOPIC PATHOLOGY

Histologic Features
- ADH is a proliferation of luminal-type cells
  - May involve terminal ductal lobular units or interlobular ducts
  - Diagnosis is based on both qualitative and quantitative assessment
  - Main differential diagnosis is between ADH and LGDCIS
    - LGDCIS requires cytologic, architectural, and size criteria to be met
    - ADH demonstrates some but not all features of LGDCIS

- **Qualitative assessment in diagnosis of ADH**
  - Architectural features
    - Most common are cribriform spaces or arched bridges; spaces often not as uniform as those seen in DCIS
    - Bridges across cribriform spaces may be thin and show streaming of cells
    - Micropapillae may be present, but generally not extensive
    - Often associated with columnar cell change
    - Focal necrosis is rarely present
  - Cytologic features
    - Cells are all luminal in type; lack expression of high molecular weight keratin 5/6
    - Cells appear to stand apart from one another with well-defined borders
    - Usually partially uniform in appearance
    - Cell populations of different morphologies may be present (cuboidal, spindle, columnar)
    - Involved spaces usually contain more than 1 cell population; monomorphic-appearing cells may merge with areas of usual type hyperplasia
    - High-grade nuclei should not be seen in ADH
- **Quantitative assessment in diagnosis of ADH**
  - Size &/or extent of involvement is used by some authorities to distinguish ADH from LGDCIS when qualitative criteria for DCIS are met
  - Different definitions required for diagnosis of DCIS have been proposed
    - At least 2 duct spaces must be involved
    - Lesion must be > 0.2 cm in size
  - Size is not a universally accepted criterion for diagnosis of ADH
    - No minimum size requirement for high-grade DCIS
  - In general, it is better to classify borderline lesions as "ADH bordering on DCIS"
    - If close to a margin, reexcision may be helpful to exclude an adjacent area of DCIS
- **Calcifications**
  - ADH is often associated with a secretory phenotype

ATYPICAL DUCTAL HYPERPLASIA

- Secretory material with membrane fragments provide a regular repeating structure for crystallization of calcifications
- Calcifications are calcium phosphate in type
- Calcium oxalate has not been described but may be present in adjacent cysts
- ○ ADH may also be associated with columnar cell change with apocrine snouts and secretions
  - Calcifications may be found in adjacent dilated lobules/cysts
- ○ Less commonly, ADH is associated with mucin production with calcifications
  - If mucinous cysts rupture, it may be difficult to distinguish the findings from invasive mucinous carcinoma
- ○ In very rare cases, focal necrosis can be seen
  - Generally too limited in extent to form mammographic calcifications
- **Distribution of ADH**
  - ○ Typically present as a single focus or involves a small area
  - ○ If multiple foci are present, foci typically differ in appearance; suggests presence of multiple different clones
  - ○ If ADH appears extensive and foci morphologically similar in appearance, diagnosis of an unusual type of DCIS should be considered
- **Examination of multiple levels**
  - ○ ADH and DCIS are often found in close proximity
  - ○ Deeper levels through paraffin blocks are often helpful to identify areas that may be diagnostic of DCIS associated with ADH
  - ○ If a specimen has not been completely sampled, additional sampling is usually warranted to seek areas of DCIS
- **ADH involving another lesion**
  - ○ ADH can be present in papillomas, fibroadenomas, sclerosing adenosis, gynecomastia, and other benign lesions
    - ADH in fibroadenoma has been termed "juvenile fibroadenoma"; however, this term has also been used for other lesions
    - ADH in papilloma has been termed "papilloma with atypia"
  - ○ Diagnosis is more complicated when underlying architecture is distorted
  - ○ Clinical significance with respect to subsequent risk of cancer is unclear
    - Areas of ADH outside lesion should be sought

ANCILLARY TESTS

Immunohistochemistry
- High molecular weight keratins 5/6
  - ○ ADH is generally negative for keratins 5/6
    - Consists of a uniform population of luminal cells expressing CK8, CK18, and CK19 only
- Estrogen receptor
  - ○ ADH typically shows uniform high levels of ER expression

DIFFERENTIAL DIAGNOSIS

Usual Ductal Hyperplasia (UDH)
- Mixed nonclonal proliferation of luminal-type cells, myoepithelial-type cells, and intermediate cells
  - ○ Cells are variable in shape (epithelioid, spindle, columnar)
  - ○ Cells vary in size
  - ○ Cells often overlap with uneven nuclear spacing
  - ○ Often show streaming or swirling pattern of growth and disorganized appearance
- Metaplastic changes in UDH can complicate interpretation
  - ○ Include apocrine metaplasia, clear cell change, and columnar cell change
  - ○ Results in cells that appear monomorphic and clonal
- Typically completely fill spaces or form irregular spaces
  - ○ Spaces are irregular in 3 dimensions (similar to spaces in a recanalized thrombus)
  - ○ Typically located peripherally
  - ○ Cells not oriented around periphery
- IHC shows mixed or "mosaic" pattern of staining with high molecular weight cytokeratin 5/6

Low-Grade Ductal Carcinoma In Situ
- Monomorphic cell population of luminal-type cells filling and distending duct spaces
  - ○ Complex architecture with micropapillary, papillary, cribriform, or solid patterns
    - Cribriform spaces are spherical in 3 dimensions
    - Uniform in size and shape and evenly distributed
    - Nuclei are oriented or polarized toward spaces
  - ○ Cells have uniform monomorphic appearance
    - Stand apart from one another
    - Cells do not overlap
    - Bridges in cribriform pattern or in arches appear rigid due to cuboidal cell shape
- Usually involves multiple duct spaces
  - ○ Rarely < 2-3 mm in size and may be very extensive

SELECTED REFERENCES

1. Wagoner MJ et al: Extent and histologic pattern of atypical ductal hyperplasia present on core needle biopsy specimens of the breast can predict ductal carcinoma in situ in subsequent excision. Am J Clin Pathol. 131(1):112-21, 2009
2. Moulis S et al: Re-evaluating early breast neoplasia. Breast Cancer Res. 10(1):302, 2008
3. Collins LC et al: Magnitude and laterality of breast cancer risk according to histologic type of atypical hyperplasia: results from the Nurses' Health Study. Cancer. 109(2):180-7, 2007
4. Ely KA et al: Core biopsy of the breast with atypical ductal hyperplasia: a probabilistic approach to reporting. Am J Surg Pathol. 25(8):1017-21, 2001
5. Page DL et al: Combined histologic and cytologic criteria for the diagnosis of mammary atypical ductal hyperplasia. Hum Pathol. 23(10):1095-7, 1992

Usual Hyperplasia, ADH, and DCIS

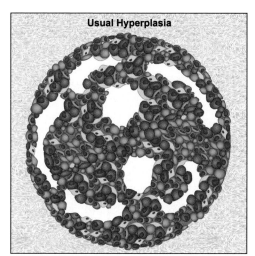

Usual Hyperplasia

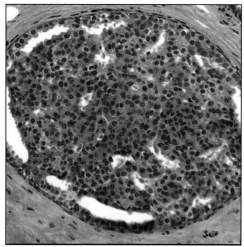

(Left) Unlike ADH and DCIS, usual hyperplasia is a polyclonal proliferation of a variety of cell types: Myoepithelial-type cells (green), luminal-type cells (red), and intermediate cell types (yellow). The cells have different shapes (epithelioid and spindled) and sizes. *(Right)* Epithelial hyperplasia is characterized by a heterogeneous cell population that often forms peripheral irregular slit-like spaces. Polarization of cells around the spaces is not typically seen.

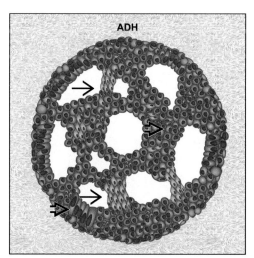

ADH

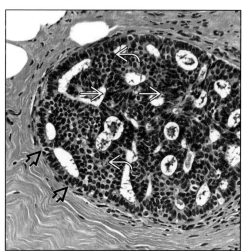

(Left) ADH is a small clonal population of luminal-type cells (purple). The cells appear more uniform in appearance than usual hyperplasia, but some variation in size and shape ⊵ and streaming of nuclei ⊟ may be present. *(Right)* ADH has some but not all the features of DCIS. Although spaces can be round, there are also slit-like peripheral spaces. Spindle cells are present in the center ➡, columnar cells at the periphery ⊵, and intermingled rounded cells ➡.

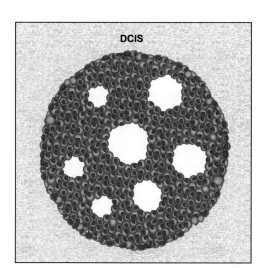

DCIS

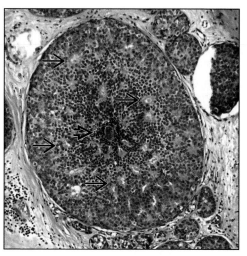

(Left) Like ADH, DCIS is a clonal population of luminal-like cells (purple). The cells are very uniform in size and shape. The spaces are very round and evenly distributed throughout the space. The cells are oriented around the spaces. *(Right)* The spaces formed by DCIS are spherical and thus usually are uniformly round in shape ➡. The cells form the spaces and are polarized around the periphery. Necrosis ⊵ is sometimes present and would be very unusual in ADH.

ATYPICAL DUCTAL HYPERPLASIA

Imaging and Immunohistochemical Features

(Left) ADH is sometimes associated with the formation of calcifications. The resulting cluster of calcifications ➡ may be detected by screening mammography. *(Right)* The calcifications ⮞ associated with ADH usually form on secretory material or mucin in the lumens formed by the ADH or by adjacent columnar cell change. Only calcium phosphate is seen in ADH, like DCIS; calcium oxalate has not been reported. The calcifications may be detected as clusters on screening mammography.

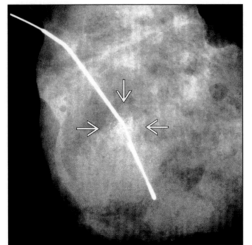
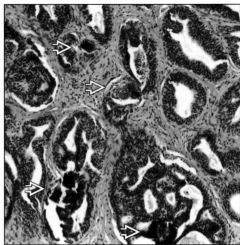

(Left) Bridges and arcades in DCIS are formed by uniform cuboidal cells resulting in a very rigid appearance ⮞. In contrast, the presence of more elongated cells in a streaming pattern ➡ is less typical of DCIS and favors classification as ADH. *(Right)* The most common architecture associated with ADH is a cribriform pattern ➡. Other patterns such as micropapillae ⮞ are also seen. Columnar cell change ➡ is often present in the same space or in adjacent spaces.

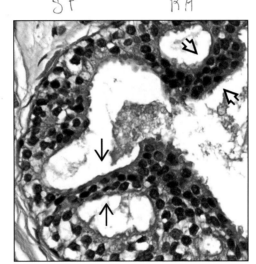
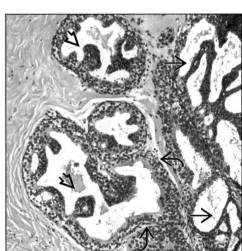

(Left) ADH is a clonal population of luminal-like cells and, therefore, is positive for luminal-type keratins ⮞ but not high molecular weight keratins. The surrounding myoepithelial cells are positive for high molecular weight keratin 5/6 ➡. *(Right)* In the normal breast, only scattered cells are ER positive, and these cells do not undergo mitosis. In contrast, ADH is diffusely ER positive ➡. There is aberrant regulation of proliferation as these cells can be mitotically active.

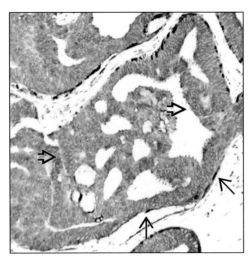
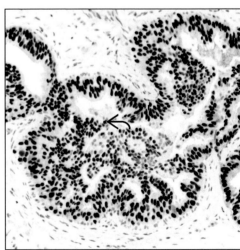

ATYPICAL DUCTAL HYPERPLASIA

Difficult Cases

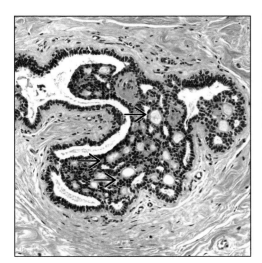

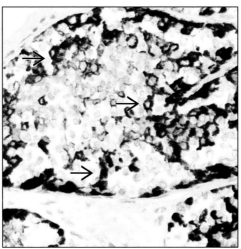

(Left) Collagenous spherulosis can mimic ADH due to the formation of cribriform spaces ➡. However, the spaces are filled with basement membrane material. IHC will demonstrate the presence of an associated myoepithelial population. (Right) Usual hyperplasia can be difficult to distinguish from ADH, particularly when there is a solid pattern. Because usual hyperplasia consists of multiple cell types, patchy positivity for high molecular weight keratins is often present ➡.

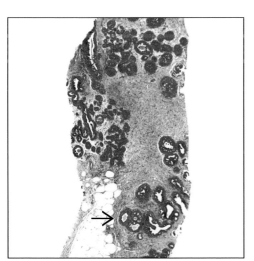

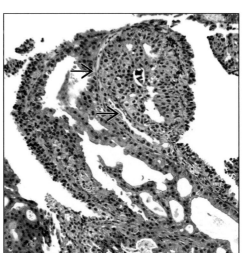

(Left) ADH ➡ is more difficult to diagnose when it involves a larger lesion such as a fibroepithelial lesion, as seen on this core needle biopsy. In this case, an excision is indicated to exclude the possibility of an adjacent area of DCIS. (Right) ADH ➡ is difficult to classify and distinguish from DCIS when found partially involving papillomas. If ADH is found only in a larger benign lesion, the significance with respect to subsequent risk of breast cancer is unclear.

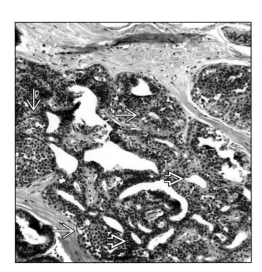

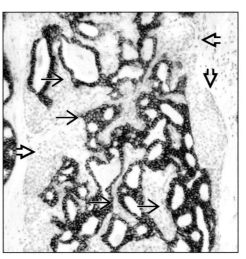

(Left) When both ADH ➡ and lobular neoplasia ➡ are present and admixed in the same location, the combination of features can closely mimic DCIS. (Right) ADH and lobular neoplasia in the same ductal space can closely resemble DCIS. An immunohistochemical study for E-cadherin reveals the 2 cell populations. The cells of ADH forming the cribriform spaces show strong membrane positivity ➡, whereas the surrounding cells of lobular neoplasia are negative ➡.

ATYPICAL LOBULAR HYPERPLASIA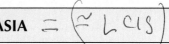

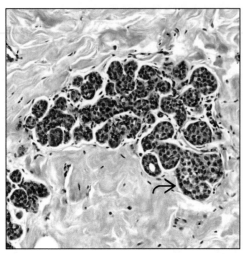

ALH is composed of a monomorphic proliferation of discohesive polygonal or cuboidal cells that are small and round. In lobules, these cells begin to fill acinar spaces, but few are widely distended ⊟.

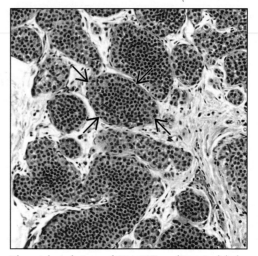

The cytologic features of ALH, LCIS, and invasive lobular carcinoma are identical. Differentiating ALH from LCIS is based on the extent of the lesion and the degree of distension ⊟ of acini.

TERMINOLOGY

Abbreviations
- Atypical lobular hyperplasia (ALH)

Synonyms
- Lobular intraepithelial neoplasia 1 (LIN1)

Definitions
- ALH is cytologically identical to lobular carcinoma in situ (LCIS) but is more limited in extent
- Term "lobular neoplasia" (LN) includes both ALH and LCIS

ETIOLOGY/PATHOGENESIS

Molecular Pathology
- The hallmark feature of ALH, LCIS, and invasive lobular carcinoma is loss of expression of the E-cadherin gene (*CDH1*)
  - E-cadherin plays a major role in intercellular adhesion and cell polarity
  - Loss of E-cadherin membrane expression can be shown by immunohistochemistry
  - Loss of expression is accompanied by E-cadherin DNA alterations in LCIS but not in ALH
    - Suggests that E-cadherin may be inactivated by means other than mutation in ALH
- ALH and LCIS share similar losses and gains of DNA
  - Loss at 16q21-q23.1 (location of E-cadherin gene)
  - Gain at 14q32.33 (site of *AKT1* gene) (involved in luminal morphogenesis)
- Genetic changes in invasive lobular carcinomas can also be found in adjacent LN
  - Evidence that LN may be a precursor lesion for invasive carcinoma
  - However, LN is a nonobligate precursor as the majority of women with ALH do not develop invasive carcinoma

CLINICAL ISSUES

Epidemiology
- Incidence
  - ALH and LCIS without invasive carcinoma are found in only 0.5–4% of breast biopsies
  - Incidental findings in biopsies performed for other indications
  - True incidence of ALH in the general population is unknown
- Age
  - ALH is more common in premenopausal women (peak incidence in mid 40s)

Site
- ALH can be multicentric and is frequently bilateral

Presentation
- Asymptomatic

Treatment
- In order to reduce risk, both breasts require treatment
  - Chemoprevention with tamoxifen reduces risk of ER-positive invasive carcinoma
  - Bilateral mastectomy reduces risk
- However, the majority of women will not develop invasive carcinoma, and most choose surveillance

Prognosis
- ALH is associated with a 4-5x increased relative risk or a 13-17% lifetime risk of developing invasive carcinoma
  - In some studies, a strong family history of breast cancer doubles risk of invasive carcinoma to 8x
  - Ductal involvement by ALH (pagetoid extension) is associated with 8x risk or a 26% lifetime risk
- LCIS has a 10x increased relative risk or a lifetime risk of ~ 30%
- Carcinomas that occur in women after a diagnosis of LN average > 10 years to diagnosis

ATYPICAL LOBULAR HYPERPLASIA

Key Facts

Terminology
- ALH is cytologically identical to LCIS but is more limited in extent
- Term "lobular neoplasia" (LN) includes both ALH and LCIS

Etiology/Pathogenesis
- The hallmark feature of ALH, LCIS, and invasive lobular carcinoma is loss of E-cadherin expression

Clinical Issues
- ALH is an incidental finding in breast biopsies performed for other indications
- ALH is considered a nonobligate cancer precursor with increased risk of developing invasive carcinoma
  ○ Relative risk is 4-5x

- Approximately 13-17% of women will develop invasive breast cancer in their lifetimes
- 60% of cancers develop in the same breast and 40% in the contralateral breast

Microscopic Pathology
- ALH is composed of a monomorphic population of polygonal or cuboidal cells that are small and round
- Cells are loosely cohesive and regularly spaced
- Overall lobular architecture is maintained
- ALH may secondarily involve other benign lesions

Top Differential Diagnoses
- Lobular carcinoma in situ
- Poor tissue preservation
- Myoepithelial cells
- Low-grade DCIS

○ Up to 1/2 of subsequent cancers show classic or variant patterns of special type histology with a good prognosis
  ▪ Likelihood of developing an invasive lobular carcinoma is 3x higher than in the general population
  ▪ However, the majority of subsequent carcinomas are not lobular in type
○ 60% of cancers that develop in women with ALH occur in the ipsilateral breast
  ▪ However, the cancers may not be at the same location in the same breast

Core Needle Biopsy
- ALH may be found as an incidental finding in a core needle biopsy
- If there is no other reason for excision, the value of excision based solely on presence of ALH is unclear
  ○ Subsequent cancers occur at other locations and in the contralateral breast
  ○ Likelihood of cancer found by excising core site is very low if there is good radiographic/pathologic correlation
  ○ Likelihood of cancer on excision is higher in the following settings
    ▪ Radiologic lesion is a mass or highly suspicious calcifications (linear &/or branching)
    ▪ Radiologic lesion may have been missed
    ▪ ALH shows atypical features, such as higher nuclear grade, or is associated with calcifications
- Consideration for additional imaging studies (such as MR) should be considered to identify the site most likely to yield invasive carcinoma prior to proceeding to surgery

IMAGE FINDINGS

Mammographic Findings
- ALH does not cause mammographically detected lesions
  ○ More commonly present in biopsies for calcifications than in biopsies for masses

○ Calcifications often present in areas adjacent to ALH

MACROSCOPIC FEATURES

General Features
- ALH and LCIS do not form gross lesions

MICROSCOPIC PATHOLOGY

Histologic Features
- ALH is composed of a monomorphic population of polygonal or cuboidal cells that are small and round
- **Architectural features**
  ○ Cells are loosely cohesive, regularly spaced, and fill and distend the acini of terminal duct lobular units (TDLUs)
    ▪ Overall lobular architecture is maintained
  ○ Cells are discohesive and cannot form cribriform spaces, micropapillae, or arcades
  ○ Calcifications are not associated with ALH
  ○ Necrosis is not associated with ALH
- **Cytologic features**
  ○ Cells are small, uniform, round, or cuboidal
  ○ Intracytoplasmic lumens (signet ring cells) may be present
  ○ Cells have low nuclear grade with inconspicuous nuclei
  ○ Mitotic figures would be highly unusual
- **Pagetoid spread**
  ○ Defined as presence of neoplastic cells between basement membrane and overlying normal epithelial cells
  ○ Can be difficult to distinguish from prominent myoepithelial cells
  ○ Can form "cloverleaf" appearance in large ducts
  ○ Increases risk of subsequent invasive carcinoma
- **ALH vs. LCIS**
  ○ Based on extent of proliferation and distention of acini in TDLUs
  ○ In ALH, neoplastic cells begin to fill acini of TDLU but with no or only mild distension of the lobule

○ In LCIS, > 50% of acini of TDLU are filled with neoplastic cells and distended
○ Distension of acini can be defined as ≥ 8 cells present across the diameter of an acinus
• **Involvement of benign lesions**
○ ALH may involve other lesions
  ▪ Sclerosing adenosis, radial sclerosing lesions, fibroadenoma, or collagenous spherulosis
  ▪ May present as a mass-forming lesion or mammographic calcifications
○ Can mimic either invasive or in situ carcinoma
  ▪ Careful attention to cytologic detail and IHC for myoepithelial cell markers and E-cadherin are helpful for correct diagnosis

ANCILLARY TESTS

Immunohistochemistry
• E-cadherin
  ○ Membrane positivity is lost in ALH
  ○ Often difficult to evaluate as, by definition, few cells are present; adjacent and intermingled luminal and myoepithelial cells can be positive
  ○ Can be evaluated best when clusters of cells are present
• Catenins
  ○ In rare cases, E-cadherin expression is present in LN but catenin expression is lost
  ○ Cells show same loss of adhesion seen when E-cadherin expression is absent
  ○ Additional studies showing abnormal loss of catenin may be helpful for classification when there is discohesive morphology but positive E-cadherin
• High molecular weight keratins
  ○ ~ 80% of LN shows weak to moderate positivity for 34βE12 cytokeratin in a cytoplasmic perinuclear pattern
    ▪ Some cases of DCIS may also be positive
  ○ Majority of LN is negative for CK5/6
    ▪ ADH and DCIS are also negative
• Estrogen and progesterone receptors
  ○ LN is positive for hormone receptors
  ○ May be useful in some cases to distinguish ALH from myoepithelial cells

DIFFERENTIAL DIAGNOSIS

Lobular Carcinoma In Situ
• ALH is distinguished from LCIS based on extent of lesion
• LCIS is diagnosed when at least 1/2 of a lobular unit is filled and distorted by neoplastic cell population
• Extent is a continuum; some cases are difficult to classify with certainty
• Some favor the term LN to include both ALH and LCIS
• However, multiple studies have shown that risk of subsequently developing breast cancer is greater for patients diagnosed with LCIS as compared to ALH

Poor Tissue Preservation
• May give the impression of a loss of cohesion of luminal cells
  ○ Discohesive cells can mimic LN
  ○ Usually involves all cells within affected area
  ○ Poor preservation may also alter expression of immunohistochemical markers
• Careful attention to quality of morphology and cytologic appearance of cells can help in making correct interpretation
• ALH should not be diagnosed if diagnostic features are not definitive

Myoepithelial Cells
• May be more prominent during menstrual cycle or if involved by metaplastic changes
  ○ Nuclei are generally smaller, rounder, and more hyperchromatic than those of ALH
  ○ Cytoplasm may be clear, whereas ALH usually has eosinophilic cytoplasm
• Appearance can mimic pagetoid spread by ALH
  ○ Cells should not be discohesive, and gaps between cells should not be seen
• IHC may be difficult to perform as there is typically a single layer of cells
  ○ Myoepithelial markers may be helpful to identify cells as myoepithelial
  ○ May be difficult to document absence of E-cadherin if only a single layer of cells is present
• ALH should not be diagnosed if diagnostic features are not definitive

Low-Grade DCIS
• Can be associated with small monomorphic cells similar to those of ALH
• Presence of secondary lumen formation or a rosette-like arrangement of cells and cellular cohesion suggests a ductal lesion rather than LN
• IHC for E-cadherin may be helpful in difficult cases
  ○ Membrane staining for E-cadherin is typically absent in LN but present in DCIS

SELECTED REFERENCES

1. O'Malley FP: Lobular neoplasia: morphology, biological potential and management in core biopsies. Mod Pathol. 23 Suppl 2:S14-25, 2010
2. Subhawong AP et al: Incidental minimal atypical lobular hyperplasia on core needle biopsy: correlation with findings on follow-up excision. Am J Surg Pathol. 34(6):822-8, 2010
3. Mastracci TL et al: Genomics and premalignant breast lesions: clues to the development and progression of lobular breast cancer. Breast Cancer Res. 9(6):215, 2007
4. McLaren BK et al: Excellent survival, cancer type, and Nottingham grade after atypical lobular hyperplasia on initial breast biopsy. Cancer. 107(6):1227-33, 2006
5. Mastracci TL et al: E-cadherin alterations in atypical lobular hyperplasia and lobular carcinoma in situ of the breast. Mod Pathol. 18(6):741-51, 2005
6. Simpson PT et al: The diagnosis and management of pre-invasive breast disease: pathology of atypical lobular hyperplasia and lobular carcinoma in situ. Breast Cancer Res. 5(5):258-62, 2003

ATYPICAL LOBULAR HYPERPLASIA

Microscopic Features and Differential Diagnosis

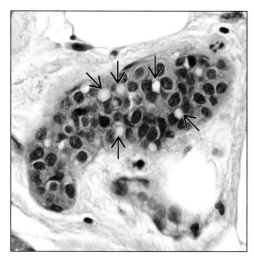

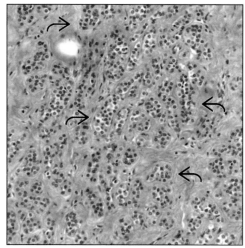

(Left) Signet ring cells may be present in ALH ⮕ just as they are in LCIS and invasive lobular carcinomas. However, signet ring cells can be seen in benign ducts and lobules, and these cells are not diagnostic of lobular neoplasia. **(Right)** ALH can involve other lesions such as epithelial hyperplasia, fibroadenomas, collagenous spherulosis, or sclerosing adenosis ⮕. The presence of a monomorphic population of cells can raise the concern for carcinoma.

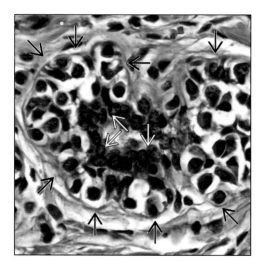

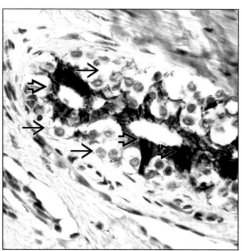

(Left) Pagetoid spread refers to the presence of lesional cells between the basement membrane ⮕ and overlying normal epithelial cells ⮕. When ALH is present as pagetoid spread, the risk for subsequent invasive carcinoma is between that of ALH and LCIS. **(Right)** Like LCIS and invasive lobular carcinoma, ALH lacks expression of the cell adhesion molecule E-cadherin ⮕. In this area of pagetoid spread, the overlying luminal cells show strong membrane immunoreactivity ⮕.

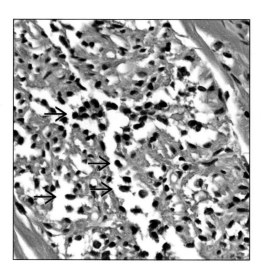

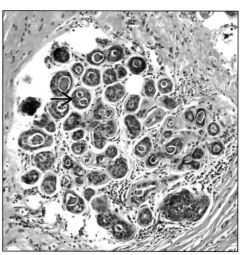

(Left) Poor fixation or crushing can cause normal epithelial cells to become rounded and dyshesive ⮕. The number of cells are generally not increased. Lobular neoplasia should not be overdiagnosed in cases with marked artifact. **(Right)** DCIS also occasionally involves lobules without causing marked distortion or unfolding of the acini. In this case, the process is distinguished from ALH by the presence of cribriform spaces ⮕, nuclear atypia, mitoses, and single cell necrosis.

Carcinomas

RISK FACTORS FOR DEVELOPING BREAST CARCINOMA

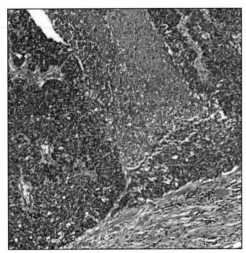

The most important risk factors for young women developing breast cancer are family history and ethnicity. The cancers are frequently poorly differentiated, highly proliferative, and ER negative.

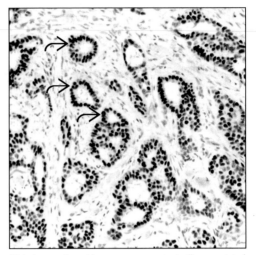

Risk factors for older women are typically associated with estrogen exposure, hormone replacement therapy, and screening. Most common are well- to moderately differentiated ER-positive ⇗ cancers.

BREAST CANCER RISK

Introduction

- Breast cancer is most common non-skin malignancy among women and is 2nd most common cause of cancer death
- All women are considered to be at risk, but level of risk varies in population
- Lifetime risk of developing invasive breast cancer ranges from 3% (for women without risk factors) to > 80% (for women with highly penetrant germline mutations)
  - ○ Average lifetime risk of developing breast cancer is 1 in 8 women (approximately 12%)
- Measuring degree of risk aids in
  - ○ Individual choices about risk reduction (e.g., chemoprevention or prophylactic surgery)
  - ○ Optimal screening strategy
  - ○ Decisions about testing for single gene mutations
  - ○ Stratification of patients for enrollment in trials
  - ○ Providing important clues into cause and biology of breast cancer
- Risk factors for developing different molecular types of breast cancer vary and are not yet well understood
- Majority of risk factors cannot be modified (e.g., age, gender, ethnicity, family history) or would be very difficult to modify (e.g., age at 1st pregnancy, age at menopause)

Breast Cancer Risk Assessment Tools

- Gail and Claus models are among most widely known examples of breast cancer risk assessment tools
  - ○ Useful to quantify magnitude of risk for individual patients
    - ▪ Not applicable for women who have been diagnosed with DCIS or LCIS
    - ▪ Different models are used for predicting risk for women with *BRCA1* or *BRCA2* mutations
    - ▪ Do not take into account increased risk due to chest wall radiation

- Gail model (http://www.cancer.gov/bcrisktool/) provides risk estimate for the next 5 years and for lifetime
  - ○ Incorporates patient age (must be 35 or older), ethnicity, age at menarche, age at 1st live birth, number of 1st-degree relatives with invasive breast cancer, number of prior breast biopsies, and diagnosis of atypical hyperplasia
  - ○ Women with risk of ≥ 1.66% in next 5 years are eligible for chemoprevention with hormonal agents
- Claus model uses information about family history
  - ○ Incorporates patient age, 1st- and 2nd-degree relatives with breast cancer, age of onset in relatives, family history of ovarian cancer
- These models perform better for predicting ER-positive cancer than ER-negative cancer

FACTORS ASSOCIATED WITH BREAST CANCER RISK

Gender

- Women are at much higher risk than men
  - ○ Only 1 of every 100 breast cancers occur in males
  - ○ Most likely due to larger pool of potential cancer precursor cells and estrogenic effects in women

Age

- Age-specific incidence rates for breast cancer increase dramatically after age 40
  - ○ Increase with age is primarily for ER-positive cancers
- Peak incidence for breast cancer among women occurs between 75-79 years
  - ○ Median age at diagnosis in USA: 61 years
- Lifetime probability of being diagnosed with breast cancer diminishes as increased age ranges are achieved
  - ○ Age 30, lifetime risk of breast cancer: 12.5%
  - ○ Age 50, lifetime risk of breast cancer: 11.1%
  - ○ Age 70, lifetime risk of breast cancer: 6.6%

RISK FACTORS FOR DEVELOPING BREAST CARCINOMA

Estrogen Exposure
- Exposure to higher levels of estrogen increases lifetime risk of developing breast cancer
- Factors that reduce risk of breast cancer
  - Late menarche, early natural menopause, or oophorectomy
  - Prolonged breastfeeding (4.3% reduction in risk for each year of breastfeeding)
  - Use of estrogen antagonists such as tamoxifen
  - Low endogenous estradiol levels
  - Obesity in premenopausal women
- Factors that increase risk of breast cancer
  - Early menarche and late menopause (early age at menarche [relative risk (RR) = 1.3], late menopause [RR =1.5])
  - Nulliparity
  - Obesity in postmenopausal women (elevated estradiol levels compared with women of normal weight)
    - Adult weight gain and abdominal fatness
    - Excess body fat may influence steroid hormone levels and inflammatory responses
  - Hormone replacement therapy (HRT)
    - After publication of the Women's Health Initiative trial in 2002, number of women using HRT decreased
    - Incidence of invasive breast carcinoma and DCIS dropped 10-15% in women over age 50 but not in younger age groups
    - Decrease occurred for ER-positive cancers
    - It is not known if HRT causes cancer, increases rate of growth of existing cancers, stimulates angiogenesis, &/or has effects on breast cancer detection
- How estrogen exposure increases breast cancer risk is unknown
  - Estrogen increases mitotic rate of breast cells
    - Increased mitogenic stimulus may increase the risk of mutation
    - Estrogen mitogenic drive may act as cancer promoter and contribute to disease progression
  - Estrogen can act as carcinogen when converted to mutagenic metabolites

Pregnancy
- Pregnancy both increases and decreases risk of breast cancer
  - Transiently increases risk of breast cancer; over many years, risk declines and eventually becomes lower than for nulliparous women (cross-over effect)
- For young women (< 20 years), protective effect predominates, and lifetime risk of ER-positive breast cancer is reduced by 1/2
  - Terminal differentiation of epithelial cells may occur, thus reducing potential pool of cancer precursors
    - Additional pregnancies further reduce risk (~ 7% per pregnancy)
  - Pregnancy permanently changes gene expression profiles of breast tissue
- For older women (> 35 years), increased risk predominates and extends for longer period of time
- Cancers diagnosed during pregnancy or in postpartum period usually present at higher stages and have poor prognosis
  - In only 1 of 3,000-10,000 pregnancies is breast cancer diagnosed during or within 1 year
- Many proposed mechanisms for the increase in risk
  - High hormonal levels could stimulate proliferation of precursor lesions, increasing risk of cancer
  - High hormonal levels may stimulate preexisting cancers to proliferate
    - However, many pregnancy-associated carcinomas are ER and PR negative
  - Stroma may become more permissive to allow lobular expansion and branching during pregnancy, which could facilitate progression from carcinoma in situ to invasive carcinoma
  - Stroma during post-pregnancy involution is similar to that of wound-healing and could promote cancer growth and metastasis

Mammographic Density
- Mammographic appearance depends on tissue composition of breast
  - Stromal tissue and glandular epithelium attenuate x-rays more than fat and increase mammographic density
- Mammographic density is strong risk factor for breast cancer
  - 4-5x greater risk in women with density in > 75% of the breast
- Density of breast tissue is influenced by age, parity, body mass index, and menopause
  - Twin studies suggest that % mammographic density, at a given age, is heritable
    - Hereditary factors may explain up to 63% of variance in breast density
  - Investigation of gene associated with breast density is an active area of research
    - Gene profile associated with density may help identify potential targets for breast cancer prevention

Family History
- 10-20% of patients with breast cancer have a 1st-degree relative with breast cancer
  - Only 1% have more than 1 affected 1st-degree relative
  - ~ 50% are thought to be due to heredity and ~ 50% due to coincidental cases in the same family
- Therefore, 5-10% of breast cancer is primarily due to inheritance of susceptibility gene(s)
  - ~ 4% of hereditary breast cancers are due to a single, highly penetrant gene
    - 2/3 are *BRCA1* or *BRCA2* germline mutations; lifetime risk is 40-80%
    - Remainder are due to *P53*, *CHEK2*, *PTEN*, and others
  - ~ 6% of hereditary breast cancers are thought to be due to combinations of genes &/or genes of lower penetrance
- Only some types of family history confer significant risk

RISK FACTORS FOR DEVELOPING BREAST CARCINOMA

- ○ 2 or more affected individuals on same side of the family with same or "related" cancers
- ○ Age of cancer diagnosis earlier than average age of onset in general population in at least 1 individual
- ○ Presence of more than 1 primary cancer in an individual (not including metastases)
- ○ History of medical conditions associated with increased risk of developing certain types of cancer
- Genetic testing is available for families with high likelihood of germline mutation
  - ○ Counseling is necessary to consider ramifications of results before requesting test
- Majority (> 85%) of women with family history will not develop breast cancer
  - ○ History of a mother developing postmenopausal breast cancer does not alter risk significantly

Radiation Exposure
- Radiation to breast during puberty increases risk of breast cancer
- Increased rates of breast cancer have been observed among female survivors of Hodgkin disease treated with mantle radiation
  - ○ Risk for breast cancer is proportional to radiation dose and age at time of treatment
  - ○ For young patients treated with > 40 Gy to chest wall, estimated cumulative breast cancer risk of 19.1% over next 30 years

Ethnicity
- Incidence and types of breast cancer vary in different ethnic groups
  - ○ White women (USA): Highest incidence of breast cancer (132 per 100,000), ~ 11% triple negative
  - ○ African-American women (USA): Lower incidence (118 per 100,000), ~ 25% triple negative, death rate 2x as high as white women
  - ○ Hispanic women (USA): Lower incidence (89 per 100,000), ~ 17% triple negative, death rate lower than for white women
  - ○ Women of Asian/Pacific Islander descent (USA): Lower incidence (89 per 100,000), ~ 11% triple negative, higher incidence of HER2-positive cancers (25-35%), lowest death rate
  - ○ Native-American women (USA): Lowest incidence (79 per 100,000), death rate lower than for white women
- Differences support major role for a genetic etiology for breast cancer
  - ○ However, incidence of breast cancer increases over several generations in groups migrating to USA, supporting an environmental role as well
- Variation in death rates is likely due to contributions from genetic susceptibility to different types of cancer and access to medical care

Pathologic Lesions
- Nashville study, the Nurse's Health Study, and the Mayo Clinic Study linked breast lesions with subsequent risk for developing invasive carcinoma
- Nonproliferative disease is not associated with increased risk of cancer

- ○ Includes mild epithelial hyperplasia, duct ectasia, and apocrine cysts
- Proliferative disease without atypia is associated with 1.5-2x increase in relative risk
  - ○ Includes moderate to florid epithelial hyperplasia, papillomas, sclerosing adenosis, radial sclerosing lesions, and fibroadenomas with complex histology
- Columnar cell change and flat epithelial atypia
  - ○ Frequently seen in association with lobular neoplasia and tubular carcinoma ("Rosen triad") or with atypical ductal hyperplasia
  - ○ Most are clonal and share same loss of 16q as atypical hyperplasia and carcinoma in situ
  - ○ Risk of subsequent invasive carcinoma is only slightly elevated
- Proliferative disease with atypia increases relative risk by 4-5x
  - ○ Atypical hyperplasia is a clonal proliferation but lacks sufficient criteria for diagnosis as carcinoma in situ
    - ■ Atypical ductal hyperplasia (ADH) and atypical lobular hyperplasia (ALH)
    - ■ ALH with pagetoid spread is associated with 8-10x increased RR
- DCIS and LCIS increase relative risk 10x
  - ○ About a 1% risk of invasive carcinoma per year
  - ○ For rare cases of non-high-grade DCIS treated with only diagnostic biopsy, subsequent invasive carcinomas most commonly occur at the same site
    - ■ Many of the cancers are diagnosed years or decades later
  - ○ No series of untreated high-grade DCIS
    - ■ Presumed that number of cases progressing to invasion would be higher
  - ○ If DCIS is treated with surgery, radiation, &/or hormonal therapy, risk of invasive carcinoma is low (< 10%)
    - ■ Subsequent invasive cancers are found at same site (1/3), at separate site in same breast (1/3), and in contralateral breast (1/3)
  - ○ Subsequent carcinomas after LCIS are more equally distributed in both breasts
    - ■ Approximately 3/5 in same breast and 2/5 in contralateral breast
    - ■ Chemoprevention reduces risk by ~ 50%

Diet and Exercise
- Lifestyle and diet have small effects on breast cancer risk
- Alcohol intake raises risk of ER-negative breast cancer at all ages
- Tobacco use is associated with small increased risk
- Exercise has been associated with small protective effect for breast cancer risk

Screening
- Does not cause breast cancer but does increase likelihood of being diagnosed with cancer
- More invasive carcinomas are detected in screened populations compared to nonscreened populations
  - ○ Estimated to be 25% of invasive cancers
  - ○ These are cancers that would not have been detected in patient's lifetime without screening

RISK FACTORS FOR DEVELOPING BREAST CARCINOMA

Pathologic Lesions and Risk of Invasive Carcinoma

Lesion	Typical Presentation	Biologic Changes	Breast at Risk	RR (% Patients)
Nonproliferative breast disease	Calcifications	Not clonal	Neither	RR 1 (3%)
Proliferative breast disease	Calcifications, lobulated mass, nipple discharge	Majority not clonal; genetic changes uncommon and not consistent	Both	RR 1.5-2 (4-6%)
Columnar cell change and flat epithelial atypia	Calcifications	Majority clonal; loss of 16q	Both	RR ~ 1.5 (4%)
Atypical lobular hyperplasia	Incidental	Loss of 16q; loss of E-cadherin	Both (3/5 ipsilateral; 2/5 contralateral)	RR 4-5 (12-15%), RR 8 (24%) with pagetoid spread
Atypical ductal hyperplasia	Calcifications	Clonal; loss of 16q	Both	RR 4-5 (12-15%)
Lobular carcinoma in situ	Incidental	Clonal; loss of 16q; loss of E-cadherin	Both (3/5 ipsilateral; 2/5 contralateral)	RR 8-10 (24-30%)
Ductal carcinoma in situ	Calcifications, mass, nipple discharge, Paget disease	Clonal; any change found in invasive carcinoma	Untreated: Ipsilateral Treated: 2/3 ipsilateral; 1/3 contralateral	Untreated, not high-grade: RR 8-10 (24-30%); untreated, high-grade: Likely higher; Treated: Lower risk (< 10%)

RR = relative risk as compared to women with no risk factors; % patients = percentage of women expected to develop breast cancer in their lifetimes.

- ○ Primarily well-differentiated ER-positive cancers
- MR detects additional foci of carcinoma in 10-30% of patients
  - ○ Significance of these very small cancers is debated
- Not currently possible to distinguish clinically important cancers from those that would not cause harm

CLINICAL IMPLICATIONS

Strategies for Breast Cancer Risk Reduction
- Numerous interventions have been used to modify breast cancer risk &/or improve detection in high-risk populations
  - ○ Risk is assessed using assessment tools and, when applicable, genetic testing
  - ○ Management of risk reduction is based on assessment of individual's risk compared with general population
  - ○ Risk reduction strategies may include lifestyle changes, screening, chemoprevention, and prophylactic surgery

Screening
- Mammographic screening reduces deaths from breast cancer in women 40-70 years old
- Women at very high risk of breast cancer (typically with *BRCA1* and *BRCA2* mutations) may undergo additional screening with MR
  - ○ MRI is not adversely affected by dense breast tissue in these (generally young) women
  - ○ Although highly sensitive, MRI is not very specific and therefore is not suitable for screening women of average risk

Pharmacotherapy/Chemoprevention
- Selective estrogen receptor modulators (SERMs) have been shown to reduce breast cancer risk
  - ○ Tamoxifen treatment will reduce risk of both recurrence and contralateral breast cancers in women with ER-positive cancers
    - ■ 5 years of tamoxifen therapy will reduce incidence of contralateral breast cancer by 47% and incidence of recurrent cancer by 42%

Prophylactic Surgery
- Prophylactic surgery reduces but does not eliminate the risk of developing cancer
  - ○ Breast tissue in subcutaneous tissue or in axilla may not be removed
  - ○ Patients can develop primary peritoneal carcinomas
- Surgical options for risk reduction include prophylactic mastectomy and salpingo-oophorectomy
  - ○ Women at markedly increased risk have greatest benefit from these procedures
    - ■ Risk usually based on presence of genetic mutations (*BRCA1, BRCA2, P53, PTEN*)
  - ○ Mastectomy reduces risk of breast cancer by 90%
  - ○ Salpingo-oophorectomy reduces risk of ovarian cancer by 85-90%
    - ■ Breast cancer risk is reduced by 50%

Lifestyle Modification
- Some lifestyle modifications will slightly reduce breast cancer risk; these changes are also recommended for other health benefits
  - ○ Reduction or elimination of alcohol and tobacco use
  - ○ Maintenance of normal weight after menopause

SELECTED REFERENCES

1. Farhat GN et al: Changes in invasive breast cancer and ductal carcinoma in situ rates in relation to the decline in hormone therapy use. J Clin Oncol. 28(35):5140-6, 2010
2. Tamimi RM et al: Evaluation of a breast cancer risk prediction model expanded to include category of prior benign breast disease lesion. Cancer. 116(21):4944-53, 2010
3. Lyons TR et al: Pregnancy and breast cancer: when they collide. J Mammary Gland Biol Neoplasia. 14(2):87-98, 2009

RISK FACTORS FOR DEVELOPING BREAST CARCINOMA

Factors Associated with Increased Risk of Breast Cancer

(Left) Dense breast tissue detected by mammography is associated with an increased risk of breast cancer. Density also decreases the sensitivity of mammography, as it makes cancers more difficult to detect. *(Right)* Breast imaging detects more cancers than are apparent clinically. This small mass ➡ grew slowly over a period of 4 years and was eventually diagnosed as a grade 2 invasive carcinoma. This may be the type of cancer that would not cause harm during the patient's lifetime.

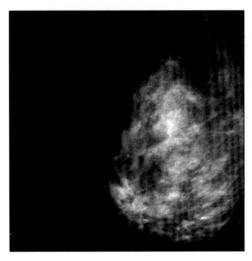
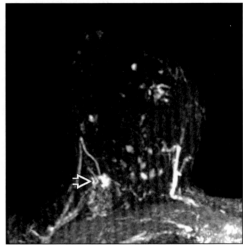

(Left) Marked nuclear atypia ➡ can be seen in epithelial cells after radiation therapy. If the breast is exposed to radiation at an early age, the risk of breast cancer is greatly increased. *(Right)* The average age for developing Hodgkin disease is 28 years. Young women undergoing mantle radiation are at high risk for subsequent breast cancer, and this risk persists for more than 25 years. This poorly differentiated breast carcinoma occurred 20 years after treatment.

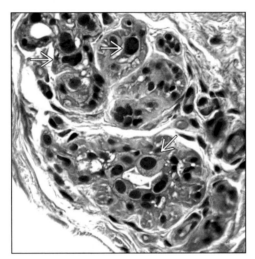
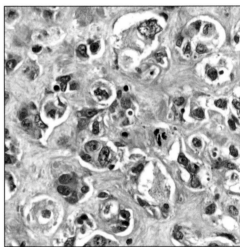

(Left) Pregnancy is a time of intense proliferation and expansion of lobular units, followed by differentiation and milk production. It is associated with an immediate increase in risk of cancer followed by an eventual decreased risk of cancer. *(Right)* The stromal remodeling allowing lobular expansion during pregnancy ➡ may facilitate the progression from DCIS ➡ to invasive carcinoma ➡ resulting in the increased incidence of cancer during or shortly after pregnancy.

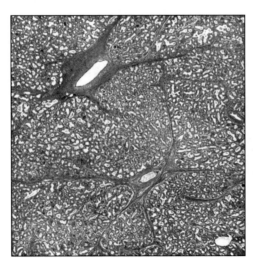
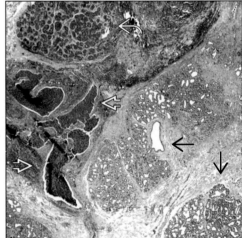

RISK FACTORS FOR DEVELOPING BREAST CARCINOMA

Lesions Associated with Risk of Invasive Carcinoma

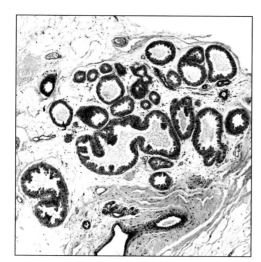

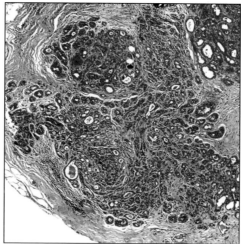

(Left) There are many changes grouped under nonproliferative breast disease, such as this cluster of small apocrine cysts, that do not increase the risk of breast cancer. *(Right)* Proliferative breast disease includes lesions that increase the number of epithelial cells, such as this case of sclerosing adenosis, as well as moderate to florid hyperplasia and intraductal papillomas. The RR of breast cancer is elevated 1.5-2x, but the great majority of women will not develop cancer.

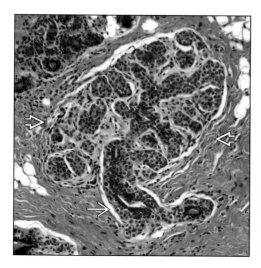

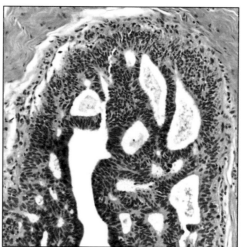

(Left) The atypical cells do not expand the lobule ⇨ and therefore would be classified as ALH rather than LCIS. ALH is associated with a RR of 4-5. However, the presence of pagetoid spread into the adjacent duct ⇨ would increase the RR to 8. *(Right)* ADH consists of a small clonal population of cells, insufficient for a diagnosis of DCIS. The RR of subsequent invasive cancer is increased 4-5x. Multiple foci of ADH with different morphologies may be present in the same specimen.

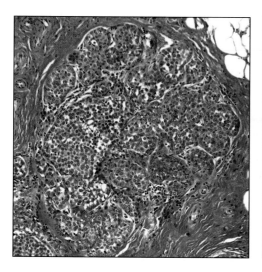

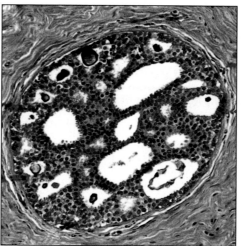

(Left) LCIS can be diagnosed if the cells fill and expand at least 1/2 of a lobular unit. The cells are morphologically identical to those of invasive lobular carcinoma. LCIS is an indicator of increased risk to both breasts and can also be a direct precursor for carcinoma. *(Right)* If untreated, many cases of DCIS will progress to invasive carcinoma. With treatment, the risk is lowered, and subsequent invasive cancers may occur in the same breast (2/3) or contralateral breast (1/3).

LOBULAR CARCINOMA IN SITU

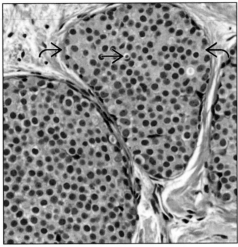

LCIS is characterized by a neoplastic proliferation of small, uniform, dyshesive cells that expand the acini of the terminal ductal lobular unit →. Signet ring cells are often present →.

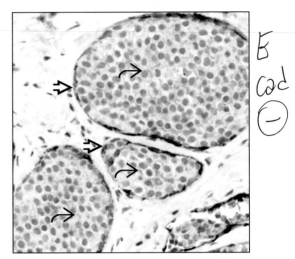

A characteristic of both in situ and invasive lobular neoplasia is the loss of E-cadherin expression in tumor cells →. The surrounding myoepithelial cells show weak E-cadherin positivity →.

TERMINOLOGY

Abbreviations
- Lobular carcinoma in situ (LCIS)

Synonyms
- Lobular intraepithelial neoplasia (LIN), includes atypical lobular hyperplasia (ALH) and LCIS

Definitions
- Neoplastic proliferation of epithelial cells lacking cell adhesion, confined to ducts and lobules, and filling and expanding at least 1/2 of 1 lobular unit

ETIOLOGY/PATHOGENESIS

Molecular Pathology
- Hallmark molecular feature of all lobular neoplasia (ALH, LCIS, and ILC) is loss of cellular cohesion
  - In > 95% of lesions, this is due to loss of expression of E-cadherin (CDH11) located on chromosome 16q
    - E-cadherin plays major role in intercellular adhesion and cell polarity
    - Cytoplasmic portion of E-cadherin is attached to actin cytoskeleton by binding β- or γ-catenin
  - Absence of E-cadherin is due to combinations of mechanisms leading to biallelic inactivation of gene
    - Allelic deletion (loss of heterozygosity 16q), CDH1 gene mutation, promoter silencing (hypermethylation)
  - In rare cases, loss of cohesion is due to defects in catenins or possibly other related proteins
    - Carcinomas have typical morphology, but nonfunctional E-cadherin is present
    - Other proteins, such as catenins, may have abnormal expression patterns
- Distribution of LCIS suggests association with germline mutation

- LCIS is not specifically associated with mutations in BRCA1, BRCA2, or CDH11 (E-cadherin)
  - Families with germline mutations in CDH11 are predominantly at risk for signet ring cell carcinomas of the stomach, with fewer cases of lobular carcinoma
- Association with other genes is being investigated

CLINICAL ISSUES

Epidemiology
- Incidence
  - 0.5-4% of breast biopsies
- Age
  - Mean age: 44-46 years; 80-90% are premenopausal

Site
- LCIS is frequently found as multiple foci within the same or both breasts
  - Up to 50% of patients have bilateral LCIS
  - Multicentric foci have been described in up to 80% of patients undergoing mastectomy for LCIS

Presentation
- Classic LCIS is incidental finding
  - Does not form palpable mass or mammographic lesion
- Variant forms of LCIS may be associated with calcifications detected by mammography

Natural History
- LCIS, ALH, and flat epithelial atypia/columnar cell change share similar molecular and cytogenetic features
  - Columnar cell change often coexists with LCIS
  - May be part of morphologic continuum in low-grade neoplasia pathway
- Genetic studies have found similar or identical mutations in LCIS and corresponding invasive lobular carcinomas

LOBULAR CARCINOMA IN SITU

Key Facts

Terminology
- Lobular carcinoma in situ (LCIS)

Etiology/Pathogenesis
- Hallmark molecular feature of in situ and invasive lobular carcinoma is loss of cellular cohesion
  - Loss of functional E-cadherin protein is most common, followed by defects in catenins

Clinical Issues
- LCIS is often found as multiple foci within either the same or both breasts
- Risk of subsequent invasive carcinoma is approximately 1% per year for both breasts
  - Higher incidence of lobular carcinomas, but majority are of no special type

- Clinical follow-up should be long-term, given extended risk for late-occurring carcinoma

Microscopic Pathology
- **Classic LCIS**
  - Solid and monotonous proliferation of small discohesive cells expanding terminal duct lobular units and small ducts
  - ER and PR positive, HER2 negative
- **Variants of LCIS**
  - Variant LCIS has morphologic and molecular features not present in classic LCIS
  - May be ER or PR negative &/or HER2 positive
  - Consistent terminology for these lesions has not yet been developed
  - Natural history and optimal treatment is unknown

- Similarities between LCIS and invasive carcinoma provide evidence that LCIS can be direct precursor of invasive carcinoma
- Natural history for variants of LCIS is unknown

Treatment
- Surgical approaches
  - Due to multicentric nature of LCIS, effective risk reduction requires bilateral mastectomy
    - However, majority of women with LCIS will never develop invasive carcinoma
- Adjuvant therapy
  - Adjuvant endocrine therapy (chemoprevention) reduces subsequent risk of ER-positive carcinomas
  - Associated with significant side effects in some women
- Surveillance
  - Women can be followed with close surveillance using imaging modalities
  - Risk of dying of breast cancer with careful follow-up is very low
- Optimal treatment for variants of LCIS is unclear
  - Some authors feel that variant forms of LCIS are better managed like DCIS

Prognosis
- Increased long-term risk of subsequent invasive carcinoma after diagnosis of classic LCIS
  - Subsequent invasive carcinomas more likely to be lobular than in general population but are most commonly of no special type
  - Magnitude of risk after variant types of LCIS is unknown but is presumed to be higher
- Risk applies to both breasts
  - Slightly greater in ipsilateral than in contralateral breast
  - Relative risk is 7-10x or about 25-30% lifetime risk
    - Corresponds to approximately 1% of patients diagnosed with invasive carcinoma per year of follow-up
  - Time to cancer from LCIS diagnosis ranges from 15-30 years

- Clinical follow-up should be long-term, given extended risk for late-occurring carcinoma
  - Some studies suggest risk for development of subsequent cancer diminishes with time whereas other studies do not

LCIS on Core Needle Biopsy
- Classic LCIS may be seen as incidental finding in core needle biopsies
- Excision is indicated for variant types of LCIS if other lesions of risk are present (e.g., ADH) or if targeted lesion may have been missed or is not well explained by pathologic findings
- Appropriate management of incidental classic LCIS on core biopsy is debated
  - In carefully selected cases, frequency of finding more significant lesions after excision is very low
  - Subsequent cancers in these patients are often not at site of core needle biopsy

IMAGE FINDINGS

Mammographic Findings
- Classic LCIS is not associated with mammographic findings
  - Usually incidental finding in biopsies performed for calcifications
    - Usually seen in coexisting sclerosing adenosis or columnar cell change adjacent to LCIS
- LCIS may grow into areas of preexisting calcifications but are not source of calcifications
- Variant forms of LCIS with necrosis &/or high-grade nuclei may be directly associated with calcifications

MR Findings
- Some lesions may show a non-mass ductal enhancement pattern or irregular enhancing mass
- However, difficult to correlate pathologic findings with MR lesions

LOBULAR CARCINOMA IN SITU

MICROSCOPIC PATHOLOGY

Histologic Features

- **Classic LCIS**
  - Solid and monotonous proliferation of small discohesive cells, expanding terminal duct lobular units (TDLUs) and small ducts
  - Criterion to distinguish LCIS from ALH is based on extent
    - At least 50-75% of acini in lobular unit must be filled and distended with no residual lumina
    - Involved lobules may be compared to uninvolved lobules to estimate degree of distension
  - 2 types of nuclei may be seen
    - Type A cells: Nuclei are small to slightly enlarged (1-1.5x size of lymphocyte), with uniform round nuclei and inconspicuous nucleoli
    - Type B cells: Nuclei are larger (2x size of lymphocyte) with more abundant cytoplasm and more prominent nucleoli
    - Type A and B cells can coexist in same lesion
  - Nuclei have a central or slightly eccentric position within the cell and show minimal pleomorphism
  - Intracytoplasmic vacuoles and signet ring cells are variably present
    - Special stains can be used to demonstrate mucin vacuoles
    - Cytoplasmic clearing can also be seen
  - Pagetoid spread in ducts (growth of cells between luminal and myoepithelial layers) may be present
    - Extensive ductal involvement can give "clover leaf" pattern
- **Variants of LCIS**
  - Recognition of E-cadherin loss as consistent feature of lobular neoplasia broadened range of lesions included within this group
    - Often associated with classic LCIS
    - Occur in older postmenopausal age group compared with classic LCIS
    - May present as mammographic calcifications or a mass
    - Many of these lesions would have been classified and treated as DCIS in the past
    - These lesions are rare, comprising < 5% of all carcinoma in situ
    - Natural history is unknown
  - Variant LCIS has morphologic features not seen in classic LCIS
    - High nuclear grade: > 3x size of a lymphocyte, irregular membrane, prominent nucleoli
    - Central necrosis, typically with calcifications
    - Abundant cytoplasm often with apocrine or plasmacytoid appearance
    - Cohesive (solid) pattern
  - Variant LCIS has molecular features not seen in classic LCIS
    - May be ER and PR negative
    - About 1/3 overexpress HER2
    - Higher proliferative rate compared with classic LCIS
    - Share genetic changes with classic LCIS (gains of 1q and losses of 16q) but have a higher number

of DNA copy number changes and more complex chromosomal rearrangements
- Associated invasive carcinomas are similar in appearance and may belong to "molecular apocrine" group of cancers
  - Consistent terminology for these lesions has not yet been developed, but suggested terms include
    - Pleomorphic LCIS
    - Carcinoma in situ with ductal and lobular features
    - Lobular intraepithelial neoplasia grade 3 (LIN3)
    - Apocrine pleomorphic lobular carcinoma in situ
    - Mammary intraepithelial neoplasia (MIN)

ANCILLARY TESTS

Immunohistochemistry

- E-cadherin
  - > 95% of cases of LCIS will lack E-cadherin
    - Some cases show weak or patchy positivity
    - Intermingled luminal and myoepithelial cells will be positive and can make interpretation of small lesions difficult
  - In cases with typical dyshesive morphology but E-cadherin positivity, IHC for other cell adhesion proteins may be helpful
  - Most common abnormal finding is cytoplasmic p120
  - Pattern can be difficult to interpret if LCIS is intermingled with residual luminal and myoepithelial cells
- High molecular weight cytokeratin
  - ~ 80% of LCIS shows weak to moderate 34βE12 positivity (cytokeratins 1, 5, 10, and 14) in cytoplasmic perinuclear pattern
    - Positivity is also seen in subset of DCIS and therefore has limited usefulness for diagnosis
  - Majority of DCIS and LCIS are negative for cytokeratins 5 and 6; usual hyperplasia typically shows positivity
    - LCIS can partially involve ducts with residual normal luminal cells, which can make interpretation difficult
- Estrogen and progesterone receptors
  - Present in > 95% of classic LCIS
    - Not usually evaluated on a clinical basis
  - May be absent in variant LCIS
- HER2
  - Absent in classic LCIS
  - Present in 10-30% of cases of variant LCIS, particularly in those with apocrine appearance
- GCDFP-15
  - Positive in > 90% of classic LCIS and 50-100% of variant LCIS

Cytogenetics

- Classic and variant LCIS
  - Relatively low numbers of DNA copy number changes compared with other morphologic types of breast neoplasia
  - Most common changes are loss of 16q (site of E-cadherin gene) and gain of 1p

LOBULAR CARCINOMA IN SITU

Immunohistochemistry

Antibody	Reactivity	Staining Pattern	Comment
34bE12	Positive	Cytoplasmic	Not a consistent finding
ER	Positive	Nuclear	May be negative in variant LCIS
PR	Positive	Nuclear	May be negative in variant LCIS
E-cadherin	Negative	Not applicable	Rare cases may be positive

- o Variant LCIS with high nuclear grade and apocrine morphology has more genomic alterations than other types of LCIS
- o LCIS associated with invasive carcinoma has more genetic alterations than pure LCIS

DIFFERENTIAL DIAGNOSIS

DCIS, Solid Pattern

- DCIS with solid pattern and low-grade nuclei can closely resemble LCIS
- Secondary spaces (microlumina) with cells polarized to lumens favors DCIS
- Cohesive growth pattern with distinct cell membranes should be present in DCIS
- In difficult cases, IHC to demonstrate presence of E-cadherin can be helpful
  - o Very rare cases of LCIS can be positive for E-cadherin, but these cases will have typical discohesive morphologic appearance of lobular neoplasia

Atypical Lobular Hyperplasia (ALH)

- ALH is cytologically identical to LCIS
- Both are negative for E-cadherin by IHC
- Distinction between ALH and LCIS is based on extent of lesion
  - o ALH is defined by its limited extent
    - Neoplastic cells only partially fill lobular acini with residual lumina present
    - Number of acini involved is < 50%
- Distinction from LCIS is subjective but important for risk stratification
  - o ALH alone confers 4-5x relative increased risk of invasive carcinoma
  - o ALH with pagetoid spread confers 8x relative increased risk of invasive carcinoma
  - o LCIS confers 10x relative increased risk of invasive carcinoma

Invasive Carcinoma

- LCIS involving sclerosing adenosis, fibroadenomas, or other benign lesions can mimic invasive carcinoma
- Architecture of underlying lesion is usually apparent
  - o Lobulocentric, swirling, back-to-back tubules are typical for sclerosing adenosis
  - o Stromal proliferation and pushing borders are seen in fibroadenomas
- Cells within benign lesion will have characteristic appearance of lobular neoplasia (uniform small cells, dyshesive pattern)
  - o IHC studies can be helpful in demonstrating presence of normal myoepithelial cell layer

- Alveolar or solid invasive lobular carcinoma can be difficult to distinguish from LCIS
  - o IHC studies can be used to confirm absence of myoepithelial cells

Artifacts Leading to Cellular Discohesion

- Poor preservation or crushing can result in rounding up of cells and loss of cohesion
  - o Usually occurs at edge of specimen or in specimen that has not been well fixed
  - o Can mimic lobular neoplasia
  - o LCIS or ALH should not be diagnosed unless cells are well preserved

Benign Cells

- Prominent myoepithelial cells with clear cytoplasm or histiocytes can mimic pagetoid spread by LCIS
  - o Cells in question will not be increased in number
  - o Similar changes in myoepithelial cells are typically seen throughout specimen
    - Histiocytes typically have abundant cytoplasm and small nuclei
  - o IHC for specific myoepithelial or histiocytic markers can be helpful in problematic cases

REPORTING CONSIDERATIONS

Key Elements to Report

- Classic LCIS
  - o Extent and margins need not be reported
- Variant LCIS
  - o Should be reported similar to DCIS including extent and margins

SELECTED REFERENCES

1. Boldt V et al: Positioning of necrotic lobular intraepithelial neoplasias (LIN, grade 3) within the sequence of breast carcinoma progression. Genes Chromosomes Cancer. 49(5):463-70, 2010
2. Carder PJ et al: Screen-detected pleomorphic lobular carcinoma in situ (PLCIS): risk of concurrent invasive malignancy following a core biopsy diagnosis. Histopathology. 57(3):472-8, 2010
3. Rakha EA et al: Clinical and biological significance of E-cadherin protein expression in invasive lobular carcinoma of the breast. Am J Surg Pathol. 34(10):1472-9, 2010
4. Rakha EA et al: Lobular breast carcinoma and its variants. Semin Diagn Pathol. 27(1):49-61, 2010
5. Brandt SM et al: The "Rosen Triad": tubular carcinoma, lobular carcinoma in situ, and columnar cell lesions. Adv Anat Pathol. 15(3):140-6, 2008

LOBULAR CARCINOMA IN SITU

Microscopic Features

(Left) LCIS expands the acinar unit of the terminal duct lobular units, but the underlying lobular architecture remains evident ➡. In contrast, DCIS typically unfolds lobules into a single large space, which then resembles a duct. The terms "lobular" and "ductal" carcinoma are based on these fundamental growth patterns of the neoplastic cells in lobules. **(Right)** Signet ring cells are commonly seen in lobular neoplasia. The cells typically have a single distinct mucin vacuole ➡.

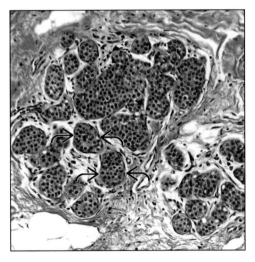
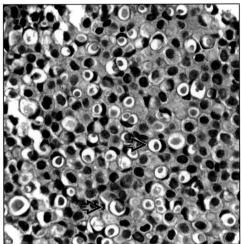

(Left) Pagetoid spread of ALH or LCIS occurs when the cells are present between the basement membrane of a duct ➡ and the overlying normal luminal cells ➡. DCIS usually displaces the luminal cells and fills the duct. **(Right)** Pagetoid spread of lobular neoplastic cells is highlighted by an immunohistochemical study showing that luminal cells ➡ and myoepithelial cells ➡ are positive for CK5/6 (brown) whereas the lobular cells ➡ are positive for CK18 (red).

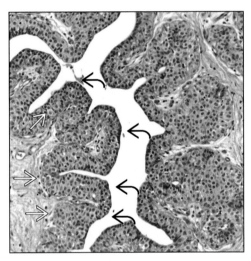
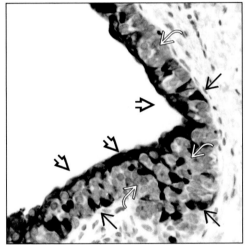

(Left) LCIS ➡ confers an increased risk of developing invasive carcinoma ➡. The cytologic features of both are identical, and they typically show identical mutations in E-cadherin. Therefore, LCIS is both a risk factor for and a biologic precursor to invasive carcinoma. **(Right)** LCIS can be associated with microinvasion, which may be difficult to detect. Immunoperoxidase studies such as CK5/6 ➡ are helpful to demonstrate the absence of myoepithelial cells in areas of invasion ➡.

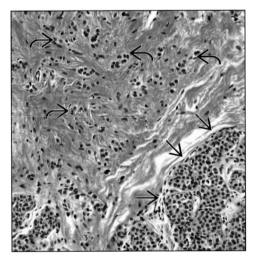
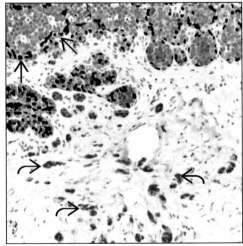

LOBULAR CARCINOMA IN SITU

Variant Microscopic Features

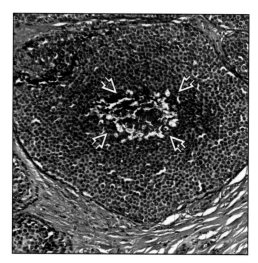

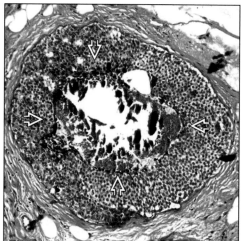

(Left) Other than the presence of central necrosis ⇉, this lesion has the cytologic features of classic LCIS and lacks E-cadherin expression. Variant types of LCIS are frequently associated with a higher rate of proliferation. (Right) Unlike classic LCIS, which is typically an incidental finding, variant LCIS is often detected by mammography. This LCIS is associated with central necrosis ⇉ and coarse calcifications. In the past, such lesions would likely have been classified as DCIS.

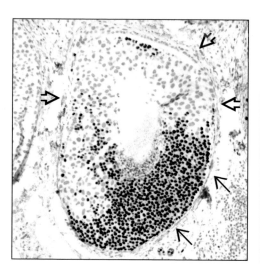

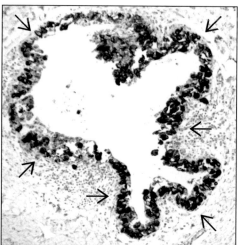

(Left) Variant LCIS is often found in association with classic LCIS. In this case, a typical ER-positive LCIS with low-grade nuclei → is present in the same duct space with ER-negative LCIS ⇾ with high-grade nuclei and central necrosis. (Right) Pagetoid spread by a variant of LCIS with apocrine features is highlighted by overexpression of HER2 →. Variant LCIS with apocrine features is frequently negative for ER and PR and has an increased number of genomic alterations.

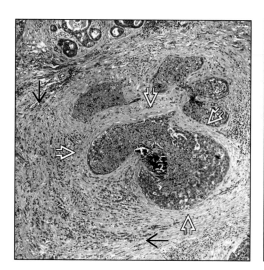

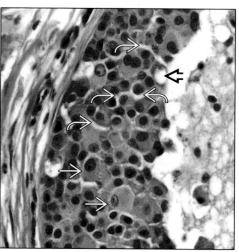

(Left) This carcinoma in situ could have been classified as comedo DCIS due to the high-grade nuclei, central necrosis, and cohesive appearance ⇉. However, both the CIS and the associated invasive carcinoma → were negative for E-cadherin. (Right) Variant forms of LCIS can be recognized by loose cellular cohesion →, rounded cell shapes, and occasional intracellular vacuoles ⇾ or signet ring cells. The cytoplasm may be abundant →, conferring an apocrine appearance.

LOBULAR CARCINOMA IN SITU

Difficult Cases

(Left) LCIS ⇶ involving sclerosing adenosis can mimic invasive cancer. Regions of adenosis will retain a lobulocentric architecture ➡ and an orderly relationship with stroma. Immunostudies to confirm the presence of myoepithelial cells may be helpful. (Right) LCIS may be present as an incidental finding in a fibroadenoma ⇶. This case was mistaken for invasive carcinoma on a core needle biopsy. The presence of a circumscribed margin ➡ was a clue to the correct diagnosis.

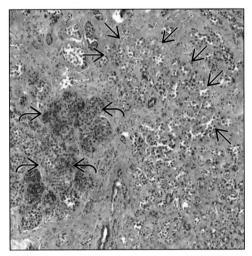
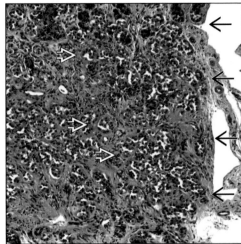

(Left) Although almost all cases of LCIS lack E-cadherin, rare cases express it but lack other cytoskeletal proteins. In this case, the catenin p120 is in an abnormal cytoplasmic pattern in LCIS ⇶ in contrast to the normal membrane pattern ➡ in the adjacent duct. (Right) LCIS involving collagenous spherulosis has a fenestrated, cribriform appearance resembling DCIS. The presence of basement membrane material ➡ in the pseudoluminal spaces is a key to the correct diagnosis.

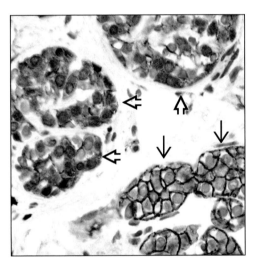
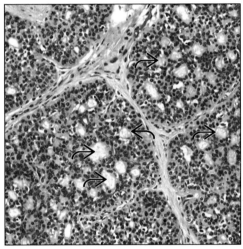

(Left) When LCIS involves other lesions, interpretation can be difficult. In this case, LCIS partially involves an area of ADH. The combination of a monomorphic population of cells and cribriform spaces closely mimics DCIS. (Right) In this case of LCIS involving ADH, areas of LCIS are E-cadherin negative ⇶ whereas the luminal cells forming cribriform spaces are E-cadherin positive ➡. The intermingling of the 2 cell populations can be mistaken for DCIS.

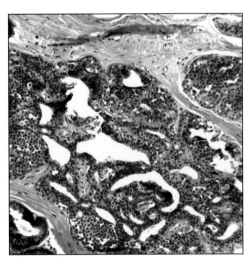
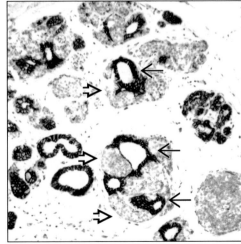

Differential Diagnosis

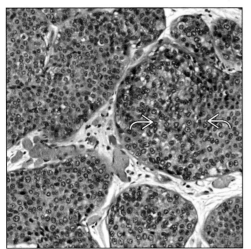

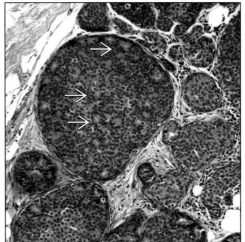

(Left) This case of DCIS has a cohesive growth pattern ⟶ and cytologic atypia that is more suggestive of a ductal than a lobular phenotype. There was a strong, diffuse membrane pattern of E-cadherin expression by IHC, supporting the diagnosis of DCIS, solid pattern, involving TDLUs. (Right) Some cases of DCIS resemble LCIS but have small microacini ⟶ recognized by polarization of the cells surrounding the spaces. These lesions are usually E-cadherin positive.

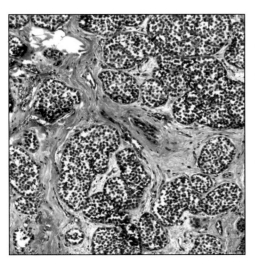

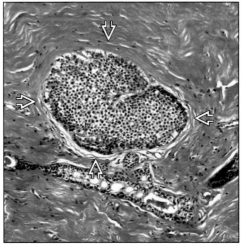

(Left) Invasive alveolar lobular carcinoma characteristically forms rounded clusters of tumor cells that can closely resemble LCIS. IHC to demonstrate the absence of myoepithelial cells in areas of invasion may be required for final classification. (Right) Lobular neoplasia can have a neuroendocrine appearance due to the presence of a uniform population of small rounded cells with dispersed chromatin. This metastatic carcinoid tumor to the breast ⟶ was mistaken for LCIS.

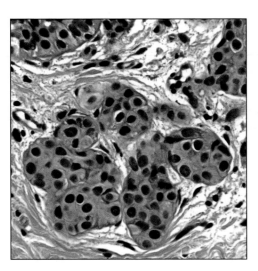

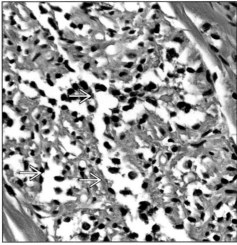

(Left) ALH is identical in appearance to LCIS but is more limited in extent, usually only partially involving lobules. Pagetoid spread can be seen in either ALH or LCIS. ALH confers a lower risk for the subsequent development of invasive carcinoma. (Right) Poor preservation of tissue can cause epithelial cells to round up and lose cohesion ⟶. These changes are most frequently seen at the edges of biopsies. LCIS should not be diagnosed if the changes could be artifactual.

DUCTAL CARCINOMA IN SITU

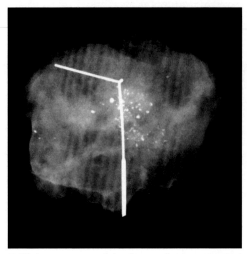

DCIS is most commonly diagnosed when clustered calcifications are detected by screening mammography. The calcifications are typically numerous and variable in size and shape.

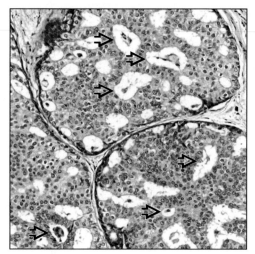

Cribriform DCIS forms sharply demarcated round spaces ⊇ distributed evenly throughout the ducts and is frequently detected due to calcifications forming on intraluminal secretory material.

TERMINOLOGY

Abbreviations
- Ductal carcinoma in situ (DCIS)

Synonyms
- Intraductal carcinoma (IDC)
  - Not recommended since the abbreviation can be confused with invasive ductal carcinoma
- Ductal intraepithelial neoplasia (DIN)
  - Only some subtypes of DIN are equivalent to DCIS

Definitions
- Clonal proliferation of epithelial cells confined to ducts and lobules with a cohesive pattern and typically E-cadherin positive

ETIOLOGY/PATHOGENESIS

Biology of DCIS
- Same molecular subtypes recognized in invasive carcinoma are also seen in DCIS
  - Luminal A (ER positive, HER2 negative): ~ 70%
  - "Luminal B HER2 positive" (ER positive, HER2 positive): ~ 10-20%
  - HER2 (ER negative, HER2 positive): ~ 20-30%
  - Triple negative (ER/PR/HER2 negative): 5-10%
- HER2 subtype is slightly more frequent and triple negative subtype less frequent in DCIS as compared to invasive carcinoma
- More biologic heterogeneity is seen in DCIS than in invasive carcinoma
- No specific differences in genetic alterations or gene expression have been found specific to invasive carcinoma that are not found in DCIS
- Changes necessary for transition to invasive carcinoma are not yet understood
  - Not all DCIS progresses to invasive carcinoma

- Possible that invasion occurs due to loss of function of normal myoepithelial and stromal cells, rather than gain of function by DCIS

CLINICAL ISSUES

Epidemiology
- Incidence
  - DCIS comprises < 5% of breast carcinomas in populations without mammographic screening
  - With screening, 20-30% of carcinomas are detected as DCIS
    - Incidence of DCIS increased after introduction of screening (1980s)
    - Majority of DCIS is diagnosed due to formation of calcifications detectable by mammography

Presentation
- Mammographic calcifications (85%)
  - Associated with either necrosis or secretory material in lumens
- Palpable mass or radiologic density (10%)
  - Usually associated with extensive high-grade DCIS with periductal stromal fibrosis
- Nipple discharge (5%)
  - Discharge is spontaneous and unilateral
  - Extensive micropapillary and papillary DCIS are the most common types
- Paget disease of nipple (< 1%)
  - Patients present with eczematous scale crust of 1 nipple
  - DCIS traverses lactiferous ducts onto nipple skin without crossing contiguous basement membranes
  - DCIS is generally high grade, and most overexpress HER2

Treatment
- Surgery is used to completely remove ductal system involved by DCIS

DUCTAL CARCINOMA IN SITU

Key Facts

Etiology/Pathogenesis
- Same molecular subtypes recognized in invasive carcinoma are also seen in DCIS
- Transition to invasion is poorly understood
  - May involve loss of function of normal myoepithelial and stromal cell rather than gain of function of tumor cells

Clinical Issues
- Incidence
  - Without mammographic screening: < 5% of carcinomas
  - With screening: 20-30% of carcinomas
- Clinical presentations
  - Mammographic calcifications (85%)
  - Palpable mass or radiologic density (10%)
  - Nipple discharge (5%)

- Natural history
  - If untreated, ~ 1% of patients per year develop invasive carcinoma at same site
  - With treatment, rate of recurrence is < 10%
  - Some recurrences are biologically related to DCIS, and some are new primary carcinomas
  - Survival rate for women with DCIS is greater than that for women without breast cancer

Top Differential Diagnoses
- Lobular carcinoma in situ
- Atypical ductal hyperplasia
- Invasive carcinoma
- Lymph-vascular invasion
- Collagenous spherulosis
- Gynecomastoid hyperplasia

  - Risk of recurrence is lower if DCIS is ≥ 0.2 cm from margins
  - Risk of recurrence after mastectomy is < 5%
- Radiation therapy reduces recurrence by ~ 50%
- Tamoxifen also reduces recurrence by ~ 50%
  - Benefit may be greater, or restricted, to ER-positive DCIS
    - Data supporting this finding is only published in an abstract of a subset analysis of NSABP B-24
    - Possibility of small effect for ER-negative DCIS not excluded due to small number of cases

Prognosis
- If untreated, approximately 1% of patients per year develop invasive carcinoma at same site
  - At 20-30 years, majority of patients remain disease free
- If treated with complete excision with negative margins and possible addition of radiation therapy &/ or hormonal therapy, risk of recurrence is < 10%
  - Approximately 1/2 of recurrences are DCIS and 1/2 are invasive carcinoma
- Lymph node metastases are very rare in cases of DCIS that have been completely examined microscopically
  - When present, usually consist of isolated tumor cells that have not been shown to have an effect on prognosis
  - If a macrometastasis is present, there is usually an undetected area of invasive carcinoma
    - Sentinel node biopsy may be performed in patients with large areas of DCIS that are difficult to completely sample
- If treated with mastectomy, risk of recurrence is < 5%
  - Local recurrence may be due to breast tissue left behind in chest wall
  - Nodal or distant recurrence may be due to undetected invasive carcinoma at time of surgery due to extensive DCIS
- Risk of dying of breast cancer after recurrence in breast is very low; most cancers are detected early and are small and node negative

  - Survival rate for women with DCIS is greater than that for women without breast cancer
  - Majority of women with DCIS have access to medical care, which is not true of women in general population
- Pathologic prognostic factors can predict likelihood of ipsilateral recurrence
  - Nuclear grade
  - Necrosis
  - Extent: Volume of breast tissue occupied by DCIS
  - Margin width
- Some recurrences are true recurrences (related to the DCIS), and some are new primary carcinomas
  - Risk of contralateral invasive carcinoma is approximately 1/2 that of ipsilateral invasive carcinoma
  - Suggests that 1/2 of ipsilateral invasive carcinomas may be due to new primary carcinomas
    - May explain why surgery with wide margins without radiation therapy does not eliminate possibility of subsequent cancer in same breast

Core Needle Biopsy
- DCIS is usually detected on core needle biopsies for calcifications
- Presence of microinvasion may influence a decision to perform a lymph node biopsy and should be documented if present
- Subsequent excisions infrequently reveal invasive carcinoma if large bore vacuum-assisted biopsies are performed and targeted lesion was calcifications and not a mass

IMAGE FINDINGS

Mammographic Findings
- Calcifications are most common presenting feature for DCIS
  - Features correlated with DCIS
    - Clustered pattern
    - Linear and branching pattern
    - Large number of calcifications

- Small size (large calcifications are more likely to be associated with benign lesions)
- Irregular or pleomorphic shape
- Increasing over time
  - 20-30% of biopsies for suspicious calcifications will reveal DCIS on excision
  - Extent of DCIS is generally greater than that suggested by distribution of calcifications
  - Grade of DCIS is not reliably predicted by shape or number of calcifications
    - However, linear and branching calcifications are often associated with comedo DCIS
  - Calcifications without a mass are rarely associated with invasive carcinoma
    - In majority of cases, if invasive carcinoma is present, then the calcifications are associated with DCIS
    - In unusual cases, calcifications are associated with secretions in tubules or with necrosis in invasive carcinoma
    - Invasive carcinoma is generally small (< 1 cm)
- DCIS sometimes forms a circumscribed mass
  - Localized area of DCIS with surrounding fibrotic stromal response can form a rounded or lobulated mass
  - DCIS involving a fibroadenoma can be detected as a circumscribed mass
  - Solid, solid papillary, or papillary DCIS can form masses

MR Findings

- Majority of cases of DCIS are associated with enhancement
  - Although sensitive, findings are not specific enough for MR to be used for screening general population
- Most common pattern is linear clumped enhancement
- DCIS is typically surrounded by collarette of small capillaries
- Associated increased blood flow is detected by MR

MACROSCOPIC FEATURES

General Features

- Most cases of DCIS cannot be seen or palpated grossly
- Cases of high-grade DCIS (typically comedo type) often have associated stromal response
  - Masses are usually firm but not hard
  - Borders are ill defined as opposed to distinct edge of invasive carcinoma
  - Color may be gray and texture gritty
- Comedo-type necrosis can be seen grossly as minute extruded plugs of necrotic cells when tissue is gently squeezed

MICROSCOPIC PATHOLOGY

Histologic Features

- **Architectural patterns**
  - Important to recognize
    - Grade is more important for prognosis; high-grade DCIS can have any architectural pattern

- Majority of cases of DCIS consist of > 1 architectural type
  - **Cribriform DCIS**
    - Cribriform lumens appear punched out and rounded in shape
    - In 3 dimensions, spaces are spherical
    - Cells should be oriented around lumen
    - Lumens are distributed evenly throughout involved duct
    - Spaces associated with hyperplasia are typically sinuous in shape and peripherally located
  - **Papillary DCIS**
    - Papillary fronds have a central fibrovascular core
    - Myoepithelial cells are present around periphery of spaces but not within papillary cores
    - Endothelial cells lining blood vessels can be apposed to base of tumor cells in thin fibrovascular cores
    - Can be difficult to distinguish endothelial cells from myoepithelial cells using IHC muscle-type markers
    - p63 is a better marker to confirm absence of myoepithelial cells in papillary lesions
  - **Micropapillary DCIS**
    - Papillae have narrow bases that expand to bulbous ends
    - Appearance has been compared to that of light bulb or drumstick
    - Papillae do not have fibrovascular cores
    - Surrounding duct usually lacks hyperplasia and is flat
  - **Comedo DCIS**
    - Central area of necrosis surrounded by rim of tumor cells
    - Strict definition of comedo DCIS requires both central necrosis and high nuclear grade
    - Calcifications are almost always present in necrotic material and are usually numerous
    - Associated mammographic finding: Clustered or linear and branching calcifications
    - Mammographic lesion is often close to actual extent of comedo DCIS
    - Associated circumferential stromal fibrosis, often with lymphocytic infiltrate
    - Some cases form a clinically palpable mass or mammographic density and can sometimes be visible as foci of necrosis in an area of firm gray-white stroma
  - **Solid DCIS**
    - Cells completely fill ductal spaces
    - Some have solid papillary pattern, as fibrovascular cores may be present within cell proliferation
    - Solid DCIS may show some morphologic overlap with LCIS
  - **Clinging DCIS**
    - Cells line spaces and do not form architectural patterns
    - Difficult to diagnose in isolation unless cells are of high nuclear grade
    - In general, more easily diagnosed architectural patterns are also present

DUCTAL CARCINOMA IN SITU

Cytologic Features

- DCIS is a clonal population, which should be reflected in morphologic appearance
- In contrast, hyperplasias consist of a mixture of luminal, myoepithelial, and intermediate-type cells
- Metaplasia makes recognition of DCIS very difficult
  - Apocrine and clear cell metaplasia impart a very uniform appearance, even in benign lesions
  - Architectural features, high-grade nuclei, necrosis, or associated similar-appearing invasive carcinoma may be necessary for definitive diagnosis as DCIS
- Nuclear grade is important feature to classify DCIS
  - Same nuclear grading system used for invasive carcinoma can be used for DCIS
  - Often a mixture of nuclear grades; highest grade present should be reported
- Mucin production can be associated with cribriform, micropapillary, papillary, or clinging DCIS
  - Calcifications may be present in mucin
  - If duct rupture, can be difficult to distinguish extravasated mucin from small foci of invasion
  - Tumor cells should not be present in extravasated mucin

Necrosis

- Presence of necrosis is often used to classify DCIS
- Comedo necrosis should involve majority of central portion of involved duct
- Focal necrosis may involve only small portion of duct
- Single cell necrosis can also be seen
- Necrosis is always associated with comedo DCIS, but varying degrees can be seen with other types

Extent of DCIS

- "Extent" refers to volume of breast tissue occupied by DCIS
  - Extent can vary from 0.2 cm to > 20 cm or all 4 quadrants of breast
  - Average extent of DCIS is 2-3 cm
- Measure of extent is useful clinically to determine
  - Likelihood of being able to achieve breast conservation with adequate margins
  - Likelihood of an area of invasion being present or being missed
- Minimal extent required for a diagnosis of DCIS (rather than ADH) has been proposed
  - 0.2 cm or 2 completely involved ductal spaces have been suggested
  - No minimal extent required for DCIS with high-grade nuclei
- Extent can only be estimated
  - Breast tissue is highly compressible
  - Shape of breast specimens changes (slumps) after excision
  - Specimen radiography also compresses and distorts shape (size) of excisions
  - Morphologic gaps in ductal involvement are reported to occur, particularly in lower grades of DCIS
  - DCIS is often removed in multiple specimens
- Multiple methods to estimate extent

- Measurement of DCIS on glass slide: Only accurate if DCIS is only present on 1 slide
  - Margins: If 2 opposing margins are positive or close to DCIS, extent can be estimated by using specimen size
  - Complete serial sequential sectioning (SSS) and mapping of sections with DCIS to give a linear measurement
  - Counting block method (CBM) multiplies number of blocks with DCIS by 0.4 cm (or average width of sliced tissue in cassettes, if known)
  - SSS correlates with CBM up to approximately 3 cm
  - Because CBM is related to volume as well as to linear dimension, it usually gives a larger estimate compared with SSS for very extensive DCIS
- Sentinel node biopsy may be performed when DCIS is extensive, particularly as part of mastectomy

ANCILLARY TESTS

Immunohistochemistry

- **Myoepithelial markers**
  - Very helpful to distinguish DCIS from invasive carcinoma and to identify microinvasion
  - Myoepithelial cells associated with DCIS may lose expression of some markers
    - p63 is marker most likely to be retained
    - May be helpful to use > 1 marker before concluding myoepithelial cells are absent
  - Myoepithelial cells may be reduced in number
    - Markers that detect cytoplasm (i.e., muscle markers, basal cytokeratin) detect more portions of the cell than nuclear marker p63
  - Myoepithelial cells may be displaced from their normal location on basement membrane
  - Double IHC for a myoepithelial marker and cytokeratin can be very helpful for detecting microinvasion
    - Focus of invasion seen on H&E may be absent on deeper level, but another focus may appear that will be difficult to recognize without keratin positivity
- **Estrogen receptor**
  - Majority of DCIS (> 80%) is positive for ER
  - ER testing may be requested to help make decisions about hormonal therapy
  - ER positive DCIS is almost always PR positive as well
- **E-cadherin**
  - DCIS expresses cell adhesion molecule E-cadherin
    - Majority of LCIS is negative for E-cadherin
    - Very rare cases of LCIS may express E-cadherin but have abnormal expression of other cell adhesion molecules
  - IHC can be useful in cases of solid carcinoma in situ difficult to classify by H&E
    - If cribriform, micropapillary, or papillary patterns are present, E-cadherin must also be present
- **HER2**
  - Approximately 20-30% of DCIS overexpress HER2
  - Routine evaluation is not usually requested by clinicians as treatment with HER2-targeted therapy for DCIS is only being used in clinical trials

o In rare cases, DCIS may overexpress HER2 whereas associated invasive carcinoma does not
  ▪ Can lead to erroneous results for gene expression profiling or FISH if DCIS is not clearly distinguished from invasive carcinoma

DIFFERENTIAL DIAGNOSIS

Lobular Carcinoma In Situ (LCIS)
- Also a monomorphic population of neoplastic cells
- Cells lack cohesion and typically do not express E-cadherin
  o In unusual cases, E-cadherin may be present, but other cell adhesion molecules are nonfunctional
- LCIS cannot form architectural structures such as papillae, micropapillae, or cribriform spaces
- Solid DCIS with low to intermediate-grade nuclei may be difficult to distinguish from LCIS
  o IHC for E-cadherin is usually helpful
- Rare cases of LCIS have high-grade nuclei &/or central necrosis
  o In the past, these cases were likely classified as DCIS
  o Absence of E-cadherin has enhanced recognition of these cases as a form of lobular neoplasia
  o Clinical outcome of these cases without treatment is not well known as most have been treated like DCIS
  o Terminology for these lesions includes "pleomorphic LCIS," "LCIS with high-grade nuclei," and "carcinoma in situ with ductal and lobular features"

Atypical Ductal Hyperplasia (ADH)
- Small clone of cells that lacks 1 criterion for classification as DCIS
- Clonal-appearing cells may not completely fill spaces
- If only a single space is involved or lesion is < 0.2 cm, classification as ADH has been recommended
- If lesion is borderline between ADH and DCIS, classification as ADH is recommended
- ADH shows similar molecular alterations as low-grade DCIS

Invasive Carcinoma
- Can invade as circumscribed nests of cells
- Arrangement is generally haphazard in stroma rather than following normal pattern of ducts and lobules
- Desmoplastic response generally extends beyond cells rather than being circumferential as in DCIS
- In difficult cases, IHC is helpful to demonstrate absence of myoepithelial cells in invasive carcinoma

Lymph-Vascular Invasion (LVI)
- Both DCIS and LVI can be present as circumscribed nests of tumor cells without a stromal response
- LVI follows vascular pattern and will be present between lobules and adjacent to veins and arterioles
  o Location of DCIS will follow normal pattern of ducts and lobules
- Some (not all) endothelial cells of lymphatics can be identified with IHC for CD31 or podoplanin (D2-40)
  o Podoplanin is also positive in some myoepithelial cells

- DCIS can be identified by IHC for p63, which will be negative in endothelial cells

Collagenous Spherulosis (CS)
- Consists of a proliferation of both luminal and myoepithelial cells
- Myoepithelial cells surround round spaces filled with basement membrane material
- Punched-out spaces mimic cribriform DCIS
  o This resemblance is more striking when CS is involved by LCIS
- IHC will reveal myoepithelial cells surrounding cribriform spaces

Gynecomastoid Hyperplasia (GH)
- Consists of an area in female breast that resembles gynecomastia of male breast
- Only ducts are present; lobule formation is absent
- Lining cells are typically hyperplastic
  o Papillae taper at ends rather than bulging (as in micropapillary DCIS)
  o Papillae form on top of a layer of hyperplasia rather than arising from a flat background

SELECTED REFERENCES

1. Pinder SE: Ductal carcinoma in situ (DCIS): pathological features, differential diagnosis, prognostic factors and specimen evaluation. Mod Pathol. 23 Suppl 2:S8-13, 2010
2. Dadmanesh F et al: Comparative analysis of size estimation by mapping and counting number of blocks with ductal carcinoma in situ in breast excision specimens. Arch Pathol Lab Med. 133(1):26-30, 2009
3. Grin A et al: Measuring extent of ductal carcinoma in situ in breast excision specimens: a comparison of 4 methods. Arch Pathol Lab Med. 133(1):31-7, 2009
4. Hilson JB et al: Phenotypic alterations in ductal carcinoma in situ-associated myoepithelial cells: biologic and diagnostic implications. Am J Surg Pathol. 33(2):227-32, 2009
5. Hughes LL et al: Local excision alone without irradiation for ductal carcinoma in situ of the breast: a trial of the Eastern Cooperative Oncology Group. J Clin Oncol. 27(32):5319-24, 2009
6. Kuerer HM et al: Ductal carcinoma in situ: state of the science and roadmap to advance the field. J Clin Oncol. 27(2):279-88, 2009
7. Lester SC et al: Protocol for the examination of specimens from patients with ductal carcinoma in situ of the breast. Arch Pathol Lab Med. 133(1):15-25, 2009
8. Maffuz A et al: Tumor size as predictor of microinvasion, invasion, and axillary metastasis in ductal carcinoma in situ. J Exp Clin Cancer Res. 25(2):223-7, 2006
9. Clingan R et al: Potential margin distortion in breast tissue by specimen mammography. Arch Surg. 138(12):1371-4, 2003
10. Lagios MD et al: Duct carcinoma in situ. Relationship of extent of noninvasive disease to the frequency of occult invasion, multicentricity, lymph node metastases, and short-term treatment failures. Cancer. 50(7):1309-14, 1982

DUCTAL CARCINOMA IN SITU

Imaging, Gross, and Microscopic Features

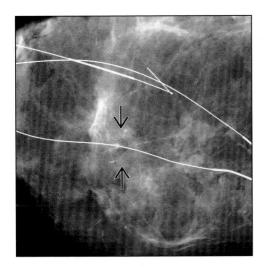
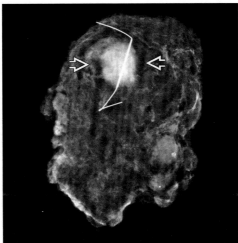

(Left) Fine linear and branching calcifications ➡ are highly correlated with DCIS. The DCIS usually has central necrosis, and the calcifications outline the underlying ductal system. (Right) DCIS rarely presents as a circumscribed or lobulated mass ⊳. The DCIS may involve an expanded ductal space (typically papillary DCIS), consist of multiple closely arranged ducts with periductal fibrosis (typically comedo DCIS), or be DCIS partially involving a fibroadenoma.

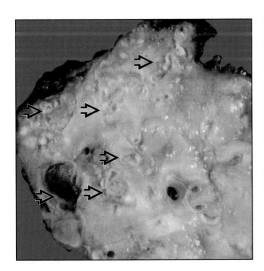
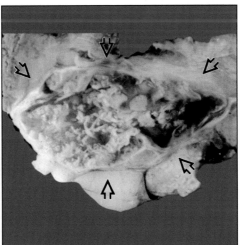

(Left) Comedo DCIS is the most common type that may be grossly visible. Numerous ducts are filled with necrotic material ⊳. With gentle compression, punctate necrotic foci may exude from the tissue (comedone-like). (Right) DCIS can expand a duct to form a mammographically and grossly visible mass ⊳. The most common type with this presentation is papillary (or solid papillary) DCIS. Encapsulated papillary carcinoma has a similar appearance but lacks myoepithelial cells.

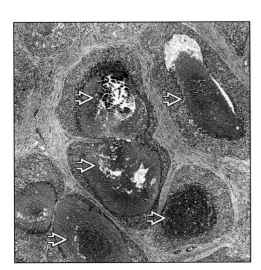
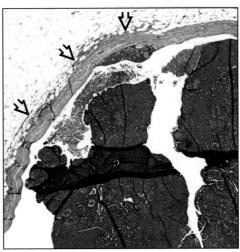

(Left) Comedo DCIS has extensive central necrosis ⊳, usually associated with numerous calcifications. The periductal fibrosis can sometimes form a mammographic density or an ill-defined palpable mass. (Right) This solid papillary DCIS is surrounded by a fibrous capsule ⊳ and forms a radiologic and gross circumscribed mass. Myoepithelial cells are present around the periphery, which distinguishes this lesion from an encapsulated (encysted) papillary carcinoma.

DUCTAL CARCINOMA IN SITU

Architectural Types

(Left) Micropapillary DCIS consists of narrow-based elongated papillae extending into the duct space. The papillae are solid without a fibrovascular core. The epithelium between the papillae is usually flat or shows minimal hyperplasia. The cells are generally well or moderately differentiated. Mucin and calcifications ⊵ may be present.
(Right) Unusual cases of micropapillary DCIS have high-grade nuclei ⊵, frequent mitoses ⊵, and necrosis ⊵.

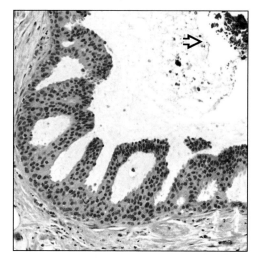 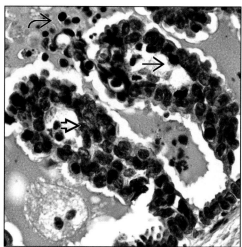

(Left) Papillary DCIS has fibrovascular cores containing blood vessels. Myoepithelial cells are absent. The endothelial cells ⊵ are often close to the basement membrane and can be mistaken for myoepithelial cells. *(Right)* Clinging DCIS consists of cells lining spaces without filling the space or forming architectural structures. This type of DCIS can be recognized with confidence in the absence of associated patterns only if the nuclei are of high grade, as in this case.

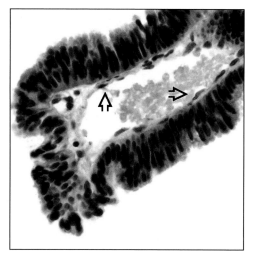 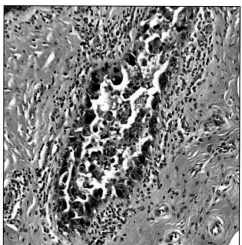

(Left) Solid DCIS can be difficult to recognize as it lacks helpful diagnostic architectural features. The main differential diagnosis is with LCIS. DCIS usually has nuclei of a higher grade and a more cohesive appearance. IHC can be helpful to demonstrate E-cadherin expression in cases of DCIS. *(Right)* This DCIS has both cribriform and solid papillary patterns. Actin positive myoepithelial cells are present at the periphery ⊵, as well as lining internal papillary cores ⊵.

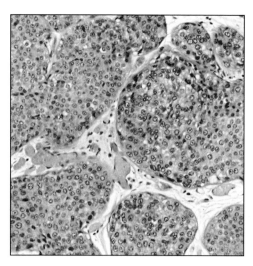 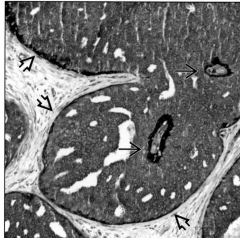

DUCTAL CARCINOMA IN SITU

Variant Microscopic Features

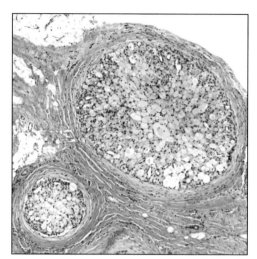

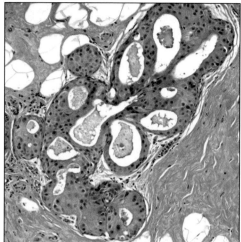

(Left) DCIS can have clear, foamy, or secretory appearing cytoplasm. The nuclei are generally small and round. This type of DCIS can be difficult to recognize in isolation if only a solid pattern is present. *(Right)* DCIS can have an apocrine appearance with enlarged nuclei and abundant eosinophilic cytoplasm. Because apocrine metaplasia gives cells a monomorphic appearance, this type of DCIS is difficult to recognize unless abnormal architecture or high nuclear grade is present.

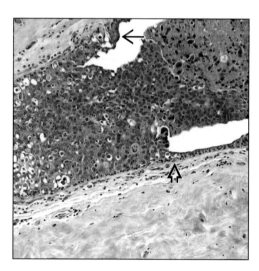

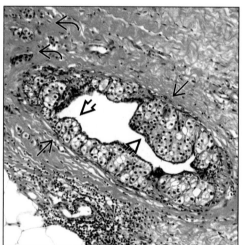

(Left) As DCIS grows into ducts and lobules, it generally overgrows and replaces the normal luminal cells ➤. Pagetoid spread preserving the overlying luminal cells is rarely seen or only seen focally at the advancing edge ➡. *(Right)* This is an unusual case of cribriform and clear cell DCIS showing an area of pagetoid spread in the breast. The tumor cells are between an intact luminal cell layer ➤ and the basement membrane ➡. There is adjacent invasive carcinoma ➘.

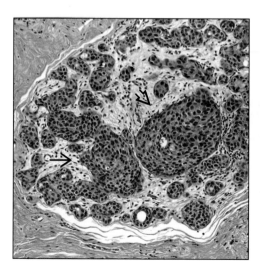

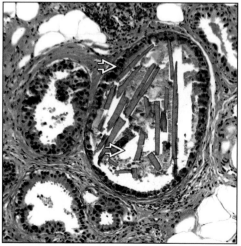

(Left) DCIS appears to be in ducts because involved lobules unfold to become large duct-like spaces. In this case, the DCIS expands the terminal duct ➡ and has started to expand and distort the acini of the lobule ➤. The entire lobule may eventually become a single circumscribed space resembling a duct. *(Right)* Crystalloids ➤ are brightly eosinophilic extracellular bodies with square or sharp borders. They are rare and have only been reported in association with DCIS.

Imaging and Immunoperoxidase Studies

(Left) The most common type of lesion associated with DCIS on MR is a pattern of clumped linear enhancement ➡. This lesion was located near a prior core needle biopsy site that had shown an area of DCIS ⊟➤. *(Right)* DCIS often is surrounded by small blood vessels as shown by this IHC study for CD31 ➡. The enhanced blood flow around ducts involved by DCIS can be detected by linear and clumped enhancement on MR. However, this finding is not specific for DCIS.

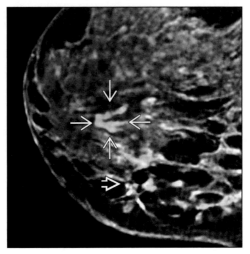
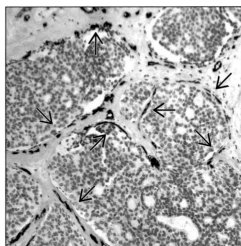

(Left) IHC is particularly helpful in the evaluation of DCIS to confirm the presence of myoepithelial cells. In this case, there is a focus of keratin positive DCIS with p63 positive myoepithelial cells ➡ adjacent to foci of keratin positive invasive carcinoma ⊟➤ without myoepithelial cells. *(Right)* E-cadherin can be useful to distinguish some cases of DCIS from LCIS when only a solid pattern is present. In this case, the cribriform spaces require the presence of E-cadherin.

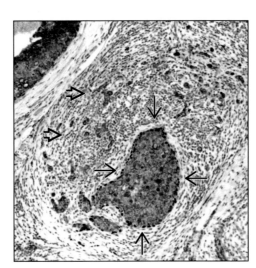
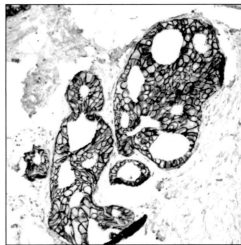

(Left) More than 80% of DCIS expresses estrogen receptor, and hormonal treatment with tamoxifen reduces the likelihood of local recurrence. The benefit may be limited to or primarily found in patients with ER-positive DCIS. *(Right)* DCIS and ADH are generally negative for high molecular weight keratins whereas myoepithelial cells are positive ⊟➤. IHC may be helpful to distinguish DCIS or ADH from usual hyperplasia in difficult cases, as ADH generally shows heterogeneous positivity.

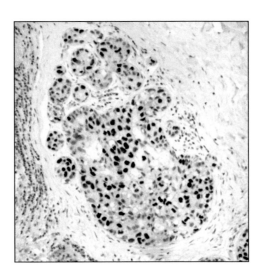
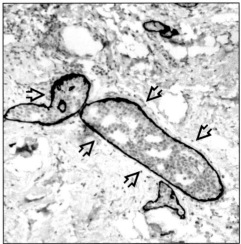

DUCTAL CARCINOMA IN SITU

Extent of DCIS

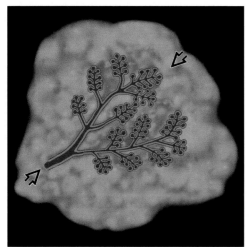

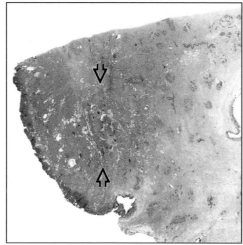

(Left) DCIS involves the duct/lobular system ⮞ in a complex pattern that can only be fully visualized microscopically. "Extent" of DCIS refers to the volume of tissue occupied by DCIS. (Right) The extent of DCIS can be measured on a single glass slide ⮞. This method is only accurate if a single block of tissue is involved. If more than 1 block contains DCIS, this method will underestimate the extent and should not be used.

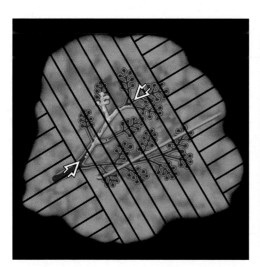

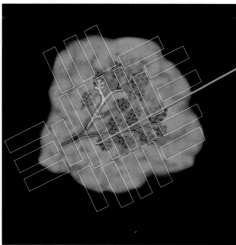

(Left) In complete serial sequential sampling, the entire specimen is processed in such a way that the location of the DCIS can be mapped. The extent is measured as the greatest linear dimension ⮞. (Right) In the block method, the entire area of DCIS is sampled as well as representative tissue from the remaining specimen. The extent of DCIS can be estimated by multiplying the number of blocks involved by the thickness of a section (approximately 0.4 cm).

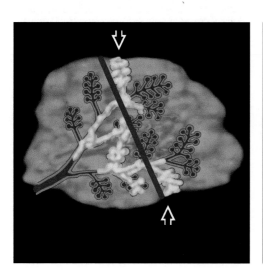

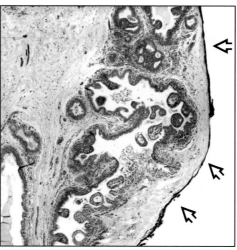

(Left) If the size of the specimen is known and DCIS involves 2 opposing margins ⮞, the size of the specimen can be used to give a measurement of extent. (Right) The extent of DCIS can only be estimated for many reasons. For example, in many cases, DCIS is removed in multiple specimens because margins are often positive or close ⮞ and DCIS is also present in subsequent margin excisions. It is difficult to determine how the extent of DCIS in more than 1 specimen could be combined.

Differential Diagnosis

(Left) Invasive carcinoma can invade as circumscribed nests of cells, and this case was mistaken for DCIS. Useful clues to the correct diagnosis are the surrounding desmoplastic stromal response and the haphazard arrangement of the tumor nests. *(Right)* IHC is useful to distinguish invasive carcinoma invading as rounded nests from DCIS. In this case, a few blood vessels are positive for calponin ⇗, but no myoepithelial cells are associated with the invasive carcinoma ➡.

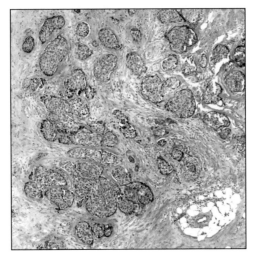
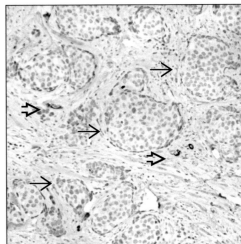

(Left) ADH lacks sufficient quantitative and qualitative criteria for DCIS. In this case, the lesion is small, there is streaming of cells across spaces ➡, and the spaces are not completely filled. Therefore, ADH is favored. *(Right)* DCIS and ADH are generally negative for high molecular weight cytokeratins, such as CK5/6, whereas usual hyperplasia is a mixture of luminal, myoepithelial, and intermediate cells with a heterogeneous pattern, as in this case.

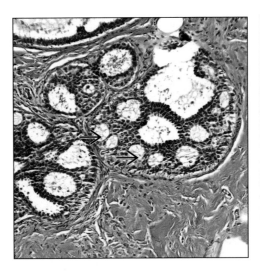
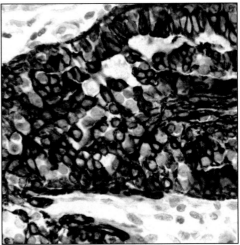

(Left) Collagenous spherulosis is a proliferation of luminal and myoepithelial cells. The latter cells line circumscribed spaces that are filled with basement membrane-like material. *(Right)* The spaces of collagenous spherulosis are lined by myoepithelial cells and filled with basement membrane material that may appear collagenous, mucinous, flocculent, or have a targetoid pattern ➡. A darkly eosinophilic cuticle often lines the spaces ⇗.

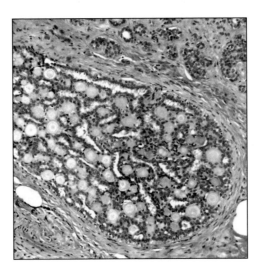
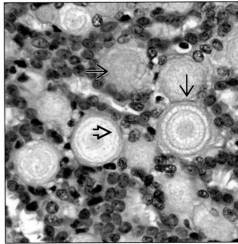

DUCTAL CARCINOMA IN SITU

Differential Diagnosis

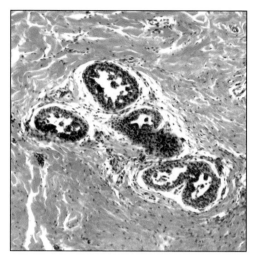
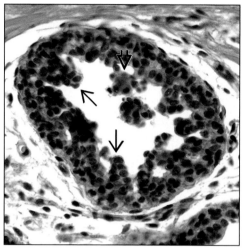

(Left) Gynecomastia or gynecomastoid hyperplasia consists of small ducts without lobule formation. The hyperplasia has the pattern of tapering and small abortive papillae that should not be mistaken for micropapillary DCIS. *(Right)* Gynecomastia or gynecomastoid hyperplasia is often associated with epithelial hyperplasia with tapering papillae ➔ or small abortive papillae ⊇ on a background of hyperplasia. The proliferation lacks the architectural atypia of micropapillary DCIS.

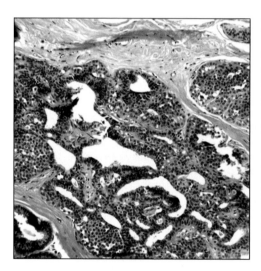
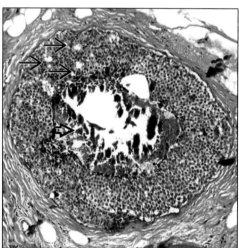

(Left) The combination of ADH and LCIS involving the same spaces can closely mimic DCIS. In this case, IHC for E-cadherin clearly demonstrates the presence of 2 separate cell populations. *(Right)* This solid proliferation of small rounded monomorphic cells with a discohesive appearance suggests LCIS. However, there is central necrosis ⊇ and possible formation of minute cribriform spaces ➔. IHC for E-cadherin can be helpful to support a diagnosis of DCIS if positive.

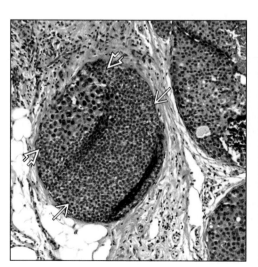
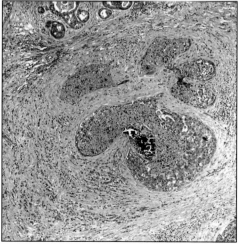

(Left) DCIS can show marked heterogeneity in morphology and in tumor markers. In this ductal space, there is 1 population of cells with high-grade nuclei ⊇ adjacent to another population of cells resembling LCIS with low-grade nuclei ➔. *(Right)* This carcinoma in situ has high-grade nuclei, a cohesive cell pattern, and central comedo necrosis with calcifications. However, the cells in the carcinoma in situ and in the associated invasive carcinoma are negative for E-cadherin.

DUCTAL CARCINOMA IN SITU, PAGET DISEASE

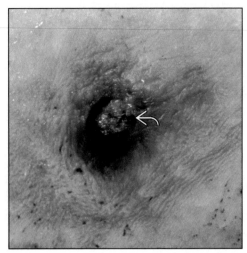

This is a typical clinical appearance of a nipple involved by mammary Paget disease. There is evidence of erythema, crusting, and scaling ➡ as well as a suggestion of focal ulceration.

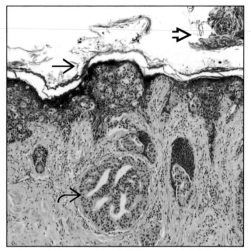

The clinical appearance of MPD is due to hyperkeratosis ➡ and loss of intercellular fluid ⇥ via the disrupted skin barrier. DCIS is typically present in the lactiferous sinuses ➡.

TERMINOLOGY

Abbreviations
- Ductal carcinoma in situ (DCIS)
- Mammary Paget disease (MPD)

Synonyms
- Paget disease of nipple
- DCIS involving nipple skin

Definitions
- Uncommon clinical presentation of breast cancer involving nipple
- MPD described by Sir James Paget (1874)
  - "An eruption on the nipple and areola ... with characteristics of ordinary chronic eczema"
    - Paget linked skin changes with later development of cancer in underlying breast
- MPD was later shown to be due to spread of carcinoma cells into nipple epidermis from lactiferous sinuses
- Pagetoid spread is presence of tumor cells between basement membrane and overlying layer of normal cells
  - In nipple skin, pagetoid spread is almost always due to DCIS with overlying squamous cells
  - In ducts and lobules, pagetoid spread is most commonly seen with LCIS with overlying luminal cells
    - Unlike LCIS, DCIS typically overgrows or pushes aside overlying luminal cells and fills ducts and lobules

ETIOLOGY/PATHOGENESIS

Pathogenesis of Paget Disease
- Remains debatable
  - In most cases, Paget cells likely originate from DCIS involving lactiferous sinuses of nipple

- Supported by finding of DCIS deeper in breast identical to Paget cells in almost all cases
  - Very rarely, Paget cells may be derived from precursor cells (Toker cells) present within nipple epidermis
    - In such cases, cancer may not be present in underlying breast
- Motility factor (heregulin-a) secreted by epidermal keratinocytes may attract Paget cells within nipple epidermis
  - Heregulin-a binds to HER2 family receptors that are overexpressed by Paget cells
- Tumor cells disrupt normal tight junctions between keratinocytes
  - Extracellular fluid can escape through skin, and this produces characteristic scale crust
    - Diagnosis can sometimes be made using cytologic preparations of skin scrapings

CLINICAL ISSUES

Presentation
- Skin lesions
  - Occur in 1-2% of women with breast cancer
  - May be limited to nipple or extend to areola
  - Scaling and redness in affected area
  - Pain and itching are frequent symptoms
  - Ulceration or serosanguineous/bloody discharge may be present in more advanced cases
  - Delay in diagnosis of MPD may be related to initial diagnosis of eczema or inflammatory skin disorder
- Underlying breast cancer found in > 95% of cases (invasive &/or DCIS)
  - No age predilection seen
  - No clinical or epidemiologic factors have been described that predispose to development of MPD
  - Up to 1/2 of patients have palpable tumor on affected side

DUCTAL CARCINOMA IN SITU, PAGET DISEASE

Key Facts

Terminology
- Mammary Paget disease (MPD)
- Uncommon clinical presentation of breast cancer involving nipple

Clinical Issues
- Occurs in 1-2% of women with breast cancer
- Clinical appearance: Scaling and redness in affected area
- Patients with palpable mass due to invasive carcinoma have worse prognosis

Image Findings
- Mammogram may be negative or show changes related to tumor in underlying breast tissue
- MR may be useful in detection of occult neoplastic disease in underlying breast tissue

Microscopic Pathology
- Adenocarcinoma cells, single and in clusters, present within keratinizing epidermis of nipple
- Tumor cells extend from lactiferous sinuses to nipple skin without crossing basement membrane
- Immunohistochemistry panel helpful in distinguishing MPD from melanoma and squamous cell carcinoma

Top Differential Diagnoses
- Carcinoma directly invading nipple skin
- Toker cell hyperplasia
- Squamous cell carcinoma in situ/Bowen disease
- Melanoma
- Clear cell change in keratinocytes

- Most of these patients have associated invasive carcinoma
- In very rare cases, invasion occurs directly from nipple skin into dermis
- Majority of cases of MPD diagnosed microscopically are not detected clinically
  - Focal nipple involvement is insufficient to produce clinically detected symptoms

Treatment
- Surgical approaches
  - Determined by presence and extent of underlying breast cancer
    - Due to nipple involvement, mastectomy is often performed
- Adjuvant therapy
  - Features of associated breast cancer, including grade and extent, dictate need for and type of adjuvant therapy

Prognosis
- Determined by presence and extent of underlying breast cancer
  - For MPD associated with underlying DCIS only, survival approaches 100% at 10 years after mastectomy
  - 10-year survival for node-negative patients with palpable invasive carcinoma is 70%

IMAGE FINDINGS

Mammographic Findings
- In early cases, imaging findings may be absent
- Skin thickening is typical finding in advanced cases
  - MPD associated with mammographic density or nipple retraction is more likely to have areas of invasion
  - Calcifications may be associated with underlying DCIS

MR Findings
- Typically shows abnormal nipple enhancement &/or ill-defined, thickened nipple-areolar complex
- MR may be useful in detection of occult neoplastic disease in underlying breast tissue
  - In setting of negative mammography, MR can facilitate treatment planning for patients with MPD

MACROSCOPIC FEATURES

General Features
- Gross changes reflect features seen clinically
  - Frequently, erythematous appearance with crusting of skin
  - Skin may show ulceration
    - However, skin preparation prior to surgery often removes gross scaling crust in surgical specimens
- Palpable mass lesion may be present in underlying breast parenchyma

MICROSCOPIC PATHOLOGY

Histologic Features
- Adenocarcinoma cells, single and in clusters, present within keratinizing epidermis of nipple
  - Clusters of Paget cells more common in basal portion of epidermis
  - Tumor cells extend from lactiferous sinuses to overlying skin without crossing basement membrane
    - Therefore, Paget disease can occur in absence of stromal invasion
- Paget cells are large and atypical in appearance, stand out from surrounding keratinocytes
  - Enlarged pleomorphic nuclei, which tend to show prominent nucleoli
  - Abundant pale or eosinophilic cytoplasm
  - Cytoplasm may contain diastase-resistant PAS positive globules consistent with mucin

DUCTAL CARCINOMA IN SITU, PAGET DISEASE

Differential Diagnosis and Special Studies

	Paget Disease	Toker Cells	Melanoma	Squamous Cell Carcinoma In Situ
CK7	+	+	-	-
CAM5.2	+	+	-	-
CK5/6	-	-	-	+
CK20	-	-	-	+
S100	+/-	-/+	+	-
HMB-45	-	-	+	-
Melan-A	-	-	+	-
HER2	+ (most cases)	-	-	-
CEA	+	-	-	-
ER/PR	- (95% of cases)	+		
Cytoplasmic mucin	+/-	-/+		

- Moderate to intense lichenoid lymphocytic infiltrates typically seen in underlying superficial dermis
  o May obscure diagnosis, should not be mistaken for dermatitis
- Varying degrees of hyperplasia and hyperkeratosis of associated epidermis
  o Inflammation, hyperplasia, and hyperkeratosis responsible for clinical appearance of lesion
  o May be associated with ulceration of epidermis
- Associated ductal carcinoma (with or without invasion) usually found in underlying breast
  o Associated DCIS is typically high grade with solid or comedo pattern

ANCILLARY TESTS

Immunohistochemistry
- Panel of immunohistochemistry stains is helpful in establishing glandular origin of Paget cells

DIFFERENTIAL DIAGNOSIS

Carcinoma Directly Invading Nipple Skin
- Subareolar tumor with infiltration of superficial dermal collagen and overlying epidermis
  o Skin ulceration is usually present
- Invasive carcinomas may involve dermis in horizontal pattern for 1-2 mm

Toker Cells and Toker Cell Hyperplasia
- Epidermally located breast ductal epithelium
  o Most common near duct orifices
  o Present in at least 70% of normal nipples when detected with immunohistochemical studies
- Benign appearance, bland nuclei, inconspicuous nucleoli
- Toker cells share some IHC features with Paget cells
  o Cells are positive for CK7, CAM5.2, and EMA but are usually negative for mucin, CEA, and HER2
- In Toker cell hyperplasia, cells are numerous and may show some nuclear atypia
  o Usually incidental finding; it would be highly unusual to be associated with clinical findings

Squamous Cell Carcinoma In Situ/Bowen Disease
- Extensive replacement of nipple epidermis by Paget cells can mimic squamous cell carcinoma in situ
- Squamous cell carcinoma in situ is not associated with underlying breast cancer
- Usually positive for high molecular weight cytokeratins (CK5/6, CK20) and negative for mucin and HER2

Melanoma
- Melanoma cells show nesting at dermo-epidermal junction
- "Buck shot" spread in overlying epidermis
- Paget cells may take up melanin pigment released by epidermal cells or melanocytes, simulating melanoma
- Immunohistochemical staining pattern is helpful for confirming diagnosis

Clear Cell Change in Keratinocytes
- Clear cell change, benign cytology, bland nuclei
- More frequently seen in basal and mid layers of epidermis

SELECTED REFERENCES

1. Lester T et al: Different panels of markers should be used to predict mammary Paget's disease associated with in situ or invasive ductal carcinoma of the breast. Ann Clin Lab Sci. 39(1):17-24, 2009
2. Park S et al: Useful immunohistochemical markers for distinguishing Paget cells from Toker cells. Pathology. 41(7):640-4, 2009
3. Di Tommaso L et al: Toker cells of the breast. Morphological and immunohistochemical characterization of 40 cases. Hum Pathol. 39(9):1295-300, 2008
4. Liegl B et al: Mammary and extramammary Paget's disease: an immunohistochemical study of 83 cases. Histopathology. 50(4):439-47, 2007

DUCTAL CARCINOMA IN SITU, PAGET DISEASE

Diagrammatic and Microscopic Features

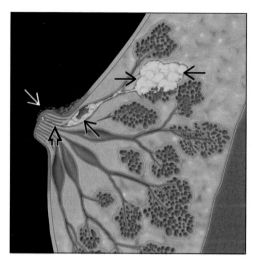

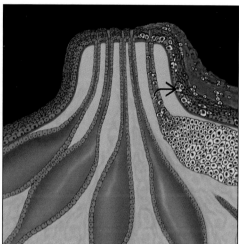

(Left) MPD is a clinical manifestation of breast cancer involving the nipple ➡. More than 95% of patients will have an underlying high-grade DCIS ➡ ± invasion. Tumor cells migrate from the underlying ducts ➡ to the epidermis of the nipple without crossing a basement membrane. (Right) Tumor cells ➡ in MPD are still contained by the basement membrane and therefore represent in situ carcinoma. These cells can move within the epidermis of the nipple and adjacent areola.

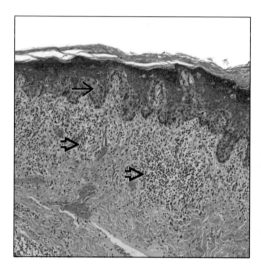

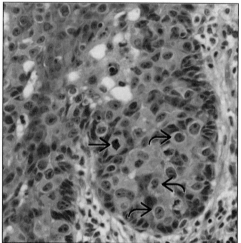

(Left) MPD is typically associated with a marked superficial dermal chronic inflammatory infiltrate ➡, which is a clue to the diagnosis. Larger pale cells can be seen in the basal portions of the epidermis ➡. (Right) At higher magnification, there is infiltration of the epidermis by pleomorphic neoplastic cells with abundant eosinophilic cytoplasm ➡. These cells are more prominent in the basal portions of the epidermis, and occasional mitotic figures may be present ➡.

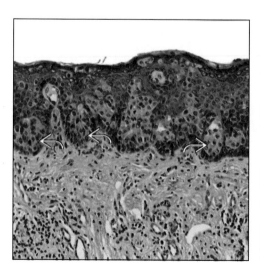

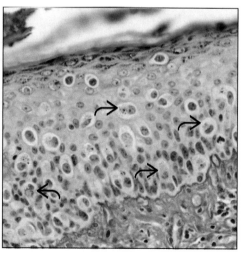

(Left) The neoplastic cells infiltrating the epidermis of the nipple will typically stand out at low power due to their abundant eosinophilic cytoplasm ➡. (Right) PAS stain with diastase digestion shows areas of cytoplasmic staining ➡ consistent with intracytoplasmic mucin. The neoplastic cells of MPD arise from an underlying adenocarcinoma. The demonstration of intracytoplasmic mucin by PAS with diastase or other histochemical stains supports the diagnosis of MPD.

Microscopic Features

(Left) *Aggregates of large pleomorphic cells with abundant pale cytoplasm in the deep dermis ⇨ are typically seen in MPD. A lymphocytic infiltrate is typically seen in the superficial dermis ⇨. (Right) In some cases, the involvement of the epidermis by the cells of MPD can be so extensive that these cases raise the possibility of squamous cell carcinoma or melanoma. In the example shown here, the overlying epidermis is almost completely replaced by neoplastic cells ⇨.*

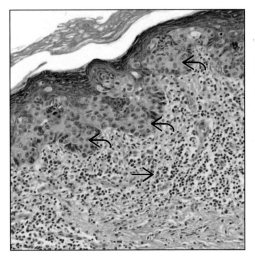
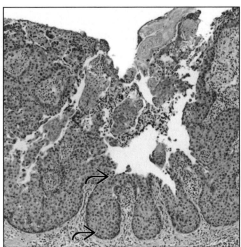

(Left) *In some cases of MPD, the intense lichenoid dermal inflammatory infiltrates and destruction of the epidermis with ulceration can obscure the underlying neoplastic nature of the disease process. (Right) Immunohistochemistry for EMA highlights the neoplastic cells within the involved nipple epidermis ⇨. Plasma cells in the inflammatory infiltrate also show staining ⇨. EMA-positive cells should not be present within the epidermis in cases of chronic inflammation.*

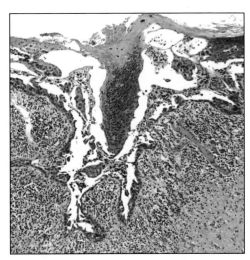
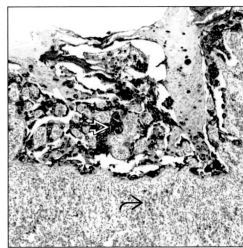

(Left) *This is an unusual case of MPD with invasion from the skin ⇨ into the underlying dermis ⇨. The nests of invasive tumor cells are obscured by the intense inflammation. (Right) The Paget cells are positive for cytokeratin (red, cytoplasmic) ⇨. The squamous cells are positive for p63 (brown, nuclear) ⇨. The area of invasion into the dermis is shown by keratin-positive tumor cells that are not associated with p63-positive myoepithelial cells or squamous cells ⇨.*

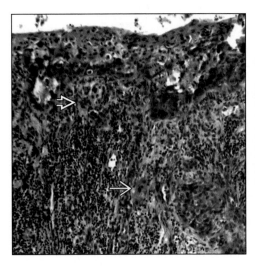
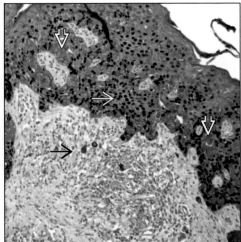

DUCTAL CARCINOMA IN SITU, PAGET DISEASE

Immunoperoxidase Studies

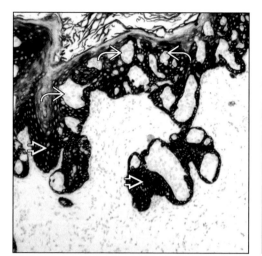

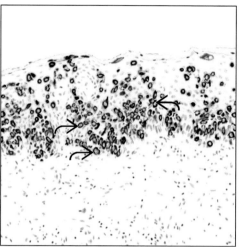

(Left) The contrast between the keratinocytes of the epidermis and the tumor cells can also be highlighted by stains for cytokeratin 5/6, which stains squamous cells ⊟. The tumor cells in the epidermis are negative ⊟. (Right) Immunostains can help establish the glandular origin of MPD and confirm the diagnosis in difficult cases. MPD will show an immunoprofile of a breast carcinoma, which is different from squamous cells. The tumor cells in this case are positive for CK7 ⊟.

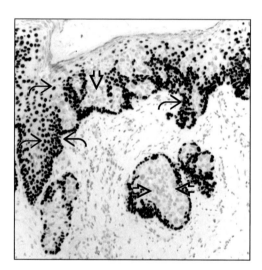

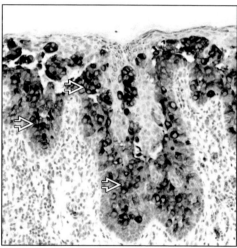

(Left) The normal squamous cells of the epidermis of the nipple will show nuclear positivity for p63 ⊟. The nests of tumor cells in this example of MPD are negative ⊟. (Right) CEA is an oncofetal protein that is expressed in fetal epithelial cells. There is marked overexpression of CEA in a number of adenocarcinomas, including those arising in the GI tract, lung, and breast. CEA expression ⊟ in this case of MPD is evidence of the glandular origin of these tumor cells.

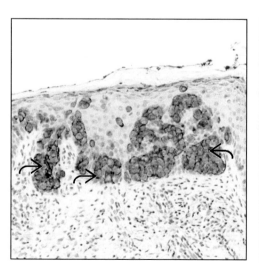

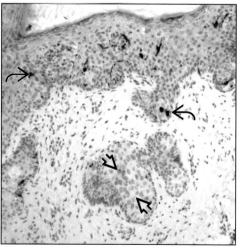

(Left) A good marker for confirming MPD is HER2, which shows strong membrane staining in tumor cells ⊟. The motility factor heregulin-a, which is secreted by epidermal cells, is a ligand for HER2 and may play a role in the pathogenesis of MPD. (Right) Markers for melanoma will also be negative in MPD. The tumor cells are negative for Melan-A ⊟. Melanocytes in the epidermis are positive ⊟ (red chromogen).

Differential Diagnosis

(Left) Eczematoid dermatitis can also present with a scaly crust and nipple irritation. In this case, there is lichen simplex chronicus-like changes and a dermal lymphocytic infiltrate. *(Right)* Invasive carcinomas can invade the overlying skin and grow within the epithelium for a short distance ➔ and mimic Paget disease. Ulceration of the skin usually occurs before there is extensive epidermal involvement.

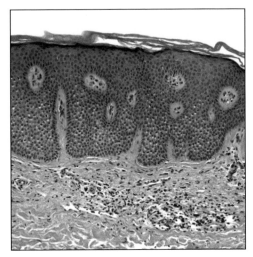
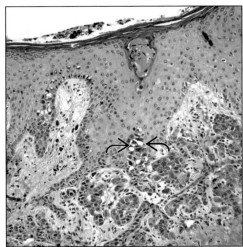

(Left) Toker cells are a normal finding and appear as intraepidermal clear cells of the nipple ➔. They are found immediately adjacent to the openings of the lactiferous ducts along the basal layer. *(Right)* Toker cells are an incidental finding in normal nipples and should not be associated with clinical changes. In this case, there was an adjacent nipple adenoma causing irritation and hyperkeratosis of the nipple ➔. Unfortunately, given the clinical appearance and large number of Toker cells ➔, the lesion was mistaken for MPD.

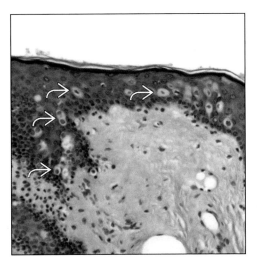
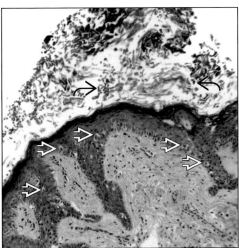

(Left) Toker cells have the immunoprofile of normal luminal cells. The majority of normal nipples will show cells positive for cytokeratin 7 ➔ and CAM5.2. *(Right)* Toker cells are also generally positive for estrogen receptor ➔ and progesterone receptor. Unlike MPD, Toker cells will be negative for CEA and HER2 and have a low proliferative rate as determined by Ki-67 expression. In contrast, MPD is usually strongly positive for CEA, HER2, and Ki-67.

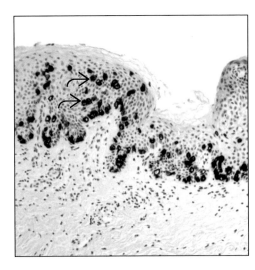
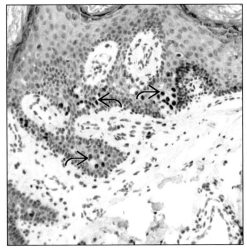

DUCTAL CARCINOMA IN SITU, PAGET DISEASE

Differential Diagnosis

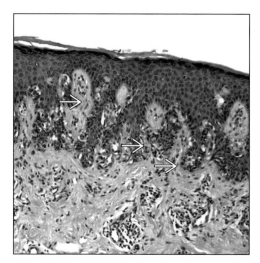
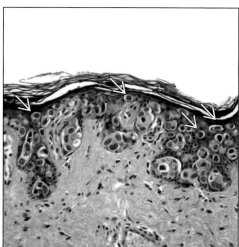

(Left) Like Paget cells, malignant melanocytes are present within the epidermis singly and as small clusters ➡. The tight junctions of the epidermal cells are not disrupted, and therefore loss of intercellular fluid and a scale crust is not typical for melanoma. *(Right)* MPD may resemble melanoma due to the the pagetoid spread within the epidermis ➡ as well as the presence of pigment granules. Paget cells may take up melanin released by epidermal cells or melanocytes.

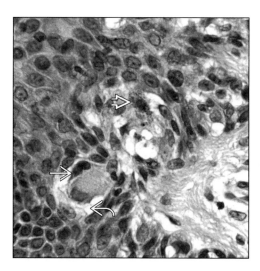
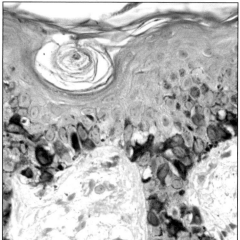

(Left) As with Paget cells, in melanoma the cells appear detached from the adjacent squamous cells ➡. The cells often contain melanin ➡, but in some cases melanin may be focal or absent. Multinucleated cells ➡ are more typical of melanoma. *(Right)* This melanoma is readily identified by immunoreactivity to mart-1. Other melanoma markers such as S100, HMB-45, or Melan-A would also be positive. These cells would be negative for cytokeratins and CEA.

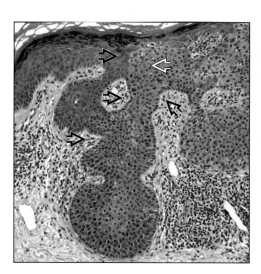
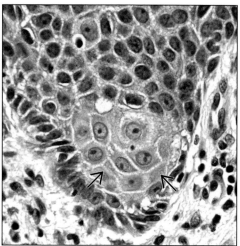

(Left) This squamous cell carcinoma in situ ➡ mimics Paget disease by being surrounded by normal squamous cells ➡. However, the cells grow in large sheets of cells (rather than individual cells) and appear cohesive. *(Right)* The cells can be identified as squamous cell carcinoma by their characteristic intercellular bridges ➡. IHC can also be used to demonstrate that the cells are positive for high molecular weight cytokeratins and negative for markers of MPD.

ENCAPSULATED PAPILLARY CARCINOMA

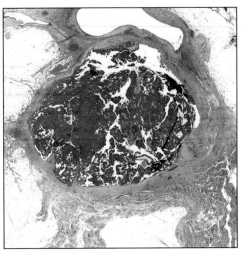

Encapsulated papillary carcinoma occurs as a well-circumscribed mass, usually located in the central breast below the nipple. Many cases are associated with nipple discharge.

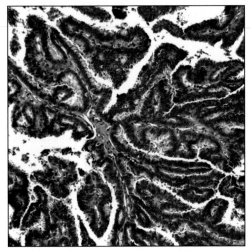

The carcinoma consists of delicate papillae with thin fibrovascular cores. The cells are often columnar in shape and monotonous in appearance.

TERMINOLOGY

Abbreviations
- Encapsulated papillary carcinoma (EPC)

Synonyms
- Intracystic papillary carcinoma
- Encysted papillary carcinoma

Definitions
- Papillary carcinoma present within single well-circumscribed cystic space

CLINICAL ISSUES

Epidemiology
- Incidence
  - 0.5-2% of breast cancers in women
    - Rare in men but more common than invasive ductal carcinoma or DCIS
- Age
  - Most common in elderly women (median: 70 years)

Presentation
- Often presents as palpable mass or circumscribed mammographic density
  - Location is usually central below nipple
  - Usually deeper in breast than large duct papillomas
- Some women present with nipple discharge

Natural History
- EPC was originally classified as DCIS
  - Lymph node metastases are rare
  - Macrometastases have been reported in rare cases; associated carcinomas are often exceptionally large
  - Cases of isolated tumor cells in nodes may be related to epithelial displacement by prior core needle biopsy
- Survival is > 95% at 10 years

- Although absence of myoepithelial cells is more compatible with classification as invasive carcinoma, clinical behavior is more similar to DCIS

MICROSCOPIC PATHOLOGY

Histologic Features
- Carcinoma is confined to well-circumscribed space
- Outer capsule is generally fibrotic with scattering of lymphocytes
  - Entrapment of epithelium within capsule may occur
- Delicate thin papillary fronds with thin fibrovascular core
- Fronds are lined by single layer of monotonous-appearing columnar cells
- Occasional globoid cells may be present
  - More abundant pale cytoplasm and rounded in shape
  - Often positive for GCDFP-15
  - Should not be misinterpreted as myoepithelial cells
- Approximately 25% of cases are associated with areas of frank stromal invasion
  - Invasive carcinoma extends beyond fibrous capsule of lesion
  - Carcinoma is generally of no special type and is not papillary in appearance

ANCILLARY TESTS

Immunohistochemistry
- Estrogen and progesterone receptors are positive in almost all cases
- HER2 is absent
- Myoepithelial markers will confirm absence of myoepithelial cells in papillary fronds and in surrounding capsule
  - p63 is most useful marker for detecting myoepithelial cells in papillary fronds

ENCAPSULATED PAPILLARY CARCINOMA

Key Facts

Terminology
- Papillary carcinoma present within single well-circumscribed cystic space
- Synonyms: Encysted papillary carcinoma, intracystic carcinoma

Clinical Issues
- 0.5-2% of breast cancers in women
- Most common in elderly women (median age: 70)
- Often presents as palpable mass or circumscribed mammographic density
- Some women present with nipple discharge
- Survival is > 95% at 10 years
- Although absence of myoepithelial cells is more compatible with classification as invasive carcinoma, clinical behavior is more similar to DCIS

Ancillary Tests
- Estrogen and progesterone receptors are positive in almost all cases
- HER2 is absent
- Myoepithelial markers will confirm absence of myoepithelial cells in papillary fronds and in surrounding capsule
- p63 is most useful marker for detecting myoepithelial cells in papillary fronds
- Collagen type IV is present around periphery of lesion

Top Differential Diagnoses
- Ductal carcinoma in situ, papillary type
- Solid papillary carcinoma
- Large duct papilloma

- o Endothelial cells often lie close to tumor cells and will also be positive for muscle markers (e.g., smooth muscle actin, calponin)
- Collagen type IV is present around periphery of lesion

DIFFERENTIAL DIAGNOSIS

Ductal Carcinoma In Situ, Papillary Type
- Usually involves multiple ductal spaces
- Myoepithelial cells will be present around periphery of involved ducts
- DCIS partially involving a papilloma may be difficult to diagnose
  - o In general, DCIS will also be present in surrounding breast tissue

Solid Papillary Carcinoma
- Growth pattern is solid with fibrovascular cores rather than cystic
- Multiple nodules are usually present, rather than single dilated space as in EPC
- If myoepithelial cells are present at periphery, lesion is classified as DCIS
  - o In some cases, myoepithelial cells are absent at periphery
  - o These cases have very favorable prognosis with only rare lymph node metastases
- Approximately 2/3 will be positive for neuroendocrine markers (chromogranin or synaptophysin)

Large Duct Papilloma
- Also occurs in central breast and often associated with nipple discharge
- Lesion grows as arborizing papillary fronds within dilated space similar to EPC
- Fibrovascular cores are generally thicker in caliber
- Cell population appears more heterogeneous; apocrine metaplasia may be present
- Well-developed myoepithelial cell layer is present within and surrounding outer portion of lesion

STAGING

AJCC T Classification
- Although absence of peripheral myoepithelial cells suggests EPC may be a type of invasive carcinoma, clinical outcome is more similar to DCIS
- If frank stromal invasion is present, T classification should be based on size of area of invasion
  - o Size should not include area of EPC
- If only a solitary circumscribed mass is present, classification as Tis (DCIS) may be most appropriate
  - o Difficulty in classifying this type of carcinoma should be described in a note

SELECTED REFERENCES

1. Koerner F: Papilloma and papillary carcinoma. Semin Diagn Pathol. 27(1):13-30, 2010
2. Esposito NN et al: Are encapsulated papillary carcinomas of the breast in situ or invasive? A basement membrane study of 27 cases. Am J Clin Pathol. 131(2):228-42, 2009
3. Seal M et al: Encapsulated apocrine papillary carcinoma of the breast--a tumour of uncertain malignant potential: report of five cases. Virchows Arch. 455(6):477-83, 2009
4. Tse GM et al: The role of immunohistochemistry in the differential diagnosis of papillary lesions of the breast. J Clin Pathol. 62(5):407-13, 2009
5. Mulligan AM et al: Metastatic potential of encapsulated (intracystic) papillary carcinoma of the breast: a report of 2 cases with axillary lymph node micrometastases. Int J Surg Pathol. 15(2):143-7, 2007
6. Collins LC et al: Intracystic papillary carcinomas of the breast: a reevaluation using a panel of myoepithelial cell markers. Am J Surg Pathol. 30(8):1002-7, 2006

ENCAPSULATED PAPILLARY CARCINOMA

Imaging and Microscopic Features

(Left) EPC typically presents as a circumscribed mass ⮞, located deep to the nipple. The lesion is often associated with nipple discharge. *(Right)* EPC grows as a papillary proliferation with well-circumscribed or lobulated margins ⮞. The surrounding capsule is often composed of reactive stroma with a few lymphocytes. DCIS, often of papillary type, may be present in the adjacent tissue ⮞. Adjacent DCIS increases the risk of local recurrence.

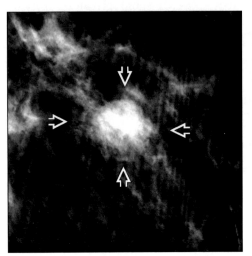
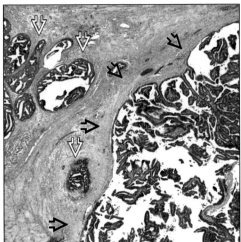

(Left) IHC demonstrates p63-positive myoepithelial cells associated with DCIS →. However, EPC is devoid of myoepithelial cells in the papillary fronds ➔ or at the periphery of the lesion ⮞. *(Right)* The fibrovascular cores are thin and delicate. The endothelial cells of blood vessels ⮞ are often very close to the base of the epithelial cells. IHC for muscle markers may be difficult to interpret as both endothelial cells and myoepithelial cells will be positive.

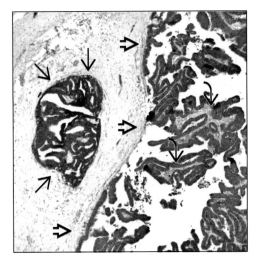
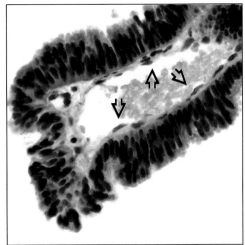

(Left) Globoid cells ⮞ are a type of epithelial cell frequently seen in papillary lesions. The cells have increased pale eosinophilic cytoplasm and a rounded contour. They are frequently positive for GCDFP-15. They should not be mistaken for myoepithelial cells. *(Right)* Papillary lesions, both benign and malignant, frequently give rise to epithelial displacement within biopsy tracks ➔. This phenomenon can make evaluation of invasion difficult in some cases. Isolated tumor cells can also be present in lymph nodes.

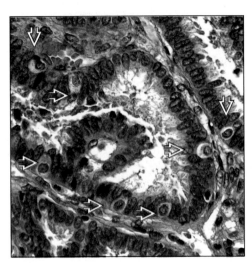
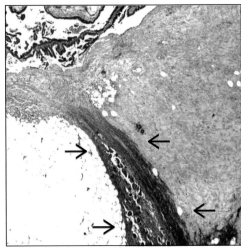

ENCAPSULATED PAPILLARY CARCINOMA

Differential Diagnosis

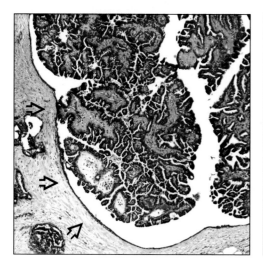

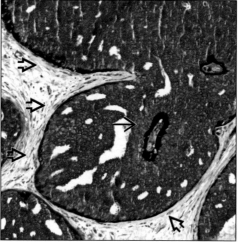

(Left) Papillary DCIS may involve a cystic space, but DCIS involving smaller ducts is almost always present in the surrounding tissue. Myoepithelial cells will be absent from the fibrovascular cores but present at the periphery ⊋. *(Right)* This DCIS has a solid papillary pattern with fibrovascular cores lined by myoepithelial cells (positive for smooth muscle actin) within ductal spaces ➡. Myoepithelial cells are also present at the periphery of the ductal spaces ⊋.

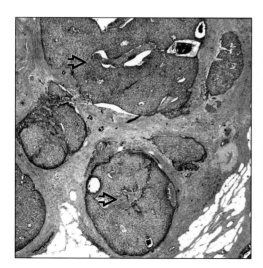

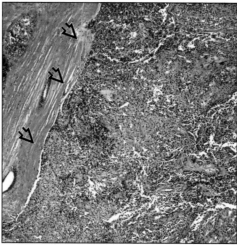

(Left) Unlike EPC, which presents as a solitary cystic mass, solid papillary carcinomas are seen as multiple circumscribed nests. Note fibrovascular cores within the central portions of the tumor cell nodules ⊋. *(Right)* Solid papillary carcinomas are often positive for neuroendocrine markers such as chromogranin or synaptophysin. Some carcinomas with this appearance have peripheral myoepithelial cells and are classified as DCIS, and others lack myoepithelial cells ⊋.

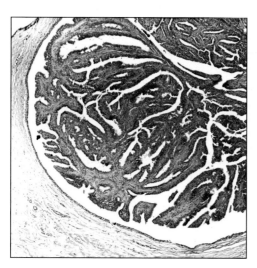

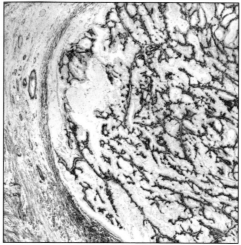

(Left) Large duct papillomas generally have broader fibrovascular cores. The cell population is more heterogeneous in appearance, and apocrine metaplasia is often present. Like EPC, these lesions are often centrally located and associated with nipple discharge. *(Right)* Papillomas have a prominent myoepithelial cell layer within the papillary fronds, as well as around the outer periphery, as seen in this study for smooth muscle actin.

DUCTAL CARCINOMA IN SITU WITH MICROINVASION

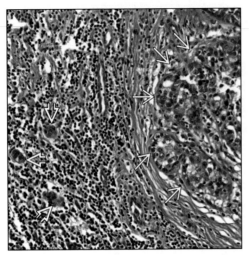
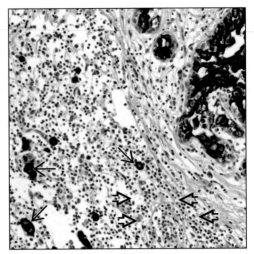

The dominant lesion in DCISM is in situ carcinoma ➡ (typically high grade) associated with microscopic foci of cancer cells ⧩ invading beyond the basement membrane into the adjacent stroma.

Frequently, stromal inflammation ⧩ surrounds the DCIS and can obscure the tumor cells. IHC for cytokeratins help identify foci of early stromal invasion ➡ and confirm the diagnosis of DCISM.

TERMINOLOGY

Abbreviations
- Ductal carcinoma in situ with microinvasion (DCISM)

Synonyms
- Microinvasive ductal carcinoma in situ
- Foci of "early stromal invasion"

Definitions
- DCIS with extension of cancer cells beyond basement membrane lining ducts and lobules
- Largest area of invasion ≤ 1 mm in size
  - DCISM has been divided into 2 types
    - Type 1: Single cells
    - Type 2: Clusters of cells

ETIOLOGY/PATHOGENESIS

Pathogenesis
- Transition from DCIS to invasive cancer is poorly understood
  - No gene expression patterns specific to invasive carcinoma have been identified
  - Loss of normal luminal cell signaling may lead to dysfunction of myoepithelial and stromal cells maintaining basement membrane
    - Myoepithelial cells associated with DCIS show abnormal loss of myoepithelial cell markers
  - Thus invasion may be primarily initiated by loss of normal function of supporting cells rather than gain of function by carcinoma
- Several studies have compared biologic properties between DCISM and DCIS
  - DCISM is characterized by higher proliferative rate and enhanced apoptosis
  - DCISM shows higher levels of expression for a number of matrix metalloproteases

CLINICAL ISSUES

Epidemiology
- Incidence
  - DCISM is an uncommon entity accounting for < 1% of all breast cancers
- Age
  - Range: 32-78 years (mean: 56.4 years)

Presentation
- Up to 50% of cases present as palpable mass
  - Imaging findings may include abnormal density with or without associated microcalcifications
  - Up to 20% patients may also experience serosanguineous nipple discharge
  - Some patients present with Paget disease of nipple
- Several studies have shown correlation between extent of DCIS and presence of microinvasion
  - High-grade DCIS with comedonecrosis is most common architectural pattern reported for DCISM
  - Presence of extensive high-grade DCIS correlates with presentation as palpable mass more commonly than DCIS without microinvasion

Prognosis
- Overall prognosis for DCISM is excellent
  - 5-year survival: 97-100%
- Outcome for patients with DCISM may depend on number of foci of microinvasion identified
  - DCISM with single focus of microinvasion consisting of single cells (type 1) usually has outcome similar to pure DCIS
  - DCISM with multiple foci of microinvasion consisting of clusters of cells (type 2) may have worse prognosis
- Lymph node metastases reported in < 10% of patients with DCISM
  - Metastases are usually micrometastases to single node

DUCTAL CARCINOMA IN SITU WITH MICROINVASION

Key Facts

Terminology

- Ductal carcinoma in situ with microinvasion (DCISM)
- 1 or more separate microscopic foci of tumor cells infiltrating into periductal stroma
- No invasive focus measuring > 1 mm in greatest dimension
- DCISM is classified as AJCC T1mi

Clinical Issues

- DCISM is uncommon, accounting for < 1% of all breast cancers
  - Up to 50% of patients present with palpable mass
  - Up to 20% of patients may also experience serosanguineous nipple discharge
- Overall prognosis for DCISM is excellent

- Outcome may depend on tumor burden and number of foci of microinvasion identified

Image Findings

- Radiographic features will be similar to pure DCIS of equivalent size and grade

Microscopic Pathology

- Typically, DCISM occurs in extensive area of high-grade DCIS
  - Periductal stromal changes are frequent finding
- Rarely, microinvasion can occur with low-grade DCIS, LCIS, or in absence of carcinoma in situ

Top Differential Diagnoses

- DCIS with cancerization of lobules
- Invasive cancer with extensive DCIS
- Artifactual displacement of tumor cells

- May be associated with large areas of DCIS that are not completely sampled, raising possibility of missed area of invasion

MACROSCOPIC FEATURES

General Features

- DCISM is generally associated with stromal response leading to abnormal gross appearance
- Tissue is usually firm but without formation of discrete mass
- Color is typically white or gray
- If comedo DCIS is present, small punctate areas of necrosis will be seen if tissue is gently squeezed
- Areas of homogeneous appearance are most likely to be associated with stromal invasion

Sections to Be Submitted

- If possible, entire area of grossly abnormal tissue corresponding to DCISM should be examined microscopically
- Additional sampling may reveal larger areas of invasion or lymph-vascular invasion

MICROSCOPIC PATHOLOGY

Histologic Features

- DCISM is defined as DCIS with ≥ 1 focus of ≤ 1 mm invasion in size
  - Foci of tumor cells penetrate basement membrane and extend into nonspecialized periductal stroma
    - Areas of microinvasion can be single focus or multiple foci
    - Tumor cells must not be attached to area of DCIS
- DCISM is usually associated with extensive area of comedo DCIS or other types of high-grade DCIS
- Periductal stromal changes are frequent
  - Periductal and perilobular dense lymphocytic infiltrates are typically present
    - Significant areas of inflammation can obscure foci of microinvasion

- Cases of high-grade DCIS with periductal inflammation should be carefully evaluated to rule out microinvasion
  - Altered periductal desmoplastic stroma response may be seen
- Microinvasion in cases of mucin-producing DCIS may be difficult to identify
  - Ducts involved by DCIS can rupture, resulting in stromal extravasation of mucin
  - Neither invasion nor microinvasion should be diagnosed unless tumor cells are present within mucin
- Morphologic patterns of microinvasive foci
  - True microinvasion will frequently adopt different morphologic appearance compared with pure DCIS
    - Invasive tumor cells beyond basement membrane often appear as single cells
    - Nests, cell clusters, or acinar formation by tumor cells will show angulated or infiltrative pattern
- Surrounding myoepithelial cells are absent in foci of true microinvasion
- In rare cases, lymph-vascular invasion can be present in DCISM
- Less frequently, microinvasion is associated with low-grade DCIS or LCIS, or, very rarely, in absence of carcinoma in situ

ANCILLARY TESTS

Immunohistochemistry

- Breast cancer biomarkers
  - ER, PR, and HER2 IHC should be attempted on all cases with unequivocal DCISM
  - Areas of microinvasion may be lost when deeper levels are examined for immunostains
    - ER, PR, and HER2 status of associated DCIS may be used as surrogate for biomarkers of invasive foci
    - Very unusual for area of microinvasion to have different pattern from associated DCIS

DUCTAL CARCINOMA IN SITU WITH MICROINVASION

Differential Diagnosis: DCISM vs. DCIS

Microscopic Features	DCISM	DCIS
DCIS grade	More commonly high grade (comedonecrosis)	Any grade
Extent of disease	More commonly extensive or multifocal disease	Any extent
Stromal response	May show periductal lymphocytic infiltrates around involved duct spaces and desmoplastic stroma (may obscure microinvasion)	Lymphocytic infiltrates and desmoplastic stroma are less common
Myoepithelial cells	Absence of myoepithelial cells in areas of microinvasion	Myoepithelial cells surround areas of DCIS
Architectural pattern	Microinvasion appears as single cells or angulated nests and glands in infiltrative pattern	Rounded contours of involved duct spaces, lobulocentric pattern

- Marker status of both DCIS and microinvasion should be reported
- Myoepithelial cell markers
  - Deeper levels and immunostudies for myoepithelial cells can be useful for confirming diagnosis of DCISM
  - Panel of myoepithelial markers (p63, calponin, smooth muscle myosin heavy chain) is recommended
    - Myoepithelial cells associated with DCIS may lose expression of 1 or more markers
  - IHC with 2 markers (e.g., keratin and p63 or keratin and smooth muscle myosin heavy chain) are useful for identifying small foci of invasive carcinoma
    - Without both markers, it may be difficult to distinguish tumor cells from reactive stromal cells or endothelial cells
    - Often, if 1 area of microinvasion is no longer present, another focus may appear in another area of slide

DIFFERENTIAL DIAGNOSIS

DCIS with Cancerization of Lobules
- Extensive lobular cancerization by DCIS may be difficult to distinguish from DCISM
  - Cancerization of lobules maintains lobulocentric pattern best seen on low magnification
  - Groups of tumor cells within lobular acini typically show rounded contours
  - Areas of branching cut tangentially can mimic microinvasion
- Cancerization of lobules can be distinguished from DCISM by presence of associated myoepithelial cells
  - DCISM will lack myoepithelial cells in areas of microinvasion

Invasive Cancer with Extensive DCIS
- Foci of invasion measuring > 1 mm should be classified as invasive breast cancer (T1a)
- If there are foci of microinvasion in addition to larger area of invasion, smaller foci should be reported as additional areas of invasion consisting of microinvasion

Artifactual Displacement of Tumor Cells
- Tumor cells of DCIS can be displaced into stroma due to prior core needle biopsy or surgical excision

- Cells will be surrounded by typical reaction around biopsy site or in needle track
  - Usual desmoplastic and lymphocytic response seen in DCISM is usually absent
- In some cases, myoepithelial cells may still be associated with tumor cells
- However, diagnosis of invasion or microinvasion should not be made if histologic appearance suggests artifactual displacement

DIAGNOSTIC CHECKLIST

Pathologic Interpretation Pearls
- Core needle biopsy
  - DCIS on core needle biopsies of masses is more likely to be associated with microinvasion
    - Presence of microinvasion on core needle biopsy may prompt lymph node sampling
    - Therefore, diagnosis of microinvasion should only be made when definitive features are present in order to avoid unnecessary lymph node evaluation

REPORTING CONSIDERATIONS

Key Elements to Report
- Size of largest focus of microinvasion
  - Number of foci of microinvasion (or number of blocks with microinvasion) should be stated
  - Note any special studies that were utilized to arrive at the diagnosis, such as immunostains for myoepithelial cells
- AJCC classification defines DCISM as T1mi
  - Sizes of multiple foci should not be added together

SELECTED REFERENCES

1. González LO et al: Expression of metalloproteases and their inhibitors by tumor and stromal cells in ductal carcinoma in situ of the breast and their relationship with microinvasive events. J Cancer Res Clin Oncol. 136(9):1313-21, 2010
2. Vieira CC et al: Microinvasive ductal carcinoma in situ: clinical presentation, imaging features, pathologic findings, and outcome. Eur J Radiol. 73(1):102-7, 2010

DUCTAL CARCINOMA IN SITU WITH MICROINVASION

Ancillary Techniques and Differential Diagnosis

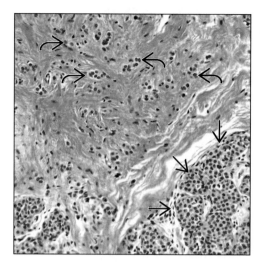

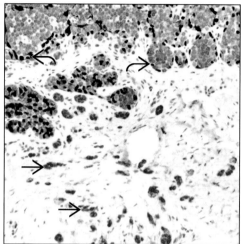

(Left) Microinvasion is most commonly associated with high-grade DCIS. On occasion, microinvasion ➡ can also be seen associated with LCIS ➡, supporting the concept that this lesion can be a precursor to invasive breast cancer in some cases. (Right) The diagnosis of microinvasion can be supported by immunostains for myoepithelial cells. Myoepithelial cells express p63 ➡ in the areas of LCIS. Areas of microinvasion ➡ express cytokeratin 18 and lack myoepithelium.

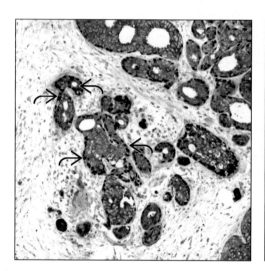

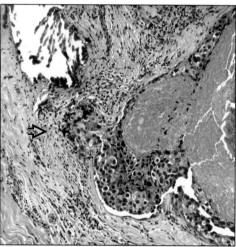

(Left) DCIS with lobular cancerization can mimic foci of microinvasion. The lesion shows a lobulocentric architecture and the small cell nests are all associated with myoepithelial cells ➡, helping to confirm the diagnosis. (Right) Tumor cells are protruding out into stroma from a breach in the basement membrane of this case of high-grade DCIS ➡. However, this finding would not be classified as microinvasion as the cells are still contiguous with the in situ carcinoma.

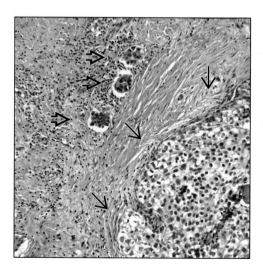

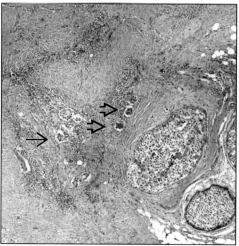

(Left) Multiple clusters of tumor cells ➡ are present in stroma adjacent to DCIS ➡. The appearance is suggestive of microinvasion. (Right) However, a lower power view shows that the tumor cells ➡ are within a biopsy site with fibrosis, giant cells, and chronic inflammation ➡. Such findings should not be classified as microinvasion. IHC sometimes confirms the presence of associated myoepithelial cells. The clinical significance of iatrogenic "microinvasion" is unclear.

HEREDITARY CANCER

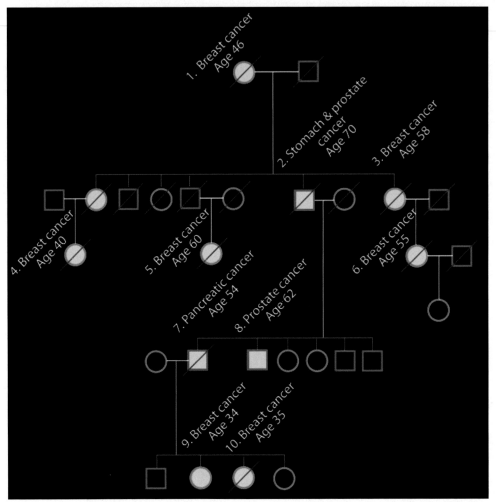

Family history is a powerful tool for detecting highly penetrant genes responsible for breast cancer susceptibility. This pedigree is very suggestive of a germline mutation due to the presence of multiple affected family members and the development of cancers at a young age. Inheritance can occur through both men and women. Genetic testing could determine if any of the currently recognized mutations are present or establish the significance of a yet undescribed mutation if it consistently maps to individuals with cancer. Some cancers in families (e.g., individual #5 who developed cancer at an older age with an unaffected parent) may be sporadic and not related to an inherited mutation.

HEREDITARY BREAST CANCER

Familial Breast Cancer
- Long recognized that many women with breast cancer also have affected relatives
  - ~ 10-25% of patients have a 1st-degree relative (parent, sister, daughter) with breast cancer
  - Having affected 1st-degree relative increases patient risk by 2-3x
  - Women whose only family history is mother developing postmenopausal cancer are not at increased risk
    - Majority of postmenopausal breast cancers are sporadic
- 5-10% of breast cancers have been linked to specific high penetrance germline mutations
  - High penetrance = RR > 10
  - Moderate penetrance = RR 2-3
  - Low penetrance = RR < 1.5
    - Penetrance may be gender dependent for associated cancers (e.g., female carriers are at higher risk for breast cancer than males)
- Remainder of familial risk is likely due to multiple genes of lower penetrance
  - Unlikely that another highly penetrant gene comparable to *BRCA1* or *2* will be identified

Most Common Germline Mutations
- Majority of germline mutations associated with breast cancer risk are involved in DNA repair pathways
  - Tissue specificity for breast cancers is not understood
  - Mutations are autosomal dominant alleles and thus can be inherited via both females and males
- *BRCA1* (**familial breast and ovarian cancer**)
  - *BRCA1* and *2* help maintain genomic stability
    - Direct role in regulation of DNA-damage responses and repair and cell cycle checkpoints
    - Inactivating mutations impair conservative DNA repair and genomic stability functions

HEREDITARY CANCER

- Cells lacking *BRCA1* & *2* functional activity prone to replication errors and genomic instability
- Accumulating DNA abnormalities enable mutations in genes essential to cell cycle check point activation
- Drives acquisition of mutations and chromosomal instability, contributing to tumor formation
  - *BRCA1* function is required for transactivation of the estrogen receptor gene promoter
    - May explain why 90% of *BRCA1*-associated carcinomas are ER(-)
  - Incidence: ~ 1 in 860
    - More common in some ethnic groups: Ashkenazi Jews, Finns, French Canadians
  - High penetrance: 45-70% lifetime risk
    - Magnitude of risk can vary for different mutations and for different types of cancers
    - Responsible for ~ 1/2 of cancers known to be due to a germline mutation (~ 2% of all breast cancers)
  - Other associated cancers
    - Ovarian (40-50% lifetime risk), fallopian tube, peritoneal, and pancreatic cancer
    - Male breast cancer (1-5% lifetime risk, but ~ 1/2 risk of *BRCA2*)
  - ~ 90% of *BRCA1* cancers share same gene expression pattern with basal-type carcinomas
    - Basal carcinomas may also have defective *BRCA1* function
  - Cancers share morphologic features
    - Mutation can be suspected in young patients (35% risk if grade 3 cancer is ER(-) and patient < 30 years of age)
- *BRCA2* (familial breast and ovarian cancer syndrome)
  - Although *BRCA2* is not structurally related to *BRCA1*, the functions of these genes are very similar
  - Incidence: ~ 1 in 740
    - More common in some ethnic groups: Ashkenazi Jews, Icelandic populations
  - High penetrance: 40-60% lifetime risk
    - Magnitude of risk can vary for different mutations and for different types of cancers
    - Responsible for ~ 1/3 of cancers known to be due to a germline mutation (~ 1% of all breast cancers)
  - Other associated cancers
    - Ovarian (10-20% lifetime risk), fallopian tube, prostate, pancreatic, gallbladder, stomach, bile duct cancers, melanoma
    - Male breast cancer: 5-10% lifetime risk; approximately 5-15% of cases are associated with *BRCA2*
  - Cancers group with luminal A type by gene expression profiling
- *CDH1* (familial gastric cancer and lobular breast cancer syndrome)
  - *CDH1* encodes the gene for E-cadherin
  - Inherited mutations increase risk for signet ring cell carcinomas of stomach and lobular carcinoma
    - Majority of women with lobular carcinomas do not have *CDH1* germline mutations

- 40-85% lifetime risk of developing gastric signet ring cell carcinoma in majority of families
  - Gastric carcinomas are more common than breast carcinomas in most affected families
  - Families developing only breast cancer have also been identified
- *PTEN* (Cowden syndrome)
  - Dual specificity phosphatase gene involved in apoptosis
  - Incidence: ~ 1 in 300,000
  - Characterized by multiple hamartomas (including trichilemmomas)
    - Breast lesions include fibroadenomas and hamartomas
  - Increased risk of breast, thyroid, and endometrial cancer
    - Women have a 25-50% lifetime risk of breast cancer
    - Men also at increased risk for breast cancer
- *TP53* (Li Fraumeni syndrome)
  - *P53* has central role in cell cycle control, DNA replication, DNA repair, and apoptosis
  - Increased risk of soft tissue sarcoma, osteosarcoma, breast cancer, brain tumors, leukemia, adrenocortical cancer (90% of patients develop some type of tumor by age 70)
    - Breast cancer is 1/3 of malignancies in affected families; found in ~ 1% of women with breast cancer < age of 40
    - ~ 55% of women will develop breast cancer by age 45 (average age at diagnosis is 36)
    - Other tumors, particularly sarcomas and brain tumors, can develop in childhood
    - 30% of tumors occur in individuals 15 years of age or younger
  - Somatic *P53* mutations are also frequently found in *BRCA1* and *2* associated carcinomas
- *ATM* (ataxia-telangiectasia carriers)
  - Serine threonine kinase that phosphorylates *TP53* and *BRCA1* in response to DNA double strand breaks
  - Incidence: 0.2-1%
  - Homozygosity results in ataxia-telangiectasia
    - Progressive cerebellar ataxia, oculocutaneous telangiectasias, immunodeficiency, and increased risk of leukemia and lymphoma
  - Heterozygosity increases risk of breast cancer
    - 11% by age 50 and 30% by age 70
- *CHEK2* (Li Fraumeni variant syndrome)
  - Cell cycle checkpoint gene involved in DNA repair
  - Incidence: 1 in 100
  - Low penetrance: 10-20% lifetime risk of breast cancer for females and males
- *STK11/LKB1* (Peutz-Jeghers syndrome)
  - Serine/threonine kinase that functions as a tumor suppressor
  - Incidence: 1 in 20,000
  - Characterized by hamartomatous gastrointestinal polyps (including small intestine) and skin pigmentation (lips and buccal mucosa)

○ Increased risk of cancers of colon, breast, stomach, pancreas, small intestine, thyroid, lung, uterus, ovaries, cervix
- *BRIP1* (FANCJ or BACH1)
  ○ DNA helicase that interacts with *BRCA1* to carry out its functions
    ▪ Mutations result in defects in DNA repair
  ○ Homozygosity results in Fanconi anemia
  ○ Heterozygosity increases risk of breast cancer
    ▪ Low to moderate penetrance

Patterns of Familial Cancer Likely to be Associated with Germline Mutations
- Affected 1st-degree relatives (mother, sister, daughter)
- Multiple relatives affected, particularly if 1st degree
- Carcinomas occurring at an early age (premenopausal)
- Individuals with history of multiple cancers
- Relatives with non-breast cancers associated with particular germline mutation
  ○ Male breast cancer for *BRCA2* or *1*
  ○ Ovarian cancers for *BRCA1* and *2*
  ○ Sarcomas for *TP53*

MICROSCOPIC FINDINGS

General Features
- Only *BRCA1*-associated and *CDH1*-associated carcinomas have specific morphologic features
- *BRCA1*-associated carcinomas
  ○ Morphology of invasive carcinomas
    ▪ Circumscribed growth pattern with pushing borders
    ▪ Dense lymphocytic infiltrate (T cell predominant)
    ▪ Geographic necrosis
    ▪ High proliferative rate
    ▪ High nuclear grade
    ▪ Syncytial growth pattern
  ○ Morphology of DCIS
    ▪ ER/PR/HER2 negative DCIS is uncommon: < 10% of all DCIS cases
    ▪ Usually has a solid pattern with high-grade pleomorphic nuclei
    ▪ Involved lobules may be associated with a dense lymphocytic infiltrate
    ▪ May be subtle with little expansion of involved lobular acini
  ○ Precursor lesions
    ▪ T-cell lobulitis has been described in prophylactic mastectomies for *BRCA1* mutations
    ▪ More common compared to women undergoing the procedure for other reasons
    ▪ Infiltrate similar to that seen associated with carcinomas
  ○ Tumor markers
    ▪ Lack hormone receptor positivity
    ▪ Lack overexpression of HER2: Both *HER2* and *BRCA1* are on long arm of chromosome 17, and loss of heterozygosity may affect both
    ▪ Majority express p53
    ▪ Majority positive for basal markers such as EGFR (HER1), cytokeratin 5/6, cytokeratin 14

○ Medullary carcinomas are overrepresented: 13% of cases vs. < 5% for all women
  ▪ Majority of women with medullary carcinomas do not have *BRCA1* mutations
○ Additional *BRCA1* carcinomas have "medullary features" but not all criteria for this diagnosis
- *CDH1*-associated carcinomas
  ○ Loss of E-cadherin prevents cell adhesion resulting in single tumor cells with rounded contours
    ▪ Many tumor cells have intracellular mucin (signet ring cells)
  ○ Gastric carcinomas and breast carcinomas can resemble each other closely
    ▪ Breast signet ring cells are more likely to have a single mucin vacuole with a central dot
    ▪ Gastric signet ring cells are more likely to have bubbly vacuolated cytoplasm
  ○ IHC may be helpful in some cases to distinguish primary and metastatic carcinomas
    ▪ Breast carcinomas are typically ER(+), PR(+), GCDFP-15(+), and MUC1(+)
    ▪ Gastric carcinomas are typically ER(-), PR(-), GCDFP-15(-), and MUC1(-), while typically CDX-2(+) and Hep-Par1(+)
- *BRCA2*-associated carcinomas
  ○ Not strongly associated with a specific morphologic appearance
    ▪ Some studies suggest higher incidence of cancers belonging to tubular-lobular group (pleomorphic lobular)
    ▪ More commonly grade 3
    ▪ Other series have not shown significant differences between *BRCA2* tumors & sporadic breast cancer
  ○ Most often ER(+), unlike *BRCA1*-associated carcinomas
    ▪ Most do not overexpress HER2

GENETIC TESTING FOR *BRCA1* & *2*

Types of Genetic Changes
- > 1,000 mutations reported for *BRCA1* and *2*
  ○ Majority are small deletions or insertions resulting in frameshift mutations, nonsense mutations, or splice site alterations
    ▪ Result in truncated or absent protein
    ▪ Less common are full-length proteins with missense mutations
  ○ Approximately 18% are large gene rearrangements or deletions not detectable by conventional mutation analysis
    ▪ Additional types of testing are required to detect these types of mutations
- Mutations distributed throughout the length of each gene
  ○ Requires full direct sequencing to exclude abnormality
    ▪ Significant expense associated with testing
    ▪ Mutations not associated with known risk may be of uncertain significance
- Specific mutations are characteristic of some ethnic groups

HEREDITARY CANCER

Syndromes Associated with Hereditary Breast Cancer

Syndrome	Gene	Clinical Features
Hereditary breast and ovarian cancer syndrome	BRCA1 (17q21)	High risk for breast cancer (50-80%); high risk for ovarian cancer (40-50%); prostate cancer, pancreatic cancer, fallopian tube cancer
Hereditary breast and ovarian cancer syndrome	BRCA2 (13q12.3)	High risk for breast cancer (50-70%); intermediate risk for ovarian cancer (10-20%); prostate cancer, pancreatic cancer, lobular histology (pleomorphic) more common in some reports
Li-Fraumeni syndrome	TP53 (17p13.1)	High risk for breast cancers (young age); risk of sarcomas, osteosarcomas, brain tumors, adrenocortical carcinoma, and leukemia
Cowden syndrome	PTEN (10q23.31)	Multiple hamartomas; breast lesions include fibroadenomas and hamartomas; increased risk of breast, thyroid, endometrial carcinomas, and others
Hereditary diffuse gastric cancer syndrome	CDH1 (16q22.1)	Risk for gastric signet ring cell carcinoma and lobular carcinoma of the breast (CDH1 encodes gene for E-cadherin)
Peutz-Jeghers syndrome	STK11/LKB1 (19p13.3)	Hamartomatous polyps of GI tract and skin pigmentation; increased risk of cancers of colon, breast, stomach, small intestine, pancreas, and others

○ Ashkenazi Jewish populations (1 in 40 individuals may be a carrier): 90% of mutations are 1 of 3 types
  ▪ BRCA1: 185delAG and 5382insC
  ▪ BRCA2: 6174delT
○ Icelandic: BRCA2: 999del5 accounts for 7% of cases
• 7% of individuals are found to have a variant of uncertain significance (VUS)
○ VUS: Genetic polymorphism that has not yet been associated with an increased risk of cancer
○ > 1,500 identified
○ More frequent in minority ethnic populations
○ Must be identified in multiple individuals to determine clinical significance
• Family testing
○ Once a mutation is identified in an individual, other family members may choose testing
○ Analysis for the specific mutation in other family members considerably less expensive

Patient Selection for Testing
• Careful patient selection important to optimize testing
○ Counseling should occur before testing to ensure patient is aware of possible implications for individual and family
• American Society of Clinical Oncology recommends that patients with > 10% mutation risk should be considered for testing
• Several models have been developed to help predict the probability of a germline mutation
○ **BRCAPRO**
  ▪ Statistical model and software for predicting individual probability for carrying a BRCA1 or BRCA2 mutation
  ▪ Based on patient age and family history of breast and ovarian cancer
  ▪ Utilizes a Mendelian approach that assumes autosomal dominant inheritance
  ▪ Available at http://astor.som.jhmi.edu/BayesMendel/brcapro.html

CLINICAL MANAGEMENT

Increased Surveillance
• Mammography at earlier age (10 years after youngest relative with cancer diagnosis) or more frequently

• MR screening more sensitive than mammography in young women with dense breasts

Surgical Risk Reduction
• Women with BRCA1 & 2 mutations are at increased risk for subsequent ipsilateral (~ 25%) and contralateral (~ 30-40%) cancer at 10 years
○ Ipsilateral cancers are likely new primary cancers rather than true recurrences
○ Recurrence does not alter survival as 2nd cancers are likely found at an early stage
• Bilateral mastectomy reduces risk by 97%
○ Not all breast tissue can be removed in all patients with acceptable cosmetic results
○ Major benefit to women prior to development of breast cancer; limited or no benefit after breast cancer diagnosis with possible distant metastases
• Bilateral salpingo-oophorectomy for mutations associated with ovarian cancer
○ Reduces risk of ovarian and fallopian tube cancer by 70-96%
○ Reduces risk of breast cancer by 50%, presumably due to decrease in hormone production
○ Reduces risk of ER(-) breast cancers for BRCA1 patients; mechanism is unknown

Chemoprevention
• Tamoxifen reduces risk of subsequent ipsilateral and contralateral cancer in breast cancer patients with BRCA1 and 2 germline mutations
• Benefit of chemoprevention for carriers without breast cancer is less clear, as few women have been studied

SELECTED REFERENCES
1. Paradiso A et al: Hereditary breast cancer: clinical features and risk reduction strategies. Ann Oncol. 22 Suppl 1:i31-6, 2011
2. Xie ZM et al: Germline mutations of the E-cadherin gene in families with inherited invasive lobular breast carcinoma but no diffuse gastric cancer. Cancer. Epub ahead of print, 2011
3. Vargas AC et al: The contribution of breast cancer pathology to statistical models to predict mutation risk in BRCA carriers. Fam Cancer. 9(4):545-53, 2010
4. Gorski JJ et al: The complex relationship between BRCA1 and ERalpha in hereditary breast cancer. Clin Cancer Res. 15(5):1514-8, 2009

BRCA1-associated Carcinomas

(Left) *An area of clumped linear enhancement* → *was detected on screening MR of a woman with a BRCA1 mutation. The area corresponded to DCIS that was not detected by mammography as no calcifications were present. MR can be a useful technique to detect cancers in young high-risk women with dense parenchyma.* *(Right)* *This DCIS detected by MR in a young woman with a BRCA1 mutation has high-grade nuclei. It is associated with a lymphocytic infiltrate and is negative for ER, PR, & HER2.*

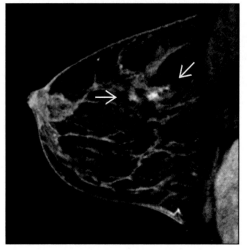
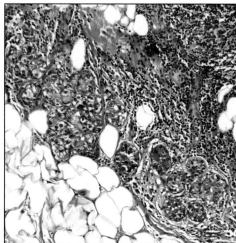

(Left) *Perilobular lymphocytic lobulitis can be seen in the breast tissue of women with BRCA1 mutations. The lymphocytes are predominantly T cells as are the lymphocytes associated with carcinomas. Benign inflammatory lesions of the breast are associated with B cells.* *(Right)* *A rapidly enlarging circumscribed grade 3 invasive carcinoma* → *with a lymphocytic infiltrate* → *negative for hormone receptors and HER2 is very suggestive of a BRCA1-associated cancer in a young woman.*

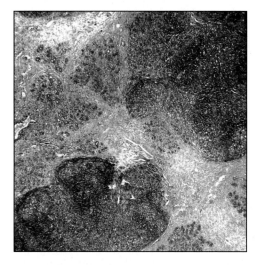
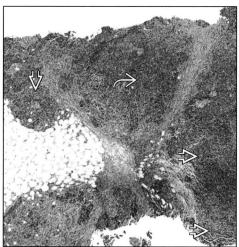

(Left) *BRCA1-associated cancers typically have a syncytial (sheet-like) growth pattern, high-grade pleomorphic nuclei, and numerous mitoses* →. *(Right)* *Carcinomas associated with BRCA1 mutations often show diffuse reactivity for CK5/6* →, *frequently have P53 mutations, and are negative for ER, PR, and HER2. Proliferation is evaluated by mitotic rate and by cell cycle markers such as Ki-67. These carcinomas cluster with basal-like carcinomas by gene expression profiling.*

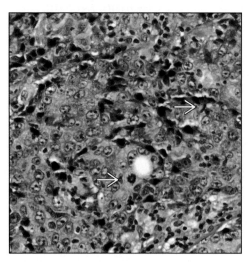
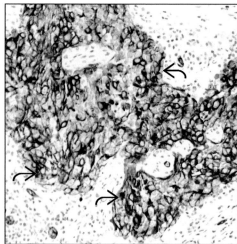

HEREDITARY CANCER

BRCA2- and CDH1-associated Breast Cancer

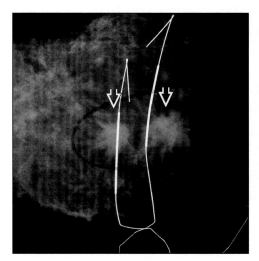

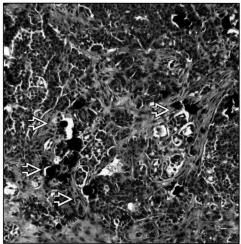

(Left) Patients with germline mutations are more likely to develop multiple cancers ➥, either synchronously or metachronously. Prophylactic mastectomy is an effective method to reduce the risk of cancer. *(Right)* Women with BRCA1 mutations and, to a lesser extent, BRCA2 mutations are at high risk for ovarian carcinomas in addition to breast cancers. The most common type is serous carcinoma, seen here as a metastasis to the breast with numerous psammoma body calcifications ➥.

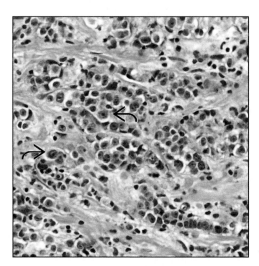

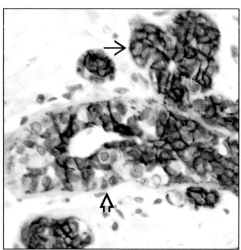

(Left) BRCA2 mutations confer a 2x higher risk of male breast cancer over BRCA1 mutations. Some studies have found a higher incidence of grade 3 lobular carcinomas. This BRCA2-associated lobular carcinoma in a male has high-grade nuclei ➥ and was negative for E-cadherin. *(Right)* Patients with germline CDH1 mutations lose expression of E-cadherin when the normal allele is inactivated. Tumor cells are negative ➥ whereas normal cells show membrane positivity ➥.

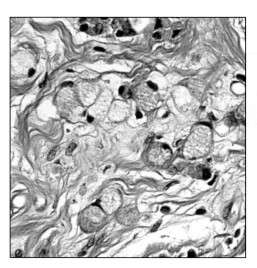

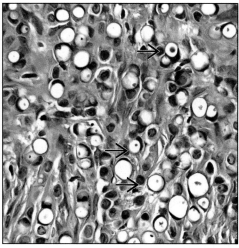

(Left) Families with germline mutations of E-cadherin are at greatest risk for gastric signet ring cell carcinomas. The cells lack adhesion and thus infiltrate as single cells with a rounded contour. The intracellular mucin has a foamy appearance. *(Right)* Individuals with germline E-cadherin mutations can develop lobular carcinomas. The signet ring cells more commonly have a single vacuole with a mucin droplet ➥, rather than the foamy cytoplasm more typical of gastric carcinomas.

CARCINOMAS WITH EXTENSIVE INTRADUCTAL COMPONENT

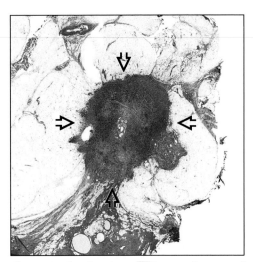

This invasive ductal carcinoma ⊳ is present in an area of fibroadipose tissue. There is no DCIS in the surrounding tissue. This carcinoma would be classified as EIC negative.

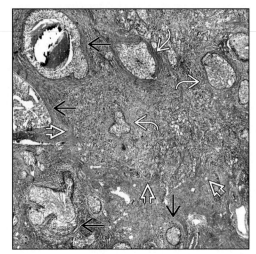

Invasive carcinomas ⊳ may be associated with extensive carcinoma in situ, both within the carcinoma ⇗ and outside the carcinoma ⇨. This carcinoma would be classified as EIC positive.

TERMINOLOGY

Abbreviations
- Extensive intraductal component (EIC)

Definitions
- Classification of extent of DCIS associated with invasive carcinomas
  - Correlated with multiple foci of invasion and margin involvement
  - Increases risk of local recurrence in absence of wide local excision

ETIOLOGY/PATHOGENESIS

Histogenesis
- Subset (25-40%) of invasive carcinomas are associated with extensive DCIS (an EIC) in adjacent tissue
  - Risk of local recurrence is diminished if all DCIS is removed surgically
  - Positive or close margins are predictors of residual DCIS in breast
  - EIC is not predictive for overall survival or distant metastasis
- Multiple foci of invasion may be present
  - EIC is the most common source of multiple synchronous invasive carcinomas
    - If EIC is present, 17% of cases have multiple foci of invasion
    - If EIC is not present, 5% of cases have multiple foci of invasion
  - Multiple carcinomas are usually similar in histologic appearance and marker studies
    - Tend to be smaller than cancers without an EIC
- Larger group (60-75%) of cancers are associated with little or no recognizable DCIS (EIC negative)
  - Triple negative cancers are in this group

- It is possible that triple negative DCIS rapidly progresses to invasion and may be overgrown by invasive component
- LCIS at margins has not been consistently shown to increase likelihood of recurrence
  - EIC is only used for DCIS
  - Studies have not specifically examined cases of LCIS with either high nuclear grade or necrosis
    - Presence of this type of carcinoma in situ at margins should be reported

EPIDEMIOLOGY

Age Range
- Women with EIC-positive carcinomas tend to be younger (40s) and premenopausal

CLINICAL IMPLICATIONS

Clinical Utility
- EIC is used to estimate likelihood of residual carcinoma in breast after excision of invasive carcinoma
- Criteria for EIC were developed for specimens in which invasive carcinoma was excised with a narrow rim of surrounding tissue
- 2 categories of EIC positive cancers
  - Category 1: Both of the following features are present
    - DCIS comprises at least 25% of area within invasive carcinoma
    - DCIS is present outside border of invasive carcinoma
  - Category 2
    - "Extensive" DCIS is present outside border of a "small" carcinoma (approximately ≤ 1 cm in size)
    - Multiple foci of invasion are present in some cases
- Some cancers do not fit well into these 2 categories

CARCINOMAS WITH EXTENSIVE INTRADUCTAL COMPONENT

- ○ If a carcinoma has < 25% DCIS within invasive carcinoma but extensive carcinoma in surrounding tissue, it should not be categorized as EIC negative
- ○ In these cases, an estimate of amount of surrounding DCIS is helpful
  - ■ For example, number of blocks with DCIS outside invasive carcinoma gives estimate of extent of DCIS
- • When invasive carcinomas are excised with wide margins, status of margins is most important for determining likelihood of residual disease
  - ○ EIC positive cancers with negative margins do not have increased likelihood of residual DCIS
- • Other definitions of EIC have also been used
  - ○ DCIS > 2 cm from edge of invasive carcinoma
  - ○ DCIS occupying area > 2-4x that of invasive carcinoma
  - ○ DCIS involves 10 or more ducts outside area of invasive carcinoma

Core Needle Biopsies

- • Attempts have been made to evaluate EIC on core needle biopsies
- • Absence of DCIS in association with invasive carcinoma increases likelihood carcinoma will be EIC negative
- • If DCIS is present, about 1/3 of carcinomas will be EIC positive
- • Mammographic calcifications, if associated with carcinoma, are better indication of extent of DCIS

IMAGING CORRELATIONS

Mammography

- • DCIS may be associated with calcifications
- • In such cases, extent of mammographic calcifications often correlates with extent of DCIS
  - ○ However, not all DCIS calcifies, and size is often underestimated

Magnetic Resonance Imaging

- • Majority of cases of DCIS are associated with increased periductal angiogenesis resulting in enhancement on MR

- • Can detect areas of enhancement surrounding invasive carcinomas that correlate with extent of DCIS
- • More accurate than mammography in predicting extent of DCIS
  - ○ Accuracy is better for high-grade DCIS than for low-grade DCIS, probably due to greater degree of angiogenesis associated with high-grade DCIS

BIOLOGIC CORRELATIONS

Predictive Markers

- • EIC may be present with any histologic type of cancer
- • No association between ER expression and an EIC
- • HER2 positive cancer (± ER expression) is most common type associated with EIC (~ 25%), compared to ER-positive/HER2-negative cancer (~ 15%) and triple negative cancer (~ 10%)

SELECTED REFERENCES

1. Sanchez C et al: Factors associated with re-excision in patients with early-stage breast cancer treated with breast conservation therapy. Am Surg. 76(3):331-4, 2010
2. Wiechmann L et al: Presenting features of breast cancer differ by molecular subtype. Ann Surg Oncol. 16(10):2705-10, 2009
3. Schnitt SJ et al: Evolution of breast-conserving therapy for localized breast cancer. J Clin Oncol. 26(9):1395-6, 2008
4. Dzierzanowski M et al: Ductal carcinoma in situ in core biopsies containing invasive breast cancer: correlation with extensive intraductal component and lumpectomy margins. J Surg Oncol. 90(2):71-6, 2005
5. Elling D et al: Intraductal component in invasive breast cancer: analysis of 250 resected surgical specimens. Breast. 10(5):405-10, 2001
6. Jing X et al: Extensive intraductal component (EIC) and estrogen receptor (ER) status in breast cancer. Pathol Int. 48(6):440-7, 1998
7. Sinn HP et al: Extensive and predominant in situ component in breast carcinoma: their influence on treatment results after breast-conserving therapy. Eur J Cancer. 34(5):646-53, 1998
8. Connolly JL et al: Evaluation of breast biopsy specimens in patients considered for treatment by conservative surgery and radiation therapy for early breast cancer. Pathol Annu. 23 Pt 1:1-23, 1988

IMAGE GALLERY

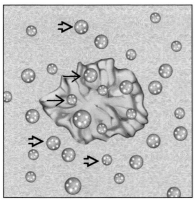 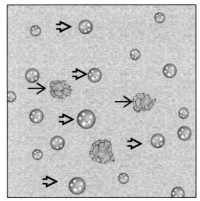 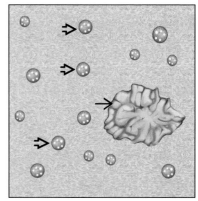

(Left) One type of EIC positive cancer has DCIS occupying at least 25% of the area of the invasive carcinoma ➡ and DCIS in the adjacent breast tissue ⏩. (Center) A 2nd type of EIC positive cancer consists of multiple small foci of invasive carcinoma ➡ associated with extensive DCIS ⏩. (Right) Some carcinomas are difficult to classify. Although there is no DCIS within the invasive carcinoma ➡, there are numerous foci of DCIS in the adjacent tissue ⏩.

INVASIVE DUCTAL CARCINOMA (ADENOCARCINOMAS OF NO SPECIAL TYPE)

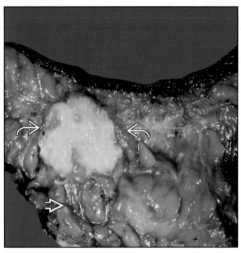

Invasive carcinomas ➡ typically form firm to hard radiodense white masses that replace radiolucent yellow adipose tissue ⬌ and thus may be detected as palpable masses or mammographic densities.

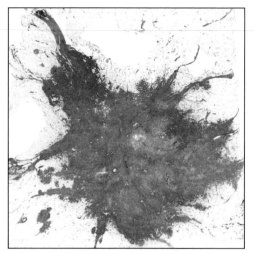

The border of an invasive carcinoma is characteristically irregular due to tumor cells infiltrating into the surrounding stroma. Less common are carcinomas with circumscribed or lobulated borders.

TERMINOLOGY

Abbreviations
- Invasive ductal carcinoma (IDC)

Synonyms
- Infiltrating ductal carcinoma
- Not otherwise specified (NOS) carcinoma
- No special type (NST) carcinoma

Definitions
- IDC includes all adenocarcinomas of the breast that are not classified as a special histologic type

ETIOLOGY/PATHOGENESIS

Classification
- IDC is a heterogeneous group of adenocarcinomas with regard to pathologic features, prognosis, and clinical outcome
  - Termed "ductal" because associated ductal carcinoma in situ expands and unfolds lobular units; thus resembles ducts more than lobules
    - In contrast, lobular carcinoma in situ expands but usually does not distort lobules; the type of associated invasive carcinoma was termed "lobular" carcinoma
  - All carcinomas are thought to arise from terminal duct lobular unit
  - Terms "ductal" and "lobular" do not indicate cell or structure of origin
- ~ 75% of invasive breast cancers
  - Remaining (~ 25%) are defined as special histologic types based on morphologic features
  - For small screen-detected cancers, ~ 60% are of special histologic type
- Therefore, most studies of "breast cancer" are primarily of IDC

- IDC can be divided into 4 major types: Luminal A, luminal B, HER2, and basal-like
  - Gene expression profiling demonstrates that each type shares global expression patterns
  - Same cancer types can be defined based on expression of ER, PR, HER2, and proliferation
  - Subtypes defined by profiling and IHC overlap by 80-85%
    - Although groups originally defined by expression profiling, convenient to use the same names to describe the very similar groups of cancers as defined by IHC
    - Here, basal-like carcinoma and triple negative breast carcinoma are described as 1 group
  - Classification by IHC has the advantage of organizing cancers according to therapeutic targets and likely response to chemotherapy
    - Some HER2 carcinomas defined by expression profiling do not overexpress HER2
    - Not yet clear if expression profiling adds sufficient additional information to warrant its use for routine classification

CLINICAL ISSUES

Epidemiology
- Incidence
  - In USA, 1 woman in 8 (~ 12%) will develop breast cancer in her lifetime
    - Highest incidence is for white women, and lowest incidence is for Native-American women
    - African-American women have a lower incidence compared to white women but higher mortality rates
    - Hispanic women have both lower incidence and lower mortality rates
- Age
  - Median at diagnosis: 61 years
    - < 15% of cases diagnosed before age 44

INVASIVE DUCTAL CARCINOMA (ADENOCARCINOMAS OF NO SPECIAL TYPE)

Key Facts

Terminology
- Invasive ductal carcinoma includes carcinomas not classified as a special histologic type
- Synonymous with "no special type" or "not otherwise specified" carcinoma

Etiology/Pathogenesis
- Heterogeneous with regard to pathologic features, prognosis, and clinical outcome
- ~ 75% of invasive breast cancers
- 4 types based on ER, PR, HER2, & proliferation
  ○ Luminal A, luminal B, HER2, and basal types
- ~ 1 in 8 women will develop breast cancer during her lifetime
- Median age at diagnosis: 61 years
  ○ < 15% diagnosed before age 44

Clinical Issues
- For women < 40, 85% detected as a palpable mass and 15% by screening
- For women > 40, 60% detected by screening and 40% as a palpable mass

Image Findings
- Masses, calcifications, and architectural distortion

Top Differential Diagnoses
- Special histologic types
- Ductal carcinoma in situ
- Sclerosing lesions
- Microglandular adenosis
- Epithelial displacement
- Other types of malignant tumors
- Metastatic tumors to the breast

- Gender
  ○ All females are at high risk for breast cancer
    ▪ Only 1 of 100 breast cancer cases occur in men

Presentation
- Patients most commonly present with a palpable mass or abnormality on screening
  ○ For women < 40, 85% of carcinomas are detected as a palpable mass and 15% on breast imaging
    ▪ Imaging may occur in this age group due to family history or as part of a work-up for a clinical finding (e.g., nipple discharge, pain, or skin changes)
  ○ For women > 40, 60% of carcinomas are detected by screening and 40% as a palpable mass
- Some cancers are not detected by mammography
  ○ Obscured by dense breast tissue
  ○ Present in unusual location and missed by routine views
  ○ Become apparent between screenings due to rapid growth ("interval" cancer)
- > 85% of palpable cancers are detected by the patient, the remainder by physician examination
  ○ Self breast examination has not been shown to decrease death rate from breast cancer
    ▪ Suggests that cancers that are capable of metastasizing will have done so by the time they become palpable
- Palpable cancers are typically larger (2-3 cm) than screen-detected (1-2 cm) cancers
  ○ Palpable cancers have a less favorable prognosis compared to nonpalpable cancers of the same size
- Uncommon presentations of breast cancer are nipple discharge, Paget disease, pain, or metastasis

Treatment
- Most patients will be treated with multiple modalities
- Surgery: Controls local disease and may be curative for localized cancers
- Radiation therapy: Reduces local recurrences and has a small effect on survival

- Endocrine therapy: Improves survival for patients with hormone-sensitive cancers
- Chemotherapy: Improves survival in subsets of patients with sensitive cancers; general correlation with higher proliferative rates
  ○ HER2-targeted therapy improves survival for carcinomas with overexpression

Prognosis
- Wide range of probable survival for IDC depending upon prognostic and predictive factors
  ○ Stage: Based on size, chest wall or skin involvement, and lymph node involvement
  ○ Grade: Modified Bloom-Richardson grade should be provided for all breast carcinomas
  ○ Subtype: Includes ER, PR, HER2, and proliferation
  ○ Lymph-vascular invasion
  ○ Response to therapy: May be evaluated if neoadjuvant therapy is used
- Gene expression profiling can also be used to determine prognosis in ER-positive IDC
  ○ Several different profiles are commercially available
  ○ Profiles are largely driven by genes related to proliferation
- Outcome is highly dependent on treatment
  ○ Reduction in the death rate from cancer is attributed to both improved detection of earlier cancers by screening and to systemic therapy

IMAGE FINDINGS

Mammographic Findings
- Masses, calcifications, and architectural distortion correlated with IDC
  ○ Vast majority of IDCs form irregular masses due to infiltration into surrounding stroma
    ▪ Only benign lesions that typically have this appearance are radial sclerosing lesions or inflammatory lesions (e.g., prior surgical sites or infections)
  ○ Less common for IDC to have circumscribed or lobulated borders

INVASIVE DUCTAL CARCINOMA (ADENOCARCINOMAS OF NO SPECIAL TYPE)

- Basal-like/triple negative cancer most likely to have this appearance
- Special histologic types of mucinous carcinoma and medullary carcinoma also have circumscribed borders
  - Calcifications are most commonly present in associated DCIS
    - IDCs detected as calcifications without a mass are typically very small (< 1 cm)
    - Calcifications are occasionally present in secretory material or necrosis in the IDC
  - Architectural distortion is uncommon finding
    - Carcinomas with this appearance are usually diffusely invasive with minimal stromal response
    - Invasive lobular carcinomas are most common carcinoma with this finding

Ultrasonographic Findings

- Borders of invasive carcinomas by ultrasound usually correlate with the shape seen on mammography
- Almost all carcinomas are hypoechoic as cancers consist of tumor cells and fibrous desmoplastic stroma
  - Very rarely, cancers can be hyperechoic due to infiltrative pattern into adipose tissue with minimal stromal response
- Not very useful as a screening modality due to low specificity
  - Most helpful to further define lesions detected by mammography or MR
  - Size by ultrasound has best correlation with gross tumor size

MR Findings

- Carcinomas are detected by MR due to quick uptake of contrast agents, resulting in rapid enhancement
- Shape of masses on imaging does not correlate well with actual borders of lesion
  - MR overestimates size in a significant percentage of patients
- MR is very sensitive (few cancers are occult by this modality) but not very specific
  - Not recommended for screening except for very high-risk populations

MACROSCOPIC FEATURES

General Features

- Majority of IDCs are very hard by palpation
  - Often "gritty" when cut
  - Cut surface is typically gray-white
- Carcinomas typically have irregular borders
  - Less common are carcinomas with circumscribed or lobulated borders

Size

- Important prognostic factor and is used for AJCC T classification
- Best determined by palpation rather than visual inspection
  - Cancers are often white (like adjacent fibrous breast stroma); can be difficult to see edges
  - Usually a palpable shelf between edge of tumor and normal breast tissue

- Extent can be determined by pinching the mass between 2 fingers

MICROSCOPIC PATHOLOGY

Histologic Features

- Histologic appearances vary according to subtype
  - Subtypes are not considered "special histologic types," as final classification depends on protein expression patterns rather than morphology
  - However, majority of cancers in each subtype have characteristic histologic features
- **Luminal A type**
  - Majority grade 1 or 2
  - Generally, pattern of well-formed tubules, cribriform nests, or papillae
  - Nuclei are small to moderate in size with minute or absent nucleoli and minimal pleomorphism
  - Mitoses are absent or rare
  - Necrosis would be very unusual
- **Luminal B type**
  - Majority grade 2 or 3
  - Tubules may be present but often less well formed; may invade as nests and sheets of cells
  - Nuclei typically high grade with prominent nucleoli
  - Mitoses are usually present and may be prominent
  - Necrosis may be present
- **HER2 type**
  - Majority grade 3
  - Usually invades as nests or sheets of cells; well-formed tubules would be unusual
  - Cytoplasm may be abundant and have apocrine features
  - Nuclei almost always high grade with prominent nucleoli
  - Mitoses are usually present and may be frequent
  - Necrosis in ~ 40%
  - Lymphocytic infiltrate in ~ 60%
- **Basal-like carcinoma/triple negative breast carcinoma**
  - Majority grade 3
  - Borders are commonly circumscribed or lobulated
  - Syncytial-like growth pattern is most common; tubule formation would be very unusual
  - Nuclei are generally high grade with prominent nucleoli
  - Mitoses usually present and often frequent
  - Central fibrosis &/or necrosis common
  - Lymphocytic infiltrate is frequently seen
- **DCIS**
  - Majority of IDCs are associated with DCIS in adjacent tissue
    - However, DCIS may be absent or very scant in basal-like/triple negative carcinoma
  - DCIS is generally similar in nuclear grade and immunoprofile to the IDC
    - Important exception: Rare cases in which DCIS is HER2 positive and IDC is HER2 negative

INVASIVE DUCTAL CARCINOMA (ADENOCARCINOMAS OF NO SPECIAL TYPE)

ANCILLARY TESTS

Immunohistochemistry

- Estrogen receptor (ER)
  - Recommended for all invasive cancers
  - Primary use: Predictive marker for likelihood of response to endocrine therapy
- Progesterone receptor (PR)
  - Recommended for all invasive carcinomas
    - Loss of PR expression can be associated with treatment with aromatase inhibitors
  - PR expression is regulated by ER signaling
    - Positive result for PR provides evidence that ER is biologically active in tumor
  - Primary use: Predictive maker for likelihood of response to endocrine therapy
- HER2
  - Recommended for all invasive cancers
  - Primary use: Predictive factor for likelihood of response to HER2-targeted therapy
- Ki-67 (MIB-1)
  - Identifies all cycling cells (cells not in G0)
  - Suggested as a method to distinguish luminal A and luminal B carcinomas
  - Cut-off of 15% positive cells identifies cancers with a high proliferative rate

DIFFERENTIAL DIAGNOSIS

Special Histologic Types of Breast Cancer

- Some breast adenocarcinomas can be subclassified into special histologic types based on morphologic appearance
  - Associated with favorable prognosis: Tubular, mucinous, papillary, medullary
  - Associated with unfavorable prognosis: Metaplastic, micropapillary
  - Some types have a characteristic clinical presentation or metastatic pattern: Lobular, inflammatory, micropapillary
- Most definitions require that at least 90% of the carcinoma be of the special type to qualify
  - Carcinomas with > 50% but < 90% special features can be classified as "mixed IDC and special type"
  - Carcinomas with focal special histologic features may be described as "IDC with special type features" (e.g., "IDC with mucinous features")

Ductal Carcinoma In Situ (DCIS)

- DCIS can closely mimic invasive carcinoma when it involves sclerosing adenosis or sclerotic stroma
- Conversely, IDC can mimic DCIS when it invades as circumscribed nests of cells in solid or cribriform pattern
- Spaces involved by DCIS generally have smooth contours and follow normal duct/lobular anatomy of breast
  - IDC more typically forms irregular nests of cells in a haphazard pattern and invading around normal structures
  - Stromal retraction is more common in IDC than in DCIS

- In difficult cases, IHC for myoepithelial markers is helpful
  - Multiple markers may be necessary as myoepithelial cells can be scant in high-grade DCIS &/or not positive for all markers
  - For muscle-type markers, stromal myofibroblasts must be distinguished from myoepithelial cells

Sclerosing Adenosis

- Usually has a lobulated or circumscribed border, back-to-back compressed glands, and evident myoepithelial cells
  - Can be easily distinguished from invasive carcinoma
- However, cases with the following features can be difficult to classify
  - Apocrine metaplasia: Can make epithelial component appear clonal and atypical
  - DCIS or LCIS: Appearance closely mimics invasive carcinoma
  - "Wandering adenosis": Acini are scattered in breast parenchyma and may surround normal structures
- IHC for myoepithelial markers is helpful as sclerosing adenosis has prominent myoepithelial cell layer

Radial Sclerosing Lesion

- Can closely mimic IDC radiologically, grossly, and microscopically
- Characterized by central zone containing well-formed glands in fibroelastic stroma
- Area surrounding central zone shows stellate scarring and contains hyperplastic glandular elements
- Myoepithelial cells are preserved
  - Along with architectural pattern at low power, establishes the diagnosis

Microglandular Adenosis (MGA)

- Rare lesion consisting of small round tubules with eosinophilic secretions, found scattered throughout breast tissue
  - No myoepithelial cells are present; MGA is most likely nonmetastasizing type of invasive carcinoma
  - MGA is negative for ER and PR
- MGA should be suspected if a lesion thought to be a well-differentiated carcinoma is negative for ER and PR
- MGA can recur locally; therefore, margins should be evaluated and reexcised if necessary
  - MGA has never been reported to metastasize; thus, lymph node biopsy is not required

Epithelial Displacement

- Benign or malignant epithelium can be displaced into stroma due to prior needle or excisional biopsies
  - Can be very prominent after biopsies of papillary lesions
- Rarely present when reexcision takes place > 1 month after the initial procedure; therefore, cells may not be viable
- Diagnosis of IDC should not be made, or only made with great caution, if the only diagnostic areas are within a site of prior biopsy changes

Other Types of Malignant Tumors

- Lymphomas and sarcomas can mimic carcinomas

INVASIVE DUCTAL CARCINOMA (ADENOCARCINOMAS OF NO SPECIAL TYPE)

Subtypes of Invasive Ductal Carcinoma

Feature	Luminal A Type	Luminal B Type	HER2 Type	Basal/Triple Negative Type
% of breast cancers	55%	15%	15-20%	10-15%
Grade	Grade 1 or 2	Grade 2 or 3	Grade 2 or 3	Usually grade 3
Special histologic types in this group	Tubular, cribriform, papillary, mucinous, grade 1 and 2 lobular		Apocrine (~ 50% overexpress HER2)	Medullary*, adenosquamous*, secretory*, adenoid cystic*, spindle cell, metaplastic
Estrogen receptor	Positive: High	Positive: May be low	Negative	Negative
Progesterone receptor	Usually positive	May be low or negative	Negative	Negative
HER2	Negative	~ 50% positive	Positive	Negative
Proliferation	Low	High	High	High
Luminal cytokeratins (CK7, 8/18, 19)	~ 100%	~ 100%		~ 85%
Basal cytokeratins or EGFR	Absent or low	Absent or low	May be present	40-85%
TP53 mutations	Low	Low	Frequent	Frequent
Extensive associated DCIS	~ 15%	~ 25%	~ 30%	~ 10%
Lymph-vascular invasion	~ 40%	~ 50-60%	~ 50%	~ 40%
Lymph node metastases	~ 45%	~ 50%	~ 60%	~ 45%
> 4 positive nodes	~ 10%	~ 20%	~ 30%	~ 15%
Time to recurrence	May be > 10 years		Usually short, < 10 years	Usually short, < 5 years
Prognosis	Favorable	Less favorable	Unfavorable (but improved with HER2-targeted therapy)	Unfavorable (but subset will have good response to chemotherapy)
Systemic therapy	Majority of patients benefit from hormonal treatment; benefit from chemotherapy less clear	May benefit from both hormonal therapy and chemotherapy	Benefit from chemotherapy and HER2-targeted therapy	Subset benefits from chemotherapy
Metastatic sites	Bone (70%), liver or lung (25%), brain (< 10%); survival with metastases possible	Bone (79%), liver or lung (30%), brain (10-15%)	Bone (60%), liver or lung (45%), brain (30%); long survival with metastases uncommon	Bone (40%), liver or lung (35%), brain (25%); long survival with metastases uncommon
Common patient characteristics	Older age, screen-detected cancers, associated with hormone replacement therapy	Younger age	Relatively more common in young women, may be more common in Asian women	Relatively more common in young women, more common in African-American and Hispanic women, typical of BRCA1-associated cancers

These basal-type carcinomas have a favorable prognosis, unlike the other members of this group.

- Other types of malignancy should be considered for tumors that are negative for hormone receptors, lack a glandular component, and are not associated with DCIS
- IHC for cytokeratin can confirm diagnosis of carcinoma
  - Many hormone-negative breast cancers are basal-like/triple negative; therefore, antibodies should include basal keratins
  - Some angiosarcomas can be keratin positive; IHC panel should be used in difficult cases
    - Podoplanin (D2-40) is positive in myoepithelial cells and some basal-like/triple negative carcinomas; therefore, not useful for identifying vascular lesions in breast

Metastatic Tumors to the Breast
- Very rare compared to primary breast carcinomas
  - Often present in adipose tissue without surrounding breast epithelium
- Patient will usually have well-known primary tumor elsewhere

  - In rare cases, breast metastasis will be the presenting lesion
- Should be considered for tumors that are negative for hormone receptors and are not associated with DCIS
  - However, metastatic gynecologic carcinomas can be hormone receptor positive
    - In these cases, comparison to the primary and IHC for Pax-8 and WT1 can be helpful
- May be impossible to distinguish a metastasis from a contralateral breast carcinoma from a new primary carcinoma unless DCIS is present in both breasts

SELECTED REFERENCES

1. Schnitt SJ: Molecular biology of breast tumor progression: a view from the other side. Int J Surg Pathol. 18(3 Suppl):170S-173S, 2010
2. Wiechmann L et al: Presenting features of breast cancer differ by molecular subtype. Ann Surg Oncol. 16(10):2705-10, 2009

INVASIVE DUCTAL CARCINOMA (ADENOCARCINOMAS OF NO SPECIAL TYPE)

IDC: Subtypes

Luminal A

Luminal B

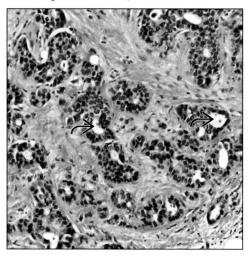
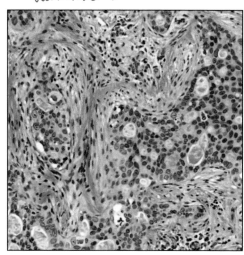

(Left) Luminal A carcinomas generally have a prominent component of well-formed tubules ➡, low-grade nuclei, and rare or absent mitoses. These carcinomas are usually strongly positive for both ER and PR. *(Right)* Luminal B carcinomas are less likely to have well-formed tubules and typically have intermediate- to high-grade nuclei. Higher rates of proliferation can be detected by Ki-67. Hormone receptors are present, but they may be at low levels. HER2 is present in 1/3-1/2.

HER2 / TRIPLE NEGATIVE

TRIPLE NEG CK5/6

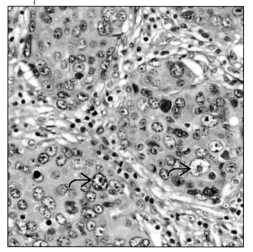
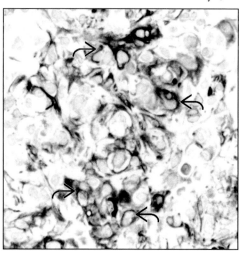

(Left) HER2-type and basal-like cancers are generally of high grade with large pleomorphic nuclei ➡ and no evidence of glandular differentiation. *(Right)* Basal-like/triple negative cancers may express basal cytokeratins such as CK5/6 ➡. The majority of these cancers would be classified as basal-like carcinomas by gene expression profiling.

HER2

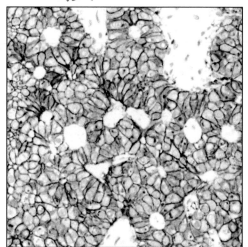
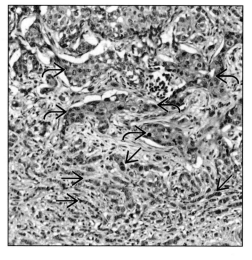

(Left) HER2-type and a subset of luminal B carcinomas overexpress HER2. It is important to identify these cancers as most patients will benefit from HER2-targeted therapy. *(Right)* Some unusual cases of IDC show a mixture of 2 distinct morphologic patterns. In this case, there are areas of no special type ➡ intermingled with invasive lobular carcinoma ➡. This type of cancer can be classified as invasive carcinoma with ductal and lobular features.

INVASIVE DUCTAL CARCINOMA (ADENOCARCINOMAS OF NO SPECIAL TYPE)

IDC: Differential Diagnosis

(Left) It can be difficult to distinguish IDC from DCIS if the latter involves a sclerosing lesion. In this case, although the nests are irregular, the very dense stroma would be unusual for IDC. *(Right)* When DCIS involves sclerosing lesions, the pattern can closely mimic IDC due to the irregular nests of tumor cells in stroma. In this case, p63-positive myoepithelial cells ⊟ can be identified at the periphery of all of the nests, confirming that no invasion is present.

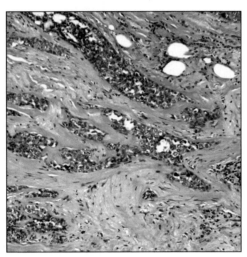
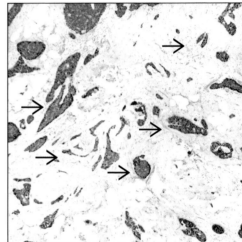

(Left) Lymph-vascular invasion can resemble IDC when the vascular spaces are completely filled by tumor. The presence of sinusoidal structures and an absent desmoplastic response are important features. In this case, it is helpful to note involvement of lymphatics around a blood vessel ⊟. *(Right)* Microglandular adenosis is a rare lesion consisting of small round tubules without myoepithelial cells. This diagnosis should be suspected if a low-grade IDC is ER negative.

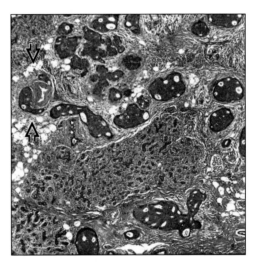
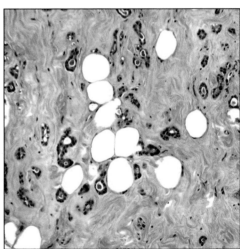

(Left) Benign and malignant epithelial cells can be artifactually displaced into the stroma after needle biopsies or surgical procedures. IDC should not be diagnosed if the only areas of stromal involvement are in an area of biopsy site changes ⊟. *(Right)* Metastases to the breast are rare but should be suspected if carcinoma in situ is absent and hormone receptors and HER2 are negative. This is a case of metastatic lung carcinoma that was positive for TTF-1.

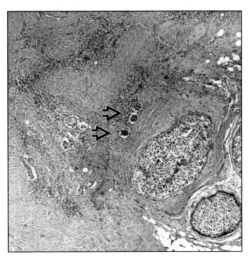
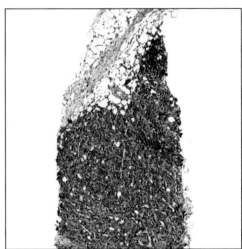

INVASIVE DUCTAL CARCINOMA (ADENOCARCINOMAS OF NO SPECIAL TYPE)

Imaging Features of Invasive Carcinoma

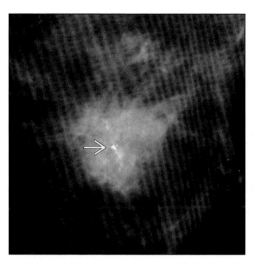
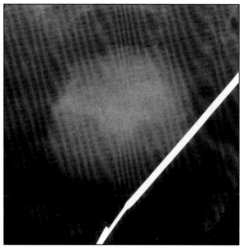

(Left) IDC consists of tumor cells and desmoplastic stroma and appears on mammography as a radiodense mass compared to the normal fibroadipose tissue. The advancing edge is typically irregular. Calcifications ➡ are often within associated DCIS. (Right) IDC in a minority of cases, particularly basal-like/triple negative, forms a circumscribed mass that mimics benign lesions. The specialized types of medullary and mucinous carcinomas also have this appearance.

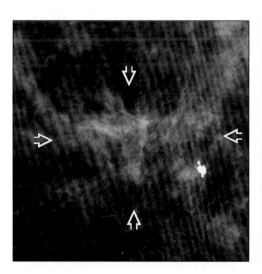
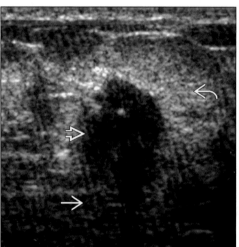

(Left) Architectural distortion is a subtle change in the texture of the breast parenchyma ➡. This finding is associated with diffusely invasive carcinomas that infiltrate into adipose tissue with a minimal desmoplastic response. (Right) On ultrasound, carcinomas are hypoechoic ➡ (black) compared to the adjacent hyperechoic ➡ (gray to white) normal tissue because adipose tissue is replaced by tumor cells. Posterior shadowing ➡ is a common feature of malignancies.

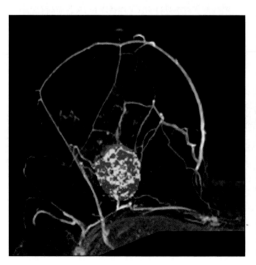
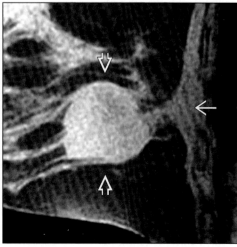

(Left) MR is a very sensitive technique for detecting breast cancers, as the majority are associated with rapid increased blood flow. It can be particularly useful in young women, as the imaging is not affected by dense breast parenchyma. The findings are not specific enough to use MR as a screening technique. (Right) MR can be used to determine the extent of carcinoma, which can be helpful in planning surgery. In this case, a large cancer ➡ shows tethering to the chest wall ➡.

INVASIVE LOBULAR CARCINOMA

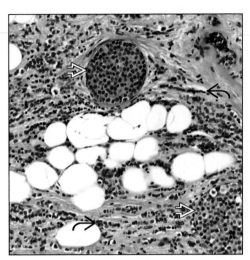

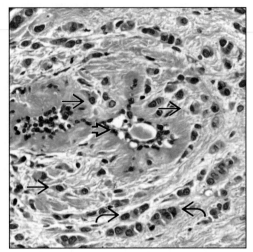

The hallmark of invasive lobular carcinoma is the presence of rounded discohesive cells with little stromal reaction ➤. Lobular carcinoma in situ ⧯ is present in the majority of cases.

The carcinoma infiltrates through stroma as individual cells ⧈ or in single files ⧈ and often forms a circumferential pattern around normal ductal structures ⧯ (termed a targetoid lesion).

TERMINOLOGY

Abbreviations
- Invasive lobular carcinoma (ILC)

Definitions
- Invasive carcinomas characterized by loss of normal cell adhesion and actin cytoskeleton regulation
  - ILC shows a specific morphologic appearance, typical diffuse pattern of tissue infiltration in breast and distant sites
    - Distant recurrence will show distinctive metastatic pattern

ETIOLOGY/PATHOGENESIS

Cell Adhesion Protein Expression
- Loss of E-cadherin gene (CDH1) expression in approximately 85% of ILC
  - E-cadherin is a calcium-dependent transmembrane protein
    - Functional role in intercellular adhesion and cell-polarity
    - Binds actin cytoskeleton through interactions with p120, α-, β-, and γ-catenin
  - Loss of E-cadherin affects cellular adhesion, motility, and possibly cell division
- Mechanism of loss of E-cadherin expression
  - 1 allele on 16q is inactivated by mutation in ~ 50-60% of ILC
  - 2nd allele is inactivated by either loss of heterozygosity or promoter hypermethylation
  - Leads to loss of E-cadherin protein expression as detected by IHC
- Expression of E-cadherin but loss of other catenin complex members occurs in approximately 15% of ILC
  - If E-cadherin is expressed, then 1 or more catenins show abnormal expression

- p120 catenin usually shows abnormal cytoplasmic staining

Gene Expression Profiling
- ILC of all grades are more similar to each other than to other breast carcinoma types
  - Majority have luminal A expression profile
- Share similar expression patterns related to cell adhesion, cell-to-cell signaling, and actin cytoskeleton signaling
- Grade 1 and 2 ILC have distinct gene expression patterns compared to grade 1 and 2 carcinomas of no special type

Germline Mutations of E-cadherin Gene
- Hereditary diffuse gastric cancer (HDGC) syndrome is due to germline mutations in E-cadherin gene (CDH1)
  - Risk of gastric carcinoma is ~ 40-80% by age ~ 80
  - Risk of ILC for females is ~ 40-50% by age ~ 80
    - Gastric signet ring cell carcinoma and ILC are morphologically similar and both lack E-cadherin expression; however, carcinomas have organ-specific gene expression patterns
    - Some families are detected by predominance of cases of ILC
- Majority of women with ILC do not have germline mutations in CDH1
  - Possibility of germline mutations in other cytoskeletal protein genes is under investigation

Genetic Changes
- ILC has fewer chromosomal abnormalities than carcinomas of no special type
- 3 frequent and consistent changes in all ILC types
  - Loss at 16q at location of E-cadherin gene (16q22.1)
  - Gains at 1q and 16p

INVASIVE LOBULAR CARCINOMA

Key Facts

Terminology

- Invasive lobular carcinomas are characterized by loss of normal cell adhesion and actin cytoskeleton regulation
  - Responsible for specific morphologic appearance, diffuse pattern of infiltration in the breast and distant sites, and characteristic metastatic pattern

Etiology/Pathogenesis

- Approximately 85% lack E-cadherin and 15% lack other cell adhesion proteins
- *CDH1* germline mutations increase risk of gastric cancer and ILC

Clinical Issues

- Most common special type of breast carcinoma: 5-15% of all breast cancers

- Majority present as irregular mass
  - Diffuse pattern of infiltration can make detection difficult by palpation or imaging in around 1/3
- Distinct pattern of metastases to serosal surfaces of GI and GYN tracts, leptomeninges, and bone
- Prognosis similar to women with carcinomas of no special type matched for grade and stage
  - Trend toward later recurrence with ILC

Top Differential Diagnoses

- Invasive carcinoma with ductal and lobular features
- Tubulolobular carcinoma
- Lymphoid infiltrates and lymphoma
- Metastatic melanoma
- Myofibroblastoma, epithelioid variant

CLINICAL ISSUES

Epidemiology

- Incidence
  - 5-15% of invasive mammary carcinomas
    - Most common special type of breast carcinoma
  - Incidence of ILC is rising, primarily among women over 50 years of age
    - Reasons for rising incidence are uncertain
    - Unlikely related to increasing use of screening mammography
    - May be linked to increased use of postmenopausal hormones
- Age
  - More common in older women (> 50 years)

Site

- More likely to be multicentric in ipsilateral breast
- Contralateral involvement may be slightly higher for ILC than for carcinomas of no special type
  - However, data is influenced by increased likelihood of bilateral mastectomy or contralateral biopsy
  - Actual risk for clinical diagnosis of contralateral carcinoma is approximately 0.5-1% per year

Presentation

- Poorly defined palpable mass or area of thickening by clinical examination
- Irregular mass or architectural distortion by imaging

Treatment

- Surgical approaches
  - Breast conservation is possible
    - Similar local control and survival if clear margins are achieved
- Adjuvant therapy
  - Majority of ILC are ER positive
    - Adjuvant endocrine therapy is usually recommended
  - Neoadjuvant studies have demonstrated that ILC is less responsive to chemotherapy than nonlobular carcinomas

Prognosis

- Prognosis similar to women with carcinomas of no special type if matched for grade and stage
  - Patients with stage I classic ILC may show better recurrence-free survival
- Prognosis is related to ILC grade
- Better prognosis for classic ILC compared with variant forms
- Trend toward late recurrence for ILC
  - Patients with ILC require long-term clinical follow-up
- ILC has distinct pattern of metastatic spread
  - Serosal and mucosal involvement of GI and GYN tracts and retroperitoneum
    - Metastatic ILC occasionally seen in GI mucosal biopsies and endometrial curettings
    - Metastatic ILC to stomach can mimic linitis plastica due to primary gastric carcinoma
    - IHC panel may be necessary to distinguish metastatic ILC (ER, GCDFP-15, and MUC1 positive) from gastric signet ring cell carcinoma (CDX-2 positive)
  - Leptomeninges and cerebrospinal fluid involvement
    - Carcinomatous meningitis is usually due to ILC
  - Bone
    - Metastatic ILC can be very difficult to detect in bone marrow due to resemblance to hematopoietic cells
    - IHC for keratin can be very helpful to determine presence and extent of involvement
  - Pleural and pulmonary metastases are less common than for other histologic types of carcinomas

IMAGE FINDINGS

Mammographic Findings

- Difficult to detect mammographically due to relatively subtle changes in density
  - Imaging findings due to lack of stromal reaction and diffuse growth pattern in many cases

INVASIVE LOBULAR CARCINOMA

- Metastases may also be difficult to image due to diffuse growth pattern
- Typical mammographic findings
  - Irregular mass
    - Solid and alveolar variants may present as circumscribed or lobulated masses
  - Architectural distortion
  - New focal asymmetry
  - Calcifications are uncommon
- Size may be underestimated by mammogram or ultrasound

MR Findings

- Irregular mass with architectural distortion
- Foci of septal enhancement
- Size may be more accurate by MR examination
- ILC can be source of false-negative MR examination

MACROSCOPIC FEATURES

General Features

- Macroscopic appearance variable
  - Majority of ILCs form discrete mass similar to carcinomas of no special type
  - Some ILC may be difficult to see grossly and are poorly defined

Size

- For subtle ill-defined carcinomas, assessment of tumor size for T staging can be difficult
  - Requires correlation between gross and histologic examination
  - Number of blocks involved can give estimate of tumor volume
    - Can be helpful for cases with multiple foci of invasion

MICROSCOPIC PATHOLOGY

Histologic Features

- ILC has distinctive cytologic features
  - Cells are round in shape due to lack of cohesion
    - Acini, papillae, or other structures requiring cell adhesion are absent
  - Nuclear grade can vary from grade 1 to grade 3; grade 2 is found in majority of ILC
  - Cytoplasmic mucin vacuoles may be present
    - If prominent, cells have signet ring appearance
    - Cells typically have single vacuole with mucin droplet whereas signet ring cells of GI tract more typically have multiple mucin vacuoles and foamy cytoplasmic appearance
    - Signet ring cells can also be seen in breast carcinomas of no special type
- Distinctive growth pattern
  - In classical growth pattern, linear arrangements of discohesive cells run in single file between collagen fascicles
    - Infiltration by bands > 2 cells across has been termed "trabecular" ILC
  - Single cells may be present

- Infiltrating cells may be orientated in circular fashion around normal ducts (targetoid, concentric, or "bull's eye" appearance)
  - Skip lesions or patchy growth pattern may be present
  - Multiple foci of carcinoma may be separated from main lesion by uninvolved breast tissue
  - Desmoplasia may be minimal or absent
    - Correlates with absence of discrete mass by imaging or by palpation in some cases
- LCIS present in 70-80% of cases
  - Nuclear grade of LCIS is usually similar to nuclear grade of invasive carcinoma
  - LCIS is more frequently associated with well- and moderately differentiated ILC
  - LCIS is less commonly seen in association with variant ILC
- Lymph-vascular is very rarely present
  - Lymph-vascular invasion associated with carcinomas of no special type is likely due to cohesive nests of tumor extending into lymphatic spaces
  - Because cells of ILC lack cohesion to each other or to vascular wall, likelihood of seeing cells in lymphatics is diminished
- **Variants of ILC according to growth pattern**
  - Classical: Most common growth pattern
    - Linear files of single cells (i.e., not alveolar or solid)
    - Some definitions also require low-grade nuclei; other definitions do not include nuclear grade
    - Of ILC with classical growth pattern, 80-90% are grade 2, 5-10% grade 1, and 5-10% grade 3
  - Alveolar
    - Tumor cells are discohesive but grow in groups of 20 or more separated by fibrovascular septae
    - Clusters of cells can resemble LCIS
  - Solid
    - Tumor cells are present in large sheets with little or no intervening stroma
    - Cells can be discohesive within mass or show single cell infiltration at edges
  - Mixed features
    - ILC showing more than 1 of above patterns
- **Variants of ILC according to cytologic appearance**
  - Signet ring cell
    - Signet ring cell morphology is prominent throughout ILC
  - Histiocytoid
    - Cells have abundant eosinophilic foamy cytoplasm
    - Cells can closely resemble histiocytes, particularly at metastatic sites or in area of inflammation
    - Cells are usually positive for GCDFP-15, correlating with apocrine appearance
  - Pleomorphic
    - Cells have larger and more irregular nuclei
    - Definition may require classical growth pattern or include solid and alveolar patterns
    - Includes ILC of both grade 2 and 3
  - Grade may be a more useful means of describing ILC as grade also includes mitotic activity

■ Mitoses are more closely correlated with prognosis than nuclear grade

Lymph Node Metastases
- Lymph node metastases due to ILC may be subtle
  - Especially true for nodes with partial involvement and scattered single cells
  - Cells can closely resemble lymphocytes or histiocytes
  - May result in false-negative intraoperative assessment of sentinel lymph node biopsy
    - Touch preps of sentinel lymph nodes may be helpful for detecting tumor cells
    - Look for cytoplasmic mucin vacuoles and signet ring cells
  - Cytokeratin stains of permanent section of sentinel lymph nodes may be helpful in some cases
    - Can aid in determining extent and evaluation of extranodal invasion
  - Metastases may be difficult to classify as isolated tumor cells, micrometastases, or macrometastases
    - If more than 200 cells are present in single cross section, metastasis should be classified as (at least) micrometastasis
    - If numerous dispersed cells are present, pathologist will need to use his/her judgment to determine if metastasis is best classified as micrometastasis or macrometastasis

ANCILLARY TESTS

Histochemistry
- Mucicarmine
  - Reactivity: Positive
  - Staining pattern
    - Mucin vacuoles

Immunohistochemistry
- E-cadherin
  - Absent in approximately 85% of ILC
    - Partial membrane positivity or cytoplasmic positivity may be present in some cases
  - Present in approximately 15% of ILC
    - Alternatively, E-cadherin is absent in some carcinomas with histologic appearance of "ductal" carcinoma
  - E-cadherin positive and negative ILC are very similar for most clinicopathologic features
    - E-cadherin positive ILC has higher frequency of lymph-vascular invasion
    - E-cadherin positive ILC is more likely to have mixed histologic pattern
- Catenins
  - E-cadherin negative ILC also lacks expression of α-, β-, and γ-catenins
    - p120 shows diffuse cytoplasmic expression
  - Majority of E-cadherin positive ILC lacks membrane expression of 1 or more catenins but may show cytoplasmic expression
    - p120 shows diffuse cytoplasmic expression in majority of cases
- Hormone receptors

  - > 90% of grade 1 and grade 2 ILC and > 80% of grade 3 ILC will be positive for ER
  - If ILC is ER negative, possibility of false-negative result or different diagnosis (e.g., metastatic melanoma or lymphoma) should be considered
- HER2
  - HER2 overexpression is very rare except for grade 3 ILC
  - Edge enhancement can be seen in some cases
    - Should not be overinterpreted as membrane positivity
  - FISH for HER2 amplification is helpful for confirmation
- Gross cystic disease fluid protein-15
  - Frequently positive, particularly in ILC with pleomorphic, apocrine, or signet ring cytologic features

DIFFERENTIAL DIAGNOSIS

Invasive Carcinoma with Ductal and Lobular Features
- Some carcinomas have heterogeneous appearance including both single cell infiltrative pattern and areas of cohesive cell growth and tubule formation
  - Single cell pattern may be prominent
  - Often associated with desmoplastic stromal response
  - Signet ring cells may be present but are uncommon
- May be associated with DCIS, LCIS, or both
- Typically show strong membrane positivity for E-cadherin and p120 catenin
- May be classified as having mixed ductal and lobular features
- Make up 3-5% of breast carcinomas
- Important to document "lobular features"
  - Metastatic pattern may be similar to ILC
  - Cells can be difficult to identify at metastatic sites

Tubulolobular Carcinoma
- Characterized by features of classical ILC in addition to small tubules
  - Single cell growth pattern in single files or targetoid configurations
  - Tubules are small (smaller than in tubular carcinomas)
- Nuclei are small and low grade
- Most tubulolobular carcinomas are positive for E-cadherin
- Rare: < 2% of all breast carcinomas
- May be considered variant of ILC or variant of tubular carcinoma
- Not synonymous for carcinomas with ductal and lobular features

Lymphoid Infiltrates and Lymphoma
- Both ILC and lymphoma can appear as single cells and linear arrays of cells in stroma
  - ILC typically has more cytoplasm than seen in lymphoma
- Presence of LCIS supports diagnosis of ILC
- IHC studies can be helpful in difficult cases

INVASIVE LOBULAR CARCINOMA

Pathologic Features of Grades 1-3 Invasive Lobular Carcinoma

Grade	Tubule Score	Nuclear Score	Mitoses Score	ER	HER2	Morphology	% of ILC
Low grade	3	1	1	Positive in > 95%	Positive in < 5%	Can resemble lymphocytes	~ 10-15%
Intermediate grade	3	Usually 2	Usually 1	Positive in > 95%	Positive in < 5%	Can resemble histiocytes	~ 70-80%
High grade	3	Usually 3	2 or 3	Positive in 80-90%	Positive in 25-50%	May be difficult to distinguish from poorly differentiated carcinomas of no special type	~ 10-15%

- o Keratin will be positive in ILC and absent in lymphoma
- o Leukocyte common antigen will be positive in lymphoma and absent in ILC
- o Rare lymphomas can be hormone receptor positive

Other Cell Types at Distant Metastatic Sites
- Stomach
  - o ILC and gastric signet ring cell carcinoma can be identical in appearance
    - ■ ILC typically has signet ring cells with single vacuole with mucin droplet
    - ■ Gastric signet ring cells typically have multiple vacuoles giving foamy appearance
  - o IHC may be necessary to identify source of carcinoma
    - ■ ILC: Usually ER, GCDFP-15, MUC1 positive and CDX-2 and Hep-Par1 negative
    - ■ Gastric: Usually CDX-2 and Hep-Par1 positive and ER, GCDFP-15, and MUC1 negative
- Bone marrow
  - o ILC can resemble hematopoietic cells
  - o Keratin studies may be necessary to determine presence and extent of metastatic carcinoma

Myofibroblastoma, Epithelioid Variant
- Presents as circumscribed mass
  - o ILC typically presents as irregular mass or architectural distortion
- Spindle cell areas are often present in addition to epithelioid cells that resemble ILC
  - o Spindle cells not seen in ILC
- Myofibroblastomas are usually positive for ER and PR
  - o IHC for keratin will be negative

Metastatic Melanoma
- Most common metastasis to breast in adult women
- Cells are discohesive and usually present as sheets of cells
  - o Appearance can mimic solid variant of ILC
- Should be suspected if LCIS is absent and tumor cells are negative for hormone receptors
- IHC for cytokeratins and melanoma markers are helpful

GRADING

Nottingham Combined Histologic Grade
- Same grading system can be used for all types of breast carcinoma

- ILC can show low, intermediate, or high histologic grades
  - o Low grade: Small low-grade nuclei, low mitotic score
  - o Intermediate grade: Larger intermediate-grade nuclei, low mitotic score
  - o High grade: Large high-grade nuclei, prominent nucleoli, &/or intermediate to high mitotic score
- Mitotic index correlates better with clinical outcome than ILC type or nuclear grade
- Solid ILC tends to have higher mitotic counts and higher grade nuclei compared to classical ILC
- Each of 3 grades show significant differences in survival

SELECTED REFERENCES

1. Rakha EA et al: Clinical and biological significance of E-cadherin protein expression in invasive lobular carcinoma of the breast. Am J Surg Pathol. 34(10):1472-9, 2010
2. Rakha EA et al: Lobular breast carcinoma and its variants. Semin Diagn Pathol. 27(1):49-61, 2010
3. van Deurzen CH et al: Nodal-stage classification in invasive lobular breast carcinoma: influence of different interpretations of the pTNM classification. J Clin Oncol. 28(6):999-1004, 2010
4. Weigelt B et al: The molecular underpinning of lobular histological growth pattern: a genome-wide transcriptomic analysis of invasive lobular carcinomas and grade- and molecular subtype-matched invasive ductal carcinomas of no special type. J Pathol. 220(1):45-57, 2010
5. Rakha EA et al: The biological and clinical characteristics of breast carcinoma with mixed ductal and lobular morphology. Breast Cancer Res Treat. 114(2):243-50, 2009
6. Rakha EA et al: Histologic grading is an independent prognostic factor in invasive lobular carcinoma of the breast. Breast Cancer Res Treat. 111(1):121-7, 2008
7. Biglia N et al: Increased incidence of lobular breast cancer in women treated with hormone replacement therapy: implications for diagnosis, surgical and medical treatment. Endocr Relat Cancer. 14(3):549-67, 2007
8. Sastre-Garau X et al: Infiltrating lobular carcinoma of the breast. Clinicopathologic analysis of 975 cases with reference to data on conservative therapy and metastatic patterns. Cancer. 77(1):113-20, 1996

INVASIVE LOBULAR CARCINOMA

Imaging and Microscopic Features

grade 1

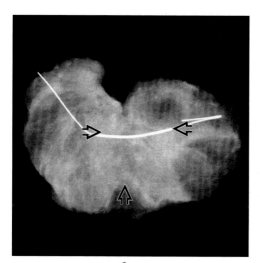

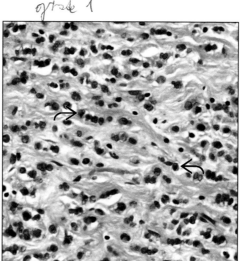

grade 2

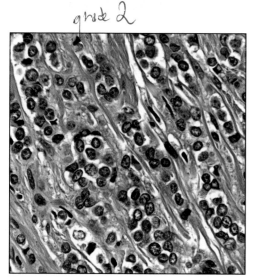

grade 3

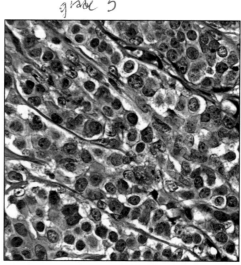

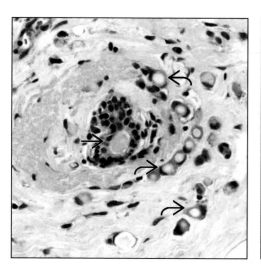

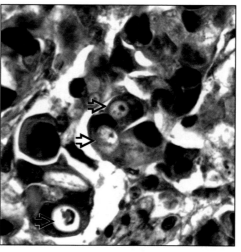

(Left) This specimen radiograph shows a subtle area of architectural distortion ⇒ corresponding to an ILC. Although the majority of ILCs present as irregular masses, the absent or minimal desmoplastic reaction can make ILC difficult to detect by palpation on physical examination or by imaging. (Right) In grade 1 ILC, the nuclei are small and uniform with inconspicuous nucleoli ➡. Mitoses are absent, and the cytoplasm is scant. The cells can be mistaken for lymphocytes if sparse.

(Left) Grade 2 ILC has larger nuclei with small nucleoli. Mitoses are generally absent. There are moderate amounts of cytoplasm and the cells can resemble histiocytes in lymph nodes. (Right) Grade 3 ILC has larger pleomorphic nuclei and mitoses and is more likely to be the solid variant. Cytoplasm can be abundant, but the cells are easily recognized as malignant. The accompanying LCIS usually has a similar appearance and may be associated with necrosis and calcifications.

(Left) Concentric infiltration around normal ducts ➡ is frequently seen in ILC. Tumor cells can contain prominent cytoplasmic mucin vacuoles ➡ giving a signet ring cell appearance. Histochemical stains for cytoplasmic mucin will be positive. (Right) Grade 3 ILC can also have signet ring cells typical of ILC harboring a single vacuole with a central mucin droplet ⇒. However, gastric-type signet ring cells (multiple vacuoles creating foamy cytoplasm) are also seen in ILC.

Variant Microscopic Features

(Left) This ILC has cells with abundant foamy cytoplasm. Some resemble gastric-type signet ring cells and others have a histiocytoid appearance. Metastasis should be considered unless there is a definite in situ component. IHC can be helpful in these cases. *(Right)* ILC can also have an apocrine appearance due to abundant eosinophilic cytoplasm. This is more common in grade 3 or pleomorphic ILC. This carcinoma had abundant mitotic figures ⊟ and overexpressed HER2.

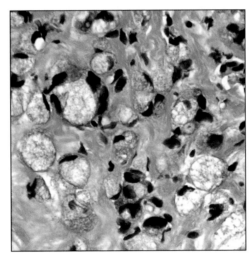 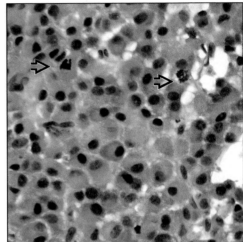

(Left) ILC can be quite subtle as the underlying breast architecture and balance of fibroadipose tissue may not be substantially altered. The increased cellularity of the stroma ⊡ is the indication that ILC may be present. The size of ILC is often difficult to determine as the extent of the tumor may not be apparent on imaging or on gross examination. *(Right)* LCIS with microinvasion is rare. In this case, a few tumor cells are present in stroma ⊟, adjacent to an area of LCIS.

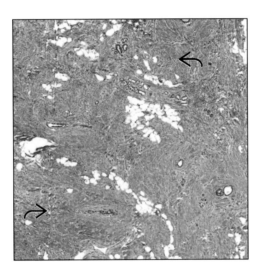 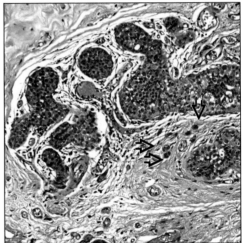

(Left) Alveolar ILC consists of clusters of at least 20 tumor cells but frequently more than this. The circumscribed nests can resemble LCIS. However, the cell nests have an infiltrative pattern and myoepithelial cells are absent. The cells are cytologically identical to the cells of classical ILC. *(Right)* Solid ILC consists of larger expanses of tumor cells than those seen in alveolar ILC. This subtype is more frequently found to be grade 3 and to have pleomorphic nuclei.

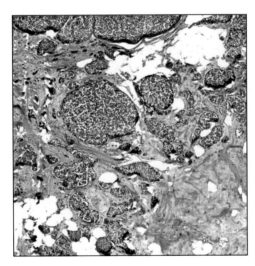 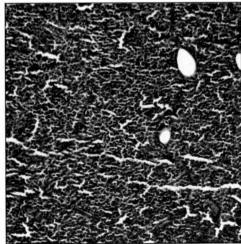

Ancillary Techniques

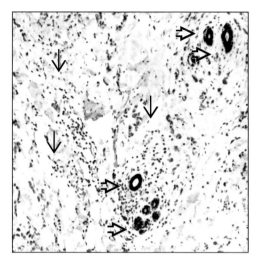

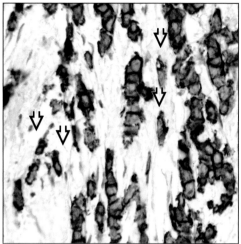

(Left) The majority of ILCs of all types lack expression of the cell adhesion molecule E-cadherin ➡. The normal ducts provide a good internal control ➡. *(Right)* Some cases of ILC (5-15%) retain E-cadherin expression, although they have the typical morphologic appearance and single cells are present ➡. These carcinomas lack or have abnormal expression of 1 or more of the catenins.

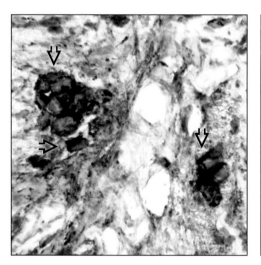

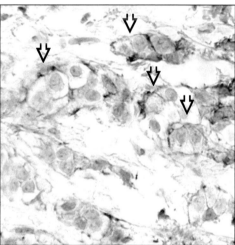

(Left) α, β, γ, and p120 catenins attach E-cadherin to the actin cytoskeleton and are normally found on the cell membrane. In cases of ILC with E-cadherin expression, catenins such as p120 ➡ are usually present in an abnormal diffuse cytoplasmic location. *(Right)* < 5% of grade 1 or 2 ILC overexpress HER2. However, some edge artifact may be present, particularly around clusters of tumor cells ➡. This finding should not be overinterpreted as membrane expression.

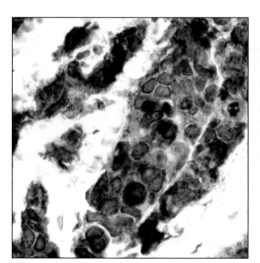

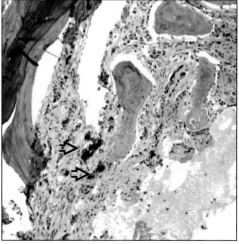

(Left) The majority of ILCs will be positive for cytoplasmic GCDFP-15, especially in apocrine, signet ring cell, and pleomorphic types. It is a useful marker to distinguish gastric and breast carcinomas. *(Right)* Keratin IHC is helpful to identify ILC at metastatic sites as the cells can mimic lymphocytes, histiocytes, or hematopoietic cells. The metastatic carcinoma in this bone biopsy specimen is keratin positive ➡.

INVASIVE LOBULAR CARCINOMA

Metastatic Lobular Carcinoma

(Left) Metastases from ILC in a lymph node can be difficult to identify as the cells are about the same size as lymphocytes ⇗ and can be dispersed as single cells and small clusters throughout the node. *(Right)* A pancytokeratin stain in this lymph node highlights metastatic tumor cells within the subcapsular sinus ⇗ and lymph node parenchyma ⇒. Cytokeratin stains can be helpful in confirming the diagnosis of nodal involvement and the extent (size) in some cases.

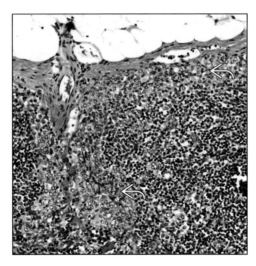
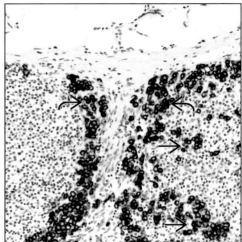

(Left) Classical ILC can show unusual patterns of metastatic dissemination, including spread to serosal surfaces or the mucosal surfaces of the GI and GYN tracts. In the case seen here, ILC has metastasized to the submucosa of the fallopian tube ⇗, beneath the overlying mucosal lining ⇒. *(Right)* E-cadherin stain shows reactivity in the attenuated mucosa of the fallopian tube ⇗, while the underlying metastatic tumor cells are negative ⇒, supporting the diagnosis of metastatic ILC.

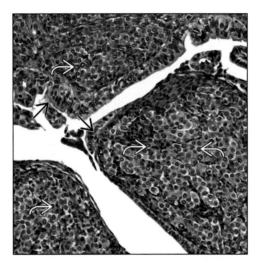
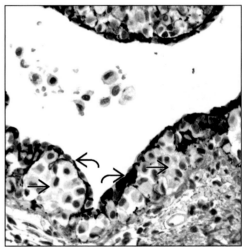

(Left) Metastatic ILC to the stomach can closely mimic gastric signet ring cell carcinoma ⇗. In some cases, the breast primary may not be clinically apparent. IHC panels can distinguish breast and gastric cancers. *(Right)* This woman had a history of ILC but was thought to be free of disease at the time of a hernia sac repair. The metastatic cells ⇗ were misinterpreted as reactive mesothelial cells. She died 2 years later of diffuse peritoneal disease undetected by imaging.

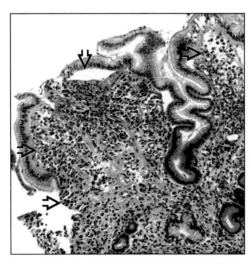
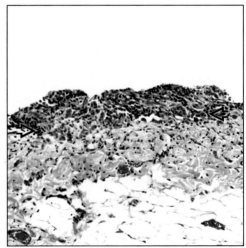

INVASIVE LOBULAR CARCINOMA

Differential Diagnosis

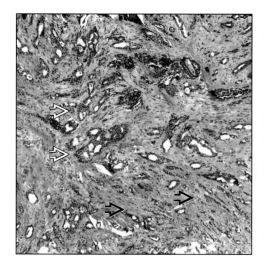

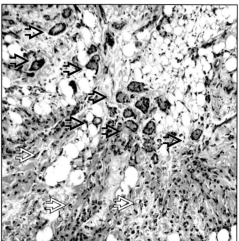

(Left) Some carcinomas show features of both ILC and carcinomas of no special type. In this carcinoma, there are areas of single cell infiltration ⊳ as well as areas with tubule formation and cribriform patterns ⊳. These carcinomas are described as having mixed features. (Right) Tubulolobular carcinomas consist of small, well-formed tubules ⊳ and single cells ⊳ and are generally E-cadherin positive. They may be considered a subtype of either ILC or tubular carcinomas.

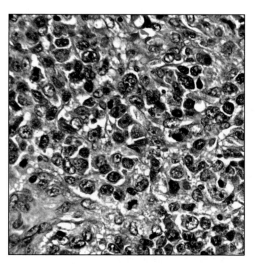

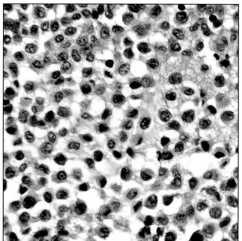

(Left) Large cell lymphomas also consist of discohesive cells and can resemble a solid ILC. Single cell infiltration may also be present. Lymphoma should be considered when LCIS is absent, particularly if hormone receptor studies are negative. (Right) Metastatic melanoma consists of sheets of discohesive cells and can mimic solid ILC. This diagnosis should be considered if LCIS is absent and the tumor cells lack hormone receptors.

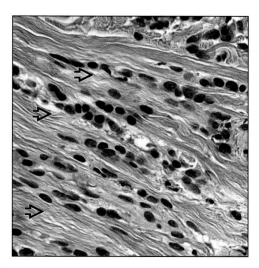

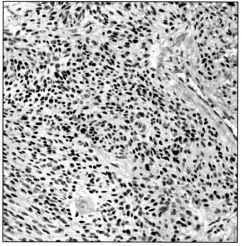

(Left) Myofibroblastomas with an epithelioid appearance ⊳ can closely mimic ILC. Important clues are presentation as a circumscribed mass (unusual for ILC), absence of LCIS, and focal areas of spindle-shaped cells. Myofibroblastoma is readily distinguished from ILC by IHC as the cells will be negative for keratins. (Right) In addition to resembling an ILC morphologically, an epithelioid myofibroblastoma is typically positive for ER and PR, as in this example.

INVASIVE LOBULAR CARCINOMA VARIANTS

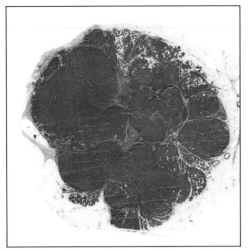

The majority of invasive lobular carcinomas invade as files of single cells. However, cytologically identical cells can grow in other patterns, such as this solid type of invasive lobular carcinoma.

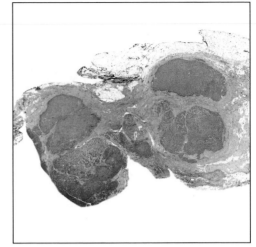

The alveolar variant of invasive lobular carcinoma invades as multiple circumscribed nests of tumor cells. The cells are discohesive due to loss or dysfunction of cell adhesion proteins.

TERMINOLOGY

Abbreviations
- Variant forms of invasive lobular carcinoma (ILC)
  - Histologic variants of ILC
    - Classical variant (ILCCV)
    - Solid variant (ILCSV)
    - Alveolar variant (ILCAV)
  - Cytologic variants of ILC
    - Pleomorphic variant (ILCPV)
    - Histiocytoid variant (ILCHV)

Definitions
- Variant forms differ from classical ILC with regard to architecture &/or cytology
  - May show substantial elements of nonlinear infiltration and growth
  - May show significant atypia with high-grade nuclei
- Focal areas of classical ILC with linear growth pattern can be found in most variant forms
- Predominant pattern (> 80%) determines histologic type of ILC

ETIOLOGY/PATHOGENESIS

Molecular Pathology
- Most ILCs, including variant types, show complete E-cadherin inactivation
  - Similar mechanisms of E-cadherin inactivation have been described in classical and variant forms of ILC
- E-cadherin gene (CDH1) has been reported to be frequently mutated in all variants of ILC
  - Remaining wild-type CDH1 allele is inactivated by loss of heterozygosity (LOH) or promoter hypermethylation at CDH1 locus (16q22.1)
- In approximately 10% of ILC, E-cadherin is expressed but cells are discohesive
  - Other components of cell adhesion, such as catenins, may be nonfunctioning

- Majority of ILC are ER/PR positive and in luminal molecular subgroup by gene profiling
  - ILCPV may display luminal, molecular apocrine, or HER2 subgroups by gene profiling

CLINICAL ISSUES

Natural History
- ILC and variant forms account for 5-15% of invasive breast cancers
  - Outcome of patients with ILC does not appear to be significantly different from that of patients with carcinomas of no special type
    - Similar prognosis when these histologic types of breast cancer are matched by stage and grade
- ILC shows proclivity for metastatic dissemination to specific anatomic sites
  - Gastrointestinal tract, uterus, meninges, ovary, serosal cavities, and bone
  - Less frequent metastasis to lung and pleura
- ILCPV shows increased tendency for local recurrence after conservative treatment compared with ILCCV

Treatment
- Treatment of all ILC and variant forms is dependent on tumor stage and parallel to treatment for IDC
- Endocrine and HER2-targeted therapies are dependent on results of biomarker studies for these factors
  - Most (but not all) ILC will be ER positive
  - Overexpression of HER2 rare (< 1%) in ILCCV
    - 48-80% of ILCPV may be HER2 positive
- In neoadjuvant studies, ILC is less likely than nonlobular carcinomas to show pathologic complete response to chemotherapy

Prognosis
- Most studies suggest that classical ILC has better prognosis than variant forms of ILC
  - Differences have not been statistically significant in many reports

INVASIVE LOBULAR CARCINOMA VARIANTS

Key Facts

Terminology

- Variant forms differ from classical ILC with regard to architecture &/or cytology
  - Show areas of nonlinear infiltration
  - Variable degree of atypia and high-grade nuclei
  - All lack cohesion either due to loss of E-cadherin or other cell adhesion molecules

Clinical Issues

- Classical ILC has better prognosis than variant forms of ILC
- Grade may be better method of subclassifying ILC and is related to variant type
  - Majority of classical ILC is moderately or well differentiated
  - Solid ILC is predominantly poorly differentiated and alveolar ILC moderately differentiated

Microscopic Pathology

- Variant forms of ILC can be classified based on differences in architectural growth pattern and cytologic features
- Architectural variants
  - Classical (55%)
  - Solid (5-10%)
  - Alveolar (5-20%)
- Cytologic variants
  - Pleomorphic
  - Histiocytoid

Top Differential Diagnoses

- Invasive ductal carcinoma
- Lymphoid neoplasms
- Metastatic melanoma

- No reproducible differences among patients with nonpleomorphic variants
- Classical ILC appears to have much more favorable prognosis than pleomorphic variant
  - ILCPV is reported to have more aggressive tumor biology and clinical behavior compared with other types
- Histologic grading of ILC (Nottingham grading system) is recommended for all tumors
  - In retrospective series, histologic grade provides strong predictor of outcome

MICROSCOPIC PATHOLOGY

Histologic Features

- **Architectural variants of ILC**
  - Variants of ILC with distinctive tissue architecture and growth patterns
- **Classical variant (55% of ILC)**
  - Linear, single file infiltrative growth pattern
    - Single rows of cells, typically no more than 1 or 2 cells wide
    - Frequent target-like concentric pattern of growth around ducts
    - Focal alveolar and solid areas may be present in < 20% of tumor
  - In some definitions of ILCCV, nuclei must be low grade (5-10% of all ILC)
  - In other definitions of ILCCV, any nuclear grade can be present
    - Grade 2 ILC comprises 80-90% of all ILC
    - Grade 3 ILCCV comprises 5-10% of all ILC
- **Solid variant (5-10% of ILC)**
  - Cells infiltrate between collagen bundles as clusters or trabeculae > 1 cell thick
    - In some cases neoplastic cells are arranged in poorly cohesive sheets and can mimic lymphoma
    - Areas of single file growth are usually present at periphery
  - 55% grade 3, 40% grade 2, and only 5% grade 1
- **Alveolar variant (5-20% of ILC)**

  - Rounded aggregates of tumor cells arranged in sheets or clusters
    - Cells are poorly cohesive with loose or "alveolar" appearance
    - Some cases may mimic LCIS but lack surrounding myoepithelial cell layer
    - Solid foci are smaller than those seen in solid variant
  - 90% are grade 2 and 10% grade 3

Cytologic Features

- **Cytologic variants of ILC**
  - Variants of ILC with typical single file growth pattern but with distinctive cytologic cellular features
- **Pleomorphic variant (10% of ILC)**
  - Tumor cells display marked nuclear pleomorphism with grade 2 or 3 nuclei
    - Nuclei may harbor single or multiple prominent nucleoli
    - Tumor cells can show abundant eosinophilic cytoplasm and apocrine appearance
    - Virtually all ILCPV are positive for apocrine marker GCDFP-15 by IHC
  - Some definitions require single cell infiltration pattern of classical ILC
  - Other definitions include any growth pattern
    - Higher grade nuclei are more common in alveolar and solid variants than in ILCCV
    - Architecture is often mixed
  - Immunohistochemical profile for ILCPV can differ markedly from ILCCV
    - HER2 overexpression and p53 nuclear expression reported in 48–80% of cases
    - 5-10% of cases will be ER and PR negative
  - Carcinomas are moderately or poorly differentiated
    - ILCPV has poorer prognosis due to higher grade and unfavorable predictive marker status in some cases
    - Prognosis is similar to carcinomas of no special type of similar grade and stage
- **Histiocytoid variant (3% of ILC)**

INVASIVE LOBULAR CARCINOMA VARIANTS

Infiltrating Lobular Carcinoma Variants

Features	Classic	Solid	Alveolar	Pleomorphic	Histiocytoid
Predominant growth pattern	Single file	Confluent sheets	Groups or round clusters	Single file	Single file
Nuclear atypia	+/-	+	+	+++	+
Cytoplasm	Scant	Scant	Scant	Abundant/eosinophilic	Foamy/pale or eosinophilic
Apocrine differentiation (GCDFP-15)	+/-	+/-	+/-	+++	+++
E-cadherin	-	-	-	-	-
ER/PR	+++	++	++	+ or -	+
HER2	-	-	-	+ or -	-

- o Cells within these tumors often have large, overtly nucleolated nuclei and copious cytoplasm
  - ▪ Overall cytomorphology may resemble macrophages; hence the term "histiocytoid"
- o Not shown to have prognostic significance

DIFFERENTIAL DIAGNOSIS

Invasive Ductal Carcinoma (IDC)
- Some cases of IDC can show single file growth pattern
  - o May mimic ILC
  - o To make distinction between IDC and ILC look for
    - ▪ Areas with trabecular growth and tumor acinar formation
    - ▪ Evidence of cohesiveness in infiltrating tumor cells
    - ▪ Association with DCIS for cases of IDC
    - ▪ Prominent desmoplastic stromal response more common in IDC
    - ▪ Loss of E-cadherin expression can be helpful in problematic cases; however, approximately 15% of ILCs express E-cadherin
- Distinction important because of potential differences in expected patterns of recurrence
- However, outcome for grade 3 carcinomas with loss of E-cadherin expression is probably related more to grade and marker expression than morphologic patterns of "lobular" or "ductal"

Lymphoid Neoplasms
- Solid variant of ILC can occasionally mimic lymphoma
  - o Sheet-like growth pattern
  - o Poorly cohesive cells
  - o Occasional cases may show plasmacytoid cytology
  - o Cytokeratin stains may be helpful in problematic cases
- Lymphoblastic lymphoma may involve mammary tissue
  - o May show prominent single file growth pattern and mimic ILC
  - o Typically seen in younger patients than ILC
  - o Nuclei appear more primitive with more frequent mitotic activity
  - o Cytokeratin stains and lymphoid markers may be helpful in problematic cases

Metastatic Melanoma
- Most common type of metastatic malignancy to breast
- Metastases can mimic grade 3 alveolar or solid ILC
  - o Cells are discohesive
  - o Usually present as circumscribed mass
- Associated carcinoma in situ will be absent
- IHC positivity for melanoma markers and negativity for cytokeratin will aid in diagnosis

DIAGNOSTIC CHECKLIST

Pathologic Interpretation Pearls
- Variants of ILC challenge pathologist to correctly assess diagnosis given wide range of morphologies
  - o Morphological and cytologic diversity implies spectrum of mammary neoplasia
    - ▪ ILC variants are unified by common molecular and cytogenetic features including loss of E-cadherin or other cell adhesion proteins
  - o Classical ILC and variant forms are remarkably similar at molecular level and should be considered as part of spectrum of carcinomas

SELECTED REFERENCES

1. Rakha EA et al: Lobular breast carcinoma and its variants. Semin Diagn Pathol. 27(1):49-61, 2010
2. Vargas AC et al: Pleomorphic lobular carcinoma of the breast: molecular pathology and clinical impact. Future Oncol. 5(2):233-43, 2009
3. Buchanan CL et al: Is pleomorphic lobular carcinoma really a distinct clinical entity? J Surg Oncol. 98(5):314-7, 2008
4. Orvieto E et al: Clinicopathologic characteristics of invasive lobular carcinoma of the breast: results of an analysis of 530 cases from a single institution. Cancer. 113(7):1511-20, 2008
5. Simpson PT et al: Molecular profiling pleomorphic lobular carcinomas of the breast: evidence for a common molecular genetic pathway with classic lobular carcinomas. J Pathol. 215(3):231-44, 2008

INVASIVE LOBULAR CARCINOMA VARIANTS

Microscopic Features

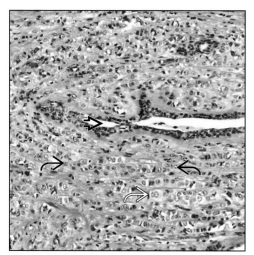

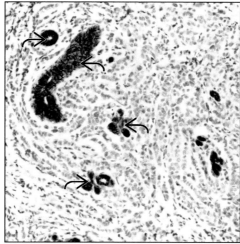

(Left) This carcinoma shows a characteristic single file growth pattern ➡ of poorly cohesive cells invading in a concentric fashion around a normal duct ⊡. While the growth pattern is typical for ILC, the cells are large and pleomorphic in appearance ➡, consistent with a pleomorphic variant of ILC (Right) Similar to classic ILC, the pleomorphic variant will show complete loss of E-cadherin staining by immunohistochemistry. Normal breast epithelium serves as a positive internal control ➡.

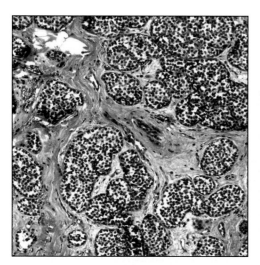

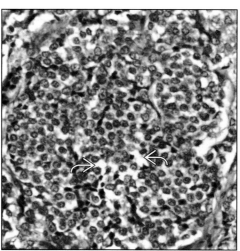

(Left) Alveolar ILC invades as nests of cells. The pattern can resemble LCIS, but myoepithelial cells are absent. (Right) The cellular aggregates of alveolar ILC are not cohesive ➡, with a loose or "alveolar" appearance. The nuclei are usually uniform with small nucleoli, and most carcinomas would be classified as grade 2.

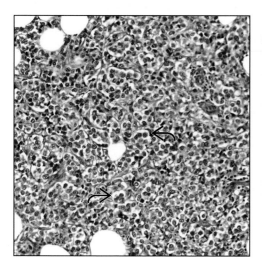

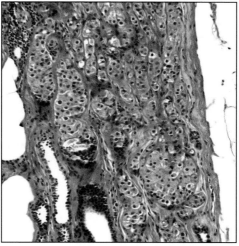

(Left) The solid variant of ILC consists of broad sheets of discohesive cells ➡ with little to no intervening stroma. Nuclei of any grade may be present. (Right) Histiocytoid ILC consists of cells with abundant eosinophilic cytoplasm. Some cases can mimic granular cell tumors. At metastatic sites, the cells may be difficult to differentiate from true histiocytes. IHC for keratin will identify the cells as carcinoma in difficult cases.

TUBULAR/CRIBRIFORM CARCINOMA

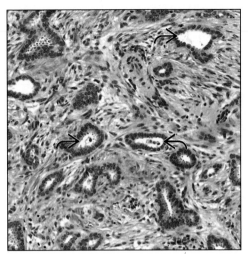

Tubular carcinoma is a special histologic type of breast cancer associated with a low metastatic potential. Favorable prognosis is restricted to tumors that consist entirely of tubular elements ➔.

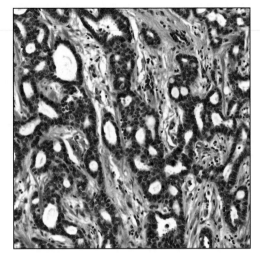

Cribriform carcinoma is often seen in conjunction with tubular carcinoma, and mixed tubular and cribriform growth patterns are frequently encountered. These carcinomas have an excellent prognosis.

TERMINOLOGY

Abbreviations
- Tubular carcinoma (TC)
- Cribriform carcinoma (CC)

Definitions
- TC and CC are very well-differentiated carcinomas that have low metastatic potential and excellent prognosis

ETIOLOGY/PATHOGENESIS

Molecular Pathology
- TC is frequently associated with
  - Low-grade DCIS (LGDCIS) (~ 90% of cases)
  - Columnar cell change (95-100% of cases)
  - Lobular neoplasia (ALH and LCIS; 15-55% of cases) ("Rosen triad")
  - In the majority of cases, columnar cell change is associated with flat epithelial atypia (FEA)
- Molecular analysis reveals similar genetic alterations shared by FEA, LGDCIS, and TC
  - Frequent loss of 16q and gain of 1q
    - May represent biological progression along low-grade breast neoplasia pathway
    - Supports a possible precursor role for LGDCIS and FEA progressing to TC
  - Associated lobular neoplasia has not been shown to share the same genetic changes
- Gene expression profiling shows that TC and CC are within the luminal A group of cancers

CLINICAL ISSUES

Epidemiology
- Incidence
  - 1-4% of breast cancers in unscreened populations
  - 10-30% of screen-detected breast cancers
- Age
  - Most common in women in their 50s to 60s undergoing mammographic screening

Presentation
- 60-70% present as nonpalpable, mammographically detected irregular masses
  - Most patients have small carcinomas (< 2 cm) and negative lymph nodes at presentation
  - More likely to be detected by mammography than other cancers
- Multicentric involvement of ipsilateral breast is present in 20-50% of patients

Prognosis
- TC and CC have excellent prognosis compared with other types of breast cancer
- Favorable prognosis restricted to TC and CC that conform to strict histologic criteria
  - > 90% of the carcinoma must consist of well-formed tubules &/or cribriform areas
- Few patients (10-20%) have positive nodes; may not impact overall survival
  - Multifocal and larger carcinomas are more likely to be associated with lymph node metastases
  - In general, only 1-3 nodes are involved

IMAGE FINDINGS

Mammographic Findings
- Small irregular mass
- Associated amorphous or pleomorphic microcalcifications in up to 50%, often due to secretory material in tubules

TUBULAR/CRIBRIFORM CARCINOMA

Key Facts

Terminology
- Tubular carcinoma (TC) and cribriform carcinoma (CC) are well-differentiated carcinomas

Etiology/Pathogenesis
- Frequently associated with low-grade DCIS, flat epithelial atypia (FEA), and LCIS
  - Similar molecular alterations shared by TC, DCIS, and FEA
  - Suggests precursor role and possible biologic progression

Clinical Issues
- 60-70% present as nonpalpable mammographically detected lesions
  - Most patients have small carcinomas and negative lymph nodes at presentation

- Pure TC and CC have excellent prognosis
  - Virtually always strongly ER positive
  - Patients may be adequately treated with adjuvant hormonal therapy alone
- Favorable prognosis restricted to tumors consisting almost entirely of tubular or cribriform patterns

Top Differential Diagnoses
- Sclerosing adenosis
- Microglandular adenosis
- Complex sclerosing lesion
- Low-grade adenosquamous carcinoma
- Syringomatous adenoma
- Well-differentiated ductal carcinomas
- Cribriform DCIS
- Adenoid cystic carcinoma

MACROSCOPIC FEATURES

General Features
- Irregular gray-white mass with retraction of surrounding tissue

Size
- Majority of TC are ≤ 1 cm, especially when mammographically detected

MICROSCOPIC PATHOLOGY

Tubular Carcinoma
- Haphazard infiltrative proliferation of well-formed glands
  - Single layer of epithelial cells
    - No surrounding myoepithelial cell layer
    - Stromal myofibroblasts apposed to base of glands can mimic myoepithelial cells on H&E and IHC
  - Cells are low grade
    - Nuclei slightly larger than normal luminal nuclei (score 1 or 2 for grading)
    - Nucleoli are small and uniform
    - Chromatin is uniform
    - Apical cytoplasmic snouts are common
    - Mitoses are rare
  - Tubules have open lumens and angulated contours with tapering ends
    - > 90% of tumor should demonstrate characteristic tubular morphology to be considered TC
    - Calcifications may be associated with secretory material in lumens
  - Desmoplastic stromal reaction should be present and may be prominent
    - Prominent stromal elastosis may be present in some cases
  - Tubules often invade around normal ducts and lobules
  - Lymph-vascular invasion is highly unusual
  - TC frequently associated with low-grade DCIS

    - DCIS typically has cribriform and micropapillary patterns
  - TC also frequently associated with columnar cell changes, FEA, ALH, and LCIS

Cribriform Carcinoma
- Haphazard infiltration of stroma by cribriform nests imparting a fenestrated appearance
  - Resembles cribriform DCIS
    - Unlike DCIS, nests of tumor cells may be found surrounding normal structures
    - CC lacks myoepithelial cells
  - CC usually associated with desmoplastic stromal reaction
  - Cytologic features are similar to those of TC

ANCILLARY TESTS

Immunohistochemistry
- Hormone receptors
  - Both TC and CC typically show high levels of ER (> 95%) and PR (> 75%) expression
  - If result is negative, test should be repeated to confirm
- HER2
  - TC and CC rarely (if ever) show HER2 overexpression or gene amplification
- Ki-67
  - Usually have a low proliferative index (usually fewer than 10% positive cells)
- Myoepithelial markers
  - IHC is often necessary to distinguish TC from other benign adenosis lesions
    - TC and CC lack myoepithelial cells
    - Benign lesions have a myoepithelial layer, which is often prominent
    - Microglandular adenosis lacks myoepithelial cells but will be negative for ER and PR
  - Muscle markers are positive in myoepithelial cells as well as in stromal myofibroblasts
    - Stromal cells apposed to base of tumor cells should not be mistaken for myoepithelial cells

TUBULAR/CRIBRIFORM CARCINOMA

Differential Diagnosis of Tubular Carcinoma

Features	Tubular Carcinoma	Sclerosing Adenosis	Complex Sclerosing Lesion	Microglandular Adenosis
Architecture/pattern	Haphazard, infiltrative growth	Nodular, circumscribed, lobulocentric	May be haphazard (confined to central region)	Nodular or diffuse
Tubular lumens	Open, similar size, angulated	Open or compressed	Open or compressed	Open, round
Luminal cells	Low grade, frequent apical snouts	Low grade, no snouts	Low grade, no snouts	Low grade, no snouts
Desmoplastic stroma	Yes, may be prominent	No	Hyalinized stroma, no desmoplasia	No
Periductal elastosis	Occasional	Usually absent	Consistent finding	Usually absent
Myoepithelial cells	Absent	Present	Present	Absent
ER/PR	+++	+	+	Negative
EMA	++	++	++	Negative
S100	Negative (luminal cells)	Negative (luminal cells)	Negative (luminal cells)	Positive (luminal cells)

DIFFERENTIAL DIAGNOSIS

Sclerosing Adenosis
- Circumscribed or nodular appearance
  - Maintains lobulocentric architecture
  - In unusual cases, portions of lesion can have infiltrative pattern into adjacent breast tissue
- Ductal structures have compressed or obliterated lumens
  - Ductal structures are usually back-to-back and typically have parallel or whirling patterns
- Myoepithelial cells are present and often prominent
  - IHC can be helpful to document myoepithelial cells
- Associated FEA, ADH, or DCIS are less common than in TC or CC

Microglandular Adenosis
- May show nodular or diffuse architecture
- Uniform, small, round luminal spaces
  - Eosinophilic secretions present in lumens
- No myoepithelial cells are present
- IHC will demonstrate that tumor cells are strongly S100 positive and ER/PR negative

Complex Sclerosing Lesion (CSL)
- Ducts can become entrapped in central fibrotic zone and closely mimic TC
  - Ducts are limited to center and do not infiltrate out into surrounding tissues
  - Stroma is densely hyalinized and lacks desmoplasia
  - Entrapped ducts have myoepithelial cell layer
- Radial sclerosing lesions can have irregular appearance radiographically and grossly

Low-Grade Adenosquamous Carcinoma
- Small well-formed tubules or solid nests of cells
- At least focal areas of squamous differentiation are present
- Negative for ER and PR

Syringomatous Adenoma (SA)
- SA arises in dermis of nipple
  - TC rarely involves dermis
- Squamoid areas will be present
- SA is negative for ER and PR

Well-differentiated Ductal Carcinomas
- TC is **not** synonymous with well-differentiated carcinomas of no special type
- Well-differentiated carcinomas can have less tubule formation, more nuclear pleomorphism, &/or increased mitotic rate
- TC has a better prognosis than other well-differentiated carcinomas

Cribriform DCIS
- DCIS with cribriform pattern may resemble invasive cribriform carcinoma
  - Invasive carcinoma often infiltrates around normal structures
  - Involved spaces may have irregular borders in contrast to usually circumscribed spaces of DCIS
- IHC will confirm presence of myoepithelial cells in DCIS

Adenoid Cystic Carcinoma (ACC)
- Both ACC and CC are invasive carcinomas with cribriform pattern
- ACC consists of both luminal and myoepithelial-type cells, whereas CC consists of only luminal-type cells
- Many of cribriform spaces in ACC are filled with basement-membrane-like material
- ACC is almost always negative for ER and PR

SELECTED REFERENCES

1. Aulmann S et al: Invasive tubular carcinoma of the breast frequently is clonally related to flat epithelial atypia and low-grade ductal carcinoma in situ. Am J Surg Pathol. 33(11):1646-53, 2009
2. Abdel-Fatah TM et al: Morphologic and molecular evolutionary pathways of low nuclear grade invasive breast cancers and their putative precursor lesions: further evidence to support the concept of low nuclear grade breast neoplasia family. Am J Surg Pathol. 32(4):513-23, 2008
3. Brandt SM et al: The "Rosen Triad": tubular carcinoma, lobular carcinoma in situ, and columnar cell lesions. Adv Anat Pathol. 15(3):140-6, 2008

TUBULAR/CRIBRIFORM CARCINOMA

Microscopic Features

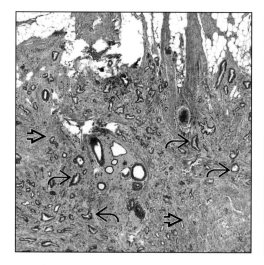

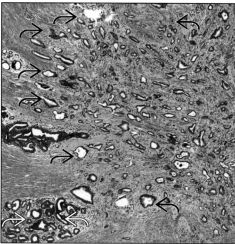

(Left) TC consists of an haphazard infiltrative proliferation of well-formed tubules with open lumens ➡. The prominent desmoplastic stromal reaction ⇉ is a helpful diagnostic feature in distinguishing TC from benign lesions and microglandular adenosis. **(Right)** The haphazard infiltrative growth pattern is not lobulocentric and is best seen at low magnification ➡. This TC is associated with foci of flat epithelial atypia ➡, which is a frequent finding.

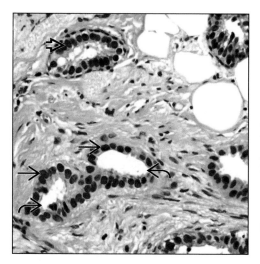

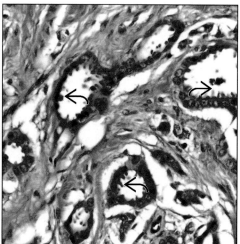

(Left) The open luminal spaces in TC demonstrate angular contours with tapering ends ➡. The neoplastic cells have low- to intermediate-grade nuclei ➡, which are of similar size to the adjacent normal luminal cells ⇉. **(Right)** The cells in TC form a monolayer and have a moderate amount of eosinophilic cytoplasm. The cells often show apical cytoplasmic snouts projecting into the luminal space ➡, which can be associated with secretions and luminal calcifications in some cases.

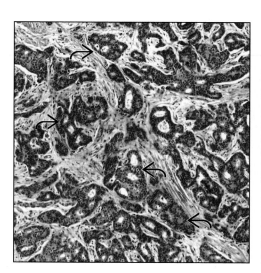

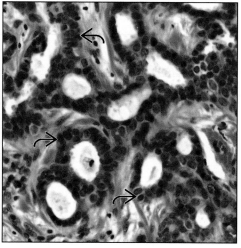

(Left) CC is characterized by a pattern of infiltrative cribriform or fenestrated nests of cells ➡ that resemble cribriform pattern DCIS. However, the nests are usually not as rounded and often invade around normal breast structures. The absence of myoepithelial cells is a helpful feature in confirming stromal invasion. **(Right)** Like TC, the cells of CC have nuclei that are small and uniform in size with inconspicuous nucleoli ➡. Mitoses are absent or very rare.

TUBULAR/CRIBRIFORM CARCINOMA

Ancillary Techniques

(Left) TC ⇨ (positive for CK18, red) can be distinguished from benign adenosis lesions by IHC to confirm the absence of myoepithelial cells in the carcinoma and their presence ⇒ (p63 and CK5/6, brown) in normal breast lobules. **(Right)** Muscle markers such as smooth muscle actin can confirm the absence of myoepithelial cells associated with TC ⇒. These studies are more difficult to interpret than p63, as both myofibroblasts ⇒ and myoepithelial cells ⇨ are positive.

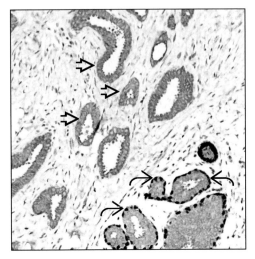 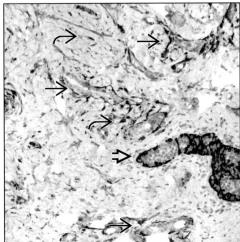

(Left) Stromal myofibroblasts are positive for muscle markers such as smooth muscle actin and can be apposed to tumor cells ⇒. These cells should not be confused with true myoepithelial cells. **(Right)** TC and CC show high levels of ER ⇒ expression, as well as PR, and will be responsive to hormonal therapy. For cases that show histologic features of TC or CC, if ER is negative, suspect a technical problem or consider an alternative diagnosis such as microglandular adenosis.

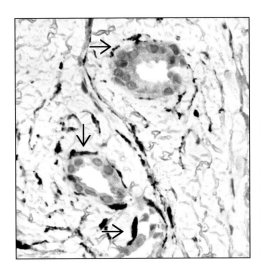 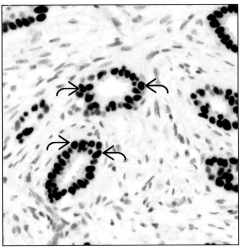

(Left) Ki-67 shows a low proliferative index ⇒ for this TC, as less than 5% of the cells show positivity. Tumors with frequent mitotic figures &/ or a high Ki-67 proliferative index should not be diagnosed as TC. **(Right)** This lesion consisted of tubules and cribriform nests of cells in the dermis. The location suggests syringomatous adenoma. However, the tumor cells, as well as the areolar smooth muscle ⇒, are strongly ER positive, favoring a carcinoma with TC and CC patterns.

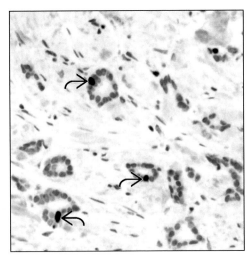 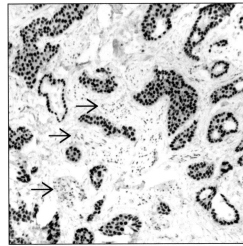

TUBULAR/CRIBRIFORM CARCINOMA

Differential Diagnosis

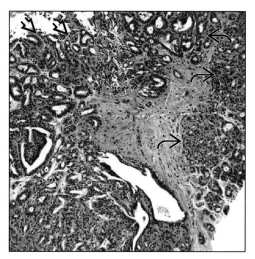

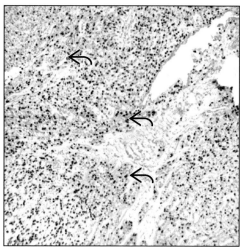

(Left) Sclerosing adenosis, when florid, can mimic TC. This differential diagnosis can be particularly problematic on core needle biopsy specimens. Look for a lobulocentric organization to sclerosing adenosis ➡ with a circumscribed or lobulated periphery ⊅. (Right) Sclerosing adenosis, unlike TC, usually has back-to-back glands with compressed lumens and a prominent myoepithelial cell layer. In this case, the myoepithelial cells are easily identified with IHC for p63 ➡.

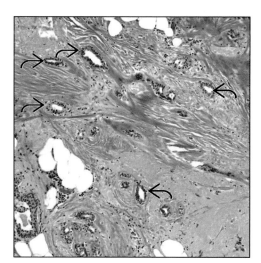

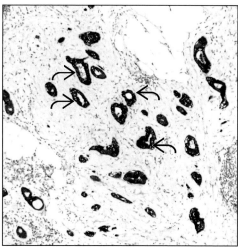

(Left) The central sclerotic zone of a radial sclerosing lesion can entrap glands and mimic the infiltrative pattern of a TC. These compressed glands ➡ are confined to the central zone and associated with a very dense stroma, unlike the loosely desmoplastic stroma typical of TC. (Right) IHC is helpful for evaluating the entrapped glands (CK18 positive, red) in the center of a radial sclerosing lesion by confirming that myoepithelial cells (p63 and CK5/6 positive, brown) ➡ are present.

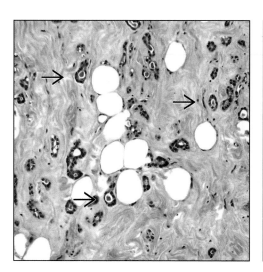

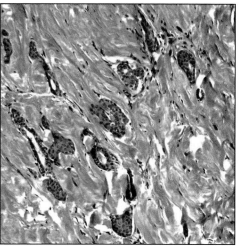

(Left) Microglandular adenosis, like TC, consists of small tubules without myoepithelial cells. Unlike TC, the tubules are round, usually have eosinophilic secretions ➡, and are not associated with desmoplasia. (Right) Syringomatous adenoma occurs in the dermis of the nipple and areola. Although small well-formed tubules are present, they are accompanied by solid nests and squamous areas. The cells will be negative for hormone receptors and are usually positive for p63, unlike TC.

TUBULOLOBULAR CARCINOMA

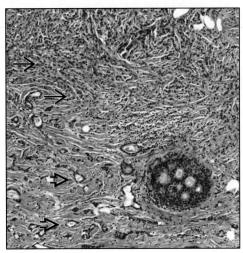

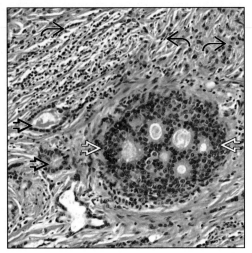

Tubulolobular carcinoma is a rare type of carcinoma composed of 2 distinct components: Well-formed tubules ⊳ and a single cell infiltrative pattern typical of invasive lobular carcinoma ⇨.

Although a lobular pattern of infiltration is present ⇨, the cells are E-cadherin positive. Tubules ⊳ and the frequent association with DCIS ⊳ also distinguish TLC from lobular carcinoma.

TERMINOLOGY

Abbreviations

- Tubulolobular carcinoma (TLC)

Definitions

- Morphologically distinct type of mammary carcinoma with 2 components consisting of minute well-formed tubules and single discohesive cells
- TLC is **not** a synonym for carcinoma with ductal and lobular features

ETIOLOGY/PATHOGENESIS

Morphologic and Phenotypic Studies of TLC

- Characterized by having both tubular ("ductal") and single cell ("lobular") morphologic components
  - Initially described as tubular variant of lobular carcinoma
  - Later studies demonstrated that TLC expresses E-cadherin and other cell adhesion molecules
  - Supports classification of TLC as variant of ductal carcinoma with lobular growth pattern
- 3-dimensional modeling of TLC and tubular carcinoma (TC)
  - Both tumor types consist of glandular structures connected by slender cords of single cells
  - Glands of TLC are connected by longer strands of single cells
    - TC has short strands of single cells that are less apparent in 2-dimensional sections
  - May account for appearance of tubular and lobular growth patterns in histologic sections
  - Morphologic appearance of loss of cohesion in presence of cell adhesion molecules is unclear
    - Catenin expression is normal in most TLCs

CLINICAL ISSUES

Epidemiology

- Incidence
  - Rare; 1-2% of invasive breast carcinomas
- Age
  - Similar to carcinomas of no special type; may be more common in older women
- Gender
  - TLC has been reported in both males and females

Presentation

- Usually presents with palpable mass
  - Less commonly found as a mass on mammographic screening

Prognosis

- Intermediate prognosis between pure TC and invasive lobular carcinoma (ILC)

IMAGE FINDINGS

General Features

- Location
  - Multifocality is present in ~ 30% of cases
    - Positive lymph nodes are found in ~ 60% of multifocal cases and ~ 30% of cases with single focus
- Size
  - Palpable mass present in 85% of patients
    - Mean size: 1.7 cm

Mammographic Findings

- Most typical mammographic finding is irregular mass
  - May also show asymmetric focal density or architectural distortion

Ultrasonographic Findings

- Mass with angulated, spiculated, or microlobulated borders

TUBULOLOBULAR CARCINOMA

Key Facts

Terminology
- Tubulolobular carcinoma (TLC)
- Not a synonym for "carcinomas with ductal and lobular features"

Etiology/Pathogenesis
- Low-grade invasive carcinoma with tubule formation and single cell lobular pattern
- Initially described as tubular variant of lobular carcinoma
- However, expression of E-cadherin supports classification as variant of ductal carcinoma
  - Reason for "lobular" appearance in presence of cell adhesion molecules has not been explained

Clinical Issues
- 1-2% of carcinomas

Microscopic Pathology
- Admixture of round tubules and single cells infiltrating in single files

Ancillary Tests
- Almost all cancers are positive for ER and PR and negative for HER2
- Positive for E-cadherin and catenins

Top Differential Diagnoses
- Tubular carcinoma
- Invasive lobular carcinoma
- Invasive carcinoma with ductal and lobular features

  - May have posterior acoustic shadowing or normal acoustic transmission

MACROSCOPIC FEATURES

General Features
- Most common gross appearance is hard, irregular, gray-tan mass, similar to carcinomas of no specific type

MICROSCOPIC PATHOLOGY

Histologic Features
- Invasive tumor shows mixed pattern of invasion with both tubules and single cells
  - Tubular component
    - Smaller than those of TC
    - Tubules are round in shape in contrast to angulated or comma shapes of TC
    - Typically lack apical snouts and are not commonly associated with calcifications
    - Cells have small uniform low-grade nuclei with inconspicuous nucleoli
    - Luminal mucin may be present
  - Lobular component
    - Infiltrates as single cells
    - Cells are rounded and appear discohesive
    - Cells have small uniform low-grade nuclei with inconspicuous nucleoli
    - May infiltrate in targetoid fashion around normal ducts
  - Proportion of tubular and lobular components in TLC is variable
    - Nearly equal components (27%), predominance of lobular component (46%), or tubular component (27%)
- Lymph-vascular invasion is uncommon
- Associated low-grade DCIS &/or LCIS is present in approximately 60% of cases
  - DCIS alone is found more often in pure TC than in TLC

- Grade is most commonly well differentiated but may be moderately differentiated
  - Tubule score may be 1, 2, or 3, depending on extent of lobular component
  - Nuclear score should be 1 or 2
  - Mitoses score should be 1

ANCILLARY TESTS

Immunohistochemistry
- **Estrogen and progesterone receptors**
  - ER positive (95%) and PR positive (79%) in majority of cases
- **HER2**
  - Not overexpressed by either IHC or FISH studies
- **E-cadherin and catenins**
  - E-cadherin displays moderate or strong complete membranous staining in all cases of TLC
  - Catenins (α, β, γ, and p120) all demonstrate strong membrane staining pattern

DIFFERENTIAL DIAGNOSIS

Tubular Carcinoma (TC)
- Lacks lobular component seen in TLC
- Tubules in TC are larger and have angulated shape
  - Often have snouts and may be associated with calcifications
- Immunoprofiles of TC and TLC are identical
- TC less likely to have lymph node metastases
- Always well differentiated
  - TLC is usually well differentiated but may be moderately differentiated
- Usually detected as small irregular mass on screening mammography
  - TLC is generally larger and often presents as a palpable mass
- Has better prognosis than TLC

Invasive Lobular Carcinoma
- Lacks tubular component of TLC

TUBULOLOBULAR CARCINOMA

Tubulolobular Carcinoma, Differential Diagnosis

Features	Tubular Carcinoma	Tubulolobular Carcinoma	Invasive Lobular Carcinoma
Nuclear grade	Low	Low	Low, intermediate, or high
Growth pattern	Tubular	Mixed tubular and lobular	Lobular
Multifocality	20-50%	~ 30% of cases	~ 50% of cases
Associated DCIS	70-90% of cases	~ 60% of cases	20% of cases
Associated LCIS	15-50%	20-30%	50-90%
Stromal reaction	Typically desmoplastic and sclerotic	Variable, may be minimal	Variable, may be minimal
ER/PR expression	Strongly positive	Strongly positive	Strongly positive except in high-grade cancers
HER2 expression	Almost always negative	Almost always negative	Almost always negative except in high-grade cancers
E-cadherin expression	Uniform strong membrane staining	Uniform strong membrane staining	Absent or aberrant staining
p120 catenin	Uniform strong membrane staining	Uniform strong membrane staining	Abnormal cytoplasmic staining
α-catenin	Uniform strong membrane staining	Uniform strong membrane staining	Absence of staining

TLC is a distinctive mammary carcinoma that shows tubular and lobular morphologic patterns but displays membranous E-cadherin/catenin complex unlike lobular carcinomas.

- Lacks E-cadherin in great majority of cases, whereas TLC is positive
  - Abnormal catenin expression is also present
    - Absence of α-catenin and uniform abnormal cytoplasmic staining for p120 catenin
- Can be of any grade, whereas TLC is almost always well differentiated
- Often associated with LCIS; only rarely associated with DCIS

Invasive Carcinoma with Ductal and Lobular Features

- 2-6% of carcinomas of no special type show focal areas with lobular single cell infiltrative pattern
  - More common than TLC
- Most important reason to note this type of carcinoma is to recognize that metastases &/or recurrences can have lobular appearance
  - Lobular pattern can be difficult to recognize at metastatic sites
    - In bone marrow, cells can resemble hematopoietic cells
    - In soft tissue, cells can resemble lymphocytes or histiocytes
    - In stomach, cells can resemble gastric signet ring cell carcinoma
    - Diffuse infiltrative pattern may not form mass evident by imaging or palpation
- "Ductal" component usually consists of solid nests and strands of tumor cells
  - Well-formed tubules are not common feature
- Most commonly of intermediate grade and can be poorly differentiated
  - TLC is almost always well differentiated
- Associated with DCIS in ~ 60% of cases, DCIS and LCIS in ~ 30%, and with LCIS alone in ~ 3%
- Immunoprofile is most commonly ER/PR positive, HER2 negative, and E-cadherin positive
  - Positivity for E-cadherin may be weaker in areas of lobular morphology

- TLC is not a synonym for "carcinomas with ductal and lobular features"
  - TLC should be reserved for well-differentiated carcinomas fitting specific morphologic criteria for this diagnosis

SELECTED REFERENCES

1. Suryadevara A et al: The clinical behavior of mixed ductal/lobular carcinoma of the breast: a clinicopathologic analysis. World J Surg Oncol. 8:51, 2010
2. Rakha EA et al: The biological and clinical characteristics of breast carcinoma with mixed ductal and lobular morphology. Breast Cancer Res Treat. 114(2):243-50, 2009
3. Abdel-Fatah TM et al: High frequency of coexistence of columnar cell lesions, lobular neoplasia, and low grade ductal carcinoma in situ with invasive tubular carcinoma and invasive lobular carcinoma. Am J Surg Pathol. 31(3):417-26, 2007
4. Esposito NN et al: The ductal phenotypic expression of the E-cadherin/catenin complex in tubulolobular carcinoma of the breast: an immunohistochemical and clinicopathologic study. Mod Pathol. 20(1):130-8, 2007
5. Günhan-Bilgen I et al: Tubulolobular carcinoma of the breast: clinical, mammographic and sonographic findings. Eur J Radiol. 60(3):418-24, 2006
6. Kuroda H et al: Expression of E-cadherin, alpha-catenin, and beta-catenin in tubulolobular carcinoma of the breast. Virchows Arch. 448(4):500-5, 2006
7. Marchiò C et al: A new vision of tubular and tubulo-lobular carcinomas of the breast, as revealed by 3-D modelling. Histopathology. 48(5):556-62, 2006
8. Qureshi HS et al: E-cadherin status in breast cancer correlates with histologic type but does not correlate with established prognostic parameters. Am J Clin Pathol. 125(3):377-85, 2006
9. Wheeler DT et al: Tubulolobular carcinoma of the breast: an analysis of 27 cases of a tumor with a hybrid morphology and immunoprofile. Am J Surg Pathol. 28(12):1587-93, 2004

TUBULOLOBULAR CARCINOMA

Microscopic Features

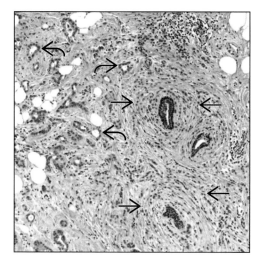
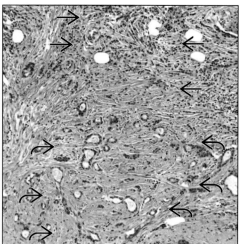

(Left) TLC is a rare, morphologically distinctive type of breast cancer consisting of 2 distinct components. One component consists of small well-formed tubules ➔. The other component consists of individual cells invading in single file ➔. **(Right)** The proportion of the tubular and lobular components in TLC is variable. In this example, the tubular (seen in the bottom of the field) ➔ and lobular ➔ components are approximately equal, which is seen in ~ 1/4 of cases.

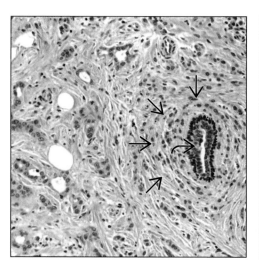
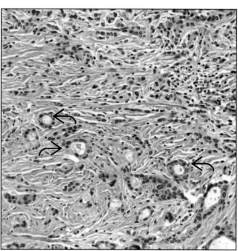

(Left) The lobular component consists of single cells with low-grade nuclei and rounded contours. They infiltrate as single cells and may form targetoid patterns ➔ around nonneoplastic ducts ➔. **(Right)** In TLC, the tubules are small and typically have a round shape ➔. In contrast, in tubular carcinoma the tubules are larger and are angulated or comma-shaped. The cells frequently have apical snouts, and calcifications may be present in the lumens.

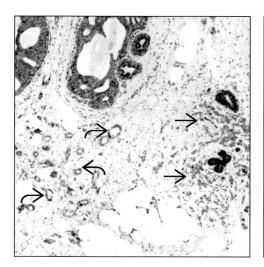
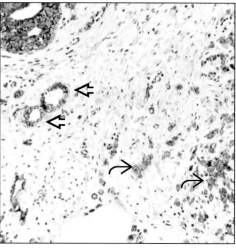

(Left) Unlike invasive lobular carcinoma, TLC is consistently positive for membranous E-cadherin and catenin complex in both the tubular ➔ and lobular ➔ components. Thus, TLC is generally not considered a subtype of lobular carcinoma. **(Right)** The presence of membrane staining for E-cadherin, as well as β- and p120 catenin, is seen in both tubules ➔ and in single cells ➔. The lack of cohesion in this component has not been explained.

MEDULLARY CARCINOMA

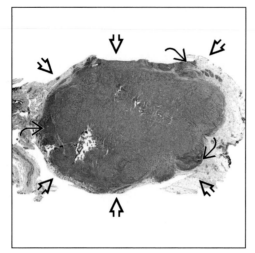

The diagnosis of medullary carcinoma requires that the carcinoma be well circumscribed ⊇ and associated with a prominent lymphoplasmacytic infiltrate ⊅.

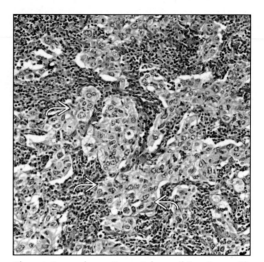

The carcinoma has a "syncytial growth" pattern with broad anastomosing sheets of tumor cells ⊵ with indistinct cell borders, pleomorphic high-grade nuclei, and frequent mitoses.

TERMINOLOGY

Abbreviations
- Medullary carcinoma (MC)

Definitions
- Rare histologic subtype of invasive breast cancer with characteristic histologic features
- "Medullary" was applied to these carcinomas in 19th century based on their gross appearance
  - "Medullary" refers to marrow of bones, signifying soft mass
  - "Encephaloid" (resembling brain) was alternative term
  - Lack of desmoplastic stroma resulting in soft consistency distinguishes MC from other carcinomas that are hard or scirrhous

ETIOLOGY/PATHOGENESIS

Molecular Pathology of MC
- Syncytial growth pattern is critical for diagnosis and is linked to prognosis
  - MC has increased expression of cell adhesion proteins including E-cadherin and β-catenin
  - Tight cell adhesion may limit tumor cell dissemination via lymphatics correlating with fewer nodal and distant metastases
- Many MC downregulate BRCA1
  - Approximately 25% of apparent sporadic MC have BRCA1 mutations
  - Approximately 2/3 of MCs without BRCA1 mutations have downregulation due to promoter methylation
  - In turn, MC accounts for 13% of breast tumors arising in BRCA1 mutation carriers
    - 30-60% of carcinomas in BRCA1 mutation carriers have medullary features

- Medullary features rare in women with BRCA2 mutations
- Gene expression profiling
  - MC is member of basal-like group of breast carcinomas
  - MC has higher level of expression of CK5/6 and higher rates of gains and losses of DNA as compared to other basal-like carcinomas
  - Most basal-like carcinomas have poor prognosis
    - MC is exception as it has more favorable prognosis compared to carcinomas of no special type when strict diagnostic criteria are applied

CLINICAL ISSUES

Epidemiology
- Incidence
  - MC represents 1-7% of all invasive breast cancers
    - Differences in incidence likely related to stringency of criteria used to make diagnosis
- Age
  - Average age at presentation: 45-52 years
    - Compared with 55 years for patients with IDC, not otherwise specified

Presentation
- Most patients present with palpable mass
  - May be soft and mobile and perceived as benign
  - Often grows rapidly
- Lymphadenopathy may be present
  - Lymph nodes may be enlarged due to hyperplasia; metastases are uncommon

Treatment
- Adjuvant therapy
  - Some medical oncologists take more conservative approach for MC due to favorable prognosis
  - However, favorable prognosis may not apply to large cancers or cancer in women with BRCA1 mutations

MEDULLARY CARCINOMA

Key Facts

Terminology
- Medullary carcinoma (MC)
  - Rare subtype of invasive breast cancer with characteristic histologic features

Etiology/Pathogenesis
- Many MCs downregulate *BRCA1* either by promoter methylation (2/3) or mutation (1/4)
- MC is member of basal-like group of breast carcinomas by gene expression profiling
  - Typically negative for ER, PRP, and HER2
  - Majority have *TP53* mutations

Clinical Issues
- MC, when strictly defined by morphologic criteria, has favorable prognosis

- Actuarial 10-year survival rates greater than 80% in some reports
- Usually presents as palpable, often rapidly growing mass
- Improved survival may be due to host immune response, syncytial growth pattern, &/or high mitotic rate leading to increased sensitivity to therapy

Top Differential Diagnoses
- Atypical medullary carcinoma (AMC)
- Carcinomas arising in women with *BRCA1* mutations
  - 13% have MC and 30-60% have carcinomas with medullary features
- Intramammary nodal metastasis
- Lymphoma

- Therefore, strict criteria should be used for diagnosis to avoid undertreating patients with poorly differentiated carcinoma of no special type

Prognosis
- MC, when strictly defined by morphologic criteria, has relatively favorable prognosis
  - Actuarial 10-year survival rates greater than 80% in some reports
  - Not yet clear if patients with *BRCA1* germline mutations and MC have same favorable prognosis
  - However, some investigators have not been able to duplicate favorable results based on alternative methods of defining MC
- Better prognosis may be linked to host immune response, syncytial growth pattern, and high mitotic rate leading to sensitivity to therapy
- Lymph node metastases are uncommon and, when present, usually involve < 4 nodes
- MC > 3 cm in size or with metastases to ≥ 4 lymph nodes does not have more favorable prognosis
  - When present, recurrence &/or death usually occurs within 5 years

Core Needle Biopsy
- Diagnosis of MC can be suggested when appropriate histologic features are present and imaged lesion is a circumscribed mass
- Final classification as MC can be made only after excision and microscopic examination of entire carcinoma

IMAGE FINDINGS

General Features
- Size
  - Typically 1-3 cm

Mammographic Findings
- Oval, round, or lobulated mass

- No specific features distinguish MC from other types of circumscribed carcinomas or benign lesions (e.g., fibroadenomas)
- Margins are often at least partially indistinct due to surrounding inflammatory infiltrate

Ultrasonographic Findings
- Round, oval, or lobular hypoechoic mass lesion
  - Margins mostly circumscribed, partially indistinct
- Thick echogenic halo is common finding

MACROSCOPIC FEATURES

General Features
- Well circumscribed with pushing borders
  - Lesions tend to have soft consistency with homogeneous white-gray cut surface
  - Areas of hemorrhage and foci of necrosis may be present in some cases
    - Necrosis, when present, usually focal and limited
  - Cancers can be mistaken grossly for fibroadenomas
    - Fibroadenomas usually bulge out from cut surface with clefts, whereas MC appears solid with only slightly raised surface

MICROSCOPIC PATHOLOGY

Histologic Features
- MC is strictly defined by presence of 5 specific morphologic features
  - 1: Predominant syncytial pattern (> 75%)
    - Neoplastic cells arranged in solid anastomosing broad sheets (at least 4 cells wide)
    - Indistinct cell borders (but not true syncytium)
  - 2: Sharply circumscribed pushing borders
    - Carcinoma cells should not invade as single cells or small nests
    - Collagenous stroma is typically very scant
    - Carcinoma may have adjacent coalescent nodules

- Border is manifestation of pushing growth pattern of carcinoma; normal epithelium and adipose tissue should not be found within carcinoma
  - 3: Moderate to frequently marked lymphoplasmacytic host inflammatory infiltrate
    - Typically involves periphery of tumor (interface of tumor and surrounding tissue)
    - Cells are predominantly T cells intermingled with plasma cells
  - 4: High nuclear grade with frequent mitoses
    - Vesicular chromatin and multiple nucleoli common
    - Multinucleated cells may be present
    - Atypical mitoses frequently present
  - 5: Absence of gland formation
- DCIS usually scant or absent
  - DCIS does not exclude diagnosis of MC
    - Absence of DCIS was earlier criterion but later shown to be unimportant
  - Adjacent lobules may appear to be colonized by tumor cells, which then coalesce with main tumor mass, resulting in multinodular appearance
    - DCIS will be negative for ER and PR
  - DCIS also associated with dense lymphoplasmacytic infiltrate
- Hemorrhage and geographic necrosis may be present
- Squamous metaplasia can be present
- Lymph-vascular invasion very unusual finding
- Lymph nodes may be enlarged and hyperplastic
  - More lymph nodes may be identified due to larger size
  - Lymph node metastases not common and, when present, usually involve only 1 or a few nodes

ANCILLARY TESTS

Immunohistochemistry
- MC almost always negative for ER, PR, and HER2
- Overexpression of p53 protein resulting from *TP53* mutation is common (60-80%)
- Cytokeratin expression includes both luminal and basal types
  - High levels of luminal CK8 and CK18
  - Frequently express basal cytokeratins CK5/6 (> 90%) and CK14
- Epidermal growth factor receptor (HER1) is positive in up to 70% of MC
- May overexpress cell adhesion molecules such as E-cadherin and β-catenin

DIFFERENTIAL DIAGNOSIS

Atypical Medullary Carcinoma (AMC)
- Some but not all features of MC
  - Associated host lymphocytic infiltration is slight to moderate
  - Circumscription of tumor in relationship to surrounding breast tissue is incomplete
    - Margins of tumor show infiltration of adjacent tissue in some areas

- Prognosis for cases classified as AMC is similar to that of nonmedullary tumors
  - AMC with sparse lymphocytic infiltrate associated with poor prognosis
- Some authors have proposed eliminating AMC
  - Alternate term is "carcinoma with medullary features," which can be used to describe appearance of many carcinomas in women with *BRCA1* mutations

Intramammary Nodal Metastasis
- Can be difficult to distinguish MC from intramammary lymph node if in upper outer quadrant of breast
- Look for evidence of node capsule or subcapsular sinus
- Look for other underlying architectural features of lymph nodes
  - However, germinal centers can be associated with MC
- Surrounding breast tissue supports diagnosis of MC
  - Adjacent DCIS would strongly support diagnosis of MC
- Look for evidence of primary carcinoma elsewhere in breast if lymph node metastasis suspected

Lymphoma
- Some MCs have marked lymphoplasmacytic infiltrates that obscure neoplastic cells
  - May mimic lymphoma in extreme cases
  - Immunostains for cytokeratin and lymphoid markers may be helpful in problematic cases

Carcinomas Arising in Women with BRCA1 Mutations
- 13% of these carcinomas classified as MC
- 60% have some medullary features; feature most often lacking is syncytial growth pattern
  - Medullary features and information about hormone receptors and HER2 have been incorporated into model predicting likelihood of germline *BRCA1* mutation

SELECTED REFERENCES
1. Rakha EA et al: The prognostic significance of inflammation and medullary histological type in invasive carcinoma of the breast. Eur J Cancer. 45(10):1780-7, 2009
2. Rodríguez-Pinilla SM et al: Sporadic invasive breast carcinomas with medullary features display a basal-like phenotype: an immunohistochemical and gene amplification study. Am J Surg Pathol. 31(4):501-8, 2007
3. Vincent-Salomon A et al: Identification of typical medullary breast carcinoma as a genomic sub-group of basal-like carcinomas, a heterogeneous new molecular entity. Breast Cancer Res. 9(2):R24, 2007
4. Farshid G et al: Morphology of breast cancer as a means of triage of patients for BRCA1 genetic testing. Am J Surg Pathol. 30(11):1357-66, 2006
5. Wargotz ES et al: Medullary carcinoma of the breast: a clinicopathologic study with appraisal of current diagnostic criteria. Hum Pathol. 19(11):1340-6, 1988
6. Ridolfi RL et al: Medullary carcinoma of the breast: a clinicopathologic study with 10 year follow-up. Cancer. 40(4):1365-85, 1977

MEDULLARY CARCINOMA

Imaging, Gross, and Microscopic Features

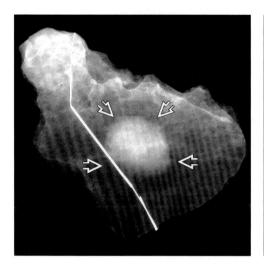

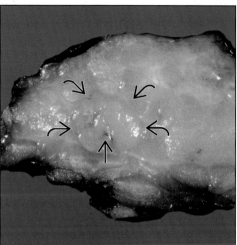

(Left) MC most commonly presents as a palpable mass. Less commonly, MC is detected on mammographic screening as a circumscribed density with sharply defined borders ➦. The appearance closely resembles a fibroadenoma. *(Right)* On gross examination, MCs are well circumscribed ➦ and have a soft to firm consistency with a homogeneous white-gray cut surface ➦. Unlike fibroadenomas that bulge outward with clefts, MC generally has a flat or slightly protruding surface.

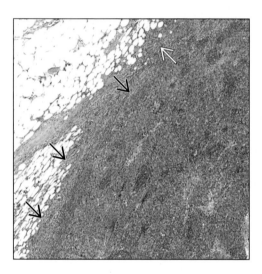

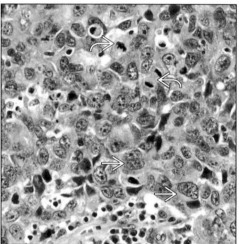

(Left) MC must have a sharply circumscribed pushing border ➦ with no invasion of single cells or small nests into the surrounding breast tissue. However, the lymphocytic infiltrate can extend into the surrounding tissue ➦. *(Right)* Despite poor prognostic features that include high-grade nuclei ➦, frequent mitotic figures ➦, and lack of hormone receptors, MC has a favorable prognosis provided strict diagnostic criteria are applied in making the diagnosis.

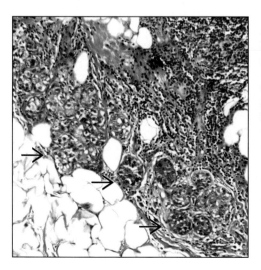

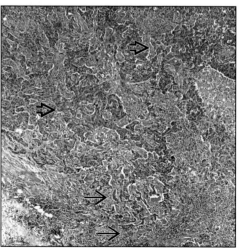

(Left) DCIS is typically absent or scant and often takes the form of tumor cells within lobules at the periphery of the carcinoma ➦ surrounded by a lymphoplasmacytic infiltrate. Areas of DCIS can form nodules that coalesce with the main tumor. *(Right)* Although this carcinoma has a partial syncytial growth pattern ➦, high nuclear grade, and an associated lymphocytic infiltrate, the presence of invasion as small nests and cords ➦ excludes the diagnosis of medullary carcinoma.

MUCINOUS (COLLOID) CARCINOMA

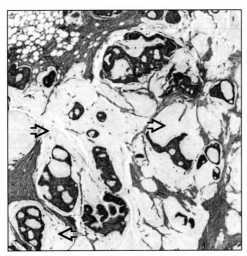

Mucinous carcinoma is a special type of invasive breast cancer characterized by abundant extracellular pools of stromal mucin production ⇨. At least 1/3 of the area involved by tumor is mucin.

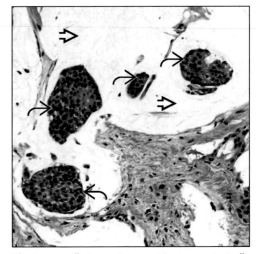

The tumor cells in mucinous carcinoma are typically low grade and are arranged in clusters and nests ➢, "floating" in pools of stromal mucin ⇨. Pure mucinous carcinoma has a favorable prognosis.

TERMINOLOGY

Abbreviations
- Mucinous carcinoma (MC)

Synonyms
- Colloid carcinoma
- Older terms: Mucoid or gelatinous carcinoma

Definitions
- Special histologic type of invasive carcinoma with distinctive features
  - Tumors are characterized by abundant extracellular pools of stromal mucin product
    - Type A MC is paucicellular and type B MC is more cellular

ETIOLOGY/PATHOGENESIS

Mucin Expression in MC: MUC Genes
- Among family of MUC genes, MC expresses predominantly *MUC2* and *MUC6*
  - MUC2 and MUC6, known as gel-forming mucins, are secreted into stroma that surrounds malignant epithelial cells
    - MUC2 and MUC6 may serve as barrier to spread of tumor cells
    - May help to explain indolent clinical behavior
    - Extracellular mucins may also increase cytotoxic T-lymphocyte activity

Gene Expression Profiling
- MC and neuroendocrine breast carcinoma (NEBC) are more similar to each other than to carcinoma of no special type
- These cancers fall within luminal type A group
- Type B MC and NEBC have essentially identical expression profiles
  - This includes type B MC with and without expression of neuroendocrine markers by IHC

CLINICAL ISSUES

Epidemiology
- Incidence
  - Uncommon tumor that accounts for 1-7% of all invasive mammary carcinomas
    - Prevalence is age-related : < 1% in women under 35, but 7% in women older than 75
- Age
  - MC tends to show older mean age at diagnosis (65.8 years)

Presentation
- Most common presentation is as a palpable mass
  - Smaller cancers may be identified as circumscribed or lobulated mass lesions on mammography

Prognosis
- Pure MC is associated with favorable prognosis
  - 10-year survival in excess of 80%
  - Patients typically have lower incidence of axillary lymph node metastasis compared with no special type carcinomas (12% of cases)
    - Axillary nodal involvement is the most important prognostic factor for these patients
- Pure MC (> 90% mucinous histology) has better prognosis than mixed tumors (carcinomas with only focal mucin production)

IMAGE FINDINGS

Mammographic Findings
- Round, oval, or lobulated density
  - Portion of margin may be indistinct
    - Irregular shape and spiculated margin may be seen in mixed tumors

Ultrasonographic Findings
- Round or oval mass lesion
  - Small lesion typically isoechoic to fat

MUCINOUS (COLLOID) CARCINOMA

Key Facts

Terminology
- Mucinous carcinoma (MC)
  - Special histologic type of invasive carcinoma with distinctive features
  - Characterized by abundant extracellular pools of stromal mucin product

Clinical Issues
- Uncommon; accounts for 1-7% of all invasive mammary carcinomas
  - Higher prevalence in older age (mean age: 65.8 years)
- Commonly presents as palpable mass or circumscribed/lobulated mass on mammogram
- Pure MC is associated with favorable prognosis
  - 10-year survival in excess of 80%
- Pure MCs have better prognosis than mixed tumors (carcinomas with only focal mucin production)

Macroscopic Features
- Soft glistening cut surface, gelatinous appearance

Microscopic Pathology
- Hallmark of MC is extracellular mucin production
  - Detached tumor cells floating in pools of mucin
  - > 90% mucinous histology (frequently, entire tumor is mucinous)
  - Tumor cells typically show low histologic grade

Ancillary Tests
- Most MCs show expression of ER and PR
- HER2 and EGFR overexpression is very uncommon
- Some MCs can show neuroendocrine differentiation

- Larger lesions or mixed tumors typically hypoechoic

MACROSCOPIC FEATURES

General Features
- Pure MC are well circumscribed
  - Cut surface is soft and typically glistening with gelatinous appearance

Size
- Can show wide range of sizes from < 1 cm up to > 10 cm
  - Median size: 2 cm

MICROSCOPIC PATHOLOGY

Histologic Features
- Pools of extracellular stromal mucin make up at least 1/3 of volume throughout tumor in pure MC
  - Delicate fibrous septae divide pools or lakes of mucin into compartments
    - Detached epithelial elements are present floating in pools of mucin
    - Mucin should surround all tumor cell nests
  - Pure MC should not contain areas of usual type of invasion of stroma in absence of mucin
    - If present, tumor should be designated as mixed mucinous/ductal
    - Pure MC has > 90% mucinous histology (frequently entire tumor is mucinous)
  - Majority of cases have low-grade nuclei and would be classified as well or moderately differentiated
    - Rare cases of poorly differentiated MC do occur (10% of total)
- Pure MC can be divided into 2 main subtypes based on architectural and cytological features
  - Mucinous type A carcinomas are paucicellular
    - Large quantities of extracellular mucin production
    - Neuroendocrine marker expression is not typical
  - Mucinous type B carcinomas are more hypercellular
    - Contain less mucin and more tumor cells

- Neuroendocrine markers and argyrophilia are present in 25%
- Older patient age
- Lower tumor nuclear grade
- Lower incidence of axillary node metastasis
- MC is often associated with DCIS component
  - DCIS may show micropapillary, cribriform, or solid patterns
    - DCIS may also demonstrate prominent mucin production

ANCILLARY TESTS

Immunohistochemistry
- Most MC will show expression of ER and PR
  - Typically tumors express high levels of both receptors
    - MC more likely to be ER (94%) and PR (81%) positive compared with carcinomas of no special type
- HER2 and EGFR overexpression is very uncommon
- Some MC can show neuroendocrine differentiation
  - Tumor cells will show expression of 1 or more neuroendocrine markers
    - Chromogranin, synaptophysin, CD56
  - MC expressing neuroendocrine markers are classified as type B by some authors
  - Tumors that are classified as type A typically do not show neuroendocrine differentiation
  - Neuroendocrine differentiation associated with better prognosis in some reports
    - Prognostic significance of neuroendocrine differentiation is not well established
    - Neuroendocrine differentiation is not considered standard prognostic feature
- Mucin expression in MC
  - MUC1, which is related to poor prognosis in gastric and colorectal cancers, is low in MC
  - Gel-forming secretory mucins (MUC2 and MUC6) are highly expressed in MC

DIFFERENTIAL DIAGNOSIS

Myxoid Fibroadenoma

- Typically seen in younger age group compared with MC
- Both present as circumscribed palpable masses or imaging densities
- Myxoid stroma associated with stromal spindle cells
- Epithelium of fibroadenoma has normal layer of myoepithelial cells, whereas epithelium of mucinous carcinoma lacks myoepithelial cells

Mucocele-like Lesion

- Characterized by cystically dilated mucin-filled ducts
  - May be associated with rupture and extravasated stromal mucin
  - Strips or clusters of epithelial cells may become detached from lining
    - May be difficult to distinguish from MC on limited biopsy samples
- Mucocele-like lesions typically show areas with linear configuration of cells lining duct space
  - Detached epithelial cell groups may be associated with myoepithelial cells
- Mucocele-like lesions may be associated with ADH or DCIS

Matrix-producing Carcinoma

- Some metaplastic carcinomas show prominent myxoid stroma
  - Will typically show areas of chondroid differentiation
    - Tumor cells located in lacunar spaces
    - Tumor cells more likely to be distributed toward periphery of lesion
    - Cells are individually dispersed or arranged in small trabeculae
- Metaplastic carcinoma with myxoid stroma is typically ER and PR negative
  - Tumors cells typically positive for basal cytokeratins (CK5/6, CK14) and p63

Invasive Micropapillary Carcinoma (IMPC)

- Tumor cells are usually present in empty-appearing spaces but may be associated with extracellular mucin
- Characteristic "inside out" papillary architecture resulting in outer apical blebs and "serrated" edge
  - Tumor cell clusters of MC usually have smooth border
- Abundant extracellular mucin is not present
- More likely to be ER and PR negative and HER2 positive
- It is important to distinguish IMPC from MC, as IMPC has poor prognosis

DIAGNOSTIC CHECKLIST

Pathologic Interpretation Pearls

- Diagnosis of mucinous carcinoma may be difficult on core needle biopsy

  - Some MCs are paucicellular with only a few dispersed clusters of tumor cells
  - Needle core may contain stromal mucin devoid of tumor cells
  - In other cases, there may be mucin-filled cysts with adjacent extravasated mucin
    - Extravasated stromal mucin without tumor cells should prompt examination of deeper levels looking for tumor cells
  - Excision for definitive evaluation should be recommended for such cases
  - Malignancy on excision is more common if lesion is mass rather than calcifications
  - Seeding of needle track by MC has been reported in rare cases

SELECTED REFERENCES

1. Begum SM et al: Mucin extravasation in breast core biopsies--clinical significance and outcome correlation. Histopathology. 55(5):609-17, 2009
2. Ishizuna K et al: A case of mucinous carcinoma of the breast in which needle tract seeding was diagnosed by preoperative diagnostic imaging. Breast Cancer. Epub ahead of print, 2009
3. Weigelt B et al: Mucinous and neuroendocrine breast carcinomas are transcriptionally distinct from invasive ductal carcinomas of no special type. Mod Pathol. 22(11):1401-14, 2009
4. Di Saverio S et al: A retrospective review with long term follow up of 11,400 cases of pure mucinous breast carcinoma. Breast Cancer Res Treat. 111(3):541-7, 2008
5. Tan PH et al: Mucinous breast lesions: diagnostic challenges. J Clin Pathol. 61(1):11-9, 2008
6. Lam WW et al: Sonographic appearance of mucinous carcinoma of the breast. AJR Am J Roentgenol. 182(4):1069-74, 2004
7. Tse GM et al: Neuroendocrine differentiation in pure type mammary mucinous carcinoma is associated with favorable histologic and immunohistochemical parameters. Mod Pathol. 17(5):568-72, 2004
8. Matsukita S et al: Expression of mucins (MUC1, MUC2, MUC5AC and MUC6) in mucinous carcinoma of the breast: comparison with invasive ductal carcinoma. Histopathology. 42(1):26-36, 2003
9. Diab SG et al: Tumor characteristics and clinical outcome of tubular and mucinous breast carcinomas. J Clin Oncol. 17(5):1442-8, 1999
10. Silverberg SG et al: Colloid carcinoma of the breast. Am J Clin Pathol. 55(3):355-63, 1971
11. Melamed MR et al: Prognostic significance of gelatinous mammary carcinoma. Cancer. 14:699-704, 1961

MUCINOUS (COLLOID) CARCINOMA

Gross and Microscopic Features

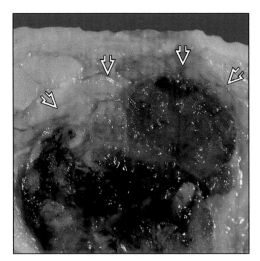

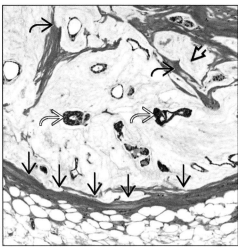

(Left) MC typically has an expansile growth pattern with pushing circumscribed or lobulated borders ⊡. The consistency is soft and gelatinous. The cut surface is generally flat and does not bulge like a fibroadenoma. (Right) The extracellular mucin of the cancer forms a well-circumscribed border ⊡. Delicate fibrous septae ⊡ divide the pools or lakes of mucin into compartments ⊡. Invasion in these tumors is in the form of nests of tumor cells ⊡ "floating" in mucin.

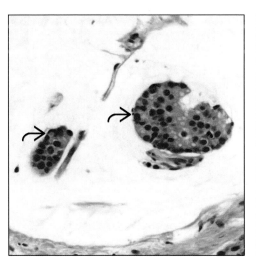

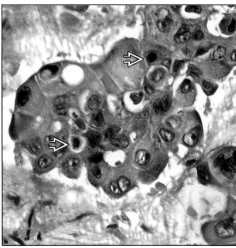

(Left) The majority of mucinous carcinomas consist of clusters and nests of tumor cells ⊡ with a low histologic grade and rare or absent mitoses. Some pathologists require grade 1 nuclei for the diagnosis of classic mucinous carcinoma. (Right) Unusual cases of MC have high-grade nuclei and frequent mitoses ⊡ and are classified as poorly differentiated. These unusual carcinomas may exhibit HER2 overexpression.

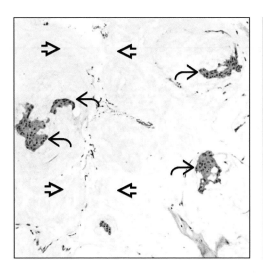

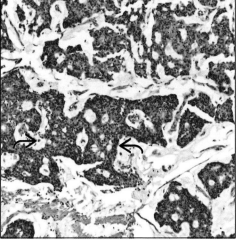

(Left) MC has been divided into 2 subtypes. Type A carcinomas are paucicellular ⊡ in a background of abundant extracellular mucin ⊡. The cells generally have low-grade nuclei, and neuroendocrine markers are absent. (Right) Type B MC is more hypercellular as seen here ⊡. However, all of the tumor cell nests should be surrounded by extracellular mucin. Type B MC occurs more frequently in older women and is more likely to be positive for neuroendocrine markers.

MUCINOUS (COLLOID) CARCINOMA

Metastasis, IHC Profile, and Core Needle Biopsy

(Left) Axillary lymph node metastasis is an important prognostic factor for MC and is associated with a more aggressive clinical course. Nests of tumor cells are seen in the subcapsular sinus ⇗ of the lymph node. The mucinous histology with extravasated mucin ⇲ can also been seen in sites of metastases. (Right) Most mucinous carcinomas show high levels of expression of both ER ⇗ and PR in tumor cells. HER2 overexpression is uncommon.

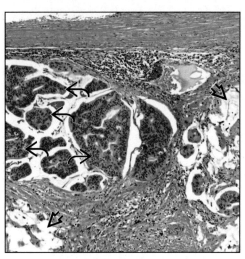
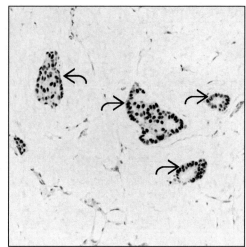

(Left) MC has a specific pattern of MUC gene expression including MUC2 and MUC6. MUC2 is seen within the tumor cells ⇗ and in the extracellular mucin ⇲. MUC2 and MUC6 are known as gel-forming mucins and may serve as a barrier to the spread of tumor cells. (Right) An immunohistochemical stain for synaptophysin shows strong reactivity in tumor cells ⇗ in this type B MC. This type of carcinoma is transcriptionally identical to solid neuroendocrine carcinoma.

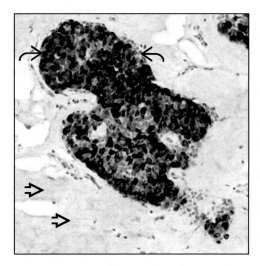
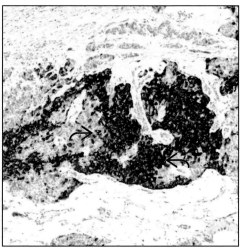

(Left) MC can be diagnostically challenging in a limited biopsy sample as tumor cells may be sparse and the carcinoma may fragment due to the mucinous matrix. In this needle biopsy, pools of extravasated stromal mucin can be seen on low power ⇗. (Right) On higher magnification, stromal mucin ⇲ and delicate fibrous septae ⇗ are seen, with rare clusters of epithelial cells ⇗. Such findings should prompt examination of deeper levels to look for tumor cells &/or a recommendation for excision.

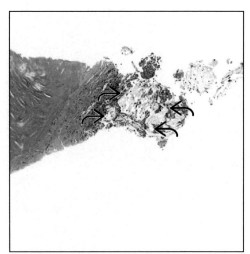
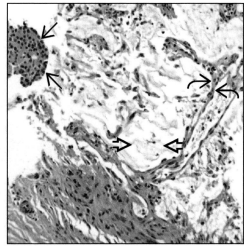

MUCINOUS (COLLOID) CARCINOMA

Differential Diagnosis

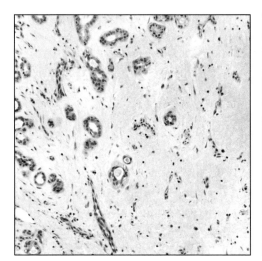 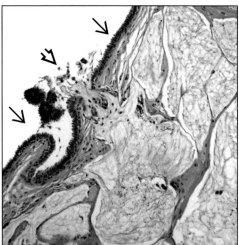

(Left) Fibroadenomas with a myxoid stroma can sometimes mimic MC. However, the epithelial elements have a normal myoepithelial layer. *(Right)* Mucinous cysts lined by benign epithelium ➡ may rupture ➡, spilling mucin into the surrounding stroma. If extensive, the mucin will form a mucocele-like lesion. Epithelial cells should not be present within the mucin pools. However, it may be difficult to distinguish such cases from MC if associated ADH or DCIS is present.

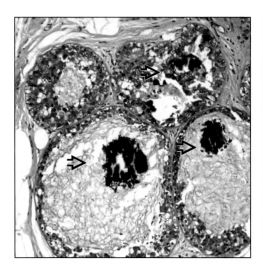 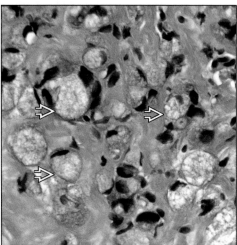

(Left) DCIS can also be associated with mucin production. The mucin may calcify ➡ and be detected on screening mammography. In some cases, it may be difficult to distinguish DCIS from MC if there is rupture or distortion of the duct spaces, particularly after core needle biopsy. *(Right)* Intracellular mucin can be seen in MC as well as in other histologic types. It is most commonly found in lobular carcinomas with a signet ring or histiocytoid appearance ➡.

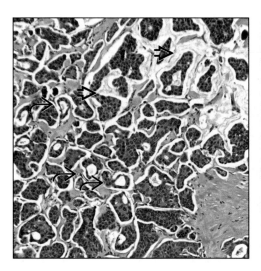 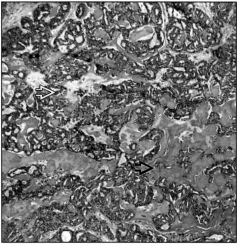

(Left) Both MC and IMPC consist of clusters of cells within spaces. In IMPC, the spaces usually appear empty but may also be associated with mucin ➡. IMPC has a characteristic "inside out" papillary pattern ➡ that is not seen in MC. It is important to distinguish these carcinomas, as IMPC has a poor prognosis. *(Right)* Metaplastic carcinomas may be associated with matrix formation that can be collagenous ➡, cartilaginous, or mucinous ➡ in appearance.

INVASIVE PAPILLARY CARCINOMA

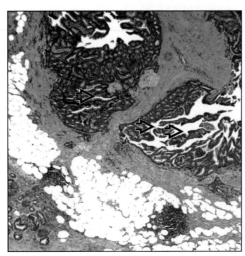

This invasive carcinoma consists of poorly circumscribed nests of cells with papillary and cribriform patterns. Fibrovascular cores ⊳ are present within the carcinoma.

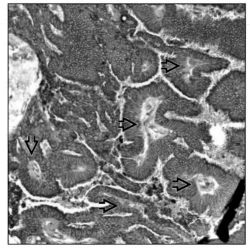

Immunohistochemical study for cytokeratin (red cytoplasmic positivity) and p63 demonstrates the complete absence of myoepithelial cells in the carcinoma, including the papillary cores ⊳.

TERMINOLOGY

Abbreviations
• Invasive papillary carcinoma (IPC)

Definitions
• Invasive carcinomas consisting predominantly of papillae with fibrovascular cores
  ○ "Papillary carcinoma" includes invasive papillary carcinoma, encapsulated papillary carcinoma, solid papillary carcinoma, papillary carcinoma in situ, and DCIS involving papilloma
  ○ These lesions are sometimes grouped together
  ○ Invasive papillary carcinoma is important to identify as risk of lymph node and distant metastases is higher than for other diagnoses

CLINICAL ISSUES

Epidemiology
• Incidence
  ○ < 2% of breast carcinomas
• Age
  ○ More common in postmenopausal women (typically 65-70 years of age)

Prognosis
• Outcome is generally better than for invasive carcinomas of no special type
  ○ Papillary carcinomas are generally ER positive and only rarely poorly differentiated
• Lymph node metastases are present in about 1/3 of cases

MACROSCOPIC FEATURES

Gross Appearance
• IPC generally has appearance similar to cancers of no special type in having an irregular border

MICROSCOPIC PATHOLOGY

Histologic Features
• Should have prominent pattern of papillae with fibrovascular cores
  ○ Papillae lack myoepithelial cells
  ○ IHC for muscle markers may be difficult to interpret as blood vessels may closely approximate basal portions of cells in fibrovascular cores
  ○ p63 is generally easier to interpret as blood vessels will be negative
  ○ Occasional tumor cells may be positive for p63
• Fibrovascular cores are thin and delicate
• Cells are monomorphic in appearance and columnar in shape
• Nuclear grade is generally low or intermediate
• Mitoses are usually infrequent
• DCIS of papillary type may be associated with carcinoma

ANCILLARY TESTS

Immunohistochemistry
• Estrogen and progesterone receptors
  ○ Majority of invasive papillary carcinomas are positive for hormone receptors
• HER2
  ○ Only rare papillary carcinomas overexpress HER2

DIFFERENTIAL DIAGNOSIS

Invasive Micropapillary Carcinoma
• Unusual type of carcinoma consisting of clusters of tumor cells in clear spaces
  ○ Tumor clusters have characteristic inverted pattern
  ○ Tumor cell clusters are likely spherules with hollow center

INVASIVE PAPILLARY CARCINOMA

Key Facts

Terminology

- Invasive papillary carcinoma (IPC)
- Invasive carcinomas consisting predominantly of papillae with fibrovascular cores
- "Papillary carcinoma" includes invasive papillary carcinoma, encapsulated papillary carcinoma, solid papillary carcinoma, papillary carcinoma in situ, and DCIS involving papilloma
- Invasive papillary carcinoma is important to identify as risk of lymph node and distant metastases is higher than for other diagnoses

Clinical Issues

- < 2% of breast carcinomas
- More common in postmenopausal women (typically 65-70 years of age)

- Outcome is generally better than for invasive carcinomas of no special type
- Papillary carcinomas are generally ER positive and only rarely poorly differentiated
- Only rare papillary carcinomas are HER2 positive
- Lymph node metastases are present in about 1/3 of cases

Top Differential Diagnoses

- Invasive micropapillary carcinoma
  - Outcome less favorable than IPC
  - Lymph node metastases are present in majority of cases
- Solid papillary carcinoma
  - Most have outcomes similar to DCIS
- Encapsulated (intracystic) papillary carcinoma
  - Most have outcomes similar to DCIS

- Frequently associated with lymph-vascular invasion and lymph node metastases; poorer prognosis compared to IPC

Solid Papillary Carcinoma

- Grows as single or multiple circumscribed nests
- Cells may be oval or spindle-shaped and have minimal nuclear atypia
- Many cases are positive for neuroendocrine markers, such as chromogranin or synaptophysin
- Fibrovascular cores are present within solid cell proliferation
  - Fronds are not separated by spaces, and growth pattern is solid
- Some cases have peripheral myoepithelial cells on IHC studies and are clearly DCIS
- Other cases lack myoepithelial cells within and at periphery of carcinoma
  - May be form of invasive carcinoma
  - However, even if myoepithelial cells are absent, prognosis is similar to DCIS
  - Small risk of lymph node metastasis
- Some cases are associated with frankly invasive carcinoma
  - Invasive carcinoma often has mucinous or neuroendocrine features

Encapsulated (Intracystic) Papillary Carcinoma

- Grows as delicate papillary fronds within a cystic space
- Myoepithelial cells are absent within and surrounding carcinoma
- About 25% of cases are associated with areas of frank stromal invasion
  - Areas of invasion are generally of no special type
- In absence of invasion beyond cyst wall, prognosis is very similar to DCIS

DIAGNOSTIC CHECKLIST

Pathologic Interpretation Pearls

- Core needle biopsy
  - Papillary neoplasms can be very difficult to classify on core needle biopsy
  - Papillary pattern of growth often results in fragmentation of specimen
  - IHC can be helpful to distinguish papillary carcinoma from benign papillomas
    - Papillomas should have well-developed myoepithelial cell layer
    - Papillary carcinomas lack myoepithelial cells
    - Can be difficult to diagnose ADH or DCIS partially involving benign papilloma
  - Detached papillae lacking myoepithelial cells may correspond to papillary DCIS, encapsulated papillary carcinoma, or invasive papillary carcinoma
  - Correlation with imaging findings can help determine most likely diagnosis
    - Irregular mass: Invasive papillary carcinoma
    - Circumscribed mass: Encapsulated papillary carcinoma or, less likely, papillary DCIS
    - Calcifications: Papillary DCIS
  - In many cases, classification should be made after excision
  - Papillary lesions are often associated with epithelial displacement within needle track
    - Papillary fragments can sometimes be seen within lymph nodes after biopsy
    - Clinical significance of papillary fragments mechanically displaced into stroma or nodes is unknown

SELECTED REFERENCES

1. Pal SK et al: Papillary carcinoma of the breast: an overview. Breast Cancer Res Treat. 122(3):637-45, 2010

INVASIVE PAPILLARY CARCINOMA

Microscopic Features

(Left) Invasive solid papillary carcinoma often has a circumscribed border ⮕. It may be difficult to distinguish this carcinoma from DCIS based on light microscopy. IHC for myoepithelial markers is helpful to confirm the absence of myoepithelial cells throughout the carcinoma. Metastases rarely occur.
(Right) Fibrovascular cores are present throughout an invasive solid papillary carcinoma ⮕. The cells are usually well to moderately differentiated, and mitoses are infrequent.

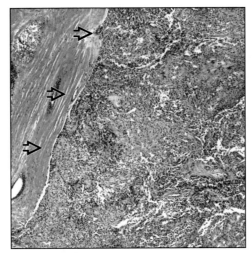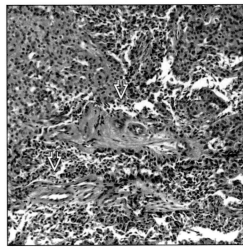

(Left) This IPC closely mimics invasive micropapillary carcinoma as the papillae are small and present in empty spaces. However, unlike micropapillary carcinoma, there are fibrovascular cores within the papillae ⮕. *(Right)* Invasive micropapillary carcinoma is composed of clusters of cells surrounding a hollow space ⮕ with the apical portion of the cells facing outward. This is an unusual carcinoma that was also associated with extracellular mucin production ⮕.

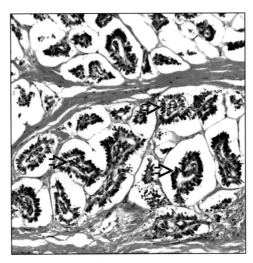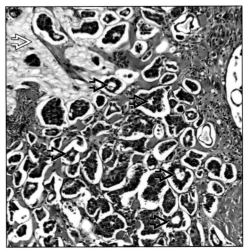

(Left) Encapsulated (intracystic) papillary carcinoma consists of delicate papillary fronds growing within a single cystic space ⮕. Myoepithelial cells are absent within the papillary cores and at the periphery of the lesion.
(Right) Papillary DCIS can involve a large cystic space but is also usually present in multiple smaller adjacent ducts. Myoepithelial cells are absent within the fibrovascular cores but are present at the periphery ⮕.

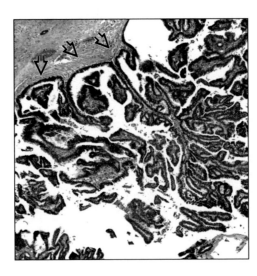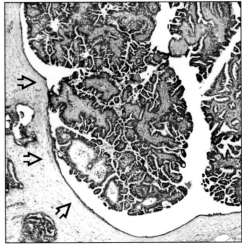

INVASIVE PAPILLARY CARCINOMA

Papillary Lesions on Core Needle Biopsy

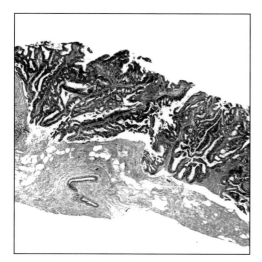

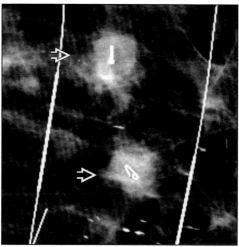

(Left) This papillary proliferation on core needle biopsy was shown to lack myoepithelial cells on IHC. The differential diagnosis includes papillary DCIS, encapsulated papillary carcinoma, and IPC. On excision, this lesion was IPC. *(Right)* This woman had 2 adjacent irregular masses ➡. Each had undergone core needle biopsies with clip placement. Both core needle biopsies showed "papillary carcinoma." The association with irregular masses makes a diagnosis of IPC more likely.

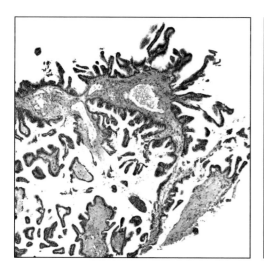

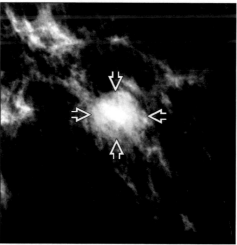

(Left) Papillary lesions frequently fragment on core needle biopsy due to their architecture. This lesion lacked myoepithelial cells. No definite stromal invasion was seen. On excision, a diagnosis of encapsulated papillary carcinoma was made. *(Right)* Specimen radiograph shows a mass ➡, which is being partially obscured by surrounding stroma. It had well-circumscribed borders on preoperative compression views consistent with the diagnosis of encapsulated papillary carcinoma.

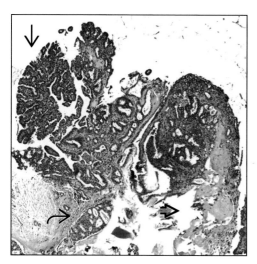

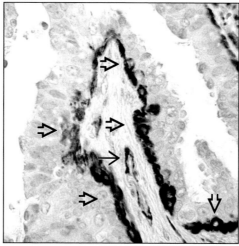

(Left) This papilloma has thick fibrovascular cores ➡ and a myoepithelial cell layer but is partially involved by papillary ➡ and cribriform ➡ DCIS. All papillomas with areas of atypia are evaluated best with excision. *(Right)* Muscle markers are very sensitive for detecting myoepithelial cells ➡. However, blood vessels are also positive ➡ and may be closely apposed to the base of the epithelial cells in IPC. p63 is usually a better choice.

INVASIVE MICROPAPILLARY CARCINOMA

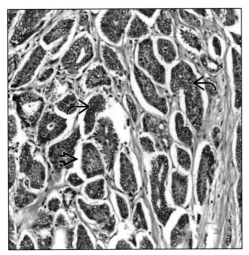

Intiltrating "pseudopapillary" clusters of tumor cells ⇗ in clear spaces ⬱ characterize invasive micropapillary carcinoma (IMPC). This unusual pattern imparts a spongy macroscopic appearance.

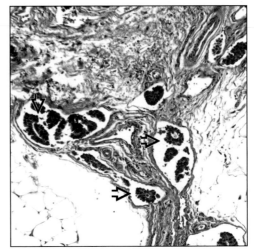

Micropapillary carcinoma is frequently associated with lymph-vascular invasion, lymph node metastasis, and local recurrence. Hollow tumor cell clusters are present within lymphatic spaces ⬱.

TERMINOLOGY

Abbreviations
- Invasive micropapillary carcinoma (IMPC)

Definitions
- Type of invasive carcinoma with distinctive pattern of tumor cell clusters growing in individual empty-appearing spaces
  - Cell clusters often have hollow core with apical aspect of cells facing outward

ETIOLOGY/PATHOGENESIS

Comparative Genomic Hybridization Studies
- IMPC exhibits losses involving short arm of chromosome 8 (8p)
- 88% show chromosomal gains of 8q
  - Findings suggest that this morphologic phenotype is related to 1 or more genes on chromosome 8
- Loss of heterozygosity reported on 17p13.1 in 80% of patients with IMPC
- *MYC* (8q24) amplification significantly associated with IMPC

MUC1 Expression
- Apical or secretory pole of cell directed toward outside of cell cluster ("reversed polarity")
  - IMPCs show MUC1 expression at periphery/surface of tumor cell clusters
    - MUC1 has inhibitory effect on epithelial/stroma interaction
  - MUC1 expression on surface may aid in detachment of tumor cells from stroma and facilitate spread

Gene Expression Profiling
- IMPCs cluster together indicating a common pattern of gene expression
- Identified as member of luminal A group of cancers

CLINICAL ISSUES

Epidemiology
- Incidence
  - Relatively rare form of infiltrating breast cancer
    - Only 3.8% of a large breast cancer series
  - Pure IMPC less frequently seen (~ 1%)
    - Mixed lesion with IMPC component more common
  - Tumors with mixed pattern including IMPC component are important to recognize
    - Prognostic significance holds true even for minor IMPC component
- Age
  - Broad age range at presentation
    - Mean: 55 years

Site
- Distribution within breast does not differ compared with other forms of carcinoma
  - More commonly multifocal (approximately 30%) compared to other carcinoma types
    - May be related to propensity for lymph-vascular invasion resulting in intramammary metastasis

Presentation
- Palpable mass; most common presentation
- Mammographic density
  - Calcifications may be associated with carcinoma
- Increased incidence of axillary nodal involvement at presentation (70-95%)
  - Lymph node metastases occur in majority of IMPC < 1 cm in size

Prognosis
- IMPC has more aggressive clinical course compared to breast cancers of no special type
  - Decreased disease-free and overall survival
- Increased incidence of local recurrence

INVASIVE MICROPAPILLARY CARCINOMA

Key Facts

Terminology
- Invasive micropapillary carcinoma (IMPC)
- Special histologic subtype of infiltrating ductal carcinoma

Clinical Issues
- Increased incidence of lymph node metastases and local recurrence
- 40-50% of patients with IMPC will present with ≥ 4 positive axillary nodes

Microscopic Pathology
- Infiltrating clusters of tumor cells surrounded by clear spaces
- Micropapillary pattern may predominate or represent minor component of tumor

- ○ Tumor likely grows as spherules rather than as micropapillae
- ○ Clusters frequently have central hollow space
- ○ Immunohistochemistry for EMA or MUC1 can support diagnosis
- Lymphvascular invasion is commonly seen
  - ○ Associated with increased nodal metastases
- IMPC of breast morphologically similar to micropapillary tumors of bladder, lung, ovary, and salivary glands

Top Differential Diagnoses
- Metastatic micropapillary carcinoma
  - ○ Finding DCIS supports diagnosis of breast primary
- Mucinous carcinoma
- Invasive ductal carcinoma with tissue retraction artifact

- ○ Recurs in ~ 22% of patients compared to ~ 12% of patients with carcinomas of no special type
- Increased incidence of lymph node metastases
  - ○ 40-50% of IMPCs will present with ≥ 4 positive axillary nodes
  - ○ Lymph node metastases are common even with smaller tumors (< 1 cm)
- Therefore, patients with IMPC are more likely to present at higher stages than patients with carcinomas of no special type
  - ○ When matched by stage, IMPC has similar survival compared to other cancer types

Core Needle Biopsy
- Micropapillary pattern on core needle biopsy is predictive of a higher likelihood of lymph node metastasis

IMAGE FINDINGS

Mammographic Findings
- Irregular or circumscribed mass
  - ○ Microcalcifications may be present

MACROSCOPIC FEATURES

General Features
- Typically firm solitary mass with ill-defined margins grossly
  - ○ Cut surface usually solid and white or white-gray
    - ■ Tumors are multifocal in about 30% of cases

Size
- Tumors range in size from 0.7-10 cm
  - ○ Median: 2.8 cm

MICROSCOPIC PATHOLOGY

Histologic Features
- "Micropapillary" may be a misnomer
  - ○ Papillae are never seen in cross section

- ○ It is likely tumor grows as hollow spherules of cells
  - ■ Similar to appearance of tumor cells in malignant effusions in cross section
  - ■ Same pattern is seen in lymphatics and in lymph nodes
- Numerous small clusters of tumor cells
  - ○ Many tumor cell clusters are hollow without fibrovascular cores
  - ○ Other clusters appear to be solid
  - ○ Peripherally located nuclei may bulge out with knobby appearance
  - ○ Apical blebs are found on outer surface of clusters
- Clusters of tumor cells are surrounded by clear spaces
  - ○ Low-power appearance resembles "fallen leaves" or has a spongy look
  - ○ 1 or only a few tumor cell clusters seen per space
  - ○ Spaces usually clear; however, scant mucin occasionally present
  - ○ Spaces surrounded by loose fibrocollagenous stroma
  - ○ May mimic lymph-vascular involvement
- Clusters of tumor cells are characterized by reversed polarity
  - ○ Apical (secretory) pole of cells is directed toward outside of cell groups (not into a lumen or central empty space)
  - ○ May contribute to ability to invade vascular lymphatic spaces
  - ○ EMA, E-cadherin, and MUC1 are positive on periphery of tumor cell clusters, highlighting reverse polarity
- Neoplastic cells are predominantly polygonal in shape or pleomorphic
  - ○ Frequently intermediate to high nuclear grade
  - ○ Nuclear pleomorphism, hyperchromasia, and macronucleoli typical
  - ○ Abundant finely granular, eosinophilic, or vacuolated cytoplasm
  - ○ Distinctive cell borders
- Micropapillary pattern may predominate (pure IMPC) or represent a minor component
  - ○ Pure IMPC is rare; 1-2% of invasive breast cancer

INVASIVE MICROPAPILLARY CARCINOMA

Immunohistochemistry

Antibody	Reactivity	Staining Pattern	Comment
ER	Positive	Nuclear	60-90% of cases
PR	Positive	Nuclear	60-70% of cases
EMA	Positive	Cell membrane	"Inside out" staining pattern, periphery of cell clusters
MUC1	Positive	Cell membrane	"Inside out" staining pattern, periphery of cell clusters
E-cadherin	Positive	Cell membrane	"Inside out" staining pattern, periphery of cell clusters
HER2	Equivocal	Cell membrane	Positive in 40-50% of cases

- o IMPC pattern more commonly seen as component of a mixed lesion with IDC of no special type
- o Proportion of IMPC pattern in carcinoma should be reported
  - ▪ Carcinoma should consist of at least 75% micropapillary pattern to be classified as IMPC
- DCIS may be present in surrounding tissue
  - o IMPC may be associated with micropapillary or cribriform DCIS
  - o Associated DCIS often has high nuclear grade

Lymphatic/Vascular Invasion

- Lymph-vascular invasion is commonly seen (1/3-2/3 of cases)
  - o Associated with increased incidence of nodal metastases
- Characteristic IMPC appearance retained in nodal metastases and lymphatic spaces
- May be difficult to distinguish lymph-vascular invasion from stromal invasion due to histologic appearance
- Lymph-vascular invasion should only be diagnosed if at a distance from main tumor and, preferably, in lymphatics associated with blood vessels

DIFFERENTIAL DIAGNOSIS

Metastatic Micropapillary Carcinoma

- Metastases from other sites should be considered; however, metastases to breast are very rare arising from an occult primary site
  - o Micropapillary carcinomas from bladder, lung, and ovary (serous) carcinoma have similar morphology
  - o All express MUC1 on surface of cell clusters
  - o Carcinomas retain site-specific markers
    - ▪ Lung IMPC: TTF-1 positive (100%), ER positive (17%), negative for other markers
    - ▪ Bladder IMPC: Uroplakin positive (92%), CK20 positive (54%), negative for other markers
    - ▪ Ovary IMPC: Pax-8 positive (100%), ER positive (92%), WT1 positive (91%), negative for other markers
    - ▪ Breast IMPC: ER positive (88%), mammaglobin positive (56%), WT1 positive (25%, usually only focally), negative for other markers
    - ▪ ER expression cannot be used to distinguish breast from ovary primary sites
- Associated DCIS supports origin in breast

Mucinous Carcinoma

- Should demonstrate abundant extracellular mucin
  - o Extracellular mucin production is unusual in IMPC but may be present focally
- Tumor cell clusters in mucinous cancer typically have smooth rather than serrated borders
  - o Spaces within clusters are lumens
- Carcinomas with micropapillary pattern and mucin production have prognosis more similar to IMPC

Invasive Carcinoma of No Special Type with Tissue Retraction Artifact

- Retraction artifact usually associated with poor tissue preservation
- Cell nests do not have inverted polarity pattern
  - o Spaces within cell clusters are luminal spaces
  - o IHC for EMA or MUC1 can be helpful to demonstrate polarization of cells; central lumens will be positive for these markers
- In 1 study, retraction artifact was poor prognostic factor, suggesting that it may be due to significant altered carcinoma/stromal relationship

SELECTED REFERENCES

1. Yu JI et al: Differences in prognostic factors and patterns of failure between invasive micropapillary carcinoma and invasive ductal carcinoma of the breast: matched case-control study. Breast. 19(3):231-7, 2010
2. Acs G et al: The presence of micropapillary features and retraction artifact in core needle biopsy material predicts lymph node metastasis in breast carcinoma. Am J Surg Pathol. 33(2):202-10, 2009
3. Lotan TL et al: Immunohistochemical panel to identify the primary site of invasive micropapillary carcinoma. Am J Surg Pathol. 33(7):1037-41, 2009
4. Marchiò C et al: Genomic and immunophenotypical characterization of pure micropapillary carcinomas of the breast. J Pathol. 215(4):398-410, 2008
5. Weigelt B et al: Refinement of breast cancer classification by molecular characterization of histological special types. J Pathol. 216(2):141-50, 2008
6. Acs G et al: Extensive retraction artifact correlates with lymphatic invasion and nodal metastasis and predicts poor outcome in early stage breast carcinoma. Am J Surg Pathol. 31(1):129-40, 2007
7. Guo X et al: Invasive micropapillary carcinoma of the breast: association of pathologic features with lymph node metastasis. Am J Clin Pathol. 126(5):740-6, 2006
8. Nassar H et al: Pathogenesis of invasive micropapillary carcinoma: role of MUC1 glycoprotein. Mod Pathol. 17(9):1045-50, 2004

INVASIVE MICROPAPILLARY CARCINOMA

Gross and Microscopic Features

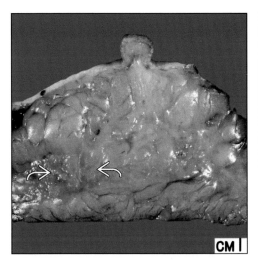

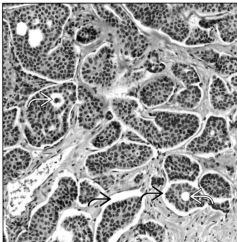

(Left) Like other invasive carcinomas, IMPC most commonly presents grossly or by imaging as an irregular firm mass ➡. IMPC can only be identified microscopically. (Right) Tumor cell clusters are found within clear spaces ➡, giving a "fallen leaf" or spongy appearance. The clusters lack fibrovascular cores ➡ and are most likely spherules in 3 dimensions, rather than micropapillae. If papillae were present, they would occasionally be seen in cross section.

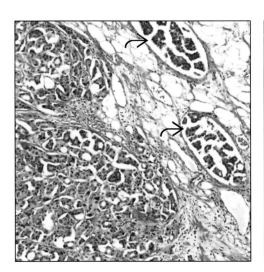

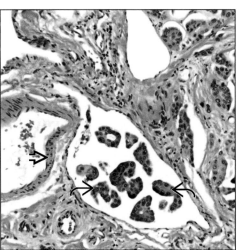

(Left) IMPC is associated with numerous foci of lymph-vascular invasion ➡, and the extent of lymphatic involvement is typically associated with multiple lymph node metastases. (Right) Tumor cell clusters are present within a dilated lymphatic space, adjacent to a small arteriole ➡. The micropapillary appearance is retained within the lymphatic space ➡. The ability of the tumor to grow as clusters within fluids may be associated with its aggressive clinical behavior.

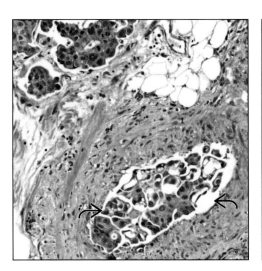

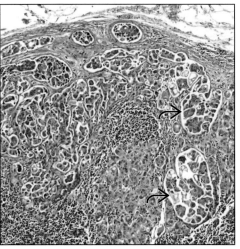

(Left) This particular IMPC demonstrates an aggressive pattern of growth with prominent lymph-vascular invasion and arterial invasion ➡, a finding that is infrequently seen with other types of breast cancers. (Right) The characteristic IMPC appearance ➡ is often retained when the tumor metastasizes to lymph nodes or other sites. IMPC is associated with a high frequency of lymph node metastases at presentation that is often disproportionate to the size of the primary tumor.

INVASIVE MICROPAPILLARY CARCINOMA

Ancillary Techniques

(Left) This unusual IMPC demonstrates marked nuclear pleomorphism ⤳ and abundant eosinophilic cytoplasm, conferring an apocrine appearance. Multiple positive axillary lymph nodes were present. *(Right)* Approximately 50% of IMPCs overexpress HER2. The "reverse polarity" of the tumor cell clusters may result in unusual partial membrane staining patterns. The HER2 IHC assay for this carcinoma showed weak apical membrane staining ⤳ and was negative for gene amplification.

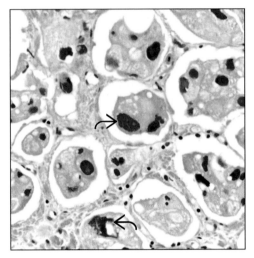 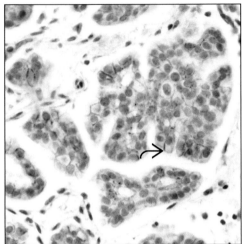

(Left) IMPC is positive for ER ⤳ in 60-90% of cases. A normal duct in the upper portion of the field also shows ER expression ⤳. *(Right)* Although most cases of IMPC are positive for PR, in this case the tumor cells are negative ⤳. A normal duct shows PR expression ⤳, confirming that the assay is working properly. Loss of PR in ER-positive carcinomas is a marker of poorer prognosis, probably due to the presence of an abnormal ER controlled gene regulatory system.

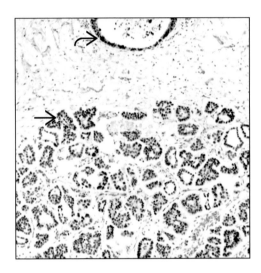 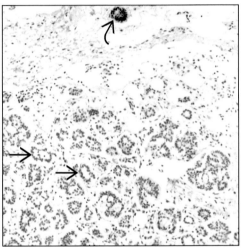

(Left) The expression of MUC1 on the stromal facing surface of the tumor cell groups ⤳ (reversed apical pattern) is a characteristic finding for IMPC, consistent with the distinctive inside-out orientation of the tumor cells. MUC1 may aid in tumor cell detachment and spread. The basal internal portions of the cells are not immunoreactive ⤳. *(Right)* EMA, in addition to MUC1, shows a reverse apical pattern with staining of the stromal-facing portion of tumor cell groups ⤳.

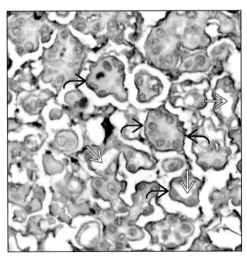 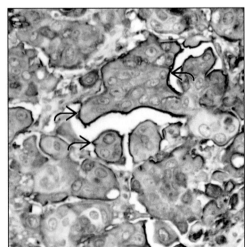

INVASIVE MICROPAPILLARY CARCINOMA

Differential Diagnosis

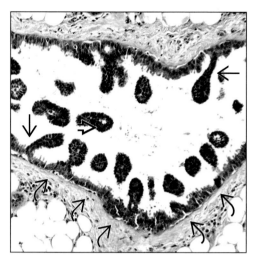

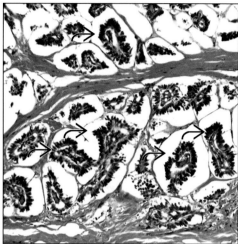

(Left) DCIS can also have a micropapillary appearance. The papillae characteristically have a narrow base ➡ and a bulbous tip ("light bulb" appearance). Like IMPC, no fibrovascular cores are seen ➡. Note myoepithelial cells around periphery ➡. (Right) This invasive papillary carcinoma resembles IMPC due to the presence of papillary fragments within clear spaces. However, fibrovascular cores with blood vessels are present ➡, unlike the empty cores seen in IMPC.

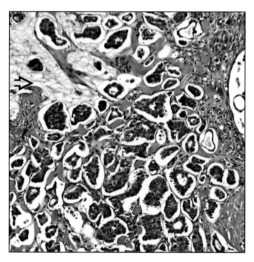

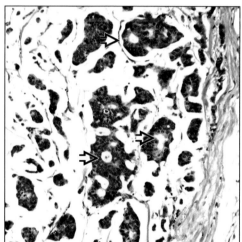

(Left) IMPC can be associated with focal extracellular mucin production ➡. It is important to distinguish IMPC from mucinous carcinoma, as the latter tumor has a favorable prognosis. (Right) Tumor cells are present as clusters in the extracellular mucin in mucinous carcinomas, rather than in individual spaces as in IMPC. The spaces within the clusters are lumens, which may contain secretory material, rather than empty central cores ➡, and the outer edges are smooth.

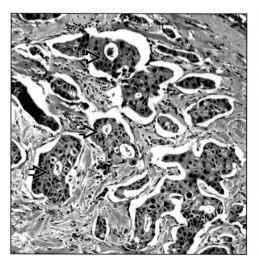

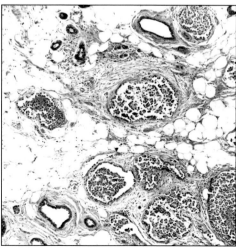

(Left) Retraction artifact can mimic the pattern of IMPC as the tumor cells are present in clear spaces. However, the apical portions of the cells face the central lumens, and secretory material may be present within the lumens ➡. The outer surfaces of the cell clusters conform to the shape of the stroma and are smooth without apical blebs. (Right) Metastatic papillary carcinomas to the breast, such as this lung carcinoma, are very rare but must be distinguished from IMPC.

METAPLASTIC CARCINOMA

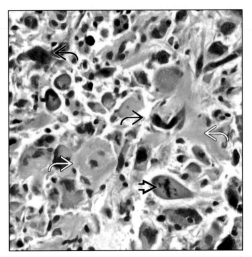

This high-grade malignant breast tumor is composed of spindle cells with pleomorphic nuclei ➔, abnormal mitotic figures ⊳, and extracellular matrix production ➔ consistent with osteoid.

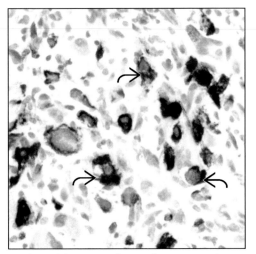

A subset of the tumor cells strongly express cytokeratin (AE1/AE3 ➔), supporting a diagnosis of metaplastic breast cancer with osteosarcomatous heterologous differentiation.

TERMINOLOGY

Abbreviations
- Metaplastic breast carcinoma (MBC)

Definitions
- MBC encompasses a diverse group of carcinomas that consist entirely, or in part, of elements that do not have the histologic appearance of adenocarcinoma
- MBC has 3 main categories
  - Carcinomas with squamous &/or spindle cells
    - Squamous cell carcinoma
    - Spindle cell carcinoma
    - Adenosquamous carcinoma
    - Low-grade carcinoma with fibromatosis-like stroma
  - Matrix-producing carcinomas
  - Carcinomas with a true malignant mesenchymal component (carcinosarcoma)

ETIOLOGY/PATHOGENESIS

Cell of Origin
- All MBCs show at least focal evidence of origin as an epithelial malignancy
  - Cytokeratin expression should be present but may be focal and only for "basal" keratins (14 and 17)
  - 1 study demonstrated that, when 2 components are present, both share the same *P53* mutation
    - Data support concept that biphasic MBC is a monoclonal tumor
- Many MBCs have features of myoepithelial differentiation
  - About 1/3-2/3 express markers typical of myoepithelial cells, including p63, smooth muscle actin, P-cadherin, maspin, or CD10
  - Myoepithelial cells can produce basement membrane material that may resemble cartilage or bone

- Myoepithelial cells can be spindled in shape and closely resemble squamous cells
  - Squamous metaplasia may occur primarily in myoepithelial cells
- Very rarely, MBC is associated with true mesenchymal differentiation
  - Sarcomatous portion of tumor should show definitive mesenchymal features
  - Monoclonality of these carcinomas supports that sarcoma component arises from malignant epithelial cells

Gene Expression Profiling
- MBC has a distinctive molecular signature, separating it from other molecular classes of breast carcinomas
  - Majority demonstrate a transcriptional profile similar to, but distinct from, basal-like carcinomas
    - Profile is most similar to a claudin-low group of carcinomas
- Discriminator genes for MBC fall into several groups
  - Decreased expression of genes related to cell adhesion and increased expression of E-cadherin repressors
    - These genes are hypothesized to play a role in the epithelial to mesenchymal transition
    - E-cadherin can be present by IHC in epithelial component and absent in matrix-producing component of MBC
  - Increased expression of genes involved in extracellular matrix formation
  - Increased expression of genes thought to be associated with stem cell-like patterns
- Expression pattern for MBC is similar to that of residual carcinoma not responding to chemotherapy
  - May indicate a gene expression pattern associated with chemoresistance

METAPLASTIC CARCINOMA

Key Facts

Terminology
- Metaplastic breast carcinoma (MBC) includes a diverse group of tumors consisting entirely, or in part, of components that do not have the histologic appearance of adenocarcinoma
- Major subtypes include
  ○ Carcinomas with squamous/spindle cell morphology
  ○ Carcinomas with matrix production
  ○ Carcinomas with a true malignant mesenchymal component

Clinical Issues
- MBCs are uncommon (< 1% of all breast cancers)
- Usually presents as large palpable mass
  ○ Lymph node metastases are less frequent compared with other carcinomas of similar size

- Prognosis is generally poor, except for some subtypes (e.g., low-grade adenosquamous carcinoma)

Ancillary Tests
- Majority are negative for ER, PR, and HER2
- Expression of cytokeratin should be present for diagnosis
  ○ Cytokeratin reactivity is often focal, and only basal types (CK14 and CK17) may be present

Top Differential Diagnoses
- Squamous cell carcinoma of the skin
- Phyllodes tumor
- Primary or metastatic sarcoma
- Epithelial/myoepithelial tumors (including adenoid cystic carcinoma and pleomorphic adenoma)

DNA Studies
- MBC has pattern of copy number gains and losses distinct from basal-like carcinomas as well as other groups
  ○ Gains of 1p/5p and loss of 3q were most common
- High frequency of mutation, amplification, and activation of *P13K/AKT* pathway genes
  ○ Changes in this pathway are uncommon in basal-like carcinomas

CLINICAL ISSUES

Epidemiology
- Incidence
  ○ Rare, < 1% of breast cancers

Presentation
- Typically presents as a large palpable mass
  ○ May be associated with rapid growth

Prognosis
- Limited prognostic data are available due to rarity of MBC
- Axillary lymph node metastases are less common in MBC compared with other cancers of similar size
  ○ Nodal metastases very uncommon for tumors showing spindle cell and squamous features
  ○ Metastatic route may be primarily hematogenous to lung and liver
- Prognosis for some types of MBC is significantly worse than for non-MBC in some studies
  ○ May be related to higher stage at presentation
  ○ Most MBCs are triple negative; thus hormonal or HER2-targeted therapy is not available
  ○ MBC may be more resistant to chemotherapy than other types of breast carcinoma
  ○ However, some low-grade subtypes of MBC have a favorable prognosis

IMAGE FINDINGS

General Features
- Size
  ○ Tumors tend to be larger compared with other types of invasive breast cancers
    ■ Mean: 2.5-4.5 cm (range: 1 to > 10 cm)

Mammographic Findings
- Lobulated or irregular mass
  ○ Usually partially circumscribed and partially indistinct
- Calcifications
  ○ Usually absent or subtle
  ○ Rarely, calcification can be prominent when associated with extracellular matrix production or ossification

MICROSCOPIC PATHOLOGY

Histologic Features
- MBC comprises a very heterogeneous group of carcinomas
- Although there are several main categories of MBC, some carcinomas can be difficult to classify due to unusual histologic patterns
- Usually associated with little or no DCIS
  ○ When DCIS is present, its presence supports classification as MBC

Squamous Cell Carcinoma (SCC)
- SCC is often located centrally in the breast
  ○ Typically adjacent to a cystic cavity
  ○ May arise in areas of squamous metaplasia secondary to inflammation
  ○ Cells that undergo metaplasia may be myoepithelial cells
  ○ In situ SCC may be present in a cyst wall or a duct
- Squamous component of MBC can range from well to poorly differentiated
  ○ May be keratinizing or nonkeratinizing

- SCC adjacent to areas of squamous metaplasia in cysts or papillomas can mimic reactive stromal cells
  o IHC may be necessary to identify spindle cells as carcinoma
- Rare acantholytic growth pattern can resemble angiosarcoma
  o Epithelium degenerates and forms pseudovascular spaces
- Lymph node metastases are rare
- Prognosis is similar to carcinomas of no special type

Spindle Cell Carcinoma
- May present as pure spindle cells or an admixture of spindle cells with epithelioid and heterologous elements
  o Appearance of spindle cell component can range from bland low-grade cytology to cells with highly pleomorphic nuclei and frequent mitoses
- Lymphocytic infiltrate is commonly present
- Frequently expresses myoepithelial markers including p63, smooth muscle actin, and muscle specific actin
- May be classified as sarcomatoid carcinoma or myoepithelial carcinoma
- Lymph node metastases are rare, but overall prognosis is generally poor

Low-Grade Spindle Cell Carcinoma with Fibromatosis-like Stroma
- Spindle cells have very bland small nuclei and resemble fibroblasts
  o Small areas with epithelioid-appearing cells may be present
- Cellularity is low
- Stromal collagen may be prominent
- Differential diagnosis often includes fibromatosis, nodular fasciitis, or reactive stromal cells
- Prognosis is favorable, but occasional distant metastases have been reported

Adenosquamous Carcinoma (ASC)
- Carcinomas composed of both adenocarcinoma and SCC
  o Can vary from low grade to high grade
  o Very rare carcinomas resemble mucoepidermoid carcinoma of the salivary glands
- Low-grade ASC is composed of well-formed glands and squamous nests
  o Glandular structures are rounded
  o Squamous nests are usually solid and can be comma-shaped; keratin pearls may be present
  o Nuclear pleomorphism is minimal, and mitoses are generally absent
  o Majority of associated spindle cells are usually reactive fibroblasts, but a few may be tumor cells
  o Usually smaller (~ 2 cm) than other types of MBC
  o Resembles syringomatous adenoma of the nipple
  o Prognosis is generally very favorable

MBC with Matrix Production (Cartilaginous or Chondroid)
- Matrix consists of homogeneous, often abundant, extracellular material
  o Can appear cartilaginous, myxoid, or collagenous

o May be basement membrane-type material or (less likely) true cartilage
o Matrix may be difficult to distinguish from mucin
  ▪ Matrix has more solid appearance with fibrillar texture
  ▪ MBC is almost always ER/PR negative whereas mucinous carcinomas are almost always ER/PR positive
- Many express myoepithelial markers
- Morphologic appearance can overlap with adenomyoepithelial carcinomas and myoepithelial carcinomas

MBC with True Malignant Mesenchymal Component
- Very rare cases of MBC can demonstrate heterologous mesenchymal differentiation
- Sarcomatous component should demonstrate definite mesenchymal features
  o Osteosarcoma (most common; may have osteoclast-like giant cells), rhabdomyosarcoma (very rare: 4 reported cases)
  o Carcinoma with melanocytic areas have also been reported (very rare: 5 reported cases)
  o Spindle cell tumors with rhabdomyosarcoma or liposarcoma are more commonly high-grade phyllodes tumors

ANCILLARY TESTS

Immunohistochemistry
- Hormone receptors
  o Majority of MBCs are negative for ER and PR
- HER2
  o HER2 overexpression is unusual (< 5%)
- Cytokeratins
  o Keratin expression is most helpful marker to establish diagnosis of carcinoma in difficult cases
    ▪ May be very focal &/or weak
  o Many MBCs only express subsets of keratins typical for myoepithelial, basal, or possible progenitor (stem) cells (cytokeratins 5/6, 14, or 17)
  o Broad-spectrum AE1/AE3 keratin cocktail does not contain keratin 14 and 17 and may not show positivity
  o Broad-spectrum keratin MNF 116 does contain keratin 17 and is more helpful in identifying MBC
  o Keratin 34βE12 contains keratin 14 and can be helpful for identifying MBC
  o Individual antibodies for keratin 14 and 17 are also available
- p63
  o Both myoepithelial cells and squamous cells show nuclear positivity for p63
  o p63 can be very useful for evaluation of spindle cell &/or squamous carcinomas
  o Stromal cells (fibroblasts and myofibroblasts) and phyllodes tumors are negative for p63
- Other myoepithelial markers
  o Many MBCs will show positivity for 1 or more myoepithelial markers
    ▪ Include smooth muscle actin, P-cadherin, CD10

METAPLASTIC CARCINOMA

Major Subtypes of Metaplastic Carcinoma

Types	Comments
Squamous cell carcinoma	Often located centrally and associated with a cystic cavity
Spindle cell carcinoma	Morphologic overlap with squamous cell carcinomas and myoepithelial carcinomas; can be difficult to detect when associated with squamous metaplasia in papilloma or cyst
Adenosquamous carcinoma	Low-grade carcinomas that are histologically very similar to syringomatous adenoma of the nipple but are present deeper in the breast
Carcinoma with fibromatosis-like stroma	Can closely mimic fibromatosis or reactive stromal proliferation
Matrix-producing carcinomas	Morphologic overlap with epithelial/myoepithelial and myoepithelial carcinomas
Carcinomas with a true malignant mesenchymal component	A recognized sarcomatous component should be present; osteosarcoma is most common

- o 2 distinct luminal-like and myoepithelial-like cell populations should not be present
  - ■ If they are, classification as an adenomyoepithelial neoplasm (e.g., adenoid cystic carcinoma or adenomyoepithelial carcinoma) may be more appropriate
- • Markers indicating a basal phenotype
  - o Majority of MBCs are negative for ER and PR, positive for EGFR &/or CK5/6, and positive for CK14 and p63
  - o This combination of markers is frequently seen in basal-like carcinomas

DIFFERENTIAL DIAGNOSIS

Squamous Cell Carcinoma of the Skin
- • Can arise from mammary skin or cutaneous appendages
- • May secondarily involve underlying breast parenchyma
  - o Clinical history may be helpful to determine origin of the carcinoma
  - o Careful examination for in situ carcinoma associated with skin or cutaneous appendages is helpful

Phyllodes Tumor (PT)
- • PT with prominent stromal overgrowth may closely resemble MBC with spindle cells
  - o May consist of pure spindle cell proliferation or show heterologous differentiation
    - ■ Association with rhabdomyosarcoma or liposarcoma is more common in PT than in MBC
  - o May be problematic on limited needle core biopsies
- • Examination of multiple sections looking for biphasic pattern is helpful
- • Stromal component of malignant PT negative for cytokeratin expression
  - o Stromal component may express CD34
- • Evidence of epithelial component by morphology or IHC helps confirm diagnosis of MBC

Primary or Metastatic Sarcoma
- • Primary sarcomas of the breast are exceedingly rare
  - o Angiosarcoma is most common primary mammary sarcoma
    - ■ Can also be secondary to prior radiation or chronic lymphedema

- • Sarcomas should be of a specific type (e.g., liposarcoma, rhabdomyosarcoma)
- • Mesenchymal differentiation in the stroma of a phyllodes tumor is more common than in primary sarcoma
- • If the sarcoma is a metastasis, a prior diagnosis of a sarcoma at a different site is usually well known
- • Important to rule out MBC or PT before diagnosing a primary sarcoma
  - o Multiple cytokeratin antibodies (including basal cytokeratins) may be necessary to demonstrate positivity in MBC

Epithelial/Myoepithelial Tumors
- • Unusual breast neoplasms composed of 2 populations of cells with distinct luminal and myoepithelial characteristics
- • Myoepithelial component can appear spindled &/or produce matrix
  - o These features can make the lesion appear to have a metaplastic or mesenchymal component
- • Adenoid cystic carcinoma (ACC) is most common member of this group
  - o Important to recognize ACC, as this carcinoma has a very favorable prognosis
- • Adenomyoepithelial carcinomas may be classified as MBC if spindle cell component is prominent &/or matrix is present
- • Pleomorphic adenoma (mixed tumor) is rarely seen in the breast but is often associated with extensive matrix production and is important to recognize as a benign tumor

SELECTED REFERENCES

1. Gwin K et al: Breast carcinoma with chondroid differentiation: a clinicopathologic study of 21 triple negative (ER-, PR-, Her2/neu-) cases. Int J Surg Pathol. 18(1):27-35, 2010
2. Hennessy BT et al: Characterization of a naturally occurring breast cancer subset enriched in epithelial-to-mesenchymal transition and stem cell characteristics. Cancer Res. 69(10):4116-24, 2009
3. Luini A et al: Metaplastic carcinoma of the breast, an unusual disease with worse prognosis: the experience of the European Institute of Oncology and review of the literature. Breast Cancer Res Treat. 101(3):349-53, 2007
4. Pezzi CM et al: Characteristics and treatment of metaplastic breast cancer: analysis of 892 cases from the National Cancer Data Base. Ann Surg Oncol. 14(1):166-73, 2007

METAPLASTIC CARCINOMA

Squamous/Spindle Cell Metaplastic Carcinoma

(Left) Epithelial cells lining cysts may undergo squamous metaplasia and can give rise to squamous cell carcinomas ⊡. In addition to the relatively well-differentiated areas, there are small nests of poorly differentiated squamous cells in the stroma ➡. (Right) p63 is a useful marker to demonstrate squamous &/or myoepithelial differentiation in tumors ⊡. DCIS can be recognized by the presence of smaller, basally located myoepithelial cells in an involved duct ➡.

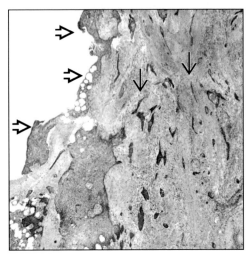
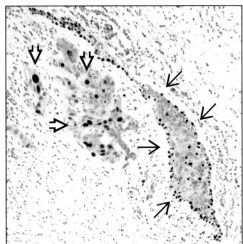

(Left) Spindle cell carcinomas can consist of a mildly cellular proliferation of bland cells in a pattern that closely resembles fibromatosis. (Right) Poorly differentiated spindle cell carcinomas are highly cellular and have markedly pleomorphic nuclei and frequent mitotic figures ➡. Extensive sampling is sometimes needed to identify areas showing epithelial differentiation. Foci of DCIS and invasive adenocarcinoma, when present, are usually seen at the periphery of the tumor.

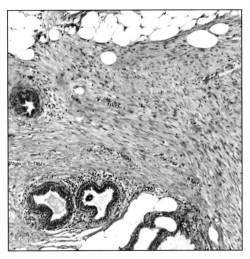
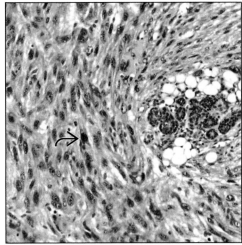

(Left) Low-grade adenosquamous carcinoma consists of well-formed tubules ➡ and squamous nests, which may be associated with keratin pearls ⊡. The pattern is very similar to syringomatous adenoma of the nipple. Although a triple negative carcinoma, the prognosis is generally quite favorable. (Right) Like other types of metaplastic carcinoma, adenosquamous carcinoma can be associated with areas of matrix production, which can have a cartilaginous appearance ⊡.

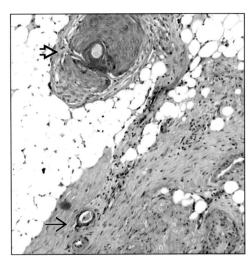
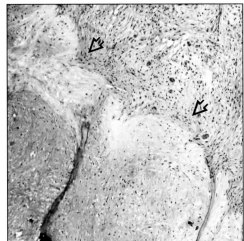

METAPLASTIC CARCINOMA

Squamous/Spindle Cell Metaplastic Carcinoma

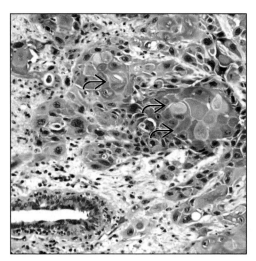

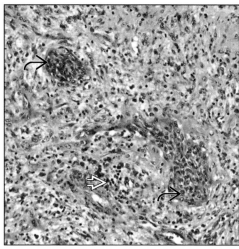

(Left) Squamous differentiation is apparent in this carcinoma due to the eosinophilic cytoplasm, defined cell borders, and intercellular bridges ➡. (Right) In this spindle cell carcinoma, epithelioid nests ➡ stand out against the neoplastic spindle cells. There is a moderate chronic inflammatory reaction present within the tumor ➡. The presence of an inflammatory reaction is a characteristic feature of MBC with spindle and squamous elements.

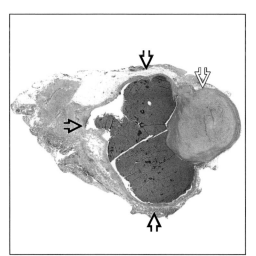

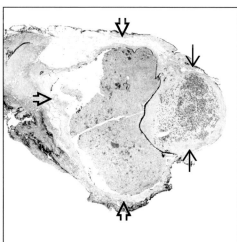

(Left) This large cyst in the breast filled with secretory material and blood ➡ is associated with a prominent spindle cell proliferation in the adjacent tissue ➡. The possibility of a squamous cell carcinoma arising in squamous metaplasia must be considered in such cases. (Right) The spindle cell proliferation ➡ adjacent to this cyst ➡ is positive for cytokeratin, identifying this lesion as a spindle cell carcinoma arising in association with squamous metaplasia.

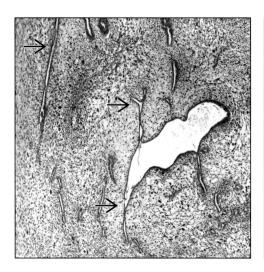

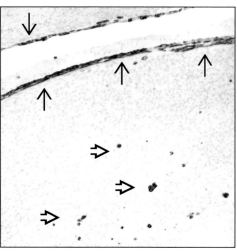

(Left) This spindle cell carcinoma surrounds normal epithelium ➡ and closely mimics the pattern of a phyllodes tumor. Small nests of epithelioid-appearing cells were present within the areas of spindle cells. (Right) This spindle cell carcinoma surrounds normal epithelium ➡ and closely resembles a phyllodes tumor. However, IHC for basal keratins revealed small nests and single cells positive for keratin ➡. Keratin positivity can be missed if basal keratins are not used.

Metaplastic Carcinoma with Matrix Production

(Left) One type of MBC is associated with abundant extracellular matrix formation ⊿. This material may be basement membrane formed by myoepithelial cells or, less likely, cartilage formation by chondroblasts. *(Right)* The matrix associated with MBC can be chondroid, mucinous ⊵, or collagenous ⊿ in appearance. Matrix can be distinguished from mucin by the use of histochemical stains, if necessary.

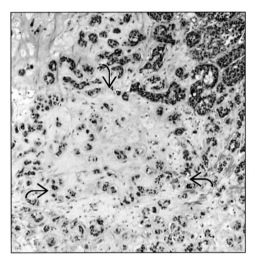
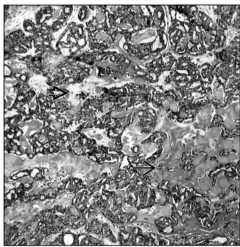

(Left) In rare cases, MBC is associated with recognizable malignant mesenchymal elements. The most common sarcomatous component is osteosarcoma. The tumor shown here demonstrates pleomorphic spindle cells with abundant extracellular osteoid matrix ⊿. The osteoid can sometimes be seen as calcification on imaging. *(Right)* This carcinoma is composed of spindle cells within an abundant extracellular matrix ⊿ and nests of highly pleomorphic epithelioid cells ⊵.

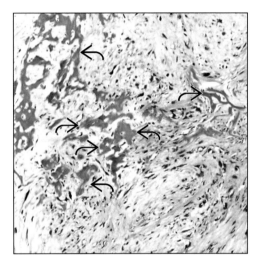
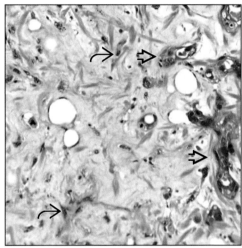

(Left) To identify keratin positivity in MBC, it is important to use antibodies to basal keratins 14, 17, & 5/6. In this case, both epithelioid and spindle cells in this matrix-producing carcinoma are positive for keratin 5/6 ⊿. *(Right)* Nuclear reactivity for p63 ⊿ in both the epithelioid and spindle cell components of this carcinoma is also helpful in identifying it as a carcinoma. p63 will not be present in other spindle cell lesions such as a phyllodes tumor or fibromatosis.

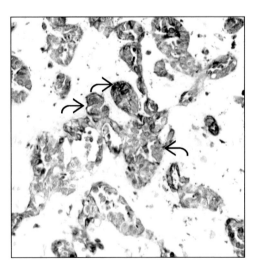
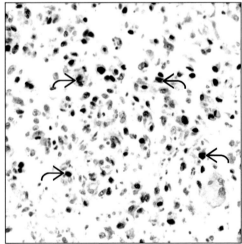

METAPLASTIC CARCINOMA

Differential Diagnosis

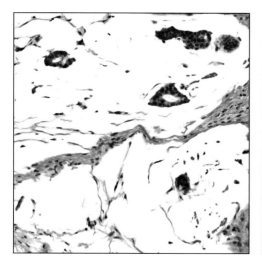

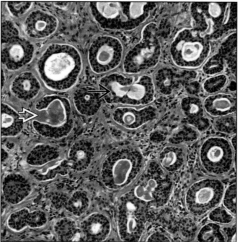

(Left) The extracellular mucin of mucinous carcinomas can sometimes resemble chondroid matrix. Matrix generally has a more fibrillar texture. Unlike MBC, mucinous carcinomas are almost always ER and PR positive and have a favorable prognosis. (Right) Adenoid cystic carcinomas are associated with matrix production that can appear collagenous ➡ or chondroid ➡. Unlike MBC, these carcinomas are composed of 2 distinct populations of luminal and myoepithelial-like cells.

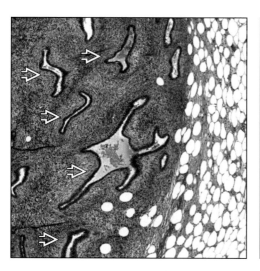

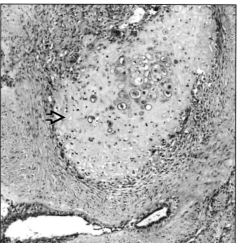

(Left) Phyllodes tumors can generally be recognized due to their close association with a component of normal nonneoplastic epithelial cells ➡. However, in cases with marked stromal overgrowth & a minimal biphasic growth pattern, IHC may be necessary to distinguish these tumors from spindle cell carcinomas. (Right) Heterologous elements, such as cartilage ➡, rhabdomyosarcoma, or liposarcoma, are more commonly observed within phyllodes tumors than found as components of MBC.

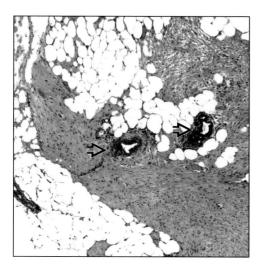

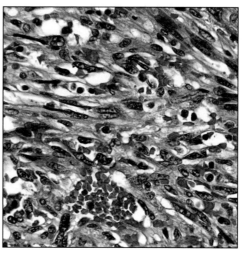

(Left) Fibromatosis consists of long sweeping fascicles of bland spindle cells that surround normal breast epithelium ➡. The possibility of a carcinoma with fibromatosis-like stroma should be excluded by IHC for keratins and p63. (Right) Angiosarcomas are the most common type of breast sarcoma. Rare acantholytic squamous cell carcinomas can form pseudovascular spaces, and IHC for epithelial and vascular markers may be required to make the correct diagnosis.

LOW-GRADE ADENOSQUAMOUS CARCINOMA

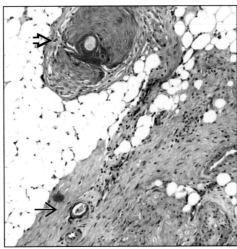

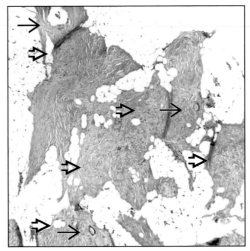

Low-grade adenosquamous carcinomas consist of well-differentiated squamous nests ⊳ as well as glands ➡. The carcinomas have a diffusely infiltrative pattern into adipose tissue.

The malignant epithelial cells are widely dispersed ➡ and accompanied by a cellular spindle cell proliferation ⊳. Some of the spindle cells are neoplastic, and some are reactive fibroblasts.

TERMINOLOGY

Abbreviations
- Low-grade adenosquamous carcinoma (LGASC)

Synonyms
- Syringomatous squamous tumor

Definitions
- Subtype of metaplastic carcinoma consisting of well-formed tubules and nests of squamous cells in background of spindle cells

CLINICAL ISSUES

Prognosis
- Generally favorable
  - Low incidence of lymph node metastases
  - Rare cases recur locally &/or metastasize
  - LGASC is example of triple negative carcinoma with good prognosis

Core Needle Biopsy
- Diagnosis can be difficult on core needle biopsy
  - Carcinoma can resemble radial sclerosing lesion
  - Squamous nests in stroma are uncommon findings in benign lesions

MACROSCOPIC FEATURES

General Features
- Generally forms irregular masses
  - LGASC may be ill defined due to diffusely infiltrative pattern into adipose tissue
- LGASCs can range from 0.5-8 cm with typical size of 2 cm

MICROSCOPIC PATHOLOGY

Histologic Features
- Consist of both glandular structures and squamous cell nests
- Nuclear pleomorphism is minimal, and mitoses are usually absent
  - Glandular structures are well formed
    - Shape of glands is rounded rather than angulated; angulated glands are more typical of sclerosing adenosis or tubular carcinoma
    - Double layer of cells is often present
    - Normal myoepithelial cell layer is not present
  - Squamous cell nests are usually solid
    - Nests may be comma- or tadpole-shaped
    - Cells may form keratin and keratin pearls
    - Small cysts filled with keratotic debris may be present
  - Surrounding stroma consists of spindle cells
    - Some of the spindle cells are neoplastic and appear to merge with epithelial cells
    - It can be difficult to distinguish reactive stromal cells from spindled tumor cells
- Carcinoma infiltrates around normal breast epithelium and into adipose tissue
  - Carcinoma often extends beyond gross or radiologic mass
  - This growth pattern is associated with risk of positive margins and local recurrence
- Lymphocytic aggregates are often present at periphery
- LGASC can be associated with higher grade carcinoma
  - Malignant spindle cell component with high-grade nuclei and mitoses may be present
- Necrosis is not a feature
- Foci of bone or cartilage formation can be present
- DCIS may be found in adjacent breast tissue
  - It can be difficult to distinguish DCIS from areas of invasion in these carcinomas

LOW-GRADE ADENOSQUAMOUS CARCINOMA

Key Facts

Terminology
- Subtype of metaplastic carcinoma consisting of well-formed tubules and nests of squamous cells in background of spindle cells

Clinical Issues
- LGASC is an example of a triple negative carcinoma with good prognosis
- Low incidence of lymph node metastases
- Rare cases recur locally &/or metastasize

Macroscopic Features
- These carcinomas form irregular masses that may be ill defined due to the diffuse infiltrative pattern into adipose tissue
- LGASCs can range from 0.5-8 cm with typical size of 2 cm

Microscopic Pathology
- Some carcinomas have been associated with sclerosing or papillary lesions or with adenomyoepithelioma

Ancillary Tests
- All LGASCs are negative for estrogen and progesterone receptors as well as HER2
- Basal cytokeratins are present in all cases
- EGFR is positive in approximately 1/2 of cases

Top Differential Diagnoses
- Syringomatous adenoma (SA) of nipple
- Metaplastic breast carcinoma
- Squamous cell carcinoma
- Sclerosing adenosis and radial sclerosing lesions
- Tubular carcinoma

- o Tumor cells can be positive for myoepithelial markers such as p63 and must be distinguished from true myoepithelial cell layer
- Some carcinomas have been associated with sclerosing or papillary lesions or with adenomyoepithelioma

ANCILLARY TESTS

Immunohistochemistry
- Hormone receptors
  - o All LGASCs are negative for estrogen and progesterone receptors
- HER2
  - o LGASCs are negative for HER2
- Basal cytokeratins
  - o Present in majority of LGASCs (cytokeratins 5/6 and 14)
  - o Epithelial cells and subset of spindle cells are positive
- EGFR (HER1)
  - o Approximately 1/2 are positive
- p63
  - o Epithelial cells are usually positive for p63, reflecting appearance of squamous cells

DIFFERENTIAL DIAGNOSIS

Syringomatous Adenoma (SA) of Nipple
- Usually presents as small subcutaneous palpable mass in nipple/areolar skin
- Histologic appearance is very similar to LGASC
  - o Cell nests and tubules infiltrate in dermis and smooth muscle of dermis
- SA is limited to dermis of the nipple-areola complex
  - o LGASC arises in breast parenchyma
  - o It may be difficult to distinguish these lesions on superficial biopsies or if LGASC invades into skin

Metaplastic Breast Carcinoma
- Many metaplastic carcinomas have areas of squamous metaplasia

- Metaplastic carcinomas with prominent squamous component could be termed "high-grade adenosquamous carcinoma"
- Nuclear pleomorphism, mitoses, necrosis, and prominent malignant-appearing spindle cell component are typical features of these carcinomas

Squamous Cell Carcinoma
- Generally forms large, centrally located masses
- Center of the carcinoma may be cystic
- Nuclear pleomorphism and necrosis are typically present
- Glandular areas are not present

Sclerosing Adenosis and Radial Sclerosing Lesions
- These lesions also consist of well-formed epithelial elements and spindled stroma
- Squamous metaplasia is less common in benign sclerosing lesions
- Benign sclerosing lesions have intact myoepithelial layer
  - o p63 may be difficult to interpret, as squamous elements in LGASC will be positive as will myoepithelial cells in benign lesions
  - o Other markers for myoepithelial cells may be more helpful

Tubular Carcinoma
- Squamoid features would be very unusual
- Carcinomas are generally more compact and do not have diffusely infiltrative pattern
- Almost all cases are positive for estrogen and progesterone receptors

SELECTED REFERENCES

1. Geyer FC et al: Genomic and immunohistochemical analysis of adenosquamous carcinoma of the breast. Mod Pathol. 23(7):951-60, 2010
2. Oo KZ et al: Infiltrating syringomatous adenoma of the nipple: clinical presentation and literature review. Arch Pathol Lab Med. 133(9):1487-9, 2009

LOW-GRADE ADENOSQUAMOUS CARCINOMA

Microscopic Features

(Left) Some of the squamous tumor cell nests form small cystic spaces filled with keratotic debris. These cells will be positive for p63, as are other types of squamous cells. *(Right)* The squamous cells can also be found in comma-shaped clusters. This pattern is also seen in syringomatous adenomas of the nipple. A mitotic figure is present ⏵, but in general mitoses are rare in low-grade adenosquamous carcinomas.

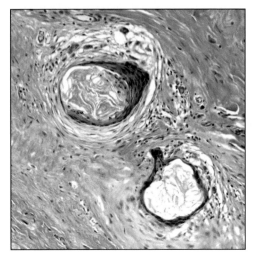
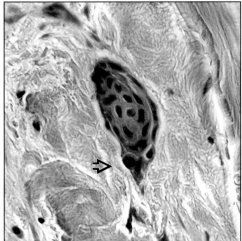

(Left) The glandular component consists of small acini lined by low-grade tumor cells. The epithelial tumor cells often blend into the surrounding spindled stromal cells ⏵. IHC studies demonstrate that some, but not all, associated spindle cells are derived from the tumor. *(Right)* A lymphocytic infiltrate is typically seen at the periphery of LGASCs ⏵. The borders of these carcinomas are often difficult to define due to sparse cellularity and the diffuse infiltrative pattern.

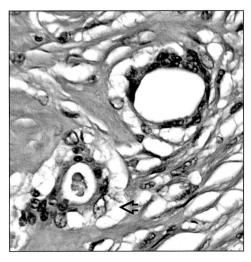
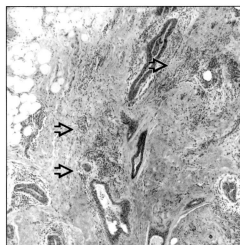

(Left) LGASC can be associated with osteocartilaginous areas ⏵. These areas are similar to the matrix production present in other types of metaplastic carcinoma. *(Right)* IHC for p63 shows positivity in many of the tumor cells, correlating with the squamous appearance of much of the tumor. Note that the pattern is not that of a normal basally located myoepithelial cell layer, which is seen in benign sclerosing lesions.

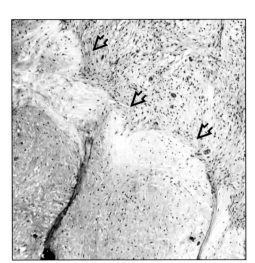
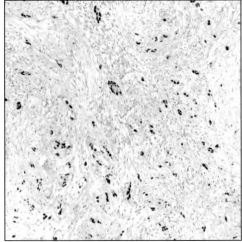

LOW-GRADE ADENOSQUAMOUS CARCINOMA

Differential Diagnosis

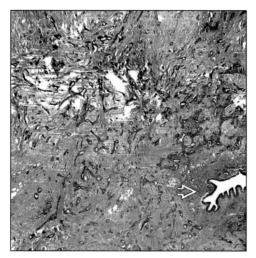

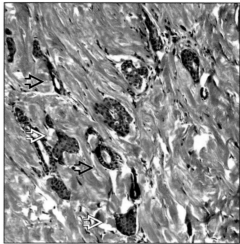

(Left) *Syringomatous adenoma has a very similar appearance to LGASC but is limited to the dermis of the nipple. Diagnosis can be difficult in superficial skin biopsies without underlying breast tissue &/or if LGASC invades into skin. In this case, the tumor cell nests infiltrate around lactiferous sinuses ➡.* **(Right)** *Like LGASC, syringomatous adenoma consists of both nests of squamous cells ➡ and small well-formed glandular elements ➡.*

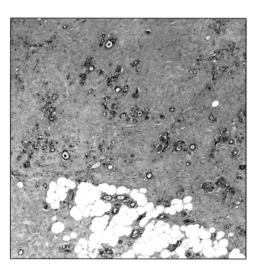

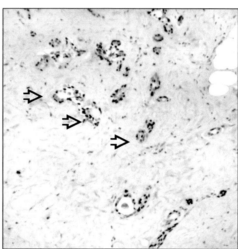

(Left) *Sclerosing lesions such as this one sometimes have a dispersed pattern and haphazard distribution in breast tissue. Unlike LGASC, the surrounding stroma usually does not have a reactive and hypercellular appearance. Squamous metaplasia is not typically present.* **(Right)** *IHC for myoepithelial cells such as this study for p63 will demonstrate a well-formed basally located myoepithelial layer ➡ associated with the tubules of sclerosing lesions.*

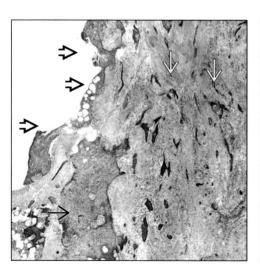

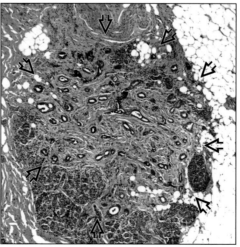

(Left) *Squamous cell carcinomas of the breast are often located centrally and surround a cystic cavity ➡. Although portions of this carcinoma resemble LGASC ➡, the majority of the carcinoma consists of poorly differentiated squamous cells ➡.* **(Right)** *Tubular carcinomas, like LGASC, are composed of small well-formed glandular elements. However, squamous areas are not present in tubular carcinoma, and the extent of the carcinoma is generally well defined ➡.*

BASAL-LIKE CARCINOMAS

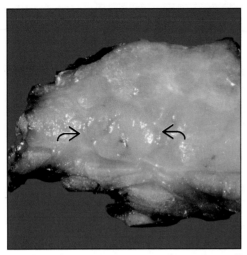

Basal like breast cancers are frequently well circumscribed ⇨ and may mimic benign lesions grossly and radiographically. The subgroup of medullary carcinomas all have this gross appearance.

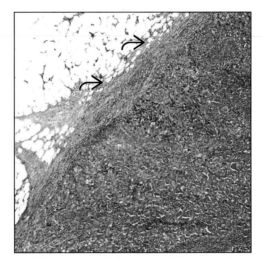

Basal-like cancers typically grow as solid masses or sheets of cells ⇨ rather than infiltrating as small nests into the surrounding breast tissue. Central fibrosis or necrosis may be present.

TERMINOLOGY

Abbreviations
- Basal-like carcinoma (BLC)
- Triple negative breast cancer (TNBC)

Definitions
- **BLC** is a type of invasive breast cancer originally defined by gene expression profiling studies

ETIOLOGY/PATHOGENESIS

Gene Expression Profiling
- 4 major types of carcinoma are identified by their patterns of gene expression
  - Luminal A (~ 55%), luminal B (~ 15%), HER2 (~ 15%), and BLC (~ 15%)
- BLC and myoepithelial cells share expression of similar groups of genes
  - Term "basal" was chosen to include myoepithelial cells as well as possible precursor or progenitor cells
  - Actual cell of origin is unknown
- Gene expression patterns characteristic of BLC include
  - Lack of hormone receptor expression (or only very rare expression)
  - Low or absent expression of HER2
  - High expression of basal cytokeratins 5, 14, and 17 (specific for BLC)
    - Cytokeratin 5/6 present in majority in most studies; however, in 1 study, only 6% of BLCs were positive, suggesting there may be variability in antibodies
    - Cytokeratin 17 present in 50% but may be focal and weak
    - Most also express luminal cytokeratins 7, 8/18, and 19
  - High expression of proliferation-related genes
  - High expression of EGFR (HER1)
    - 45-75% positive

- Less common in non-BLC
  - Expression of other proteins: C-Kit (CD117), VEGF, cyclin-E, fascin, α B-crystallin
- p53 overexpression present in 50-60%
  - Mutations of *TP53* are more common compared to all breast cancers
- CD117 (C-Kit): Majority of positive cancers are BLC
  - Positive in ~ 45% of BLC
  - Does not correlate with mutations indicative of sensitivity to tyrosine kinase inhibitors
  - Not all cancers with increased mRNA levels have increased protein expression

BRCA1, BLC, and Hereditary Breast Cancer
- Majority of breast cancers occurring in *BRCA1* mutation carriers are in BLC group
  - *BRCA1* has many functions
    - DNA repair of double-strand breaks by homologous recombination: Cells that lack *BRCA1* must rely on other less reliable modes of repair and are genetically unstable
    - Cell cycle regulation, checkpoint control
    - Transcriptional control, ubiquitination, chromatin remodeling, and regulation of apoptosis
    - Required for transactivation of the ER gene promoter: Loss may result in ER negativity
  - Genetic instability results in replication errors
    - Result in accumulation of chromosomal abnormalities
    - Enables mutations in genes essential to cell cycle checkpoint activation
    - Accumulating mutations predispose to tumor formation
  - *BRCA1* defects are postulated to be initiating oncogenic events in hereditary and sporadic BLC
    - Mammary stem cells demonstrate a basal-like gene expression profile
- Many sporadic BLCs also have altered *BRCA1* activity and loss of function
  - About 10-20% show methylation of gene promoter

BASAL-LIKE CARCINOMAS

Key Facts

Terminology
- Triple negative breast cancer (TNBC)
- Basal-like carcinoma (BLC)
  - Lack of hormone receptor expression
  - Low expression of HER2
  - High expression of basal cytokeratins 5, 14, & 17
  - High expression of proliferation-related genes
- TNBC increasingly used as surrogate for BLC
  - Most but not all BLCs fall into the TNBC category

Clinical Issues
- Approximately 15% of infiltrating carcinomas of the breast
  - *BRCA1*-associated cancers are usually BLC
  - More frequent in premenopausal African-American women
- Most BLCs demonstrate an aggressive clinical course

- Increased risk for early relapse/recurrence
- Increased risk for visceral organs & CNS recurrence
- No role for endocrine- or HER2-targeted therapies
  - Most patients receive aggressive multiagent chemotherapy
  - Tumors may be hypersensitive to DNA-damaging agents

Microscopic Pathology
- BLC has distinctive morphologic features
  - Circumscription with pushing borders
  - Pleomorphic tumor cells, syncytial-like growth
  - High nuclear grade
  - Areas of geographic necrosis
  - Brisk lymphocytic stromal reaction

- About same percent of non-BLCs show methylation of *BRCA1*
- Some BLCs show decreased *BRCA1* mRNA
- Mutations in *BRCA1* gene are rare in sporadic BLC
- Role of *BRCA1* in BLC and link between sporadic and hereditary tumors are still unclear

CLINICAL ISSUES

Epidemiology
- Incidence
  - 10-15% of invasive breast carcinomas
- Age
  - More common in younger patient population
    - Range: 47-55 years
    - Patients more likely to be premenopausal

Treatment
- Adjuvant therapy
  - No role for endocrine- or HER2-targeted therapy due to lack of expression of hormone receptors and HER2
  - Most patients treated with aggressive multiagent chemotherapy
    - Hypersensitivity to DNA-damaging agents due to abnormal DNA repair function
    - Anthracyclines and platinum agents
    - BLC may show resistance to mitotic spindle poisons (taxanes)
  - BLC often shows response after neoadjuvant chemotherapy
    - About 15% demonstrate pathologic complete response
    - Some of these patients may be cured
    - Patients without pathologic complete response to neoadjuvant chemotherapy have poor prognosis

Prognosis
- Most BLCs demonstrate aggressive clinical course and poor prognosis

- Decreased disease-free interval, disease-specific survival, and overall survival compared with other breast cancers
  - Increased risk for early relapse/recurrence
  - Increased risk for visceral organs & CNS recurrence
- However, some carcinomas within this group have exceptionally good prognosis
  - Adenoid cystic carcinoma, secretory carcinoma, low-grade adenosquamous carcinoma, and (to some extent) medullary carcinoma
  - In these cancers, histologic classification is more important than expression profiling classification
- Other special histologic types of BLC share same poor prognosis
  - Metaplastic carcinoma, spindle cell carcinoma
- Poor prognosis may be due to overexpression of genes promoting proliferation and migration
  - EGFR activates signaling pathways involved in cell proliferation
  - α B-crystallin, a heat shock protein, inhibits apoptosis
  - Fascin, a cell motility protein, promotes tumor cell invasion
  - VEGF promotes angiogenesis
- BLC has specific pattern of metastases
  - Higher incidence of metastasis to brain (central nervous system) and lung
    - Metastases to these sites have poorer prognosis
  - Less likely to metastasize to bones or lymph nodes

Core Needle Biopsies
- Patients may be diagnosed with BLC on core needle biopsy
- It is important to document hormone receptor positivity in normal breast tissue when possible as an internal control and to include appropriate controls to ensure accuracy
- Repeat studies on subsequent excisions are helpful to confirm negative results and evaluate possible tumor heterogeneity

IMAGE FINDINGS

Mammographic Findings
- Often ill-defined oval, round, or lobulated mass lesion
  - Partially circumscribed, partially indistinct margins
  - Calcifications uncommon
- BLC may grow rapidly
  - Tumors are overrepresented among "interval breast cancers" (cancers becoming clinically evident between annual mammograms)

Ultrasonographic Findings
- Hypoechoic mass, oval or lobulated
  - May show pseudocystic component due to necrosis in larger lesions

MACROSCOPIC FEATURES

General Features
- Partially circumscribed or lobulated mass lesion
- Extensive necrosis may impart a cystic appearance

MICROSCOPIC PATHOLOGY

Histologic Features
- Most BLCs have distinctive morphologic features
  - Circumscription with pushing borders
  - Sheets of pleomorphic tumor cells, syncytial-like growth pattern
  - High nuclear grade
  - High mitotic index
  - Areas of geographic necrosis or fibrosis
  - Brisk lymphocytic stromal reaction; may be related to cytokine production by tumor cells
- BLCs with medullary-like features
  - Prominent lymphoplasmacytic infiltrate
  - Syncytial growth pattern
  - Associated with better prognosis compared with all BLCs
- BLC with central fibrotic focus of > 30% associated with poorer prognosis compared with all BLCs
- Special histologic types with same gene expression profile as BLC have specific morphologic features
  - Medullary carcinoma
  - Metaplastic carcinoma
  - Adenoid cystic carcinoma
- Basal-like DCIS has also been described
  - DCIS is usually scant or absent adjacent to BLC
  - DCIS negative for ER, PR, and HER2 comprises only 8% of all cases of DCIS
  - Almost all have high nuclear grade and are often associated with necrosis
  - Almost all show expression of basal cytokeratins

ANCILLARY TESTS

Surrogate IHC Tests to Identify BLC
- Gene expression profiling requires fresh or frozen tissue and is not available for majority of breast cancers

- Panels of IHC markers have been developed to identify BLC as defined by gene expression profiling
  - Triple negative (negative for ER, PR, and HER2)
    - ~ 70% specific as some TNBC are not BLC
    - ~ 90% sensitive as majority of BLC are TNBC
    - Does not identify 15-45% of BLC that are not TNBC
  - Triple negative and positive for either cytokeratin 5/6 or EGFR ("5-marker method" or "core basal classification")
    - Any immunoreactivity for cytokeratin 5/6 or EGFR is considered a positive result
    - 100% specific
    - 76% sensitive
  - Triple negative and positive for cytokeratin 14 and cytokeratin 34bE12 (includes cytokeratins 1, 4, 10, 14) and EGFR
    - 100% specific
    - 78% sensitive
    - CK5/6 was not used in this particular study as < 10% of cases were positive and EGFR positivity was not specific for BLC
    - Suggests that it may be difficult to reproduce BLC classification across institutions due to differences in IHC results
  - Triple negative and positive for 1 basal cytokeratin, EGFR, &/or C-Kit (CD117)
    - 100% specific
    - 76% sensitive
  - Compared with TNBCs that are negative for CK5/6 and EGFR, BLC (defined by expression of CK5/6 or EGFR) shows the following
    - More likely to be high grade (87% vs. 64%)
    - Occurs more frequently in patients < 40 years of age (19% vs. 10%)
    - Decreased 10-year breast cancer survival (57% vs. 67%)
- **Best method to identify BLC with relevant biologic, predictive, and prognostic correlations has not yet been determined**

DIFFERENTIAL DIAGNOSIS

Triple Negative Carcinoma (TNBC)
- Defined by the absence of ER, PR, and HER2 by IHC
  - Comprises 10-15% of all breast cancers
- 50-80% of TNBCs are BLCs by expression profiling
  - Therefore, these 2 categories of cancer have substantial overlap but are not identical
- Subtypes in 20-50% of TNBCs that are not BLC have been identified
  - "Multiple marker negative breast cancer" lacks expression of basal markers
    - May be well or moderately differentiated
    - Expresses cytokeratin 8 or other "luminal" keratins
  - "Claudin negative breast cancer"; low expression of basal markers and genes involved in tight junctions and cell adhesion
- Cancers that are TNBC and BLC have features described for BLC
  - High histologic grade and high proliferative rate

BASAL-LIKE CARCINOMAS

Pathologic Features of BRCA1-related Tumors, TNBC, and BLC

Tumor Features	BRCA1-associated	BLC	TNBC
Grade	Majority grade 3	Majority grade 3	Typically grade 3
Tumor/parenchymal interface	Pushing borders	Pushing borders	Typically pushing borders
Proliferation index	High	High	High
Host lymphocytic response	Typically brisk and extensive	Typically brisk and extensive	Typically brisk
Geographic areas of necrosis	Present	Present	Present
DNA copy # changes/aneuploidy	Aneuploid	Aneuploid	Typically aneuploid
ER status	Negative (80-90%)	Negative (80-90%)	Negative by definition
HER2 status	Negative (80-90%)	Negative (> 90%)	Negative by definition
P53 status	Frequent P53 mutations	Frequent P53 mutations	Frequent P53 mutations
BRCA1 status	Mutation, loss of function	Diminished expression (~ 20%)	May show diminished expression
Basal cytokeratin expression	~ 80% (can be focal and weak)	~ 80% (can be focal and weak)	40-80% (may be focal)
Patterns of metastases	Visceral and CNS more frequent	Visceral and CNS more frequent	Visceral and CNS more frequent
Prognosis	Aggressive, increased incidence of early recurrence	Aggressive, increased incidence of early recurrence	Typically aggressive, early recurrence
Chemotherapy sensitivity	Increased sensitivity to DNA-damaging agents	Increased sensitivity to DNA-damaging agents	Increased sensitivity to DNA-damaging agents

- o Metastases more frequent to brain and lung than to bone and lymph nodes
- o Risk of early recurrence within 5 years and death
- Cancers that are TNBCs but not BLCs have different features
  - o Lower incidence of TP53 overexpression compared with BLC
  - o Do not have increased incidence of brain and lung metastases and decreased incidence of lymph node metastases
  - o Better overall survival compared with BLCs
    - Non-BLC may have increased response to chemotherapy compared with BLC (defined by IHC)
- TNBC is more common in some ethnic groups
  - o 20-25% of carcinomas in African-American women are TNBC, compared with 10% in all women
  - o 17% of carcinomas in Hispanic women are TNBC
- Factors that reduce risk of breast cancer in general increase risk for TNBC
  - o 1st childbirth at an early age increases risk
  - o Multiparity increases risk
- TNBC includes special histologic types of breast cancer
  - o Medullary, adenosquamous, secretory, metaplastic (including spindle cell), squamous cell, adenoid cystic
  - o In these subtypes, histologic classification may be more important than immunoprofile for predicting clinical behavior

Non-Breast Malignancies
- If malignant tumor of the breast is ER, PR, and HER2 negative and lacks an in situ component, other types of tumors should be considered
  - o Melanoma is most common metastatic tumor to the breast
  - o Angiosarcoma is most common sarcoma and can have an epithelioid appearance
  - o Lymphomas can be high grade and mimic carcinomas

SELECTED REFERENCES

1. Molyneux G et al: The cell of origin of BRCA1 mutation-associated breast cancer: a cautionary tale of gene expression profiling. J Mammary Gland Biol Neoplasia. 16(1):51-5, 2011
2. Haupt B et al: Basal-like breast carcinoma: a phenotypically distinct entity. Arch Pathol Lab Med. 134(1):130-3, 2010
3. Thike AA et al: Triple-negative breast cancer: clinicopathological characteristics and relationship with basal-like breast cancer. Mod Pathol. 23(1):123-33, 2010
4. Rakha EA et al: Triple-negative breast cancer: distinguishing between basal and nonbasal subtypes. Clin Cancer Res. 15(7):2302-10, 2009
5. Rakha EA et al: Triple-negative/basal-like breast cancer: review. Pathology. 41(1):40-7, 2009
6. Cheang MC et al: Basal-like breast cancer defined by five biomarkers has superior prognostic value than triple-negative phenotype. Clin Cancer Res. 14(5):1368-76, 2008
7. Lin NU et al: Sites of distant recurrence and clinical outcomes in patients with metastatic triple-negative breast cancer: high incidence of central nervous system metastases. Cancer. 113(10):2638-45, 2008
8. Schneider BP et al: Triple-negative breast cancer: risk factors to potential targets. Clin Cancer Res. 14(24):8010-8, 2008
9. Voduc D et al: Basal and triple-negative breast cancers: impact on clinical decision-making and novel therapeutic options. Clin Breast Cancer. 8 Suppl 4:S171-8, 2008
10. Carey LA et al: Race, breast cancer subtypes, and survival in the Carolina Breast Cancer Study. JAMA. 295(21):2492-502, 2006
11. Hicks DG et al: Breast cancers with brain metastases are more likely to be estrogen receptor negative, express the basal cytokeratin CK5/6, and overexpress HER2 or EGFR. Am J Surg Pathol. 30(9):1097-104, 2006

Histologic Features of Basal-like Carcinoma

(Left) The typical BLC demonstrates a characteristic growth pattern with circumscribed or pushing borders that are sharply defined at the interface with the surrounding breast parenchyma ➟. *(Right)* The presence of extensive geographic necrosis ➟ is a common feature. These areas can be prominent and may give rise to a cystic appearance on ultrasound examination. Carcinomas with extensive necrosis have a higher rate of response to chemotherapy.

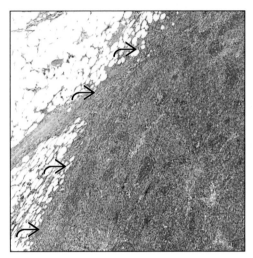
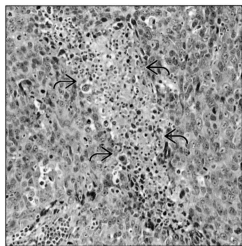

(Left) BLC is often associated with a marked lymphoplasmacytic infiltrate ➟ that may include germinal centers. In some cases, differential diagnosis of an upper outer quadrant mass may include metastasis to an intramammary lymph node. *(Right)* High-grade pleomorphic tumor cells arranged in syncytial-like sheets are typical of BLC. Frequent mitotic figures are usually readily apparent ➟ while indicators of proliferation by IHC such as Ki-67 will also be highly expressed.

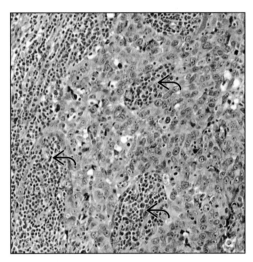
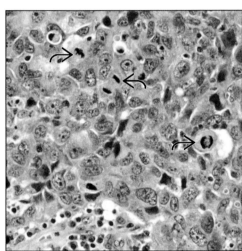

(Left) TNBC is also typically of high grade and has a high mitotic rate ➟. The majority are also BLC. It is not yet clear if it is clinically important to identify TNBC that is not BLC. *(Right)* IHC can be used to identify TNBC most likely to be BLC. This carcinoma is positive for EGFR in a membrane pattern ➟ and was also positive for basal cytokeratins 5/6. It is highly likely that it would be classified as BLC by gene expression profiling. This method will not identify BLC that is not TNBC.

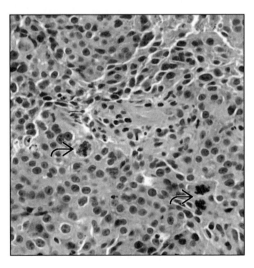
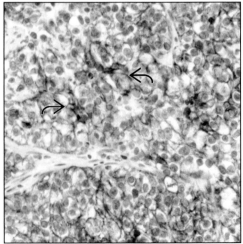

BASAL-LIKE CARCINOMAS

Special Types of Basal-like Carcinomas

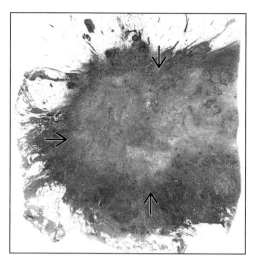

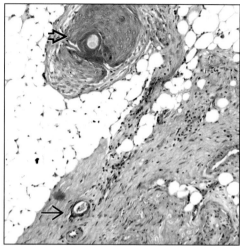

(Left) Carcinomas with a central fibrotic focus ⇥ are typically high grade and negative for ER, PR, and HER2. Extensive central necrosis is also sometimes seen. Most will be BLC. *(Right)* Low-grade adenosquamous carcinoma is characterized by squamous cell nests with keratin formation ⇥ in addition to well-formed tubules ⇥. ER, PR, and HER2 are not expressed and proliferation is low. Unlike other types of TNBC, this special histologic type has a good prognosis.

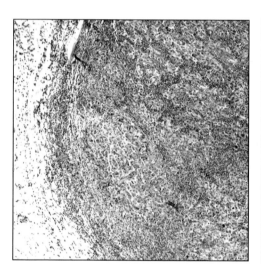

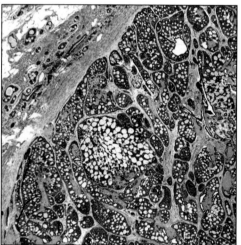

(Left) Medullary carcinomas cluster with BLC by GEP. However, prognosis is more favorable than BLC in the absence of specific strict histologic criteria for this diagnosis. BRCA1-associated carcinomas often have medullary features, but the relationship to prognosis in this setting is not yet clear. *(Right)* Adenoid cystic carcinomas are composed of 2 populations of luminal-like and myoepithelial-like cells. Although they cluster with BLC by GEP, prognosis is very favorable.

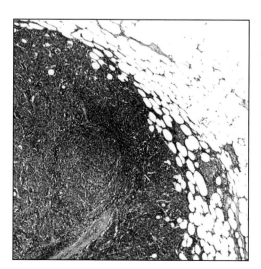

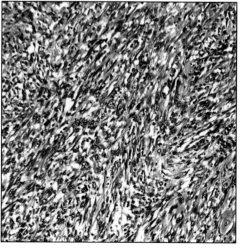

(Left) BRCA1-associated cancers are usually high grade and often associated with a dense lymphocytic infiltrate. They cluster with BLC by GEP. Some BLC may have reduced BRCA1 function although specific mutations are rare. *(Right)* Metaplastic carcinomas, including spindle cell carcinomas, also cluster with BLC by GEP. They often have morphologic or tumor markers suggestive of squamous or myoepithelial differentiation, including frequent expression of p63 and basal keratins.

ADENOID CYSTIC CARCINOMA

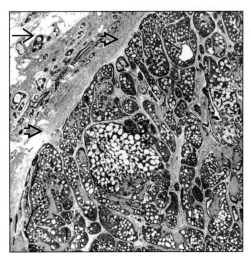

Adenoid cystic carcinoma usually presents as a circumscribed mass ⇒ consisting of rounded nests of tumor cells. Smaller tumor cell nests infiltrate into breast tissue at the periphery ⇒.

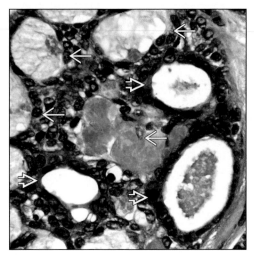

ACC consists of 2 cell types. Luminal-like cells line spaces that appear empty or filled with secretions ⇒. Myoepithelial-like cells surround basement membrane-type material ⇒.

TERMINOLOGY

Abbreviations
- Adenoid cystic carcinoma (ACC)

Definitions
- Invasive carcinoma composed of 2 cell populations: Luminal-like cells and myoepithelial-like cells
- Rare; only 0.1% of breast cancers

CLINICAL ISSUES

Presentation
- Most frequently presents as palpable circumscribed or lobulated mass below the nipple
  - Some carcinomas are tender
- Rarely presents as mammographic mass; may be lobulated or irregular
- Most patients are women; rare cases are reported in men
  - Average age: 50-65 years

Prognosis
- Excellent prognosis
  - 90-100% survival at 10 years
  - Local recurrence: 6% of patients
  - Axillary lymph node metastasis: 3% of patients
  - Distant metastasis and death: 3% of patients
    - Most common site is lung; also reported to bone, liver, brain, and kidney
- These carcinomas will score as having a poor prognosis using either 21 gene recurrence score or 70 gene prognosis profile
  - Therefore, histologic type is more important than gene expression profiling in predicting outcome for ACC

MACROSCOPIC FEATURES

General Features
- Firm, white, circumscribed or ill-defined mass
  - Microscopic extent of tumor may be greater than appreciated grossly due to minimal stromal response associated with peripheral infiltrating tumor nests

MICROSCOPIC PATHOLOGY

Histologic Features
- 3 histologic patterns
  - Cribriform: Most common pattern
  - Reticular-tubular: Tumor cells are surrounded by predominant component of stroma
  - Solid: Myoepithelial cells predominate with few luminal-type cells
- Large cribriform spaces are lined by myoepithelial-type cells
  - Spaces are filled with basement membrane-type material that can be collagenous, myxoid, or mucinous
- Luminal-type cells can form solid nests or small tubules with true lumens
  - Lumens may be empty or filled with flocculent secretions
- Grading has been suggested but does not correlate well with clinical outcome
  - I: No solid elements
  - II: < 30% solid elements
  - III: > 30% solid elements
- Some cases are associated with microglandular adenosis

ADENOID CYSTIC CARCINOMA

Key Facts

Terminology

- Invasive carcinoma composed of 2 cell populations: Luminal-like cells and myoepithelial-like cells
- Rare; only 0.1% of breast cancers

Clinical Issues

- Excellent prognosis: 90-100% survival at 10 years
- Most frequently presents as palpable circumscribed or lobulated mass
- These carcinomas will score as having poor prognosis using either 21 gene recurrence score or 70 gene prognosis profile
  - Therefore, histologic type is more important than gene expression profiling in predicting outcome for adenoid cystic carcinomas

Microscopic Pathology

- 3 histologic patterns
  - Cribriform: Most common pattern
  - Reticular-tubular: Tumor cells are surrounded by predominant component of stroma
  - Solid: Myoepithelial cells predominate with few luminal-type cells
- Grading has been suggested but does not correlate well with clinical outcome

Top Differential Diagnoses

- Invasive cribriform carcinoma
- Adenomyoepithelial carcinoma
- Ductal carcinoma in situ, cribriform type
- Collagenous spherulosis
- Cylindroma

ANCILLARY TESTS

Immunohistochemistry

- Immunoperoxidase studies demonstrate 2 distinct cell populations
  - Luminal-type cells: Positive for cytokeratin 7 or CAM5.2, some positive for C-Kit (CD117), rarely positive for ER or PR
    - It is unknown if activating mutations in C-Kit that would predict sensitivity to tyrosine kinase inhibitors are present
  - Myoepithelial-type cells: Usually positive for p63, smooth muscle actin, cytokeratin 5/6, laminin

Cytogenetics

- Same t(6;9)(q22-23;p23-24) was found in 4 of 4 breast adenoid cystic carcinomas
  - This translocation creates a fusion between *MYB* and *NFIB* transcription factor genes

DIFFERENTIAL DIAGNOSIS

Invasive Cribriform Carcinoma

- Cribriform spaces are empty or filled with secretory material
- Almost all cribriform carcinomas are positive for ER and PR
- Myoepithelial-like cells are not present

Adenomyoepithelial Carcinoma

- ACC is subtype of adenomyoepithelial carcinoma with specific histologic features
- Adenomyoepithelial carcinomas have multiple cell types, but 2 distinct cell populations may not be present
- Solid or spindle cell patterns are typical
- Stromal production by myoepithelial-like cells is usually minimal or absent
- Carcinoma may invade as ragged sheets and individual cells instead of circumscribed nests

- Lymph-vascular invasion or perineural invasion may be present
- Tumor necrosis may be present

Ductal Carcinoma In Situ, Cribriform Type

- Almost all cribriform DCIS is ER and PR positive
- Myoepithelial cells are limited to periphery
- Cribriform spaces are empty or filled with secretory material

Collagenous Spherulosis (CS)

- Usually a small incidental finding and easily distinguished from ACC; however, they may be difficult to distinguish on core needle biopsy
- In 1 report, CS was shown to not have C-Kit (CD117) tubules present
  - ACC may also be negative for CD117
- Positivity for smooth muscle myosin heavy chain and calponin was more common in CS

Cylindroma

- Also composed of both myoepithelial and epithelial cells
- Tumor is well circumscribed, and tumor cell nests fit together in jigsaw-like pattern
- Nests of cells are surrounded by thick basement membrane
- Nuclear atypia and mitoses are absent
- These tumors are benign and do not metastasize
- Some cases are associated with Brooke-Spiegler syndrome

SELECTED REFERENCES

1. Da Silva L et al: Molecular and morphological analysis of adenoid cystic carcinoma of the breast with synchronous tubular adenosis. Virchows Arch. 454(1):107-14, 2009
2. Persson M et al: Recurrent fusion of MYB and NFIB transcription factor genes in carcinomas of the breast and head and neck. Proc Natl Acad Sci U S A. 106(44):18740-4, 2009
3. Weigelt B et al: Refinement of breast cancer classification by molecular characterization of histological special types. J Pathol. 216(2):141-50, 2008

ADENOID CYSTIC CARCINOMA

Imaging and Microscopic Features

(Left) ACC usually appears as a circumscribed mass by imaging ⊵. However, the actual extent of the carcinoma is often underestimated. Adjacent smaller tumor nests can extensively infiltrate into the adjacent stroma without a desmoplastic response. *(Right)* The most common pattern of ACC consists of rounded nests with a cribriform pattern. Some spaces are filled with basement membrane material that can be collagenous ⊵ or myxoid ➡. Other spaces are empty or contain secretions ⊵.

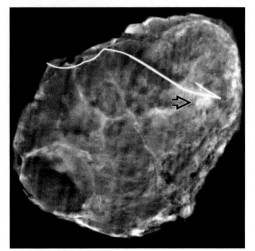
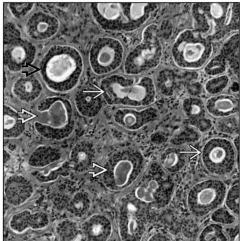

(Left) In the reticular-tubular pattern of ACC, the collagenous basement membrane material predominates and surrounds the epithelial cells. *(Right)* In the solid pattern, many nests of cells consist predominantly of myoepithelial-like ⊵ cells with few or no luminal-like cells. However, in focal areas, both cell types should be present ➡.

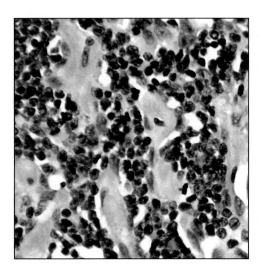
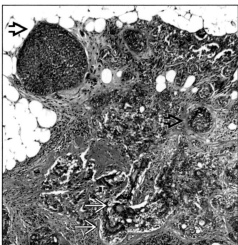

(Left) The tubules formed by luminal-like cells may be positive for CD117 ⊵, as well as luminal-type cytokeratins. The surrounding myoepithelial-like cells are negative for these markers ➡. *(Right)* The myoepithelial-like cells are positive for myoepithelial markers such as p63. The tubules formed by luminal-like cells are negative for these markers ➡.

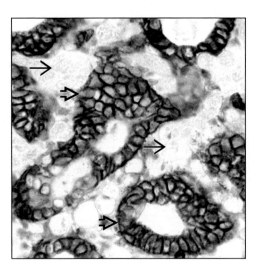
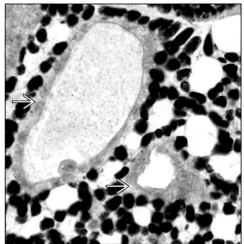

ADENOID CYSTIC CARCINOMA

Microscopic Features and Differential Diagnosis

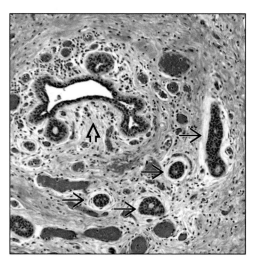

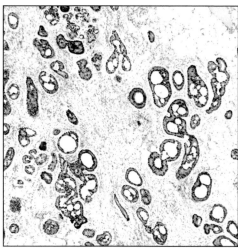

(Left) The minimal stromal reaction around the areas of invasive carcinoma can make it difficult to distinguish ACC from DCIS. In this case, the pattern of small nests of tumor cells ➡ infiltrating around a normal duct ➡ demonstrates that the tumor cells are part of the invasive carcinoma. **(Right)** In ACC, myoepithelial cell markers are often not helpful to distinguish DCIS from invasive carcinoma, as many of the tumor cells will be positive (as seen here for p63).

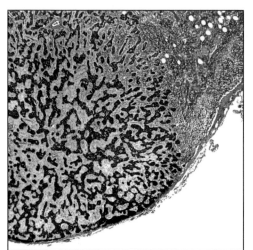

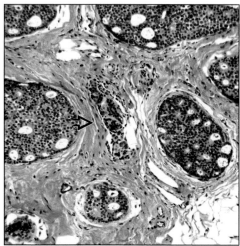

(Left) ACC rarely metastasizes to lymph nodes or to distant sites. When metastases do occur, both cell types are present, as can be seen in this node. **(Right)** Invasive cribriform carcinoma can resemble ACC or cribriform DCIS. In this case, the carcinoma reveals its invasive pattern by surrounding a normal lobule ➡. The cribriform spaces are empty or filled with secretions, and only 1 cell type is present. Almost all cribriform carcinomas are strongly ER and PR positive.

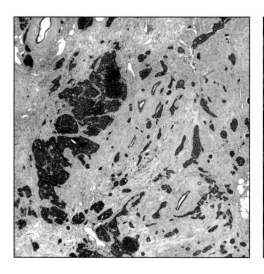

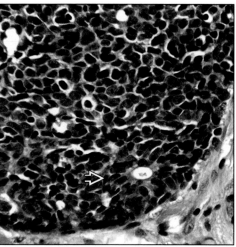

(Left) This is a carcinoma with an almost exclusively solid pattern with few luminal cells forming tubules. Although there is heterogeneity for luminal and myoepithelial markers, 2 distinct cell populations are not present. This carcinoma would be better classified as an adenomyoepithelial carcinoma. **(Right)** In this carcinoma with a solid pattern, only very rare luminal type cells forming tubules are present ➡. The tumor cells had features of both luminal and myoepithelial cells.

SECRETORY CARCINOMA

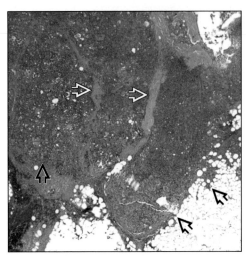

Secretory carcinomas may invade as irregular nests of tumor cells ⊳, as in this case, or be present as circumscribed masses. Hyalinized bands ⊳ or central areas of fibrosis are common.

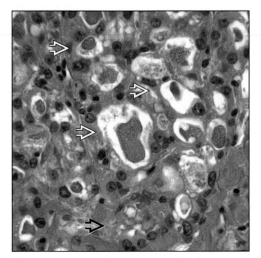

The name "secretory" derives from the characteristic feature of distinct eosinophilic material in tumor lumens ⊳ and the bubbly cytoplasm ⊳. The material is positive for PAS and Alcian blue.

TERMINOLOGY

Synonyms
- Juvenile breast carcinoma (this name is discouraged as majority of cases occur in older patients)

Definitions
- Very rare type of breast cancer characterized by specific translocation and occurring over wide age range from children to adults

CLINICAL ISSUES

Epidemiology
- Incidence
  - Very rare type of invasive breast carcinoma (< 0.2% of breast carcinomas)
- Age
  - Occurs over wide range: < 5 years to > 80 years (median: 25 years)

Presentation
- In young women and men, carcinoma is generally in subareolar location due to presence of breast tissue at this site
- Not associated with pregnancy or lactation, although histologic appearance mimics lactating breast tissue

Treatment
- Majority of patients have been treated surgically with excision of breast and lymph nodes
- Too few patients to determine benefit of chemotherapy and radiation
  - Rare patients with metastatic secretory carcinoma who received chemotherapy progressed during treatment

Prognosis
- Majority of patients remain free of disease after surgical excision

- About 30% of patients have axillary lymph node metastases
- Local recurrences can occur in residual breast tissue or in chest wall many years after initial surgery
- In rare cases, systemic metastases have resulted in death of patient
  - Only 5 cases with distant metastases have been reported

IMAGE FINDINGS

Mammographic Findings
- May appear as circumscribed or irregular densities
  - Calcifications may be present
- No specific imaging features

MACROSCOPIC FEATURES

General Features
- Gross tumors are firm and lobulated or circumscribed
  - No gross features that are specific for secretory carcinoma

MICROSCOPIC PATHOLOGY

Histologic Features
- Generally grows as nests of cells
  - Separated by thick fibrous bands giving lobulated appearance
    - Less frequently, carcinoma has irregular invasive pattern into adjacent stroma
- 3 main growth patterns are recognized
  - Solid
  - Microcystic ("honeycomb")
  - Tubular
- Cells typically have uniform round nuclei with minimal pleomorphism and small nucleoli
- Mitoses are absent or infrequent

SECRETORY CARCINOMA

Key Facts

Clinical Issues

- Very rare type of invasive breast carcinoma (< 0.2% of breast carcinomas)
- Occurs over wide age range: < 5 years to > 80 years (median: 25 years)
- Majority of patients have been treated surgically with excision of breast tumor and lymph nodes

Microscopic Pathology

- Characterized by proliferation of tubules containing characteristic eosinophilic secretory material
- Cells have typical bubbly or granular cytoplasm and are strongly positive for S100
- These carcinomas have characteristic balanced translocation, t(12;15)(p13;q25), resulting in *ETV6-NTRK3* gene fusion product

- Same translocation occurs in pediatric mesenchymal cancers (congenital fibrosarcoma and congenital cellular mesoblastic nephroma) and adult acute myeloid leukemia
- Majority of secretory carcinomas are negative for ER, PR, and HER2
- Although secretory carcinomas have immunohistochemical similarities to basal-like carcinomas, genetic/molecular relationship with this group is unclear

Top Differential Diagnoses

- Invasive ductal carcinoma of other types
- Lactational changes in normal breast tissue
- Granular cell tumor
- Microglandular adenosis (MGA)
- Cystic hypersecretory carcinoma (CHC)

- Cytoplasm has typical bubbly (vacuolated) or granular cytoplasm due to secretory material
  - Cells are positive for periodic acid-Schiff and Alcian blue
  - Signet ring cells may be present
  - Some carcinomas have apocrine appearance
- Tumor cell lumens contain characteristic dense eosinophilic secretory material
  - Also positive for periodic acid-Schiff and Alcian blue
- May be associated with DCIS
  - Papillary and cribriform types of DCIS are most common
  - Same gene translocation found in secretory carcinomas is also present in associated DCIS
  - Central comedo-like necrosis is uncommon but may occur
  - Associated DCIS is histologically similar to invasive carcinoma
  - IHC for myoepithelial cells may be necessary to distinguish circumscribed nests of invasive carcinoma from DCIS

ANCILLARY TESTS

Immunohistochemistry

- Majority of secretory carcinomas are negative for ER
  - About 1/2 of cases are reported to be positive for PR
- Majority of secretory carcinomas are negative for HER2
- Secretory carcinomas are strongly positive for S100 (nuclear and cytoplasmic)
  - Also positive for CEA and smooth muscle actin (~ 80%)
- Negative for GCDFP-15 and nuclear p63
  - Cytoplasmic p63 positivity may be present
- Secretory carcinomas express some markers typical of "luminal" carcinomas
  - Cytokeratin 8/18 positive in ~ 100% (but may be weak and focal)
  - E-cadherin positive in ~ 100%
- Secretory carcinomas express markers typical of basal-like carcinomas

- Basal cytokeratin 5/6 positive in ~ 80%
- Basal cytokeratin 14 positive in ~ 30%
- EGFR (HER1) positive in ~ 50%
- CD117 (C-Kit) positive in ~ 70% (but may be weak and focal)
- Although secretory carcinomas have immunohistochemical similarities to basal-like carcinomas, genetic/molecular relationship with this group is unclear

Molecular Studies

- Secretory carcinomas have characteristic balanced translocation: t(12;15)(p13;q25), which results in a *ETV6-NTRK3* gene fusion product
  - *ETV6* (TEL) encodes *E26* transformation-specific (ETS) transcription factor active in hematopoiesis and angiogenesis
  - *NTRK3* encodes neurotrophic tyrosine receptor kinase 3, which is predominantly expressed in central nervous system
- Same translocation occurs in pediatric mesenchymal cancers
  - Congenital fibrosarcoma and congenital cellular mesoblastic nephroma
  - Translocation may be seen in adult acute myeloid leukemia
  - This translocation has not been reported in other types of breast cancer
- Loss of heterozygosity (LOH) is not seen at 17p13 (the *P53* gene locus); LOH is present at this site in 47% of breast carcinomas of no special type
- Comparative genomic hybridization shows 2.0 alterations per carcinoma including gains of 8q or 1q and losses of 22q
- Results of molecular profiling tests (such as Oncotype DX [Genomic Health; Redwood City, CA]) should be interpreted with caution
  - Validity of results has not been determined in rare tumor types such as secretory carcinoma

SECRETORY CARCINOMA

DIFFERENTIAL DIAGNOSIS

Invasive Ductal Carcinoma of Other Types
- Other types of breast carcinomas can have granular eosinophilic &/or vacuolated cytoplasm
  - Apocrine carcinomas, acinic cell carcinomas
- Immunohistochemical pattern of negativity for ER, PR, HER2, and GCDFP-15 and positivity for S100
  - Helpful to support the diagnosis of secretory carcinoma
- In some cases, it may be helpful to confirm diagnosis of secretory carcinoma with molecular studies for translocation

Lactational Changes in Normal Breast Tissue
- Occur in breast tissue with normal underlying architecture
  - Occasionally, these changes are pronounced and form circumscribed masses ("lactational adenomas")
- Solid, cribriform, and infiltrative patterns are not present
- During pregnancy and lactation, lumens appear empty as secretory products are water soluble and dissolve during processing
- Luminal eosinophilic secretions seen in secretory carcinoma are not present

Granular Cell Tumor
- Solid variant of secretory carcinoma can resemble granular cell tumor
- In most cases, tubule formation with intratubular secretions will exclude diagnosis of granular cell tumor
- Immunohistochemical studies can be used to confirm cytokeratin expression in secretory carcinomas
- Both granular cell tumors and secretory carcinomas are strongly positive for S100

Microglandular Adenosis (MGA)
- MGA and secretory carcinomas have several features in common
  - Characterized by tubules containing dense eosinophilic material
  - Typically negative for ER, PR, and HER2 and strongly positive for S100
  - Have invasive pattern but do not (MGA) or rarely (secretory carcinoma) metastasize or cause death of patient
- MGA is usually not confused with secretory carcinoma due to absence of solid and cribriform growth patterns
- In 1 reported case of MGA, t(12;15) translocation characteristic of secretory carcinoma was not found

Cystic Hypersecretory Carcinoma (CHC)
- Consists of grossly evident cystic spaces filled with densely eosinophilic secretory material
  - Spaces are lined by cells with pleomorphic hyperchromatic nuclei and scant cytoplasm
  - Bland nuclei and abundant foamy cytoplasm of secretory carcinomas are not typical
- Majority of cases of CHC are in situ carcinomas
  - Rare associated invasive carcinomas are poorly differentiated and have solid growth pattern

- Invasive carcinoma lacks secretory features of in situ carcinoma
- Nuclei may be centrally clear (similar to papillary thyroid carcinoma)

DIAGNOSTIC CHECKLIST

Clinically Relevant Pathologic Features
- Very rare variant of invasive breast cancer
  - Very wide age range for presentation
  - May occur in adolescents or in young children

Pathologic Interpretation Pearls
- Secretory carcinoma will have characteristic morphologic appearance, immunophenotype, and molecular alterations
  - Bubbly or granular cytoplasm
  - Negativity for ER, PR, HER2, and GCDFP-15; positivity for S100
  - Balanced translocation, t(12;15)(p13;q25), that results in *ETV6-NTRK3* gene fusion product
- Immunohistochemistry and molecular studies may be helpful to confirm diagnosis

SELECTED REFERENCES

1. Geyer FC et al: Microglandular adenosis or microglandular adenoma? A molecular genetic analysis of a case associated with atypia and invasive carcinoma. Histopathology. 55(6):732-43, 2009
2. Lambros MB et al: Genomic profile of a secretory breast cancer with an ETV6-NTRK3 duplication. J Clin Pathol. 62(7):604-12, 2009
3. Laé M et al: Secretory breast carcinomas with ETV6-NTRK3 fusion gene belong to the basal-like carcinoma spectrum. Mod Pathol. 22(2):291-8, 2009
4. Arce C et al: Secretory carcinoma of the breast containing the ETV6-NTRK3 fusion gene in a male: case report and review of the literature. World J Surg Oncol. 3:35, 2005
5. Bratthauer GL et al: Antibodies targeting p63 react specifically in the cytoplasm of breast epithelial cells exhibiting secretory differentiation. Histopathology. 47(6):611-6, 2005
6. Ozguroglu M et al: Secretory carcinoma of the breast. Case report and review of the literature. Oncology. 68(2-3):263-8, 2005
7. Diallo R et al: Secretory carcinoma of the breast: a distinct variant of invasive ductal carcinoma assessed by comparative genomic hybridization and immunohistochemistry. Hum Pathol. 34(12):1299-305, 2003
8. Rivera-Hueto F et al: Long-term prognosis of teenagers with breast cancer. Int J Surg Pathol. 10(4):273-9, 2002
9. Herz H et al: Metastatic secretory breast cancer. Non-responsiveness to chemotherapy: case report and review of the literature. Ann Oncol. 11(10):1343-7, 2000
10. Maitra A et al: Molecular abnormalities associated with secretory carcinomas of the breast. Hum Pathol. 30(12):1435-40, 1999

SECRETORY CARCINOMA

Microscopic Features

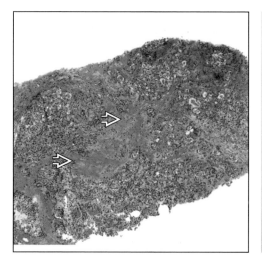

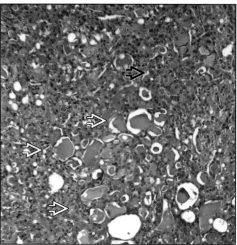

(Left) This core needle biopsy shows irregular nests of tumor cells in a dense stroma. Note the thick bands of dense fibrosis ⮞ separating nests of tumor cells, a characteristic feature of secretory carcinoma. *(Right)* This carcinoma has both microcystic ⮞ and solid ⮞ patterns. The lumens are filled with characteristic eosinophilic secretory material. Some cases mimic lactating breast, but true lactation has empty spaces as milk is water soluble and does not survive processing.

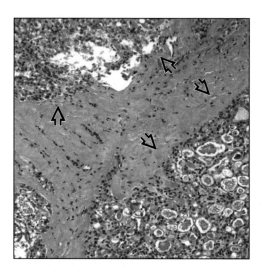

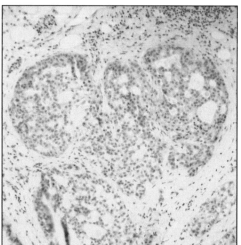

(Left) The nests of tumor cells can appear well circumscribed ⮞ and surrounded by dense tissue. IHC studies for myoepithelial cells may be necessary to distinguish invasive carcinoma from DCIS. *(Right)* Secretory carcinomas are typically negative for ER (as seen here), PR, and HER2. Nevertheless, these carcinomas have a favorable prognosis. The results of some prognostic tests, such as Oncotype DX, are likely to be inaccurate for this rare tumor type.

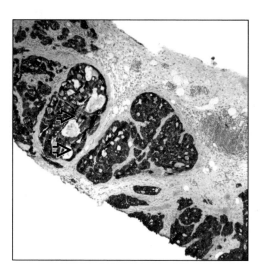

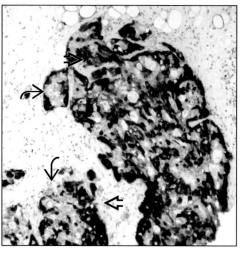

(Left) Tumor cells are positive for cytokeratin (AE1/AE3; red cytoplasm). No myoepithelial cells are identified using p63 (brown nuclei), showing that the circumscribed nests of cells are invasive carcinoma. Focal cytoplasmic positivity for p63 is present ⮞. This finding has been reported in cells with a secretory phenotype. *(Right)* Secretory carcinomas are strongly positive for S100. This carcinoma shows marked heterogeneity with both positive ⮞ and negative ⮞ cells.

HER2 POSITIVE CARCINOMA

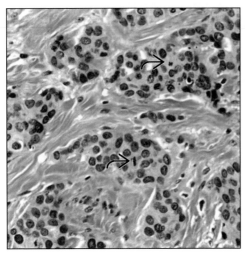

HER2 overexpression is most frequently associated with carcinomas of high nuclear grade that typically show increased mitotic activity ⤳ and are of no special histologic type ("ductal").

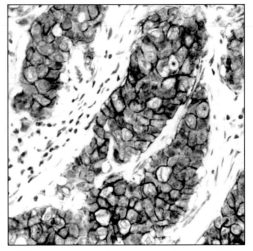

HER2(+) carcinomas demonstrate an intense "chicken wire" pattern of membrane positivity (the nucleus and cytoplasm are unstained) that is typically uniformly distributed throughout the tumor.

TERMINOLOGY

Abbreviations
- HER2 positive breast cancer (HER2+BC)

Synonyms
- HER2 (human epidermal growth factor receptor, HER-2/neu, c-erbB2, NEU, NGL, TKR1, CD340, ERBB2)

Definitions
- Carcinomas characterized by overexpression of HER2: 15-20% of all breast carcinomas

ETIOLOGY/PATHOGENESIS

HER2+BC Biology
- HER2 encodes a 185 kDa membrane tyrosine kinase growth factor receptor located on chromosome 17q12
  - Member of family of genes that includes epidermal growth factor receptor (EGFR or HER1)
- Gene amplification results in increased mRNA and protein overexpression
  - HER2 overexpression likely plays role in carcinogenesis and tumor formation
  - Majority of HER2+BC continues to express HER2 with recurrence (lymph node and distant metastases)
- HER2 overexpression increases receptor activation and HER receptor family signaling
  - Signaling promotes angiogenesis, proliferation, cell survival, invasion, and metastasis
- Adjacent genes are coamplified with HER2
  - Carcinomas vary in number of genes amplified; at minimum 6 genes (and likely several dozen) are coamplified
  - Only a subset of these genes show overexpression of protein products

- Variations in number of coamplified genes may explain some differences in response to HER2-targeted therapy
- HER2+BC also frequently displays amplification of other DNA segments
  - 70% of these carcinomas amplify at least 1 other DNA segment
  - CEP17 (chromosome 17 centromere enumeration probe) sequences are amplified in 10-20% of these carcinomas
  - True chromosome 17 polysomy (duplication of entire chromosome) is rare: Only 1-2% of cancers
  - Relationship of CEP17 amplification to HER2 overexpression is unclear

Gene Expression Profiling
- Molecular subtypes of breast cancer include luminal A, luminal B, HER2, and basal-like cancers
  - HER2+BC by gene expression studies are ER negative (10-20% of cancers)
  - ER(+) luminal B carcinomas (15-20% of cancers) overexpress HER2 in up to 50% of cases
    - ER positive but often at lower levels than in luminal A carcinomas
    - HER2 downregulates PR, and many of these carcinomas lack PR expression
    - Some studies using IHC to classify breast cancers have defined all luminal B carcinomas as HER2 positive
    - However, up to 50% of luminal B carcinomas by gene expression studies are HER2 negative
- HER2 expressing carcinomas detected clinically are included in luminal B and HER2 groups
  - These patients show similar benefit from HER2-targeted therapy in clinical trials
- Approximately 1/2 of HER2 carcinomas are ER positive and 1/2 ER negative
- HER2 expression profile includes increased expression pattern for HER2 as well as other adjacent coamplified genes

HER2 POSITIVE CARCINOMA

Key Facts

Clinical Issues

- 15-20% of breast carcinomas overexpress HER2
  - All newly diagnosed invasive breast cancers should be evaluated for HER2
  - IHC, FISH, and CISH methods have received FDA approval
- HER2+BC is associated with poorer prognosis
  - Higher incidence of lymph node metastases
  - Distant metastases are often to visceral sites and brain
- HER2-targeted treatment is available
  - HER2+BC shows the highest responses to neoadjuvant therapy
- HER2 status also may be predictive for response for different types of chemotherapy and endocrine therapy

- Some HER2+BC is resistant to treatment or develop resistance to treatment
  - May be due to varying numbers of coamplified genes in different cancers or due to heterogeneity of HER2 overexpression

Microscopic Pathology

- Majority of HER2+BC are of no special type ("ductal" carcinomas)
  - Other subtypes that can be HER2(+) are apocrine carcinoma, invasive micropapillary carcinoma, and inflammatory carcinoma
- Usually poorly differentiated and have high proliferative rate
- Extensive DCIS and multiple foci of invasion are more common than in other subtypes

CLINICAL ISSUES

Epidemiology

- Incidence
  - HER2+BC reported in 15-20% of patients
- Age
  - HER2+BC patients are younger (~ 53 years) than the average woman with breast cancer (~ 61 years)
    - HER2+BC is not associated with *BRCA1* or *BRCA2*
- Gender
  - HER2+BC is less common in males than in females
- Ethnicity
  - No significant differences in HER2+BC rates in different ethnic populations have been reported

Laboratory Tests

- HER2 overexpression can be documented by evaluation of DNA, mRNA, and protein assays
  - DNA analysis for gene amplification is usually evaluated by fluorescent in situ hybridization (FISH)
    - Chromogenic in situ hybridization (CISH) is alternative technique
    - 2nd probe often used to evaluate number of copies of centromere 17
    - Criteria for gene amplification utilize total number of genes or ratio of genes to number of centromere copies
    - In majority of cases, both methods of evaluation yield same interpretation
    - If the 2 methods give discordant results (usually due to increased centromere copies), it is not yet clear whether these carcinomas respond to HER2-directed therapy
  - HER2 mRNA level is evaluated and reported as part of Oncotype DX assay (Genomic Health; Redwood City, CA)
    - Should not be used to select patients for targeted therapy
  - Protein overexpression is analyzed by IHC
    - Correlation between IHC and FISH results is > 90%

- Rare carcinomas may overexpress protein due to mechanisms other than gene amplification
- It is easier to detect heterogeneity in HER2 expression and discordant expression patterns for DCIS and invasive carcinoma using IHC
- IHC, FISH, and CISH methods have received FDA approval for assessing HER2 status in clinical practice
- If HER2(+) is discordant with histologic features (e.g., carcinoma is well differentiated or subtype unlikely to show overexpression), repeat &/or additional studies should be considered

Natural History

- HER2+BC is associated with poor prognosis
  - Higher rate of recurrence and mortality in patients with newly diagnosed breast cancer who do not receive any adjuvant systemic therapy
    - Early recurrence more commonly seen compared with HER2 negative disease
  - Small carcinomas (< 1 cm) with negative nodes have worse prognosis if HER2(+)
  - HER2+BC has worse prognosis if also ER(+)
    - May be due to higher incidence of lymph node metastases and lower response rates to therapy
- Metastatic HER2+BC usually also overexpresses HER2
  - In rare cases, recurrent or metastatic disease lacks HER2 expression
    - Likely due to heterogeneity of expression in primary carcinoma with possible selection of subclones after treatment
    - For example, residual disease after neoadjuvant treatment with HER2-targeted therapy can lack expression in up to 1/3 of cases
- HER2+BC more likely to spread early to major visceral sites (brain, lungs, liver, adrenals, ovaries)
  - With HER2-targeted therapy, progressive visceral disease significantly diminished
  - CNS metastases more common after treatment with HER2-targeted therapy
    - May be related to inability of trastuzumab to cross blood-brain barrier

HER2 POSITIVE CARCINOMA

Treatment
- Adjuvant therapy
  - HER2 positivity may be associated with relative, but not absolute, resistance to endocrine therapy
    - Effect may be specific to selective estrogen receptor modulator therapy, such as tamoxifen
  - HER2 status may be predictive for either resistance or sensitivity to different types of chemotherapies
    - HER2 positivity is associated with response to anthracycline therapy
    - Anthracycline sensitivity may be secondary to coamplification of *HER2* with topoisomerase II α (*TOP2A*)
    - *TOP2A* amplification occurs in about 1/3 of HER2+BC and is associated with ER(+)
  - HER2-targeted therapy has demonstrated remarkable efficacy in both metastatic and adjuvant settings
    - Trastuzumab (humanized monoclonal antibody) targets an extracellular epitope of HER2 receptor
    - Trastuzumab improves response, time to progression, and survival when used alone or with chemotherapy in metastatic breast cancer
    - Adjuvant trastuzumab given during &/or after chemotherapy results in significant improvement in disease-free and overall survival
    - Lapatinib (small molecule tyrosine kinase inhibitor) improves outcome in patients with advanced disease in combination with chemotherapy
  - **Only patients with HER2+BC are candidates for HER2-targeted therapy**
    - HER2 is a useful marker for therapeutic decision making for patients with breast cancer
    - HER2(+)/ER(-) carcinomas have best response to neoadjuvant therapy
    - HER2(+)/ER(+) carcinomas have lesser response to neoadjuvant therapy, and response is related to degree of ER expression

MICROSCOPIC PATHOLOGY

Histologic Features
- Majority are invasive carcinomas of no special histologic type ("ductal carcinomas")
  - Majority have high nuclear grade and DNA aneuploidy
  - Necrosis present in ~ 40%
  - Lymphocytic infiltrate in ~ 60%
  - More likely to harbor *P53* mutations
  - High mitotic rate and proliferation index
  - Lymph-vascular invasion more common
  - More likely to be associated with extensive DCIS and multiple foci of invasion
  - Lymph node metastasis and > 4 lymph node metastases more common
- Some subtypes of breast carcinoma have higher rates of HER2 positivity
  - Apocrine carcinoma: ~ 50%
  - Inflammatory carcinoma: 40-50%
  - Invasive micropapillary carcinoma: 30-50%

- Some subtypes of breast carcinoma do not overexpress HER2 or have very low rate of HER2 positivity (< 5%)
  - Tubular carcinoma
  - Mucinous carcinoma
  - Invasive papillary carcinoma
  - Triple negative carcinomas (including medullary carcinoma, basal-like carcinoma, adenoid cystic carcinoma, low-grade adenosquamous carcinoma, and metaplastic carcinoma)
- Frequency of HER2 expression in invasive lobular carcinoma is dependent on grade
  - Well- and moderately differentiated lobular carcinomas: < 5%
    - Edge enhancement can mimic appearance of HER2 positivity
    - FISH should be used to confirm amplification
  - Poorly differentiated lobular carcinomas: 50-80%
    - Many of these carcinomas have apocrine features
- HER2(+) DCIS
  - Number of cases of DCIS overexpressing HER2 is reported to be from 20-80%
    - Higher incidence of HER2 overexpression compared with invasive breast cancer
  - HER2 overexpression associated with high nuclear grade and comedo necrosis
  - HER2(+) DCIS may be more likely than lower grade DCIS to be detected by mammography due to calcifications
- HER2(+) DCIS is more commonly associated with invasion
  - Associated invasive carcinoma is usually also HER2(+)
  - In rare cases, invasive carcinoma is negative for HER2
    - May yield incorrect results for some assays unless only invasive component is analyzed
    - Some assays may require microdissection
  - Treatment is based on HER2 status of invasive carcinoma
- DCIS involving nipple skin (Paget disease of nipple) is HER2(+) in > 90% of cases
  - Toker cells, which can be mistaken for Paget disease, are usually negative for HER2
  - Rare cases of atypical Toker cell hyperplasia can show weak HER2 positivity

DIFFERENTIAL DIAGNOSIS

HER2 Negative Breast Cancer
- Very important to identify the subset of cancers overexpressing HER2 to optimize appropriate treatment
- Testing for HER2 should be performed with appropriate quality control
  - Repeat or additional studies using a different test should be utilized as appropriate
- Some cancers are difficult to classify as HER2 positive or negative
  - Carcinomas with borderline expression
    - HER2 expression is a continuum and is not bimodal

HER2 POSITIVE CARCINOMA

Clinical Profile for HER2 Positive Breast Cancer

Tumor Features	HER2 Positive Carcinomas
Patient age	Younger age at presentation
Most likely histologic types	Poorly differentiated invasive ductal carcinoma (no special type), poorly differentiated (pleomorphic) lobular carcinoma, apocrine carcinoma, invasive micropapillary carcinoma, inflammatory carcinoma
Histologic grade	Moderate to poorly differentiated (typically higher nuclear grade)
ER status	~ 50% ER(-) (HER2 molecular subtype), and ~ 50% ER(+) (luminal B molecular subtype)
Proliferation	Higher proliferation by mitotic score or Ki-67 proliferative index
Nodal status	Higher incidence of lymph node metastases (> 4 lymph nodes more common)
LVI	Lymph-vascular invasion more common

Clinical Profile for HER2 Negative Breast Cancer

Tumor Features	Lower Histologic Grade	Higher Histologic Grade
Most likely histologic types	Tubular carcinoma, mucinous carcinoma, invasive papillary carcinoma, well- to moderately differentiated lobular carcinoma, low-grade adenosquamous carcinoma	Medullary carcinoma, basal-like carcinoma, triple negative carcinoma
ER status	Most will be ER positive (except low-grade adenosquamous)	Most will be ER negative
Proliferation	Lower proliferative index by mitotic score or Ki-67 expression	High proliferative index by mitotic score or Ki-67 expression

- Carcinomas with expression close to the cut-offs for test interpretation may have variable results on repeat testing
  - Carcinomas with heterogeneity of expression
    - Majority of HER2+BC show diffuse strong expression throughout the carcinoma
    - At least 30% of the carcinoma must show expression by IHC to be classified as HER2 positive
    - In rare cases, < 30% of carcinoma shows overexpression
  - Response of these carcinomas to targeted therapy requires investigation

DIAGNOSTIC CHECKLIST

Clinically Relevant Pathologic Features

- All newly diagnosed invasive breast carcinomas should be evaluated for HER2 overexpression
  - HER2 status identifies a subset of carcinomas with more aggressive tumor biology and clinical course
    - Patients with HER2+BC have worse prognosis and are candidates for specific therapies that target HER2
    - HER2(+) tumors tend to be higher grade and occur in younger patients
- Role of anti-HER2 therapy in HER2+BC is well established
  - Accurate HER2 testing is essential before initiation of appropriate breast cancer treatment
  - HER2 status, either gene copy number or protein expression level, is best predictive marker available for assessing response to trastuzumab and lapatinib
    - Both IHC and FISH have been clinically validated in prospective randomized trials to predict benefit from HER2-targeted therapy
    - Whether power of these predictive markers is the same in advanced and early-stage cancers is unclear

HER2-Targeted Therapy and Resistance

- Not all HER2+BC will respond to HER2-targeted therapy
  - De novo and acquired resistance is significant clinical problem
    - Mechanisms of resistance to trastuzumab therapy are poorly understood
  - Better understanding of predictors of response/ resistance and strategies to treat tumors that are refractory to HER2-targeted therapy is crucial
    - May provide framework for developing new therapeutic strategies to overcome resistance
    - May help to prolong duration of response and decrease treatment-related toxicity
- Novel HER2-targeted agents are being developed and evaluated
  - May represent important step in management of HER2-targeted refractory breast cancer

SELECTED REFERENCES

1. Bhargava R et al: Semiquantitative hormone receptor level influences response to trastuzumab-containing neoadjuvant chemotherapy in HER2-positive breast cancer. Mod Pathol. 24(3):367-74, 2011
2. Bhargava R et al: Breast cancer molecular class ERBB2: preponderance of tumors with apocrine differentiation and expression of basal phenotype markers CK5, CK5/6, and EGFR. Appl Immunohistochem Mol Morphol. 18(2):113-8, 2010
3. Staaf J et al: High-resolution genomic and expression analyses of copy number alterations in HER2-amplified breast cancer. Breast Cancer Res. 12(3):R25, 2010
4. Mittendorf EA et al: Loss of HER2 amplification following trastuzumab-based neoadjuvant systemic therapy and survival outcomes. Clin Cancer Res. 15(23):7381-8, 2009
5. Hicks DG et al: HER2+ breast cancer: review of biologic relevance and optimal use of diagnostic tools. Am J Clin Pathol. 129(2):263-73, 2008

HER2 Expression in Subtypes of Breast Carcinoma

(Left) The majority of this carcinoma shows no overexpression of HER2 ⇨, but approximately 1/3 is HER2 positive ⇨. Heterogeneity in expression may result in discordant results between core needle biopsies and excisions or pre- and post-therapy analyses. (Right) Heterogeneity in HER2 expression is seen in this lymph node metastasis with both positive ⇨ and negative ⇨ areas. The absence of uniform expression may be a source of resistance to HER2-targeted therapy.

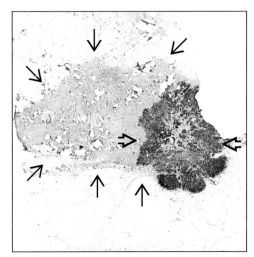 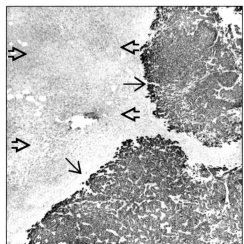

(Left) Some histologic types of carcinoma such as apocrine carcinoma (shown), invasive micropapillary carcinoma, and inflammatory carcinoma are more likely to overexpress HER2 than ductal carcinomas are. (Right) Some histologic types of breast cancer rarely, if ever, overexpress HER2. These include tubular carcinoma, papillary carcinoma, mucinous carcinoma, and triple negative carcinomas (including medullary carcinoma). This is a rare mucinous carcinoma showing overexpression.

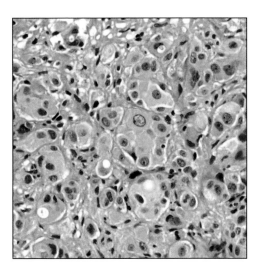 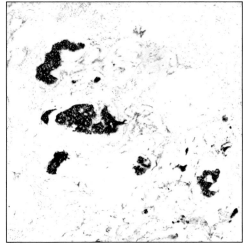

(Left) Well- and moderately differentiated invasive lobular carcinomas rarely overexpress HER2. Due to the discohesive cells, enhancement at the edges can occur and should not be overinterpreted as positivity. FISH studies will confirm the absence of amplification. (Right) Poorly differentiated invasive lobular carcinomas overexpress HER2 in 50-80% of cases. This carcinoma lacked E-cadherin expression in both the invasive and in situ components but strongly expressed HER2.

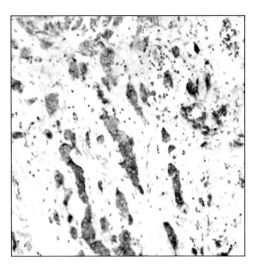 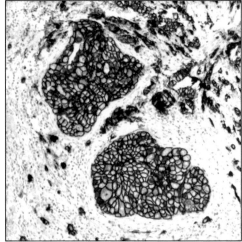

5

HER2 POSITIVE CARCINOMA

HER2 Expression in Carcinoma In Situ

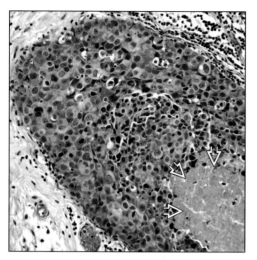

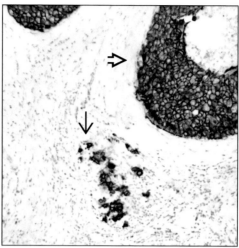

(Left) HER2 overexpression in DCIS ranges from 24-38% and is more common in cases with high nuclear grade and necrosis ➤. High-grade DCIS is more likely to be detected as mammographic calcifications, and this may explain why HER2(+) is more common in DCIS than in invasive carcinoma. (Right) HER2 positive DCIS ➤ is more likely to be associated with invasion ➤ than HER2 negative DCIS. The foci of invasion are also usually HER2 positive. The DCIS is often extensive.

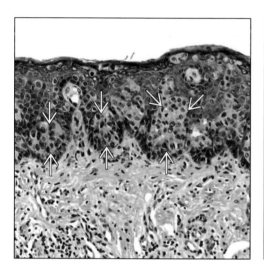

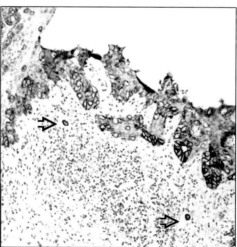

(Left) DCIS involving nipple skin (Paget disease of the nipple) ➤ is often detected due to disruption of the normal tight junctions of the keratinocytes, resulting in exudation of intercellular fluid and a scale crust. 80-90% of cases overexpress HER2. (Right) In this case of Paget disease of the nipple, the Paget cells are strongly positive for HER2. There is early stromal invasion of the dermis by tumor cells ➤.

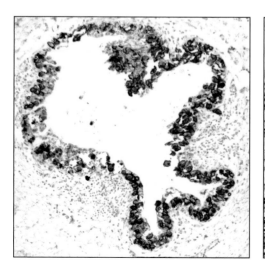

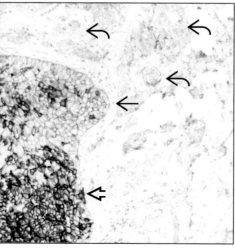

(Left) LCIS is generally negative for HER2 expression. This was an unusual case of an E-cadherin negative LCIS, present predominantly as pagetoid spread that was positive for HER2. (Right) This DCIS shows heterogeneity for HER2 with strongly positive ➤ and weakly positive ➤ areas. The associated invasive carcinoma is HER2 negative ➤. Without microdissection, erroneous results could be obtained from assays such as the 21-gene recurrence score.

HER2 in Metastases and FISH/CISH Studies

(Left) A 41-year-old woman was treated for HER2(+) breast cancer 2 years previously and was doing well until she developed a cough and progressive respiratory symptoms. She underwent bronchoscopy and transbronchial biopsy, which showed metastatic carcinoma in submucosal lymphatics ➡. (Right) This pulmonary metastasis was detected by transbronchial biopsy (respiratory mucosa ➡) and retains the HER2 overexpression ➡ that was present in the patient's primary breast carcinoma.

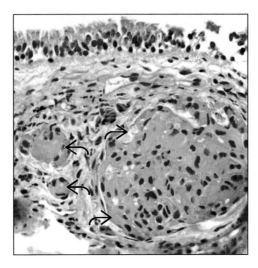
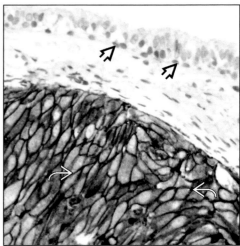

(Left) A 52-year-old woman presented with an ER-negative and HER2-positive invasive carcinoma. She was treated with chemotherapy and trastuzumab. Trastuzumab was discontinued due to congestive heart failure. She developed liver metastases ➡, diagnosed by needle biopsy 2 years later. (Right) The metastatic tumor in this liver biopsy shows HER2 overexpression ➡. HER2(+) carcinomas are more likely to recur at major visceral sites including the lung and liver, as well as the CNS.

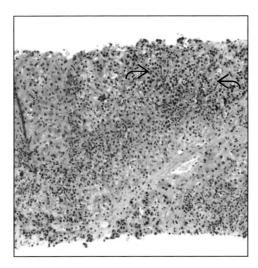
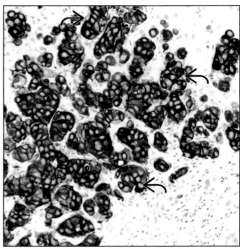

(Left) This FISH assay demonstrates an abnormal number of HER2 genes as detected by positivity for a red probe ➡. In contrast, each cell has on average only 2 copies of the green probe ➡ identifying the chromosome 17 centromere. (Right) CISH uses light microscopy and is an alternative to FISH for evaluating the number of HER2 gene copies. This dual-CISH shows an increased number of HER2 genes (red probes ➡) and a normal number of centromeric sequences (CEP17 blue spots ➡).

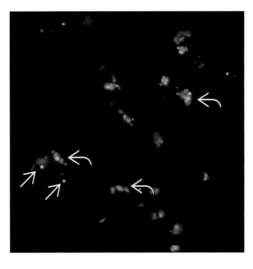
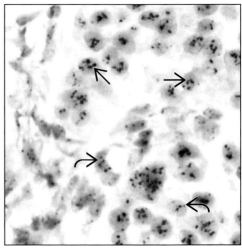

HER2 POSITIVE CARCINOMA

Microscopic Features

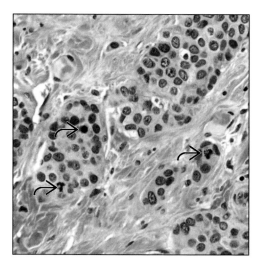 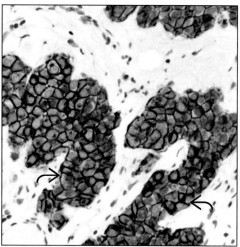

(Left) The majority of HER2(+) breast cancers are high-grade carcinomas of no special type ("ductal") with increased mitotic activity ➡. These cancers are more frequent in young (premenopausal) patients. (Right) HER2(+) breast cancer shows an intense membrane staining pattern ➡ that is typically uniform throughout the invasive tumor. More than 95% of cancers with this pattern of staining will show HER2 gene amplification by FISH.

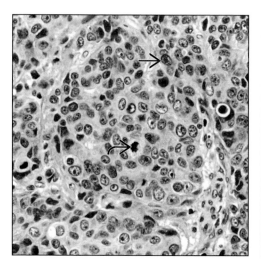 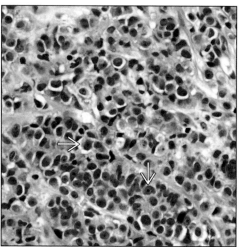

(Left) HER2(+) breast cancer can be identified by gene expression profiling. These cancers have a high nuclear grade ➡, about 1/2 are ER &/or PR negative, and they have a high proliferative rate ➡. Cancers with these features are more likely to overexpress HER2. (Right) Well- and moderately differentiated invasive lobular carcinomas are most typically HER2 negative. In contrast, poorly differentiated invasive lobular carcinoma ➡ can be HER2 positive in over 50% of cases.

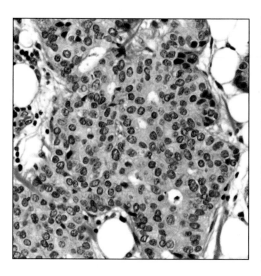 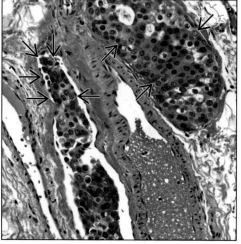

(Left) This moderately differentiated carcinoma overexpresses HER2 and is also ER positive. This type of cancer is usually classified in the "luminal B" group and is a type of ER-positive cancer that may benefit from HER2-targeted therapy. (Right) In addition to histologic grade, HER2+BC has a number of other associated morphologic correlates. Lymph-vascular invasion ➡ and multiple lymph node metastases are typically more common in HER2+BC compared with HER2(-) carcinomas.

INFLAMMATORY CARCINOMA

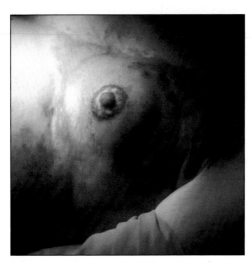

Inflammatory breast carcinoma is a type of cancer characterized by erythema, edema (peau d'orange), induration, warmth, and tenderness of mammary skin, which can closely mimic an infectious process.

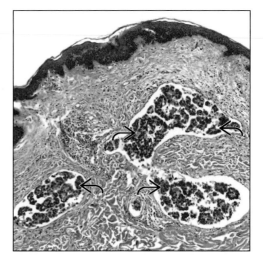

The key pathologic finding is the presence of dermal lymph-vascular invasion ➔. Lymphatic obstruction by tumor emboli is responsible for the clinical appearance. True inflammation is absent.

TERMINOLOGY

Abbreviations
- Inflammatory breast carcinoma (IBC)

Definitions
- IBC is defined by clinical presentation of disease
  o Diffuse erythema and edema involving 1/3 or more of breast skin
    ▪ Gives rise to "peau d'orange" appearance (skin of orange/orange peel)
    ▪ Clinical appearance results from tumor emboli within dermal lymphatic spaces
    ▪ Term "inflammatory" refers to clinical appearance of skin, which mimics inflammation
    ▪ Significant inflammatory infiltrate is not a feature of this type of carcinoma

ETIOLOGY/PATHOGENESIS

Biology of IBC
- Gene expression profiling has demonstrated marked transcriptional heterogeneity among IBC samples
- Studies have been limited by
  o Small numbers of cancers due to rarity of the disease
  o Differing definitions of IBC
  o Diffuse pattern of infiltration leading to large stroma/tumor cell ratio in samples
- IBC includes basal (20-40%), HER2 (20-40%), and luminal A and B subtypes
  o Suggests that independent gene sets are responsible for molecular subtype and specific characteristics of IBC
- 1 group has reported nuclear factor-κB (NF-κB) hyperactivation and augmented insulin-like growth factor signaling
  o Associated with increased tumor cell invasion, angiogenesis, and metastatic potential

- o It is unclear if this expression pattern is related to absence of ER expression or specifically to IBC
- Specific genes responsible for clinical behavior of IBC have not yet been identified but are under active investigation

CLINICAL ISSUES

Epidemiology
- Incidence
  o 1-5% of all breast cancer cases
    ▪ Time-trended data from SEER database suggest incidence may be increasing
- Ethnicity
  o Slightly more common in African-American women

Presentation
- Patients usually present with symptoms of warmth, swelling, induration, and erythema of mammary skin
  o May be initially diagnosed as mastitis or cellulitis and treated with antibiotics
    ▪ Breast infections rare outside lactational period, and carcinoma should be suspected
- Palpable mass may not be present, making diagnosis more difficult
  o Up to 30% of patients will not have palpable mass; when present, mass is often ill defined
  o Some patients will have palpable axillary nodes; however, this finding is also common in true inflammatory conditions
- Involved breast may enlarge rapidly over a period of weeks
- Up to 15% may present with bilateral involvement
  o This is likely due to cancer metastasizing to contralateral breast
- Non-IBC can recur as IBC ("secondary IBC")

Treatment
- Options, risks, complications
  o Neoadjuvant chemotherapy is standard of care

INFLAMMATORY CARCINOMA

Key Facts

Terminology

- Inflammatory breast carcinoma (IBC)
  - Characteristic clinical presentation of edema and erythema of > 1/3 of breast skin

Clinical Issues

- 1-5% of all breast cancer cases
- May be initially misdiagnosed as mastitis or cellulitis and treated with antibiotics
- IBC associated with high risk of locoregional and distant recurrence
- Neoadjuvant chemotherapy is standard of care for IBC, followed by mastectomy and radiation
- Poor prognosis: Median overall survival is 2.9-4.2 years (5-year survival 30%)
- Classified as T4d in AJCC cancer staging

Microscopic Pathology

- Prominent dermal lymph-vascular invasion that obstructs lymphatic outflow causing clinical symptoms
  - True inflammation is not present or is only incidental to carcinoma
- Diffusely infiltrative pattern without formation of discrete mass by palpation or imaging
- IBC is more likely to be negative for ER and PR and overexpress HER2 than non-IBC

Top Differential Diagnoses

- Infection (mastitis, cellulitis, abscess)
- Locally advanced carcinoma with skin invasion
- Occult IBC
- Leukemia and lymphoma

- Goal is to eliminate micrometastatic disease and reduce tumor burden, making tumor more amenable to surgery and radiation
- Response to neoadjuvant chemotherapy provides information on prognosis
- Pathologic complete response predicts for better outcome
- However, 1/2 of patients with pathologic complete response will subsequently recur
- Surgical approaches
  - Mastectomy following neoadjuvant chemotherapy, if there has been response to treatment
    - Sentinel node biopsy may not be accurate; axillary dissection is recommended
  - Breast conservation not appropriate due to skin involvement and high risk for local recurrence
- Adjuvant therapy
  - Endocrine therapy and targeted therapy, such as trastuzumab, depending on marker status of patient's tumor
- Radiation
  - After mastectomy, radiation therapy to the chest wall and regional lymph nodes is recommended

Prognosis

- IBC is associated with aggressive clinical course and poor prognosis
  - Approximately 30% of patients present with distant metastases, compared to < 10% of all breast cancer patients
  - Median overall survival for IBC patients is 2.9-4.2 years
    - 5-year survival rate about 30%
    - Lower survival rates among African-American women and those with ER negative tumors
- Current targeted therapy (e.g., HER2-directed treatment) has resulted in improved survival in some patients

IMAGE FINDINGS

Mammographic Findings

- Skin thickening
- Diffuse increase in breast density compared with contralateral breast
- Trabecular thickening

Ultrasonographic Findings

- Skin thickening
- Diffuse increased echogenicity and dilated lymphatics due to edema

MACROSCOPIC FEATURES

General Features

- Gross appearance of mastectomy can be highly variable
  - Skin changes include thickening, erythema, induration
  - Underlying primary tumor may be indistinct clinically, radiologically, and by gross inspection
- For some cases, large tumors measuring up to 12 cm have been reported
  - When a gross lesion is identified, most will be centrally located in breast

MICROSCOPIC PATHOLOGY

Histologic Features

- Invasive carcinomas of no special type are most common; lobular histology is reported in < 10%
  - Approximately 2/3 are poorly differentiated, 1/3 moderately differentiated
  - Carcinomas typically have diffusely infiltrative pattern, often without prominent desmoplastic response
    - Correlates with frequent absence of a discrete mass by palpation or imaging
  - Prominent permeation of vascular spaces

INFLAMMATORY CARCINOMA

- Particularly localized within dermis and subdermis of mammary skin
- Tumor emboli are usually present throughout breast, in addition to dermis
  - Mammary skin changes
    - Dilated lymphatic spaces and small capillaries
    - Edema and diffuse thickening of papillary and reticular dermis
  - In some patients with clinical appearance of IBC, dermal lymph-vascular invasion (LVI) may not be seen on skin biopsy
    - If skin biopsy is small (e.g., a punch biopsy), dermal LVI may be missed
    - At least 2 skin punch biopsies (2-8 mm) are recommended
    - Multiple deeper levels may be helpful to look for small foci of LVI
    - If true inflammation is seen on skin biopsy (e.g., cellulitis), then diagnosis is unlikely to be IBC
    - Dermal LVI may not be seen after neoadjuvant therapy, particularly if skin changes resolved during treatment

ANCILLARY TESTS

Immunohistochemistry
- Hormone receptors: More likely to be negative as compared to non-IBC (60% ER negative; 80% PR negative)
- HER2 protein overexpression is more common in IBC (40-50%) than in non-IBC (15-20%)
- Overexpression of p53 occurs in 60-80% of IBC
  - These cancers have worse prognosis compared to IBC without p53 overexpression
- IBC exhibits prominent angiogenesis
  - High microvessel density seen with CD31 staining
  - Overexpression of angiogenic factors such as VEGF

DIFFERENTIAL DIAGNOSIS

Infection (Mastitis, Cellulitis, Abscess)
- Mammary infection can mimic IBC clinically
- Mastitis typically develops rapidly over a few days
  - Erythema is associated with tenderness and typically occupies a wedge-shaped quadrant of breast
  - Patient feels unwell and may have fever and leukocytosis
  - Symptomatic improvement should occur within 24-48 hours of initiating antibiotics

Locally Advanced Carcinoma with Skin Invasion
- Large carcinomas may directly invade into skin and cause skin ulceration
- Associated IBC-like skin changes may or may not be present
- Focal dermal LVI may be present adjacent to area of skin invasion
- This type of cancer should not be classified as IBC

Occult IBC
- Some patients will have dermal LVI without clinical signs of IBC
  - Referred to as "occult IBC" by some authors
  - Likely due to more limited dermal LVI as compared to typical IBC
  - If skin changes are present, but involve < 1/3 of the skin, carcinoma is classified as T4b
  - Occult IBC has better prognosis as compared to IBC, but worse prognosis compared to patients without dermal LVI

Leukemia and Lymphoma
- Leukemic infiltration of breast usually occurs at late stage of disease
  - Breast involvement is rarely initial presentation of disease; both breasts may be affected
  - These patients will typically have systemic symptoms
  - Examination of peripheral blood smear usually confirms diagnosis
- Lymphoma may present as axillary adenopathy
  - Obstruction of lymphatic outflow can cause breast edema and enlargement, mimicking IBC
  - Lymph node biopsy will provide correct diagnosis

STAGING

AJCC Classification
- IBC, defined as diffuse erythema and edema (peau d'orange) involving ≥ 1/3 of the skin, is classified as T4d
  - Invasive carcinoma must be confirmed by biopsy
  - Dermal LVI need not be confirmed pathologically but is present in > 80% of cases if an adequate biopsy is performed
- Cancers with < 1/3 involvement of skin are classified as T4b
- Cancers with dermal LVI, but without clinical skin involvement, are assigned a T class according to tumor size

SELECTED REFERENCES

1. Dawood S et al: International expert panel on inflammatory breast cancer: consensus statement for standardized diagnosis and treatment. Ann Oncol. 22(3):515-23, 2011
2. Bertucci F et al: Gene expression profiling of inflammatory breast cancer. Cancer. 116(11 Suppl):2783-93, 2010
3. Zell JA et al: Prognostic impact of human epidermal growth factor-like receptor 2 and hormone receptor status in inflammatory breast cancer (IBC): analysis of 2,014 IBC patient cases from the California Cancer Registry. Breast Cancer Res. 11(1):R9, 2009
4. Lerebours F et al: NF-kappa B genes have a major role in inflammatory breast cancer. BMC Cancer. 8:41, 2008

INFLAMMATORY CARCINOMA

Microscopic Features

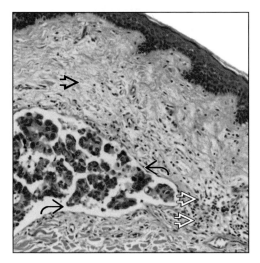

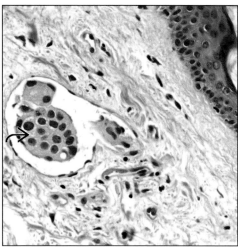

(Left) In addition to tumor cell emboli within dilated dermal lymphatics ➔, edema ⮕ and thickening of the dermis are typically present. A minimal chronic inflammatory infiltrate may be present ➔. **(Right)** Dermal lymphatic spaces are dilated and contain clusters of tumor cells ➔, usually with high-grade nuclei. Extensive lymphatic obstruction is likely responsible for the clinical presentation of these patients.

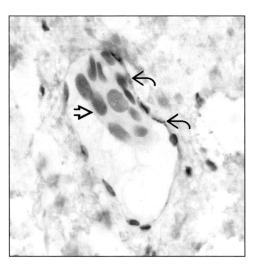

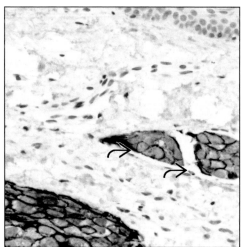

(Left) In most cases, the presence of tumor cells ⮕ within lymphatic spaces is readily apparent on H&E. For problematic cases, staining for podoplanin can help to highlight lymphatic endothelial cells ➔. **(Right)** HER2 overexpression ➔ is present in about 1/2 of cases of IBC. However, all breast cancer molecular subtypes, including basal and luminal types, have been reported with a clinical presentation of IBC and all have an associated aggressive clinical course.

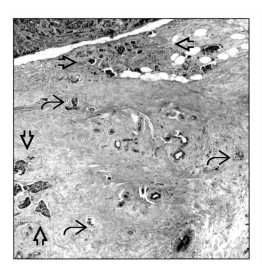

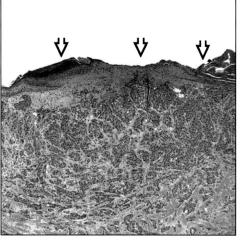

(Left) Carcinomas with a clinical presentation of IBC often have a diffusely infiltrative pattern with minimal desmoplasia and widely dispersed tumor cells ⮕. Multiple foci of LVI are present within the breast ➔ in addition to the dermal LVI. **(Right)** Locally advanced carcinomas can invade the skin and cause skin ulceration ⮕. Although such cancers can be associated with skin changes and even focal adjacent dermal LVI, they should not be classified as IBC.

INVASIVE APOCRINE CARCINOMA

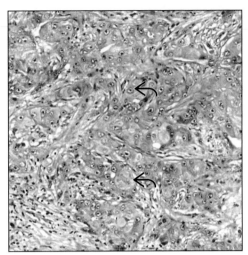

Apocrine carcinoma is a morphologically distinct type of invasive breast cancer characterized by large cells with a low nuclear to cytoplasmic ratio and abundant eosinophilic granular cytoplasm ➡.

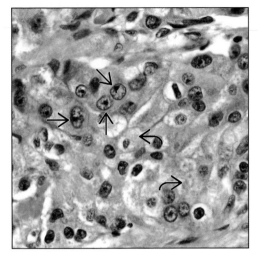

The cytoplasm is abundant with a coarsely granular eosinophilic appearance ➡. The nuclei are large and pleomorphic with prominent nucleoli ➡. The growth pattern is typically solid in type.

TERMINOLOGY

Abbreviations
- Invasive apocrine carcinoma (IAC)

Definitions
- Breast carcinoma with characteristic morphologic appearance resembling apocrine sweat glands in at least 90% of tumor cells, closely linked with androgen receptor expression

ETIOLOGY/PATHOGENESIS

Androgen Metabolism in IAC
- Majority of breast cancers (70-80%) express androgen receptor (AR)
  - Highest expression is seen in ER/PR/HER2 positive cancers (~ 80%), followed by ER/PR positive, HER2 negative cancers (~ 60%) and ER/PR negative, HER2 positive cancers (~ 50%); lowest expression is in ER/PR/HER2 negative cancers (~ 35%)
    - HER2 may induce AR transactivation through MAP kinase pathway
  - IAC expresses AR in 56-100% of cases
    - AR expression may help distinguish IAC from basal-like cancers that are also "triple negative"
- Expression of AR is also frequent in benign apocrine lesions
  - Growth of cutaneous apocrine glands is stimulated by androgens
- Enhanced metabolism of testosterone precursors has been reported in IAC
- Altered androgen metabolism may play a role in pathogenesis and tumor progression

Gene Expression Profiling
- Molecular studies indicate that invasive apocrine carcinomas may represent distinct subgroup of breast cancers

- IAC is characterized by gene expression pattern largely driven by expression of AR
  - Majority AR positive; AR may be potential therapeutic target
  - About 1/2 negative for ER, PR, and HER2; however, IAC does not cluster with basal-like group
  - About 1/2 negative for ER and PR but HER2 positive
    - Tumors overlap significantly with HER2 group as defined by intrinsic gene classification
    - Gene expression data suggests link between HER2 signaling and molecular apocrine phenotype
  - Gene signature includes increased expression of numerous genes with role in metabolism

Association with Benign Apocrine Lesions
- Apocrine glands normally occur in skin
  - Breast evolved from skin appendages and, thus, has many features in common
- Cells with functional apocrine characteristics have been described in fetal breast tissue
- Apocrine change is commonly seen in cysts in adult breast tissue and may arise from fetal cells or from metaplasia
- Benign apocrine lesions express AR and are negative for ER and PR
- Apocrine change without atypia has not been consistently linked to increase in risk of breast cancer
  - Difficult to define atypia in apocrine lesions
  - Lesions with high-grade nuclei, cribriform architecture, &/or necrosis would be considered atypical
    - Additional studies will be necessary to show that these changes increase risk of invasive cancer
- Some apocrine lesions show loss of heterozygosity and other genetic changes, supporting that some are clonal lesions and may be nonobligate precursors of apocrine carcinomas
  - Atypical apocrine proliferations are found more commonly in breasts with apocrine carcinomas

INVASIVE APOCRINE CARCINOMA

Key Facts

Terminology
- Invasive apocrine carcinoma (IAC)
- Term is reserved for cases in which nearly all tumor cells show prominent apocrine features

Etiology/Pathogenesis
- Molecular studies indicate that IAC may represent a distinct subgroup of breast cancers
- Characterized by gene expression pattern largely driven by expression of androgen receptor (AR)

Clinical Issues
- Pure IAC incidence varies from < 1% up to 4%
  - Variability due to lack of well-defined diagnostic criteria
- IAC does not have any specific epidemiologic, clinical, or imaging features

- Prognosis appears to be similar to carcinomas of no special type
- Expression of AR may lead to therapeutic strategies in future

Ancillary Tests
- Tumor cells are usually positive for AR, negative for ER and PR, and about 1/2 overexpress HER2

Top Differential Diagnoses
- Apocrine metaplasia or DCIS involving adenosis
- Granular cell tumor
- Cutaneous apocrine carcinoma (sweat gland carcinoma of the skin)
- Other special types of invasive carcinoma (oncocytic, lipid-rich, histiocytic, sebaceous)

CLINICAL ISSUES

Epidemiology
- Incidence
  - Pure IAC incidence varies from < 1% up to 4%
    - Variability due to lack of well-defined diagnostic criteria
- Age
  - No consistent differences compared with carcinomas of no special type
- Ethnicity
  - Not reported to be associated with family history or ethnic groups

Presentation
- No characteristic clinical or radiographic features that differ from other types of breast carcinomas

Treatment
- Adjuvant therapy
  - Currently no specific treatment based on classification as IAC
  - Altered androgen metabolism may be therapeutically useful in future

Prognosis
- No consistent difference in prognosis as compared to matched carcinomas of no special type in majority of studies

MICROSCOPIC PATHOLOGY

Histologic Features
- IAC has characteristic nuclear and cytoplasmic features that should be present in > 90% of tumor cells
  - Nuclei
    - Round &/or pleomorphic, large vesicular nuclei
    - Prominent, often multiple nucleoli
    - Some carcinomas have lower nuclear grade
  - Cytoplasm
    - Abundant, nuclear to cytoplasm ratio 1:2 or greater

    - Eosinophilic and finely granular most common; some may have foamy or clear cytoplasm
    - Sharply defined cell borders
  - Carcinomas with focal apocrine appearance are common (approximately 30% of carcinomas of no special type) and should not be classified as IAC
- Growth pattern
  - Majority grow as sheets of cells without tubule formation ("no special type")
    - May be reported as "invasive ductal carcinoma with apocrine features"
  - Subset of IACs grow in lobular pattern and are E-cadherin negative
    - Usually poorly differentiated ("pleomorphic" lobular)
    - Includes some lobular carcinomas described as "histiocytoid"
    - May be reported as "invasive lobular carcinoma with apocrine features"
- Associated carcinoma in situ usually has an apocrine appearance
  - Apocrine DCIS can be difficult to recognize in isolation as it can be difficult to distinguish metaplasia from a clonal neoplastic proliferation
  - High nuclear grade, necrosis, and atypical architectural patterns (e.g., cribriform spaces) are useful in recognizing apocrine DCIS

ANCILLARY TESTS

Histochemistry
- PAS-diastase
  - Reactivity: Positive
  - Staining pattern
    - Cytoplasmic

Immunohistochemistry
- Androgen receptor
  - Tumor cells are usually positive
    - In 1 study, 92% of benign and 72% of malignant apocrine lesions were strongly positive for AR
- Estrogen and progesterone receptors

INVASIVE APOCRINE CARCINOMA

Apocrine Carcinoma of the Breast

Tumor Cell Feature	Apocrine Carcinoma
Cytologic appearance	Eosinophilic granular cytoplasm (nuclear:cytoplasmic ratio 1:2 or greater)
Nuclear features	Large pleomorphic nuclei (grade 2 or 3) often with prominent nucleoli
Histologic growth pattern	Most commonly sheets of cells without tubule formation; lobular growth patterns can also be seen
Estrogen and progesterone receptor expression	Typically negative
Androgen receptor expression	Typically positive (56–100% of cases)
GCDFP-15 expression	Typically positive (> 75% of cases)
HER2 protein overexpression	50% of cases
p53 protein immunoreactivity	46–50% of cases
Gene expression analysis	Apocrine molecular signature defined by gene expression profiling overlaps with HER2(+) tumors, characterized by expression of AR and genes with roles in metabolism

- Tumor cells are frequently negative for ER and PR
- May be positive for ER-β but negative for ER-α
- HER2
  - HER2 protein overexpression is present in 50% and associated with gene amplification
- Gross cystic disease fluid protein-15 (GCDFP-15)
  - > 75% of cancers show cytoplasmic reactivity for GCDFP-15 (15 kDa glycoprotein of cystic breast disease)
  - 23% of nonapocrine breast carcinomas are also positive for GCDFP-15, including most lobular carcinomas
    - Therefore, GCDFP-15 expression is not specific for apocrine differentiation

DIFFERENTIAL DIAGNOSIS

Granular Cell Tumor (GCT)

- Both IAC and GCT have abundant granular eosinophilic cytoplasm
- IAC has greater nuclear pleomorphism than GCT does
- GCT is cytokeratin negative and strongly positive for S100 protein
  - IAC is strongly cytokeratin positive and may or may not be S100 positive

Apocrine Metaplasia or DCIS Involving Adenosis

- Apocrine-appearing cells in adenosis can mimic IAC
- Borders of adenosis are usually circumscribed or lobulated
- Immunoperoxidase studies for myoepithelial cells may be helpful in problematic cases
  - Adenosis will have well-defined myoepithelial layer

Cutaneous Apocrine Carcinoma (Sweat Gland Carcinoma of the Skin)

- Breast evolved as modified skin appendage and, therefore, shares many characteristics with skin glands
- Sweat gland carcinomas of skin can have same appearance and immunoprofile as apocrine breast carcinomas
- Most important distinguishing feature is location of carcinoma (i.e., dermis vs. deep in breast tissue) and involvement of breast ducts and lobules with in situ carcinoma
  - Sweat gland carcinomas are much less common than IAC of the breast

Other Special Types of Invasive Carcinoma

- Several types of carcinoma are characterized by abundant cytoplasm
  - Oncocytic carcinoma: Abundant granular eosinophilic cytoplasm due to numerous mitochondria
  - Histiocytoid carcinoma: Foamy clear cytoplasm due to secretory vacuoles
  - Sebaceous carcinoma: Finely vacuolated cytoplasm
  - Lipid-rich carcinoma: Abundant microvacuolated, foamy, or clear cytoplasm due to lipids
- It is important to recognize these histologic variants to distinguish them from benign cells and non-breast tumors
- Histologic features may overlap with apocrine carcinoma
- Prognosis and therapy for all these types are based on standard prognostic and predictive markers; it is not necessary to perform special tests to attempt to distinguish these special types of carcinoma

SELECTED REFERENCES

1. Bhargava R et al: Breast cancer molecular class ERBB2: preponderance of tumors with apocrine differentiation and expression of basal phenotype markers CK5, CK5/6, and EGFR. Appl Immunohistochem Mol Morphol. 18(2):113-8, 2010
2. Lopez-Garcia MA et al: Breast cancer precursors revisited: molecular features and progression pathways. Histopathology. 57(2):171-92, 2010
3. Niemeier LA et al: Androgen receptor in breast cancer: expression in estrogen receptor-positive tumors and in estrogen receptor-negative tumors with apocrine differentiation. Mod Pathol. 23(2):205-12, 2010
4. Vranic S et al: EGFR and HER-2/neu expression in invasive apocrine carcinoma of the breast. Mod Pathol. 23(5):644-53, 2010
5. O'Malley FP et al: An update on apocrine lesions of the breast. Histopathology. 52(1):3-10, 2008
6. Weigelt B et al: Refinement of breast cancer classification by molecular characterization of histological special types. J Pathol. 216(2):141-50, 2008

INVASIVE APOCRINE CARCINOMA

Microscopic Features

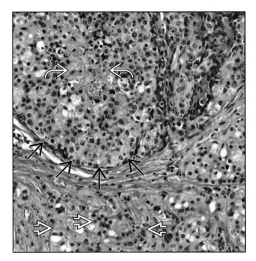

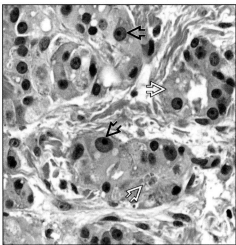

(Left) IAC ⇨ is often associated with apocrine DCIS ➡, which can be difficult to distinguish from hyperplasia with apocrine metaplasia. In this case, necrosis is present ➡. *(Right)* Strict histologic criteria for IAC include large cells with abundant eosinophilic granular cytoplasm ➡, a nuclear to cytoplasmic ratio of 1:2 or greater, and large vesicular nuclei with prominent nucleoli ➡ in > 90% of the cancer. IHC for AR and GCDFP-15 can be supportive of the diagnosis.

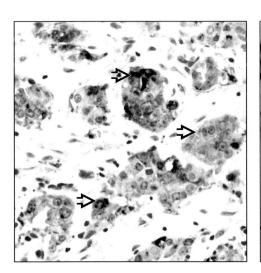

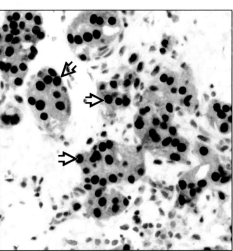

(Left) The majority of IACs show strong cytoplasmic positivity for GCDFP-15 ➡ throughout the tumor. However, positivity is not sufficient for the diagnosis as some carcinomas without the typical apocrine appearance are also GCDFP-15 positive. *(Right)* IAC frequently shows marked expression of androgen receptor ➡ as a characteristic feature. Altered androgen metabolism may play a role in the pathogenesis of these tumors and disease progression.

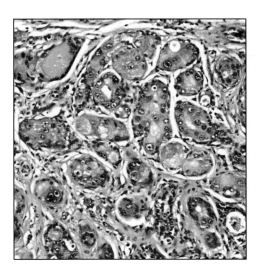

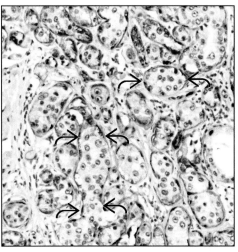

(Left) Apocrine DCIS can involve sclerosing adenosis and closely mimic an invasive carcinoma. A low-power search for a lobulocentric architectural organization can be a helpful diagnostic feature. For problematic cases, immunostains can confirm the presence of myoepithelial cells and exclude invasion. *(Right)* This lesion is confirmed to be a case of apocrine DCIS involving sclerosing adenosis by a calponin stain that highlights the surrounding myoepithelial cells ➡.

NEUROENDOCRINE/SMALL CELL CARCINOMA

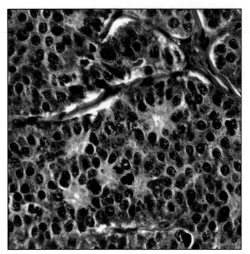

Histologic features of neuroendocrine differentiation include an organoid growth pattern with uniform epithelioid cells having moderate amounts of cytoplasm, dispersed chromatin, and rosette formation.

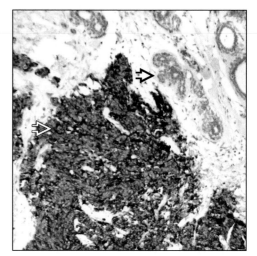

Neuroendocrine breast carcinoma must express a neuroendocrine marker such as chromogranin in ≥ 50% of tumor cells ➡. Normal breast epithelial cells are negative for these markers ➡.

TERMINOLOGY

Abbreviations
- Neuroendocrine breast carcinoma (NEBC)
  - Solid neuroendocrine breast carcinoma (SNEBC)
  - Small cell/oat cell breast carcinoma (SCOCBC)
  - Large cell neuroendocrine breast carcinoma (LCNEBC)

Synonyms
- Invasive carcinoma with endocrine differentiation (argyrophilic carcinoma)
- Mammary carcinoma with endocrine features

Definitions
- WHO classification recognizes 3 categories of neuroendocrine breast carcinoma
  - Solid neuroendocrine breast carcinoma
  - Small cell/oat cell breast carcinoma
  - Large cell neuroendocrine breast carcinoma
- Carcinomas must have "morphologic features similar to those of neuroendocrine tumors of both gastrointestinal tract and lung"
  - Tumors must express at least 1 neuroendocrine marker in > 50% of cells to qualify
- Some carcinomas with typical morphologic appearance will not express neuroendocrine markers
- Alternatively, not all carcinomas that express neuroendocrine markers have a distinctive morphologic appearance
- This is a heterogeneous group of carcinomas; not all cases will easily fit into 3 groups as defined by WHO

ETIOLOGY/PATHOGENESIS

Biology of NEBC
- Gene expression profiling analysis of NEBC
  - NEBC belongs to luminal A subgroup

- SNEBC has transcriptional pattern identical to type B mucinous carcinoma (hypercellular type)
- This association is present whether or not mucinous carcinomas express neuroendocrine markers
- Type A mucinous carcinomas (paucicellular) cluster in separate but related group

CLINICAL ISSUES

Epidemiology
- Incidence
  - NEBCs comprise 2-5% of breast carcinomas
- Age
  - NEBC has same age distribution as carcinomas of no special type; median age at diagnosis is 61 years

Presentation
- NEBC usually presents as palpable mass or mammographic density
  - Calcifications have not been associated with these tumors
- Very rare breast carcinomas produce ectopic hormones
  - Human chorionic gonadotropin, calcitonin, adrenocorticotrophic hormone, parathormone, and epinephrine have been reported
  - Clinical symptomatology from these hormones is very rare

Treatment
- Not altered by presence of neuroendocrine markers

Prognosis
- Information is limited due to small numbers of patients and varying definitions of NEBC
- In small studies, SNEBC, especially if associated with solid papillary pattern or mucin production, has better prognosis
- In 1 study, LCNEBC had worse prognosis compared to matched controls with carcinomas of no special type

NEUROENDOCRINE/SMALL CELL CARCINOMA

Key Facts

Terminology

- WHO classification recognizes 3 categories of NEBC
  - Solid neuroendocrine carcinoma: Most common
  - Large cell neuroendocrine carcinoma
  - Small cell/oat cell carcinoma: Very rare
- Carcinomas must have typical histologic features and express at least 1 neuroendocrine marker in > 50% of cells to qualify
  - However, this is a heterogeneous group of carcinomas and not all will easily fit into these 3 groups

Etiology/Pathogenesis

- Gene expression profiling has shown that solid neuroendocrine carcinoma has transcriptional pattern identical to type B mucinous carcinomas (cellular mucinous carcinomas)

Clinical Issues

- 2-5% of breast carcinomas
- Information on prognosis is limited due to small numbers of patients and varying definitions of NEBC
- Solid neuroendocrine carcinoma, especially if associated with solid papillary pattern or mucin production, has better prognosis
- Other types may have worse prognosis

Top Differential Diagnoses

- Primary carcinoid tumor of breast
- Metastatic carcinoid tumor
- Metastatic small cell carcinoma
- Breast carcinomas of no special type
- Alveolar lobular carcinoma

IMAGE FINDINGS

Radiographic Findings

- No specific imaging features

MACROSCOPIC FEATURES

General Features

- No specific gross features

MICROSCOPIC PATHOLOGY

Histologic Features

- Histologic types of NEBC are recognized in WHO classification
  - Solid neuroendocrine breast carcinoma (SNEBC)
    - Most common type of NEBC
    - Tumors form circumscribed or lobulated masses that may be solitary or multiple
    - Cell nests may be separated by delicate septae; some have solid papillary pattern
    - Cell type can vary from spindled to epithelioid
    - Peripheral palisading and rosette formation may be present
    - About 25% are associated with at least focal extracellular mucin or intracellular mucin
  - Small cell/oat cell breast carcinoma (SCOCBC)
    - Very rare type of breast carcinoma; most are poorly differentiated
    - Cancers form irregular masses
    - Cell morphology is identical to small cell carcinoma of lung
    - Cells have scant cytoplasm and hyperchromatic nuclei
    - Crush artifact is common
    - Some carcinomas will be intermingled with carcinoma of non-small cell type
    - Identification of a similar in situ component is helpful to exclude metastasis to the breast
    - DCIS should resemble the invasive carcinoma
  - Large cell neuroendocrine breast carcinoma (LCNEBC)
    - 2nd most common type of NEBC; usually moderately or poorly differentiated
    - Moderate to abundant cytoplasm
    - Vesicular to finely granular chromatin
    - High mitotic rate
    - Focal areas of necrosis are frequent
- DCIS with neuroendocrine features has also been described
  - Solid papillary or organoid growth patterns are typical
  - Unusual are cribriform or comedo patterns
  - Identification useful to exclude metastasis from another site

ANCILLARY TESTS

Histochemistry

- Grimelius: Silver stain
  - Reactivity: Positive
  - Staining pattern
    - Cytoplasmic; fine black granules
  - Identifies argyrophilia in breast cancers
  - Correlates with neurosecretory granules as seen by electron microscopy and detected by antibodies to chromogranin

Immunohistochemistry

- Estrogen and progesterone receptors
  - SNEBC: > 90% positive
  - SCOCBC and LCNEBC: 50-60% positive
- HER2
  - Very rare in any type of NEBC
- Neuroendocrine markers
  - By definition, at least 50% of tumor cells must be positive for at least 1 neuroendocrine marker
    - WHO definition does not specify which neuroendocrine markers should be used
  - Chromogranin-A or -B and synaptophysin are markers considered most sensitive and specific

NEUROENDOCRINE/SMALL CELL CARCINOMA

- Granins are components of neurosecretory granules
- Synaptophysin is glycoprotein found in presynaptic vesicles
- Other markers are less specific: Neuron-specific enolase, N-cellular adhesion molecule/CD56, Leu-7/CD57, bombesin, neurofilament triplet protein

Electron Microscopy

- Neurosecretory (dense core) granules are present in cytoplasm
  - Round membrane-bound vesicles with dense central core
  - Chromogranin and Leu-7/CD57 are found in matrix of granules

DIFFERENTIAL DIAGNOSIS

Primary Carcinoid Tumor of Breast

- Existence of primary carcinoid tumor of breast is not accepted by all
- Carcinoid syndrome due to ectopic hormone production has not been reported
- Although alternative primary site was not found in all reported cases of breast carcinoid tumors, extent of work-up has not been clearly reported in all cases
  - Primary carcinoid tumors at other sites can be quite small and difficult to detect
- Diagnosis of primary carcinoid tumor of breast should be made with great caution
  - Metastatic carcinoid tumor should always be considered

Metastatic Carcinoid Tumor

- In approximately 50% of cases, breast mass is presenting symptom of occult carcinoid tumor
- Majority of patients have symptoms of carcinoid syndrome
- Carcinoid tumors can closely mimic LCIS, low-grade DCIS, and well-differentiated invasive carcinomas
  - Carcinoid should be suspected when low-grade malignancy is ER and PR negative
- Carcinoid tumor is more likely to be strongly positive for chromogranin than breast NEC
- Identification of in situ component is helpful to demonstrate that NEC has arisen in the breast

Metastatic Small Cell Carcinoma

- SCOCBC can be histologically identical to small cell carcinoma of the lung
- 1st evidence of lung carcinoma as breast mass is unusual
- Majority of lung small cell carcinomas will be positive for TTF-1
  - However, rare breast NEBCs have also been reported to be TTF-1 positive
- Lung small cell carcinomas are usually CK7 negative, but breast SCOCBC is often positive

Breast Carcinomas of No Special Type

- Can be focally positive for neuroendocrine markers (10-20%)

- Not all such cancers have histologic features suggesting neuroendocrine differentiation
- In contrast, some cancers can have histologic features of neuroendocrine differentiation but lack expression of neuroendocrine markers
- Diagnosis of NEBC should not be made unless carcinoma has both typical histologic features and > 50% of cells are positive for at least 1 neuroendocrine marker
- If neuroendocrine markers are focally present, there is no known prognostic significance
- Metastatic breast carcinoma should be suspected in patients with history of breast cancer diagnosed with "neuroendocrine tumor" at another site
  - Metastatic breast cancer can closely mimic carcinoid tumors in lung and liver
    - Commonly positive for ER and PR
  - Comparison of primary carcinoma and metastasis, as well as neuroendocrine studies on primary carcinoma, can be helpful for correct classification

Alveolar Lobular Carcinoma

- Can mimic NEBC due to uniform small round cells and nested pattern
- Areas of single cell infiltration favor invasive lobular carcinoma
- Absence of E-cadherin and neuroendocrine markers support diagnosis of lobular carcinoma

SELECTED REFERENCES

1. Christie M et al: Primary small cell carcinoma of the breast with TTF-1 and neuroendocrine marker expressing carcinoma in situ. Int J Clin Exp Pathol. 3(6):629-33, 2010
2. Klingen TA et al: Thyroid transcription factor-1 positive primary breast cancer: a case report with review of the literature. Diagn Pathol. 5:37, 2010
3. Righi L et al: Neuroendocrine differentiation in breast cancer: established facts and unresolved problems. Semin Diagn Pathol. 27(1):69-76, 2010
4. Wei B et al: Invasive neuroendocrine carcinoma of the breast: a distinctive subtype of aggressive mammary carcinoma. Cancer. 116(19):4463-73, 2010
5. Ersahin C et al: Thyroid transcription factor-1 and "basal marker"--expressing small cell carcinoma of the breast. Int J Surg Pathol. 17(5):368-72, 2009
6. Shahrokni A et al: Breast metastasis of small bowel carcinoid tumor misdiagnosed as primary breast cancer. Ann Saudi Med. 29(4):320-1, 2009
7. Weigelt B et al: Mucinous and neuroendocrine breast carcinomas are transcriptionally distinct from invasive ductal carcinomas of no special type. Mod Pathol. 22(11):1401-14, 2009
8. Upalakalin JN et al: Carcinoid tumors in the breast. Am J Surg. 191(6):799-805, 2006
9. Shin SJ et al: Small cell carcinoma of the breast: a clinicopathologic and immunohistochemical study of nine patients. Am J Surg Pathol. 24(9):1231-8, 2000

NEUROENDOCRINE/SMALL CELL CARCINOMA

Microscopic Features

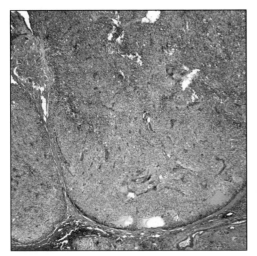

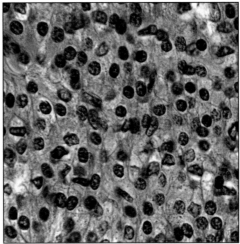

(Left) Solid NEBC grows as a single or multiple well-circumscribed or lobulated masses. Some cancers have a solid papillary pattern with thin fibrovascular septae, and about 25% have focal mucin production. (Right) The cells of solid NEBC have uniform rounded nuclei, small nucleoli, and moderate amounts of cytoplasm. Mitoses are infrequent. Most carcinomas are either well or moderately differentiated.

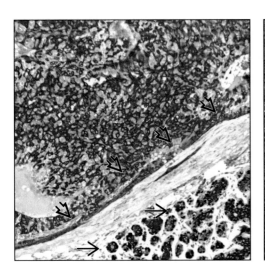

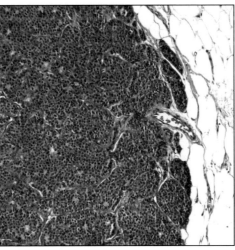

(Left) IHC is helpful to distinguish solid NEBC from DCIS. This invasive carcinoma is positive for cytokeratin (red cytoplasmic staining), but no nuclear positivity for p63 is seen at the tumor edge ➡. Myoepithelial cells positive for p63 are present in the adjacent normal lobule ➡. (Right) NEBC can also consist of multiple nests of tumor cells separated by thin fibrous septae. The border is often circumscribed or lobulated.

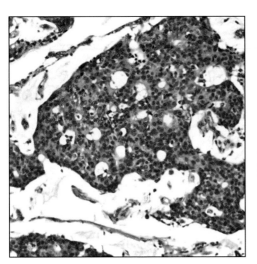

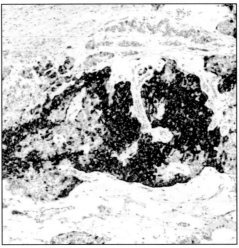

(Left) Type B mucinous carcinomas share histologic features with solid NEBC. Gene expression profiling has shown that both types of carcinoma are transcriptionally very similar. (Right) This type B mucinous carcinoma shows strong positivity for synaptophysin in > 50% of the tumor cells. In contrast, it is unusual for type A mucinous carcinomas to be positive for neuroendocrine markers. They are probably closely related but different tumor types.

NEUROENDOCRINE/SMALL CELL CARCINOMA

Microscopic Features and Differential Diagnosis

(Left) Very rare breast carcinomas have the same histologic appearance as small cell carcinoma of the lung. There is very scant cytoplasm, smudged chromatin, and nuclear molding. Mitotic figures are frequent ⇨. *(Right)* Some cases of SCOCBC can resemble small cell carcinoma of the lung and also be positive for TTF-1. In addition, ER may be negative. It may not be possible to distinguish such carcinomas from a metastasis unless DCIS with a similar appearance is also present.

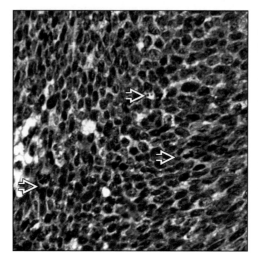

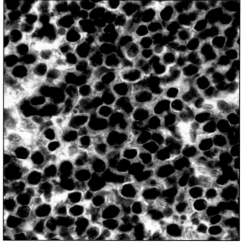

(Left) This is a carcinoma with high-grade pleomorphic nuclei, frequent mitoses, and an infiltrative invasive pattern. There are extensive areas of necrosis ⇨. *(Right)* This degree of positivity for chromogranin in a carcinoma would be insufficient for a diagnosis as NEBC. However, a carcinoma does not need to show positivity in > 50% of tumor cells for all neuroendocrine markers to qualify; this finding need only be true for 1 neuroendocrine marker.

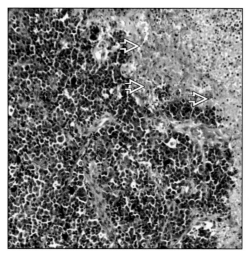

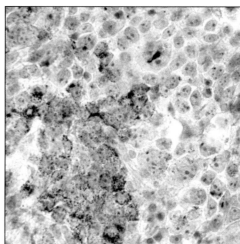

(Left) Synaptophysin was strongly positive in almost all of the tumor cells. This carcinoma does not fit into the WHO definition of NEBC due to the lack of typical morphologic features of a neuroendocrine neoplasm. *(Right)* Alveolar lobular carcinoma can resemble a NEBC due to its small round uniform cells and nested appearance. The presence of single cell invasion ⇨ favors a diagnosis of lobular carcinoma. IHC could also support the diagnosis if negative for E-cadherin.

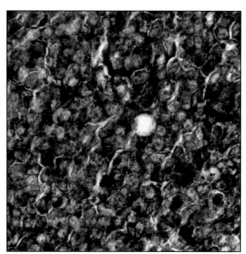

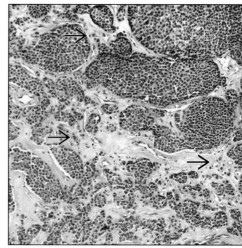

NEUROENDOCRINE/SMALL CELL CARCINOMA

Metastatic Neuroendocrine Tumors

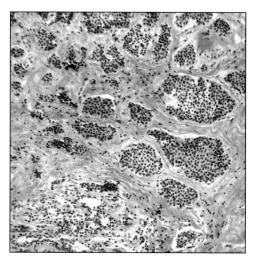
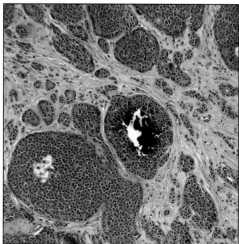

(Left) Carcinoid tumors in the breast can closely mimic a low-grade invasive carcinoma. The absence of ER and PR as well as DCIS should raise the possibility of carcinoid. True primary carcinoid tumor of the breast is not well described; metastasis is more likely. *(Right)* Metastatic carcinoid may also be mistaken for DCIS due to the nested pattern. This case of metastatic carcinoid tumor presented as mammographic calcifications. IHC can confirm the absence of myoepithelial cells.

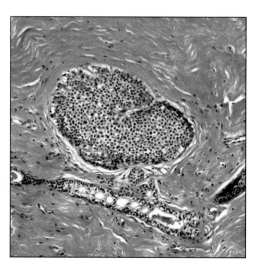
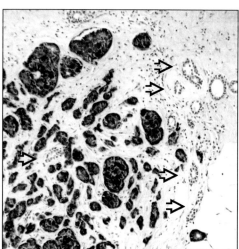

(Left) Metastatic carcinoid can also resemble LCIS due to the uniform rounded cells and nested pattern. IHC would confirm the absence of ER and PR, as well as the absence of myoepithelial cells. *(Right)* Carcinoid tumors will be strongly positive for neuroendocrine markers such as chromogranin as in this case. Normal breast epithelium is negative for neuroendocrine markers ➤. Thus, the cell of origin of breast neuroendocrine tumors is unknown.

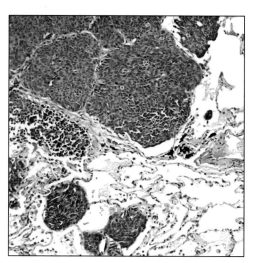
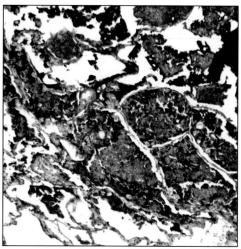

(Left) This patient presented with a lung mass, which was biopsied. The tumor had a neuroendocrine appearance, and a diagnosis of atypical carcinoid was considered. However, the patient had a prior history of breast carcinoma. *(Right)* Additional IHC studies showed that the tumor was strongly positive for chromogranin but also ER and PR. The patient's prior breast carcinoma had an identical immunoprofile. A diagnosis of metastatic breast carcinoma was rendered.

LOCALLY RECURRENT CARCINOMA

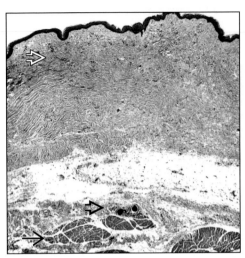

Reconstructions after mastectomy consist of skin ⊟ and skeletal muscle ⊟; recurrent carcinoma ⊟ in this location carries a dire prognosis, as it is an indicator of treatment-resistant cancer.

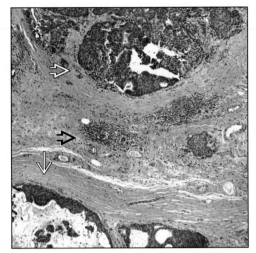

In this chest wall excision there is normal breast ⊟, DCIS ⊟, and invasive carcinoma ⊟. Therefore, this could be a new primary cancer, which has a better prognosis than a true recurrence.

TERMINOLOGY

Definitions
- Subsequent carcinoma in breast after breast-conserving therapy or in chest wall after mastectomy, following prior diagnosis of breast carcinoma
  - True recurrences (TR) due to failure to eradicate carcinoma by initial treatment
  - New primary cancers (NP) not clonally related to first carcinoma

ETIOLOGY/PATHOGENESIS

Types of Recurrent Carcinoma
- **After breast-conserving therapy**
  - May be DCIS or invasive carcinoma
  - Approximately 1/3 of cases will be NP
  - Location, histologic type, and tumor markers can help determine if cancer is TR or NP
  - Recurrent DCIS has favorable prognosis
    - About 1/2 of recurrent cases after diagnosis of DCIS will again be DCIS and 1/2 invasive carcinoma
  - Recurrent invasive carcinoma after initial diagnosis of invasive carcinoma has less favorable prognosis
    - If TR, then carcinoma is resistant to therapy given to patient and prognosis is generally poor
    - If NP, prognosis is more favorable as carcinoma may be sensitive to treatment
    - If patient has developed new invasive carcinoma due to residual DCIS, effect on prognosis is less clear
    - This finding suggests original DCIS was resistant to treatment
- **After mastectomy**
  - Majority of cases are due to TR and occur in chest wall or skin
    - Prognosis generally poor because majority of patients eventually develop distant metastases

  - Recurrent carcinoma likely arose from foci of lymph-vascular invasion
  - In rare cases, NP may occur due to residual normal breast tissue remaining after surgery
    - Impossible to remove all breast tissue in all patients because breast tissue can be present in subcutaneous tissue over anterior chest wall and can extend into axilla
    - Important to evaluate "chest wall" excisions for residual normal breast tissue &/or DCIS
    - NP occurring in residual breast tissue likely has better prognosis than TR

CLINICAL ISSUES

Epidemiology
- Incidence
  - Ipsilateral breast recurrence after breast-conserving therapy: 5-10% at 5 years and 10-15% at 10 years
  - Chest wall recurrences after mastectomy: < 5%

Presentation
- TR in breast often presents in same manner as original carcinoma
  - Carcinomas presenting as mammographic calcifications often recur as calcifications
  - Carcinomas presenting as palpable masses or mammographic densities usually recur as masses
- Recurrences after mastectomy often present as subcutaneous skin nodules
  - Nodules are commonly associated with prior surgical scar
- TR is more likely to be diagnosed at shorter intervals than NP
  - 1-5 years: ~ 80-90% of recurrences are TR
  - 5-10 years: ~ 50-60% TR and ~ 40% NP
  - 10-15 years: ~ 30% TR and ~ 70% NP

LOCALLY RECURRENT CARCINOMA

Key Facts

Terminology

- Subsequent carcinoma in breast (after breast-conserving therapy) or in chest wall (after mastectomy) following prior diagnosis of breast carcinoma
- True recurrent carcinoma is due to failure of initial treatment to eradicate carcinoma
- New primary carcinomas are not clonally related to 1st carcinoma

Etiology/Pathogenesis

- **After breast-conserving therapy**
- True recurrences are most common in 1st 5 years
  - Prognosis is generally poor, as carcinoma is resistant to treatment, and majority of patients develop distant metastases

- New primaries are more common 10 years and beyond after initial diagnosis
  - Prognosis is generally favorable because carcinoma may be sensitive to therapy
- **After mastectomy**
- Majority of cases are true recurrences of original invasive carcinoma present in chest wall or skin
- Prognosis is generally poor because majority of patients eventually develop distant metastases
- In rare cases, new carcinomas may arise from residual normal breast tissue remaining after surgery

Ancillary Tests

- DNA-based assays are more accurate in determining whether cancer is true recurrence or new primary cancer

---

- In rare cases, cancer that did not present as inflammatory carcinoma recurs as inflammatory carcinoma
- Axillary nodal recurrences also occur but are uncommon

Prognosis

- Highly dependent upon type of recurrence
  - Recurrence as DCIS can be treated with surgery and radiation
    - Unlikely to have impact on prognosis
  - Recurrence as invasive carcinoma varies in prognosis
    - TR has poor prognosis (indicator of treatment-resistant cancer)
    - The shorter the interval to recurrence (measure of growth rate of cancer), the worse the prognosis
    - Majority of patients with TR will develop distant metastases; risk is 3-4x higher than patients without local recurrence
    - NP has more favorable prognosis depending on stage of cancer
    - Patients with NP are at higher risk for contralateral cancer

Risk Factors for TR

- Young age
  - More likely to have ER negative carcinomas
- Molecular subtypes of breast cancer have different risks of local recurrence at 10 years
  - Luminal A has lowest risk (8%) followed by luminal B (10%)
  - HER2 (ER negative) has highest risk (21%) if not treated with HER2-directed therapy
  - Basal-like (triple negative and EGFR or cytokeratin 5/6 positive) has the 2nd highest risk (14%)
  - Effective systemic therapy may decrease likelihood of TR
- 21-gene recurrence score assay (Oncotype DX [Genomic Health; Redwood City, CA]) is predictive for local recurrence in patients with ER-positive cancer without lymph node metastases

  - 10-year locoregional recurrence was 4% if score was low, 7.2% if score was intermediate, and 15.8% if score was high
- Extensive lymph-vascular invasion
- Extensive intraductal component (EIC)
- Skin involvement by cancer
- Multiple cancers
- Extensive nodal involvement
- Margins positive for DCIS or invasive carcinoma
  - Most patients with positive margins will undergo additional surgery
  - TR can occur in patients with initial negative margins
    - Lymph-vascular invasion can be source of TR
- Omission of radiation therapy for women undergoing breast conservation

Risk Factors for NP

- Young age
  - More likely to have germline mutations, putting these women at higher risk for multiple cancers
  - Also at higher risk for contralateral carcinomas
- Omission of whole breast radiation
  - Radiation may also treat precursor lesions elsewhere in breast
  - Not yet known if partial breast irradiation will result in relative increase in NP at other sites in breast

ANCILLARY TESTS

Methods to Distinguish TR from NP

- Location in breast
  - 70-90% of recurrences occur in same area of breast
    - However, relative locations of 1st and 2nd cancers are often difficult to define
    - Breast imaging can be helpful if surgical changes at prior cancer site
    - NP can also occur in same general location as prior carcinoma
  - Microscopic features may help to identify prior surgical site

- Hyalinized scar tissue may be present; however, it may be difficult to distinguish scar from dense breast stroma
  - Suture material may be present; however, in majority of cases suture material will have been resorbed
  - In majority of cases, definite prior surgical site will not be evident by histologic features
- Histologic type of cancer
  - TR generally has same appearance as original carcinoma
  - If 2nd carcinoma has different morphology, it is more likely to be NP
  - However, majority of breast cancers are of no special type and it may not be possible to make this distinction on morphology
- Tumor markers: ER, PR, HER2
  - Markers usually do not change in TR
    - However, majority of breast cancers are ER/PR positive and HER2 negative
    - Therefore, same marker pattern does not necessarily indicate cancer is TR
  - PR loss (or selection for PR negative cells) can occur if patient has been treated with aromatase inhibitor
  - HER2 loss (or selection for HER2-negative cells) can occur after trastuzumab (Herceptin) treatment
  - If major change in markers (e.g., ER positive/HER2 negative to ER negative/HER2 positive) then cancer is likely NP
- Ploidy by flow cytometry
  - Concordance of ploidy between primary carcinomas and synchronous lymph node metastases is only 77%
  - Therefore, this method may misclassify many cases
- PCR-based loss of heterozygosity (allelic imbalance) assay
  - Can be performed on formalin-fixed paraffin-embedded tissue
  - Microsatellite alleles in tumor suppressor genes are frequently lost in carcinomas
  - Each carcinoma has characteristic pattern of loss
  - Sensitive assay to identify carcinomas arising from same clone of malignant cells
  - Results show that 30-45% of cancers are misclassified as TR or NP using other methods
- DNA breakpoint and DNA copy number alterations
  - Requires frozen tissue
  - Assumes genetic changes in cancers are relatively stable over time
  - Can be used to establish clonality of cancers
  - Will probably give similar results to PCR-based allelic imbalance assays but may be more difficult to perform

DIFFERENTIAL DIAGNOSIS

Angiosarcoma
- Patients receiving radiation therapy are at increased risk for angiosarcoma
  - However, actual incidence of angiosarcoma is very low

- Angiosarcomas can appear epithelioid and resemble poorly differentiated breast cancer
  - IHC panel may be necessary to distinguish angiosarcoma from recurrent carcinoma
    - Angiosarcomas may be keratin positive; some poorly differentiated breast cancers may only be positive for basal keratins
    - Angiosarcomas and some breast carcinomas will be positive for podoplanin (D2-40)

Scar Tissue
- Occasionally scar tissue at prior surgical site will appear to increase in size
- Traumatic neuromas can form small masses in breast or in subcutaneous tissue
- Degenerating/regenerating muscle fibers can mimic pleomorphic malignant cells
- Excision may be necessary to exclude recurrent carcinoma

REPORTING CONSIDERATIONS

Key Elements to Report
- When possible, prior carcinoma should be compared to current carcinoma
  - Statement should be made on likelihood of carcinoma being TR or NP
- If recurrence is after mastectomy
  - Report residual normal breast tissue, if present
  - Report DCIS, if present
    - Some invasive carcinomas in non-breast tissue form circumscribed masses
    - Myoepithelial markers may be necessary to distinguish DCIS from lymph-vascular invasion or solid nodules of invasive carcinoma

SELECTED REFERENCES
1. Buist DS et al: Diagnosis of second breast cancer events after initial diagnosis of early stage breast cancer. Breast Cancer Res Treat. 124(3):863-73, 2010
2. Mamounas EP et al: Association between the 21-gene recurrence score assay and risk of locoregional recurrence in node-negative, estrogen receptor-positive breast cancer: results from NSABP B-14 and NSABP B-20. J Clin Oncol. 28(10):1677-83, 2010
3. McGrath S et al: Long-term patterns of in-breast failure in patients with early stage breast cancer treated with breast-conserving therapy: a molecular based clonality evaluation. Am J Clin Oncol. 33(1):17-22, 2010
4. Panet-Raymond V et al: Ipsilateral breast tumor recurrence after breast-conserving therapy. Expert Rev Anticancer Ther. 10(8):1229-38, 2010
5. Rudloff U et al: Nomogram for predicting the risk of local recurrence after breast-conserving surgery for ductal carcinoma in situ. J Clin Oncol. 28(23):3762-9, 2010
6. Voduc KD et al: Breast cancer subtypes and the risk of local and regional relapse. J Clin Oncol. 28(10):1684-91, 2010
7. Bollet MA et al: High-resolution mapping of DNA breakpoints to define true recurrences among ipsilateral breast cancers. J Natl Cancer Inst. 100(1):48-58, 2008

LOCALLY RECURRENT CARCINOMA

Microscopic Features

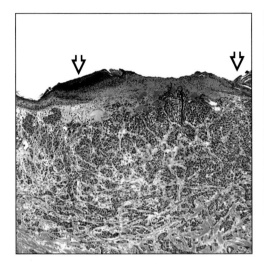

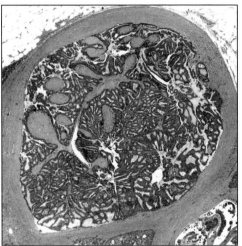

(Left) Recurrence with skin invasion and ulceration ⊳ is a particularly dreaded outcome. Prior to modern treatment modalities, the majority of women with breast cancer died with locally advanced disease involving the chest wall. (Right) Recurrent carcinomas in the chest wall can look deceptively well circumscribed. This carcinoma is present in adipose tissue from a flap reconstruction. No normal breast tissue was present, and no myoepithelial cells were detected by IHC.

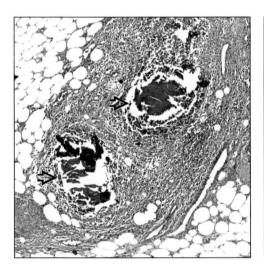

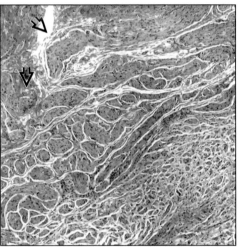

(Left) It is difficult to identify a prior tumor site months to years after surgery. Suture material ⊳ is biodegradable and only rarely persists. Dense breast tissue can be difficult to distinguish from scar tissue. The location using clinical and radiologic information may be the only means to determine if cancer has recurred at the same site. (Right) Traumatic neuromas ⊳ can be an indicator of prior surgery. This one presented as a skin nodule in the prior mastectomy scar.

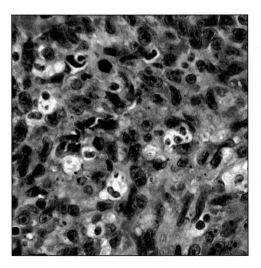

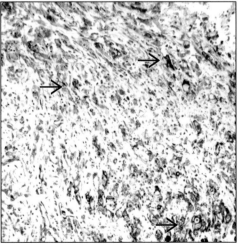

(Left) Patients are at risk for recurrent carcinoma as well as treatment-associated angiosarcoma. This patient had a history of a poorly differentiated triple negative carcinoma and presented with extensive disease in her breast and axilla. (Right) This malignancy was originally diagnosed as angiosarcoma as the tumor cells were negative for keratin and positive for podoplanin (D2-40) ⇥. However, this was a basal-like carcinoma positive for basal-type keratins and podoplanin.

INTRODUCTION: PROGNOSTIC AND PREDICTIVE FACTORS

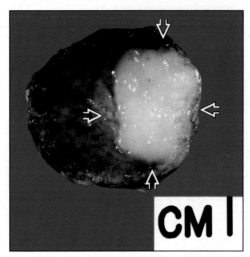

For patients without distant metastases, regional lymph node involvement ➡ is the most important prognostic factor. The likelihood of survival diminishes with each additional positive node.

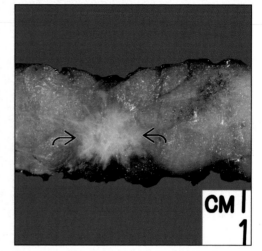

The size of invasive carcinoma ➡ is the next most important prognostic factor. The size used for staging should incorporate clinical, radiologic, gross, and microscopic information.

TERMINOLOGY

Definitions
- **Prognostic factors**
  - Predict patient clinical course in terms of risk of disease recurrence and death
  - Provide information about patient outcome based on
    - Patient-related factors: Age, menopausal status, performance status, comorbidities
    - Tumor-related factors: Lymph node staging, tumor size, grade, histologic type, lymph-vascular invasion
  - Extensively clinically validated as useful in determining probability of local &/or distant disease recurrence
    - Basis for clinical risk assessment and decisions on the need for adjuvant systemic therapy
    - Prognostic factors are robust in terms of their ability to predict disease recurrence
    - Prognostic factors are less accurate/successful at predicting patient response to systemic adjuvant therapy
  - Prognostic factors are important whether evaluated prior to therapy or after neoadjuvant therapy
    - After treatment, response to treatment and amount of residual disease are important prognostic factors
    - AJCC staging both before and after treatment provide significant prognostic information, especially in combination
  - Prognostic factors are clinically most useful in helping to identify a subset of patients with small (< 2 cm), node-negative cancer who may benefit from systemic therapy
- **Predictive factors**
  - Predict the likelihood that patient will benefit from adjuvant treatment regimens including
    - Hormonal therapy

- Chemotherapy
- Biologic and targeted therapies
  - Provide information on the likely outcome following a specific treatment regimen
  - Development of new treatment regimens and novel targeted agents has led to a shift from risk assessment to treatment responsiveness
    - Better patient selection for specific treatments
    - Improved patient response rate
    - Reduction of toxicity from therapies that will be unlikely to be of benefit
  - Some factors, including ER, PR, and HER2, are both prognostic factors and predictive factors

CLINICAL IMPLICATIONS

Major Pathologic Prognostic Factors
- Used for AJCC/UICC TNM staging (7th edition, 2010)
  - Used to combine patients into groups with similar likelihood of survival
  - Majority of factors are determined by readily available standard techniques
  - Useful to compare patients over time and in diverse locations
    - Essential for grouping patients for clinical trials and other studies
  - Include local extent of cancer in the breast, regional lymph node metastasis, and distant metastasis
  - Staging is prognostically important for carcinomas prior to treatment and after neoadjuvant treatment
- Patients are divided into 5 stages with different survival rates at 10 years
  - Stage 0: DCIS; > 95% survival
    - Without screening, this group is very small (< 5% of breast cancers)
    - In screened populations, 20-30% of carcinomas are DCIS
  - Stage I: Invasive carcinomas < 2 cm with negative nodes or only micrometastases; > 90% survival

- - Approximately 50% of patients with invasive carcinoma
  - Incidence has increased with screening
  - Stage II: Invasive carcinoma up to 5 cm with 1-3 lymph node metastases or carcinoma > 5 cm with negative nodes; ~ 60% survival
    - Approximately 30% of patients with invasive carcinoma
    - Incidence has decreased with screening
  - Stage III: Locally advanced disease (skin ulceration or chest wall invasion or inflammatory carcinoma) ± lymph node metastases or metastases in ≥ 10 lymph nodes; ~ 40% survival
    - Only 5-10% of patients
    - Incidence has decreased due to greater awareness and earlier detection
  - Stage IV: Distant metastases; < 10% survival
    - Only 5-10% of patients
    - Incidence has not changed substantially over time
    - Likely a subset of carcinomas that metastasize early prior to possible detection by screening
- **Size of invasive carcinoma (AJCC T1-3)**
  - Size of an invasive carcinoma is an independent prognostic factor
    - Does not include associated carcinoma in situ
    - Correlated with likelihood of lymph node metastasis
    - Clinical, radiologic, gross, and microscopic information should be used to determine best size for T classification
    - Palpable carcinomas have worse prognosis compared with nonpalpable carcinomas, detected by screening, of same size
  - Tumor size directly correlates with number of involved lymph nodes and an increased risk of recurrence
    - For node-negative patients, tumor size is routinely used to make adjuvant treatment decisions
    - Patients with carcinomas ≤ 1 cm have an excellent prognosis, and selected patients have little benefit from systemic therapy
  - AJCC T classification separates majority of carcinomas by size
  - T1 carcinomas are ≤ 2 cm in size
    - T1mi: ≤ 0.1 cm (microinvasion)
    - T1a: > 0.1 cm but ≤ 0.5 cm
    - T1b: > 0.5 cm but ≤ 1 cm
    - T1c: > 1 cm but ≤ 2 cm
  - T2: > 2 cm but ≤ 5 cm
  - T3: > 5 cm
  - T4: Tumor of any size with direct extension to chest wall or skin involvement or inflammatory carcinoma
- **Regional lymph nodes (AJCC N1-3)**
  - Prognosis diminishes with each additional lymph node metastasis
    - N0: Negative nodes, 82.8% 5-year survival
    - N1a: 1–3 positive nodes, 73% 5-year survival
    - N2a: 4–9 positive nodes, 45.7% 5-year survival
    - N3a: 10 or more positive nodes, 28.4% 5-year survival
  - Prognosis is dependent on size of the metastasis

- - Macrometastases measure > 2 mm and have prognostic significance
  - Isolated tumor cells (< 0.2 cm or < 200 cells) & micrometastases (between isolated tumor cells & macrometastases) have very small effect on prognosis compared to node-negative women
  - Total number of positive nodes includes macrometastases and micrometastases but not isolated tumor cells
  - Patients with only micrometastases are classified as stage I in AJCC 7th edition manual
  - Subset (10-30%) of node-negative patients eventually develop distant metastases
    - Some of these carcinomas may metastasize to nodal basins that are generally not sampled (e.g., internal mammary nodes)
    - Other carcinomas may metastasize primarily via blood vessels (e.g., spindle cell carcinomas)
  - Lymph nodes are removed or sampled primarily for prognostication
    - Removal of positive lymph nodes has little or no effect on survival
- **Distant metastases (AJCC M1)**
  - Generally detected clinically or radiologically
    - Patients with indeterminant findings may undergo biopsy for confirmation
    - M1 metastases are detected by clinical or radiologic means &/or are pathologically shown to be > 0.2 mm
    - M0 (i+) metastases are detected by microscopy or other tests and are ≤ 0.2 mm; are not evident clinically or radiologically or by symptoms or signs
  - Patients with M1 (stage IV) disease have a poor prognosis, < 10% survival at 10 years
    - Patients who present with distant metastases at a long interval after diagnosis have a better prognosis
    - Indicative of a carcinoma with a slower growth rate
  - Most common sites of metastasis are bone, lung, brain, and liver
    - Bone is most common site and, in ER-positive cancers, may occur many years after diagnosis
    - Brain metastases are relatively more common in HER2-positive cancers and triple negative cancers
  - Pathologic M0 can only be defined at autopsy
    - For living patients, only clinical M0 is applicable
  - MX was eliminated as a term in the AJCC 7th edition
- **Skin involvement, chest wall involvement, or inflammatory carcinoma (AJCC T4)**
  - Extensive skin &/or chest wall involvement originally identified in patients with very large locally advanced carcinomas who would not benefit from surgery
    - Current prognosis is improved with better surgical and adjuvant treatment
    - Difficult to study as these patients are now quite uncommon
  - T4a: Extension to chest wall

INTRODUCTION: PROGNOSTIC AND PREDICTIVE FACTORS

- Does not include adherence to or invasion of pectoralis muscle
  ○ T4b: Skin involvement
    ▪ Ulceration of skin: Does not include ulceration due to a prior surgical procedure or Paget disease of the nipple
    ▪ Small superficial carcinomas with ulceration are unlikely to have the poor prognosis associated with large ulcerating carcinomas (but do have increased likelihood of lymph node metastases)
    ▪ Satellite skin nodules: Invasive carcinoma in skin not contiguous with the main carcinoma; generally due to extensive lymph-vascular invasion
    ▪ Edema (including peau d'orange) is not sufficient for diagnosis of inflammatory carcinoma; this finding cannot be determined in surgical excisions and is rarely used for staging
  ○ T4c: Features of both T4a and T4b
  ○ T4d: Inflammatory carcinoma
    ▪ Defined by clinical sign of diffuse erythema and edema (peau d'orange) involving 1/3 or more of skin of the breast
    ▪ Correlates with a type of carcinoma characterized by extensive dermal lymph-vascular invasion
    ▪ Pathologic finding of dermal lymph-vascular invasion has a poor prognosis, but in absence of clinical signs is insufficient for classification as inflammatory carcinoma

Additional Pathologic Prognostic Factors

- Important for prognosis but not currently incorporated into AJCC staging
- **Histologic grade**
  ○ Used to stratify breast cancer patients into favorable (well-differentiated) and less favorable (poorly differentiated) outcome groups
  ○ A number of different breast cancer grading systems have been clinically validated
  ○ Nottingham combined histologic grade (Elston-Ellis modification of Scarff-Bloom-Richardson grading system) is recommended by the College of American Pathologists, the American Joint Commission on Cancer, and the European Working Group on Breast Screening Pathology
    ▪ Grade is based on evaluation of glandular (acinar)/tubular differentiation, nuclear score, and mitotic score
    ▪ Adherence to strict morphologic criteria is needed for reproducibility so that grade is reliably useful as a prognostic factor
  ○ Grade 2 cancers may be a mixture of grade 1 and 3 cancers
    ▪ Proliferative rate may be used to reclassify grade 2 cancers
  ○ Extensive necrosis (> 1 high-power field) identifies grade 3 cancers with a particularly poor prognosis
    ▪ Necrosis is predictive of a good response to chemotherapy
- **Lymph-vascular invasion (LVI)**
  ○ Peritumoral LVI has prognostic significance for risk of local and distant recurrence

- Recurrence for stage I disease with LVI is ~ 38% compared with 22% in its absence
  ○ Closely associated with lymph node metastases but is an independent factor
    ▪ Prognosis is diminished if both LVI and nodal metastases are present
  ○ Currently unnecessary to distinguish small capillaries from lymphatics using IHC markers
    ▪ Both have prognostic significance
- **Special histologic types of invasive carcinoma**
  ○ Some histologic types of breast cancer have a generally better prognosis compared with carcinomas of no special type ("ductal carcinomas")
  ○ Strict criteria in diagnosis of these special types of breast cancer are important to maintain prognostic significance
    ▪ Should fulfill criteria in > 90% of the carcinoma
  ○ Group with a better prognosis, as most are associated with being well to moderately differentiated, ER/PR positive, and HER2 negative
    ▪ Tubular carcinoma, tubulolobular carcinoma, mucinous (colloid) carcinoma, papillary carcinoma, cribriform carcinoma, lobular carcinoma
  ○ Group with a favorable prognosis due to unknown biologic reasons; carcinomas in this group are important to recognize as they fall within the triple negative subset of breast cancers
    ▪ Medullary carcinoma, adenoid cystic carcinoma, low-grade adenosquamous carcinoma, secretory carcinoma
  ○ Other special types of breast carcinoma have an unfavorable prognosis
    ▪ Metaplastic carcinoma, invasive micropapillary carcinoma
- **ER and PR expression**
  ○ Both prognostic and predictive factors
    ▪ Weak prognostic effect is seen in absence of hormonal therapy
    ▪ Any hormone receptor expression is associated with better survival than if no expression is present (defined as immunoreactivity in < 1% of cells)
  ○ Follow-up studies suggest that pure prognostic effect of ER and PR may not persist long-term
    ▪ ER and PR may predict for more indolent tumors with longer time to recurrence
  ○ ER and PR expression are powerful predictive factors for patients likely to benefit from endocrine therapy
  ○ ER-positive/PR-negative carcinomas are more likely to be grade 2 or 3, be larger, have a higher proliferative rate, and have a higher recurrence score by Oncotype DX (Genomic Health; Redwood City, CA)
    ▪ Disease-free survival and overall survival are lower
- **HER2 expression**
  ○ Overexpression is associated with a worse prognosis and more aggressive disease
  ○ HER2 may have a predictive role for response to anthracycline-based chemotherapy
  ○ HER2-targeted therapy is available

INTRODUCTION: PROGNOSTIC AND PREDICTIVE FACTORS

- Herceptin is humanized monoclonal antibody against extracellular portion of HER2 receptor
- Lapatinib is dual tyrosine kinase inhibitor that interrupts HER2 growth receptor pathway
  - HER2 overexpression by IHC or FISH is predictive factor for benefit from HER2-targeted therapy
- **Proliferation**
  - Proliferative rate of breast cancer is associated with overall survival and disease-free survival
  - Highly proliferative carcinomas are associated with better response to chemotherapy
  - Proliferation can be measured in variety of ways
    - Mitotic count: Included as part of histologic grade
    - Immunohistochemical markers including Ki-67 (MIB-1), cyclin-D, cyclin-E, p27, p21
    - S-phase fraction by flow cytometry
    - Gene expression profiling: mRNA levels of proliferation-related genes may be increased
  - Good correlation between different methods
    - ~ 50% of carcinomas have low proliferation by any measure, and ~ 50% have higher rates of proliferation
  - Proliferative rates are a continuum and are not bimodal
    - Cut-off point for "low" and "high" rates may be difficult to define
  - Optimal method to measure proliferation and to use results for clinical management has not yet been determined
- **Gene expression profiling**
  - Multiple groups have identified expression of sets of genes that are correlated with prognosis
    - Examples include Oncotype DX, MammaPrint (Agendia; Irvine, CA), and the Rotterdam signature
  - Most useful for ER-positive, HER-negative cancers
    - Majority of ER-negative &/or HER2-positive cancers would be classified as high risk
  - All identified profiles include genes related to proliferation
    - Proliferation appears to be strongest prognostic factor for ER-positive cancers
    - Unclear whether profiling adds clinically significant information after proliferation has been taken into account
  - This technique may be more useful to determine profiles predicting response to specific therapeutic agents

Methods of Combining Prognostic Factors

- Prognostic indices for individual patients may be obtained by combining multiple prognostic factors
  - Each factor is weighted according to its prognostic importance
- **Nottingham Prognostic Index (NPI)**
  - Includes lymph node status, tumor size, and grade
    - NPI = 0.2 x tumor size (cm) + lymph node status + grade (1, 2, or 3)
    - Lymph node status: 1 = node negative; 2 = 1-3 positive nodes; 3 = 4 or more positive nodes
  - 5 prognostic groups can be identified using scores with different 5-, 10-, and 15-year survivals
    - Excellent (scores < 2.41): 97%, 91%, 84%

- Good (2.41-3.41): 93%, 82%, 74%
- Moderate I (3.41-4.4): 85%, 73%, 63%
- Moderate II (4.41-5.4): 75%, 55%, 46%
- Poor (> 5.4): 42%, 26%, 18%
- **Flanagan Prognostic Index**
  - Uses nuclear grade, mitotic count, ER (H-score), PR (H-score), HER2
    - RS = 13.424 + 5.420 (nuclear grade) + 5.538 (mitotic count) - 0.045 (ER H-score) - 0.030 (PR H-score) + 9.486 (HER2)
  - Predicts Oncotype DX recurrence score with R^2 = 0.66
  - Including tubule formation, patient age, or tumor size did not improve results
- **Tang Prognostic Index**
  - Uses tubule formation, mitotic rate, PR, HER2, luminal A, and luminal B
    - Recurrence score (RS) = 17.489 + 2.071 (tubule formation) + 2.926 (mitosis) - 2.408 (PR) - 1.061 (HER2) + 7.051 (luminal A) + 29.172 (luminal B)
    - Luminal A = ER positive/HER2 negative
    - Luminal B = ER positive/HER2 positive
    - HER2 and triple negative carcinomas were not included in group tested
    - Mitosis = score (1, 2, 3)
    - PR = Allred score (0, 2, 3, 4, 5, 6, 7, 8)
    - HER2 = score (0, 1, 2, 3)
  - Correlates with Oncotype DX recurrence score with R^2 = 0.65
- **Geradts Prognostic Index (Breast Cancer Prognostic Score [BCPS])**
  - Includes ER, PR, HER2, and the 3 components of tumor grade
    - BCPS = 40.0 - 5.3 (ER Allred score) - 2.7 (PR Allred score) + 13.0 (HER2 score) + 2.3 (tubule score) + 2.4 (nuclear score) + 6.5 (mitotic score)
    - HER2 score (for either IHC or FISH): 1 = negative; 2 = equivocal; 3 = overexpressed
  - Correlates with Oncotype DX recurrence score with R^2 = 0.42
    - 56% of cases were given same low/intermediate/high risk classification
- **IHC4 (Cuzick)**
  - Includes ER, PR, Ki-67, and HER2
  - Details are not yet published (Cuzick J et al: Cancer Res. 69(24 Suppl) a74, 2009 [abstract])
  - Correlates well with Oncotype DX recurrence score
- **Eden Prognostic Index**
  - Includes grade, tumor size, patient age, angioinvasion, ER (% of cells), PR (% of cells), and lymphocytic infiltrate
    - F = 1 (grade) + 0.51 (size in cm) - 0.14 (age in years) + 1.2 (angioinvasion status) - 0.011 (ER) - 0.00026 (PR) - 0.34 (lymphocytic infiltrate) + 3.0
  - F > 0 identifies patients with a poor prognosis
  - Index was developed using a group of node-negative patients; therefore, node status could not be included
  - Index is not predictive for ER-negative cancers
  - Provides similar results to the Amsterdam 70-gene signature (MammaPrint)
- **Adjuvant! Online**

INTRODUCTION: PROGNOSTIC AND PREDICTIVE FACTORS

Summary of Breast Cancer Prognostic and Predictive Factors

Feature	Prognostic	Predictive	Comment
Lymph node metastasis	+++	+/-	Most significant prognostic indicator of disease recurrence and survival for patients without distant metastases; node-positive patients usually receive systemic therapy
Tumor size	+++	+/-	2nd most important prognostic factor and is routinely used to make decisions on adjuvant treatment (tumors > 1-2 cm warrant consideration of adjuvant therapy, distant recurrence rate may be > 20%)
AJCC stage	+++	+/-	Important to compare groups of patients over time and in different locations as well as to identify similar patients for clinical trials
Histologic grade	++	+/-	Particularly important for clinical decisions on adjuvant treatment for node-negative patients with borderline tumor size
Lymph-vascular invasion	++	+/-	Primarily used to make adjuvant treatment decisions for lymph node-negative patients with borderline tumor sizes
Special histologic types	++	+/-	Special histologic types of carcinoma may have better or worse prognosis than carcinomas of no special type ("ductal" carcinomas)
ER, PR	+/-	+++	ER and PR expression are weakly prognostic but are strongly predictive for patient benefit from endocrine therapy
HER2	+	+++	HER2 overexpression is both a prognostic indicator of aggressive disease and predictive for response from HER2-targeted therapy
Proliferation	+++	+++	Carcinomas with high proliferative rate have worse prognosis but are more likely to respond to chemotherapy
Gene expression profiling	+++	++	Most applicable for ER-positive, HER2-negative carcinomas

○ Includes patient age, menopausal status, comorbidities, tumor size (cm), number of positive nodes, ER (positive or negative), and grade

○ Web-based tool is available at www.adjuvantonline.com

○ Predicts 10-year breast cancer survival and efficacy of adjuvant therapy

○ Should not be used for tubular carcinoma, papillary carcinoma, medullary carcinoma, or inflammatory carcinoma

○ Underestimates survival in women younger than age 40 and overestimates survival for women with LVI

• **St. Gallen Consensus Criteria (2009)**

○ Criteria have changed over time with each successive conference

○ High-risk groups (patients for whom chemotherapy would be recommended)

■ HER2-positive cancers: Chemotherapy is recommended for all patients but may not be required if cancer is < 1 cm, nodes are negative, and no LVI is present

■ Triple negative cancers: Chemotherapy is recommended for all patients but may not be required if cancer is < 1 cm, nodes are negative, no LVI is present, and cancer is not medullary carcinoma, apocrine carcinoma, or adenoid cystic carcinoma

■ ER-positive, HER2-negative cancers: Chemotherapy is recommended for all patients with cancers with lower ER and PR levels, grade 3, high proliferation (e.g., > 30% Ki-67 positive cells), 4 or more positive nodes, extensive LVI, tumor size > 5 cm, or high scores on multigene assays

○ Low-risk group for ER-positive, HER2-negative carcinomas

■ Endocrine therapy alone might be considered for cancers with higher ER and PR levels (> 50%), grade 1, low proliferation (e.g., ≤ 15% Ki-67 positive cells), negative nodes, LVI not extensive, ≤ 2 cm, or low score on multigene assays

SELECTED REFERENCES

1. Duraker N et al: The prognosis of tumors with only microscopic skin involvement without clinical T4b signs is significantly better than T4b tumors in breast carcinoma. Breast J. 17(1):47-55, 2011
2. Weaver DL et al: Effect of occult metastases on survival in node-negative breast cancer. N Engl J Med. 364(5):412-21, 2011
3. Geradts J et al: The oncotype DX recurrence score is correlated with a composite index including routinely reported pathobiologic features. Cancer Invest. 28(9):969-77, 2010
4. Tang P et al: A lower Allred score for progesterone receptor is strongly associated with a higher recurrence score of 21-gene assay in breast cancer. Cancer Invest. 28(9):978-82, 2010
5. Weigelt B et al: Molecular profiling currently offers no more than tumour morphology and basic immunohistochemistry. Breast Cancer Res. 12 Suppl 4:S5, 2010
6. Garassino I et al: Outcome of T1N0M0 breast cancer in relation to St. Gallen risk assignment criteria for adjuvant therapy. Breast. 18(4):263-6, 2009
7. Gwin K et al: Complementary value of the Ki-67 proliferation index to the oncotype DX recurrence score. Int J Surg Pathol. 17(4):303-10, 2009
8. Harms K et al: Prognosis of women with pT4b breast cancer: the significance of this category in the TNM system. Eur J Surg Oncol. 35(1):38-42, 2009
9. Koscielny S et al: Impact of tumour size on axillary involvement and distant dissemination in breast cancer. Br J Cancer. 101(6):902-7, 2009
10. Natarajan L et al: Time-varying effects of prognostic factors associated with disease-free survival in breast cancer. Am J Epidemiol. 169(12):1463-70, 2009
11. Flanagan MB et al: Histopathologic variables predict Oncotype DX recurrence score. Mod Pathol. 21(10):1255-61, 2008

Prognostic Factors Used in AJCC Staging

IV

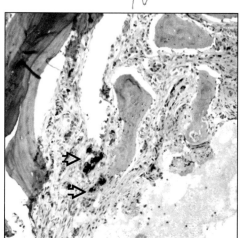

T4a

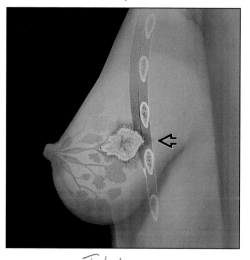

(Left) Patients who present with distant metastases are classified as having stage IV disease and have a particularly poor prognosis. The most common site of metastasis is to the bone, and IHC for markers such as mammoglobin ⊡ *can be used to identify small tumor deposits. (Right) Carcinomas that invade through the pectoralis muscles into the chest wall* ⊡ *are classified as T4a. If the carcinoma only invades into the pectoralis, T classification is based on tumor size.*

T4b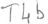

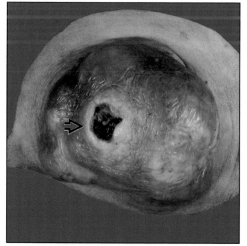

T4b

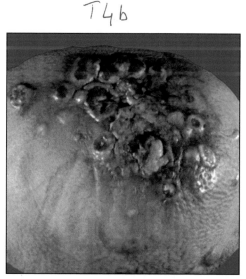

(Left) Skin ulceration ⊡ *is typically associated with very large locally advanced carcinomas and is classified as T4b. Ulceration due to prior surgical procedures or Paget disease of the nipple is not included. (Right) Satellite skin nodules are clinically apparent tumor deposits located at some distance from the primary carcinoma (i.e., not due to direct extension) and are classified as T4b. They are usually associated with dermal LVI and are a form of intramammary metastasis.*

T4d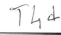

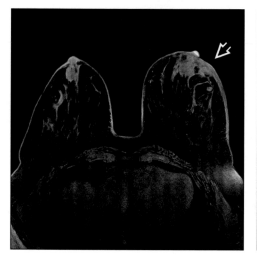

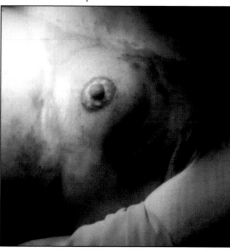

(Left) This carcinoma is associated with marked skin edema ⊡ *but did not have the clinical signs of inflammatory carcinoma. Although skin edema is included in the definition of T4b, it cannot be evaluated in surgical specimens and is rarely used for staging. (Right) Inflammatory carcinoma is defined by the presence of erythema and edema involving at least 1/3 of the breast. It is classified as T4d. The clinical appearance is due to extensive dermal LVI plugging the vasculature.*

Additional Prognostic Factors

(Left) Histologic grade incorporates 3 features. This well-differentiated carcinoma has good tubule formation, low nuclear grade ⟶, and a low mitotic index. These cancers are generally ER/PR positive, slow growing, and have an excellent prognosis. *(Right)* This poorly differentiated carcinoma grows as sheets of cells, has high-grade nuclei, and has a brisk mitotic rate ⟹. This type of carcinoma generally has a poor prognosis although a subset will respond well to chemotherapy.

LG BR-PR ⊕

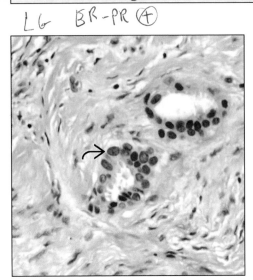

HG

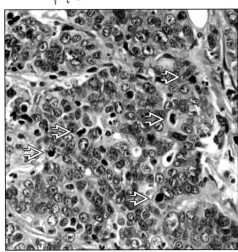

(Left) Lymph-vascular invasion ⟶ is associated with increased likelihood of lymph node involvement as well as disease recurrence. Prognosis is diminished if both LVI and nodal metastases are present. *(Right)* Inflammatory carcinoma presents clinically with skin edema (peau d'orange) and breast swelling as a result of tumor emboli within dermal lymphatics ⟶ and is associated with a very poor prognosis. The carcinomas are often diffusely invasive and do not form a palpable mass.

LVI

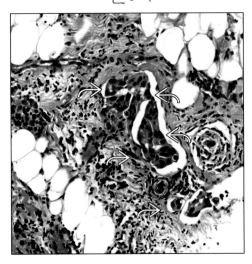

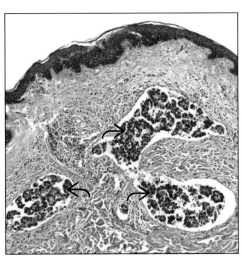

(Left) Special histologic types of invasive breast cancer have prognostic significance. Tubular carcinoma, as seen here, has an excellent prognosis. *(Right)* Some special histologic types of carcinoma have a prognosis that would not be predicted by other features. For example, adenoid cystic carcinomas of the breast have a very favorable prognosis although these cancers are ER/PR- and HER2-negative and would score as high-risk carcinomas by gene expression profiling.

Tubular

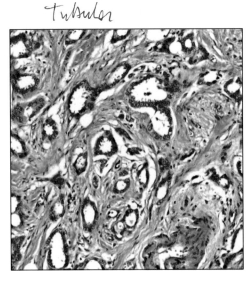

ACCs

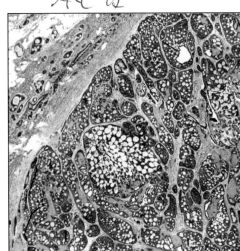

INTRODUCTION: PROGNOSTIC AND PREDICTIVE FACTORS

Predictive Factors

ER ⊕

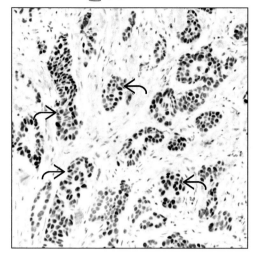

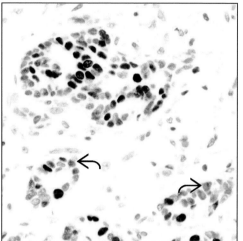

(Left) ER expression by invasive cancers ➔ is weakly prognostic and associated with a more indolent clinical course of disease without adjuvant treatment. ER expression is strongly predictive for a clinical benefit from adjuvant endocrine therapy. *(Right)* Carcinomas with a lower level of ER expression showing only moderate to weak staining in a few cells ➔ often have a higher proliferative rate and may benefit from the addition of chemotherapy to adjuvant hormonal treatment.

HER 2 ⊕

Necrosi)

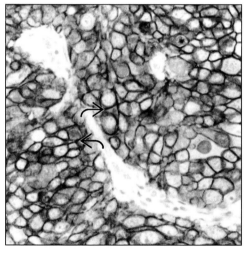

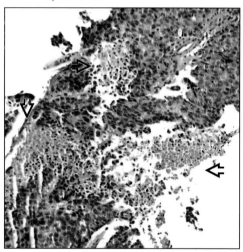

(Left) This carcinoma shows the characteristic circumferential "chicken wire" membrane staining of HER2(+) breast cancer ➔. HER2 overexpression is associated with a more aggressive clinical course, younger age at presentation, and, most important, it predicts benefit from HER2-targeted therapies. *(Right)* Extensive necrosis ➔ in a poorly differentiated carcinoma is associated with a worse prognosis but is also predictive of a greater likelihood of response to chemotherapy.

Mitoses

Ki 67

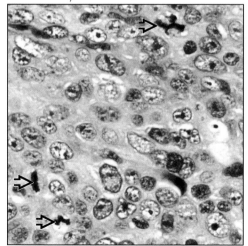

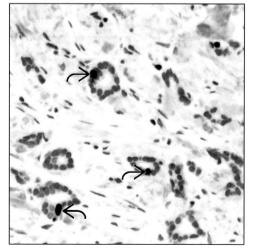

(Left) Proliferation is an important prognostic factor and can be determined using several different methods. The enumeration of mitoses in cancers ➔ is used for histologic grading and correlates well with other measures of proliferation. *(Right)* Ki-67 (MIB-1) is often used as a measure of proliferation. This well-differentiated carcinoma shows < 5% positive cells ➔, which would predict for little if any benefit from adjuvant chemotherapy added to hormonal therapy.

SIZE AND MULTIPLE FOCI

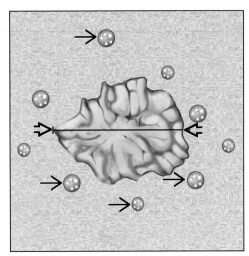

Size is a very important prognostic factor and refers to the greatest linear dimension of an invasive carcinoma ➡. Surrounding carcinoma in situ ➡ is not included in the measurement.

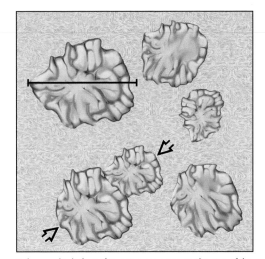

When multiple foci of invasion are present, the size of the largest carcinoma is used for AJCC T classification ➡. The modifier "m" is added to indicate the presence of multiple carcinomas.

INTRODUCTION

Size of Invasive Cancer

- Important independent prognostic factor for both node-negative and node-positive patients
  - Size is defined as greatest linear dimension of an invasive carcinoma
  - Adjacent carcinoma in situ is not included in determination of size
- Cancers grow at very different rates
  - Some cancers grow very slowly or appear stable in size for many years
    - Typically well-differentiated ER positive cancers
  - Other cancers grow rapidly
    - Most common in young women
    - In older women, may be detected as "interval cancers": Cancers detected by palpation in time between mammographic screening
    - Typically poorly differentiated ER negative cancers
- Typical size of cancers detected by palpation is 2-3 cm
  - Screening by patient self breast examination does not decrease number of breast cancer deaths
  - Suggests that by the time a carcinoma is palpable, carcinomas capable of metastasizing will have already done so
- Nonpalpable invasive carcinomas detected by screening are much smaller in size
  - Average size of carcinomas associated with a mammographic density is about 1 cm
  - Average size of carcinomas detected as mammographic calcifications (without an evident mass) is 0.6 cm
  - More often well differentiated, tubular type, and ER positive
  - Screen-detected cancers have better prognosis than palpable cancers of same size
- Important to carefully identify node-negative carcinomas ≤ 1 cm in size

- These patients have an excellent prognosis and may not require systemic therapy
  - Majority of patients with carcinomas > 1 cm will be offered systemic therapy
- Lymph node metastases are closely correlated with size
  - Likelihood of nodal metastases increases rapidly from cancer size 0-4 cm and then levels off at ~ 70-90%
  - Some very large carcinomas do not metastasize to axillary lymph nodes
    - May metastasize using blood vessels or via lymphatics to internal mammary nodes
    - Some carcinomas reach very large size without metastasis, likely due to as yet unidentified biologic factors

Multiple Invasive Cancers

- 10-40% of patients have more than 1 focus of invasive carcinoma in same breast at time of diagnosis
  - Incidence increases with more extensive imaging workup (including MRI) &/or detailed pathologic evaluation
    - MRI finds additional foci of cancer in 10-30% of patients
- Patients with multiple cancers are more likely to have family history of breast carcinoma, have lobular carcinomas, and are at greater risk for contralateral carcinoma
- Terms "multifocal" and "multicentric" have been used to describe cases of multiple cancers but have been defined in different ways
  - Do not always specify whether carcinoma in situ is included in the definition
  - Some definitions only include grossly identified invasive carcinomas, whereas others include microscopic carcinomas
- Multifocal is generally defined as > 1 focus of invasive carcinoma within 1 quadrant
  - May refer to carcinomas in "close proximity"

SIZE AND MULTIPLE FOCI

- ○ Has also been used for any case with 2 or more foci
- Multicentric has multiple definitions
  - ○ ≥ 2 foci in different quadrants of breast
  - ○ ≥ 2 foci a certain distance apart, which can be from 2-5 cm
  - ○ Foci involving different ductal systems
  - ○ ≥ 2 biologically independent cancers
- "Multicentric" and "multifocal" are not useful terms unless specifically defined
  - ○ Difficult to apply to most pathology specimens
  - ○ Do not address the underlying biology responsible for the multiple foci of invasion
- Multiple invasive cancers are associated with greater incidence of lymph node metastases
  - ○ Each cancer has an independent risk of metastasis; thus, overall risk is increased
  - ○ Multiple foci of invasion do not diminish survival as compared to a single focus of invasion, if adjusted for number of lymph node metastases
- 5 etiologies for multiple foci of invasion
  - ○ **Extensive DCIS**
    - Most common setting in which multiple invasive carcinomas arise
    - Carcinomas are usually very similar to each other with respect to grade, histologic type, and tumor markers
    - In unusual cases, there is marked heterogeneity in underlying DCIS leading to heterogeneity in associated invasive carcinomas
    - HER2 positive carcinomas are more commonly associated with extensive DCIS with multiple foci of invasion
  - ○ **Invasive carcinoma with extensive lymph-vascular invasion (LVI) and intramammary metastases**
    - Usually a single large carcinoma associated with multiple smaller carcinomas arising from foci of LVI
    - Carcinomas arise from same malignant clone of cells and are usually identical in grade, histologic type, and tumor markers
  - ○ **Biologically separate carcinomas**
    - Rare occurrence
    - Cancers are usually widely separated and not associated with same area of DCIS
    - Carcinomas may differ in grade, histologic type, and tumor markers
    - Patients with germline mutations may have multiple synchronous carcinomas; in these women, carcinomas may be similar as they share same mutation
  - ○ **Carcinomas after neoadjuvant chemotherapy**
    - After a marked response, residual carcinoma is often present as multiple foci scattered over a fibrotic tumor bed
    - Extent of invasive carcinoma can be difficult to quantify by size
    - Size of largest contiguous focus is used for AJCC T classification
    - Cellularity of carcinoma averaged over tumor bed is used in many systems for classifying response to treatment
  - ○ **Carcinomas with satellite foci**
    - Usually seen as a large central carcinoma surrounded by multiple smaller satellite carcinomas within a few mm
    - Likely due to infiltration along fibrovascular septae resulting in a false impression of separate carcinomas in 2 dimensions
    - Most commonly seen with invasive lobular carcinomas

METHODS OF EVALUATION

Breast Imaging: Size
- Imaging can be very helpful in determining size of carcinomas in some situations
  - ○ Small cancers that have previously undergone needle biopsy can be difficult to evaluate
    - Overestimates can occur if biopsy sites are included
    - Underestimates can occur if a substantial portion of the carcinoma has been removed
- Size prior to core needle biopsy may be more accurate than residual size in excisional specimen
- Ultrasound, in general, provides measurement closest to size by gross examination
- MRI may overestimate size by including adjacent DCIS or benign enhancing tissue

Breast Imaging: Number of Foci
- Imaging often shows multiple separate densities that correlate with multiple invasive carcinomas
- Size and distance between carcinomas can sometimes be determined best by imaging

Gross Examination: Size
- Majority of carcinomas are associated with a desmoplastic response and will be hard to palpation
  - ○ Most carcinomas are white or tan and blend in with normal fibrous breast stroma
    - Visual appearances can be misleading and result in overestimating size
  - ○ Size by palpation is more accurate
    - Most carcinomas have a distinct edge or shelf at junction with adjacent breast stroma
    - Edges of carcinoma can be pinched between 2 fingers to determine extent of invasive component
- Minority of carcinomas diffusely invade in fibroadipose tissue and it may be difficult to determine extent grossly
  - ○ Submitting cassettes in an organized fashion (e.g., 1 every cm) allows microscopic mapping of carcinoma

Gross Examination: Number of Foci
- Helpful to determine the number and spatial relationship of masses by imaging prior to processing the specimen
- Size of each gross mass and its relationship (distance from) other masses, as well as from margins, should be recorded
- Tissue between separate masses should be submitted to evaluate whether or not they represent portions of a single large carcinoma

Microscopic Examination: Size

- Gross size should always be confirmed microscopically
  - Some cancers, particularly lobular carcinomas, have diffusely invasive pattern and may be larger than apparent on gross examination
  - Some patients have dense stroma and borders of cancer may be difficult to determine
  - Prior core needle biopsy sites can result in stromal fibrosis and inflammation that can make tumor size difficult to measure
  - Size can only be determined by measuring from a glass slide in small (generally < 1 cm) carcinomas

Microscopic Examination: Number of Foci

- Microscopic examination of tissue between 2 grossly apparent cancers is useful to determine if 1 or 2 separate cancers are present
- Foci of invasion identified microscopically can only be identified as separate areas of invasion if tissue is designated as being away from grossly apparent carcinomas

DIFFICULT SPECIMENS

Core Needle Biopsy Followed by Excision

- Size of invasive carcinoma on core needle biopsy gives lower limit of the size of cancer
  - In majority of cases, size of cancer in excision will be larger
  - However, if size in excision is smaller, size on core should be used for T classification
  - Size on core can be helpful to evaluate reliability of negative results on core for ER, PR, or HER2
    - If size on core is very small compared to entire cancer, repeat studies on excision may be helpful
- Size of cancer in core should not be added to size in excision
  - Ideally, core site will pierce center of cancer and size can be determined grossly &/or microscopically
  - If residual carcinoma is only present at 1 side of a biopsy cavity, pre-core needle biopsy size will be difficult to determine
  - In some cases, pre-core needle biopsy size by imaging may be best determination of size

Cancer Transected by Excision

- It is unusual for a palpable carcinoma to be transected by surgeon
- Nonpalpable carcinomas (e.g., small or diffusely invading) may be transected
  - Extensive carcinoma will be present at margin
  - Focal invasive carcinoma at margin does not usually correlate with residual invasive carcinoma as biopsy cavity in patient is usually cauterized for several mm
- Adding sizes of a transected carcinoma in 2 specimens may overestimate actual size
  - Correlation with imaging studies may be helpful to determine most likely actual size
  - Minimal and maximal tumor sizes can be estimated based on 2 sections of cancer

Diffusely Invasive Carcinomas

- Some carcinomas have diffusely invasive pattern and either do not form a palpable mass or form an ill-defined mass
  - Subset of invasive lobular carcinomas can have appearance of innumerable small invasive foci throughout a specimen
  - Carcinomas associated with clinical presentation of inflammatory carcinoma are often difficult to define grossly
- Size may not be available from imaging or gross examination
- Estimates of size may be provided
  - Number of blocks with invasive carcinoma
  - Number of foci
    - Minimal size estimate based on size of the largest contiguous focus
  - Size based on involvement of opposing margins

REPORTING CRITERIA

Size

- Size for AJCC T classification is largest focus of invasive carcinoma
  - Sizes of multiple carcinomas should not be added together
- When it is not possible to provide a specific size, a note explaining reason for uncertainty is helpful
  - Estimate of smallest &/or largest possible size is often helpful
- Correlation with imaging may be suggested if studies are not available to pathologist

Multiple Cancers

- Report the presence, number, and size of multiple foci of invasion
  - Modifier "m" is used to signify that multiple foci of invasive carcinoma are present; the number of foci can also be indicated
- Grade and histologic type should be reported for each focus if different
- Distance between foci should be reported
- Report findings that could be etiology of the multiple cancers
  - Extensive carcinoma in situ, lymph-vascular invasion, satellite foci, or biologically separate carcinomas

SELECTED REFERENCES

1. Weissenbacher TM et al: Multicentric and multifocal versus unifocal breast cancer: is the tumor-node-metastasis classification justified? Breast Cancer Res Treat. 122(1):27-34, 2010
2. Yerushalmi R et al: Does multicentric/multifocal breast cancer differ from unifocal breast cancer? An analysis of survival and contralateral breast cancer incidence. Breast Cancer Res Treat. 117(2):365-70, 2009

SIZE AND MULTIPLE FOCI

Difficulties in Classification of Multiple Carcinomas

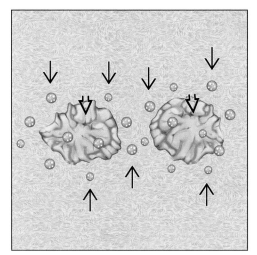

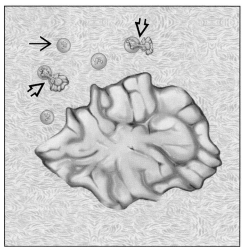

(Left) The most common etiology for multiple invasive carcinomas ⊋ is an area of extensive carcinoma in situ ⊅ associated with more than 1 area of invasion. The invasive carcinomas are generally similar in histologic type, grade, and tumor markers. *(Right)* Some carcinomas are associated with extensive lymph-vascular invasion ⊅. These foci can give rise to smaller foci of invasion (intramammary metastases) ⊋ that are identical in appearance to the primary carcinoma.

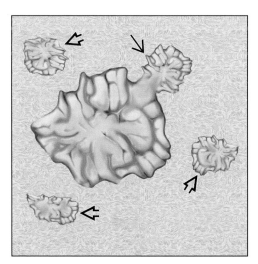

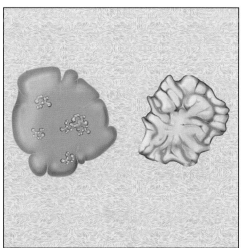

(Left) Smaller satellite foci ⊋ are sometimes seen around the border of an invasive carcinoma. The satellite foci are likely connected to the main carcinoma in another plane of section ⊅ via invasion down fibrovascular septae. *(Right)* Rarely, a patient may have 2 biologically independent carcinomas. They may differ in histologic type, grade, and tumor markers. The carcinomas are not associated with the same area of carcinoma in situ and are usually located far apart.

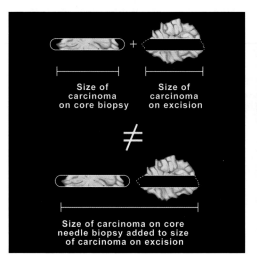

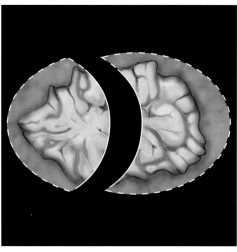

(Left) Core needle biopsies can complicate the determination of size. The size in the core should not be added to the size of the carcinoma in the excision. In some cases, the pre-biopsy imaging size may provide the best estimate of actual size. *(Right)* Invasive carcinomas, particularly if diffusely invasive, may be transected during excision and extensively involve the margins. This complicates size determination, as adding together the size in each specimen can overestimate size.

AJCC T4 CARCINOMAS (CHEST WALL OR SKIN INVOLVEMENT)

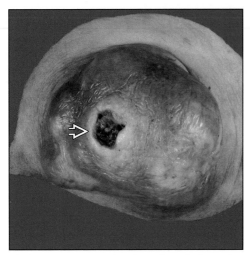

This large cancer, occupying almost the entire breast, has caused ulceration of the skin and nipple ➪. In the past, this was the typical type of cancer that would be classified as AJCC T4b.

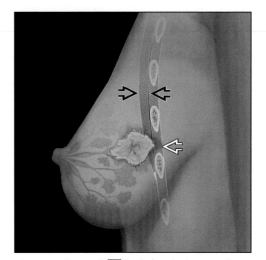

The pectoralis muscle ➪ lies below the breast and may be invaded by deep-seated cancers. However, a cancer must penetrate beyond this muscle into the chest wall ➪ in order to be classified as T4a.

TERMINOLOGY

Definitions
- Carcinomas with skin or chest wall involvement classified as T4 by AJCC/UICC
  - Chest wall involvement (T4a)
    - Carcinoma invading into skeletal muscle of chest wall beyond pectoralis muscle
  - Skin involvement (T4b)
    - Invasion into skin with ulceration
    - Satellite skin nodules
    - Skin edema or peau d'orange ("skin of an orange"): Due to tethering of the skin by Cooper's ligaments causing pitting of the swollen skin
  - Inflammatory breast carcinoma (T4d)
    - Superficial dermal lymphatic involvement with erythema and swelling (peau d'orange)
    - Classified as T4d by AJCC/UICC
- Term "locally advanced breast carcinoma"
  - Includes all T4 tumors and some large T3 carcinomas (AJCC stages IIIA and IIIB)

ETIOLOGY/PATHOGENESIS

Etiology
- Incidence of carcinomas with noninflammatory chest wall and skin invasion (T4a, b, c) increases with age
  - Delays in diagnosis in older patients may allow carcinomas to reach larger sizes
  - Do not have biologic features of increased aggressiveness
- Incidence of inflammatory carcinomas (T4d) increases to age 50 and then levels off
  - More likely to be poorly differentiated and hormone receptor negative
  - Likely have specific biological profile that promotes early lymph-vascular dissemination

EPIDEMIOLOGY

Incidence
- Inflammatory carcinomas: 1-5% of breast carcinomas
- T4b carcinomas: Approximately 1% of carcinomas
- T4a and T4c carcinomas exceedingly rare (< 1%)
- Carcinomas with skin involvement but not classified as T4 make up 2-3% of carcinomas

Age Range
- T4a, b, c: Mean age is 10 years older than usual for women with breast carcinoma (i.e., 70s rather than 60s)
- T4d: Occurs in women at younger mean age (40s to 50s)

CLINICAL IMPLICATIONS

Prognosis
- Patients whose prognosis was so poor that surgery was not beneficial were originally classified as having T4 cancers
  - Majority of these patients had very large bulky local disease
- With current chemotherapy and radiotherapy, patients with carcinomas that respond to treatment may become candidates for surgery
  - Smaller carcinomas with only skin ulceration have better prognosis than other T4 carcinomas

MACROSCOPIC FINDINGS

Specimen Handling
- Skin
  - If skin invasion, carcinoma will be fixed to skin
  - Take sections of carcinoma closest to skin and any skin ulceration

AJCC T4 CARCINOMAS (CHEST WALL OR SKIN INVOLVEMENT)

- ○ If satellite skin lesions are present, take sections to demonstrate there is no direct connection with main carcinoma
- Chest wall
  - ○ Deep margin of specimens should be examined to determine if muscle is present
    - ▪ In majority of cases, any muscle present will be pectoralis (chest wall invasion does not include this muscle)
    - ▪ Take sections to demonstrate relationship of carcinoma to muscle
  - ○ If true chest wall invasion, ribs and serratus muscle will be resected
    - ▪ Bones should be examined for direct invasion
- Inflammatory carcinoma
  - ○ Majority of patients will have received neoadjuvant chemotherapy
  - ○ May be difficult to determine location and extent as these carcinomas are typically diffusely invasive
  - ○ If clip marks prior biopsy site, this should be found and sampled
  - ○ In cases without gross or radiologic correlate, sections taken every cm across specimen, including samples of skin, may be necessary

MICROSCOPIC FINDINGS

T4a: Extension to Chest Wall

- Carcinoma must invade into serratus muscle between ribs
- Correlation with radiologic findings may be necessary to demonstrate true chest wall invasion
- Specimens will typically contain portions of ribs
  - ○ Ribs should be radiographed and sectioned to determine if carcinoma has invaded into bone

T4b: Ulceration of Skin

- Carcinoma invades into and through skin causing ulceration
- Invasion into epidermis without ulceration is not included
- Associated Paget disease with erosion is not included
- Carcinomas that would otherwise be classified as stage I or II have better prognosis compared to the typically very large carcinomas with this finding

T4b: Satellite Skin Nodules

- Must be detected clinically
  - ○ Microscopic satellite skin nodules are not classified as T4b
- Skin involvement cannot be due to direct invasion by main carcinoma
- Nodules are generally associated with dermal lymph-vascular invasion and are a form of intramammary metastasis

T4b: Edema of Skin

- Skin edema (peau d'orange) can be detected clinically or radiographically
- Edema cannot be reliably identified either grossly or microscopically in surgical specimens
- Criterion is rarely used for classifying carcinoma as T4

T4c: T4a and T4b

- Includes carcinomas with both chest wall and skin invasion

T4d: Inflammatory Carcinoma

- Defined by clinical appearance of characteristic edema and erythema involving at least 1/3 of breast
  - ○ These findings cannot be assessed reliably in surgical specimens
- Pathologic correlate is dermal lymph-vascular invasion
  - ○ Dermal lymph-vascular invasion without clinical findings is insufficient for classification as T4d

DIFFERENTIAL DIAGNOSIS

Chest Wall Invasion Not Classified as T4

- Carcinoma invading into pectoralis muscle
  - ○ Surgically resectable with removal of this muscle
  - ○ Removal of deeper muscles requires chest wall excision including ribs

Skin Involvement Not Classified as T4

- Carcinoma directly invading into skin without ulceration
  - ○ Classified according to size
  - ○ Skin invasion is associated with 2x higher frequency of lymph node metastases
    - ▪ May be due to access to greater number of lymphatics in skin
    - ▪ However, survival at 10 years is similar for size-matched carcinomas with or without skin invasion
- Paget disease of nipple
  - ○ Caused by DCIS involving nipple skin
  - ○ Skin erosion can occur with extensive skin involvement
  - ○ Not considered skin ulceration that would be classified as T4b
- Edema due to inflammation
  - ○ Patients may develop inflammatory conditions of breast after surgical procedures (e.g., infections)
  - ○ Edema due to true inflammation is not a criterion for classification as T4
- Dermal lymph-vascular invasion without clinical signs of inflammatory carcinoma
  - ○ Poor prognostic finding but not sufficient for classification as inflammatory breast carcinoma
- Dimpling or nipple retraction
  - ○ Can be caused by carcinomas shortening Cooper ligaments

SELECTED REFERENCES

1. Güth U et al: Breast cancer with non-inflammatory skin involvement: current data on an underreported entity and its problematic classification. Breast. 19(1):59-64, 2010
2. Massidda B et al: Molecular alterations in key-regulator genes among patients with T4 breast carcinoma. BMC Cancer. 10:458, 2010
3. Harms K et al: Prognosis of women with pT4b breast cancer: the significance of this category in the TNM system. Eur J Surg Oncol. 35(1):38-42, 2009

AJCC T4 CARCINOMAS (CHEST WALL OR SKIN INVOLVEMENT)

Carcinomas with Skin Involvement

(Left) Carcinomas that directly invade into and ulcerate the skin ⇨ are classified as T4b. The associated carcinoma is generally large and locally advanced. In the unusual case of a small superficial cancer with ulceration, the prognosis is not as poor. *(Right)* Carcinomas that invade into the skin without ulceration ⇨ are classified based on size and do not qualify as T4b. However, cancers with skin invasion are associated with a higher frequency of lymph node metastases.

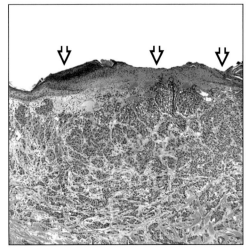
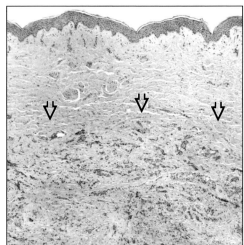

(Left) Invasive carcinomas can invade into the dermis and can mimic Paget disease in a superficial biopsy ⇨. However, a scale crust is generally absent and there will be an underlying palpable mass. If there is no skin ulceration, the cancer is not classified as T4b. *(Right)* Paget disease is due to DCIS involving nipple skin. It is typically associated with a scale crust, and skin erosion can occur in extensive cases. However, these skin changes do not affect the T classification.

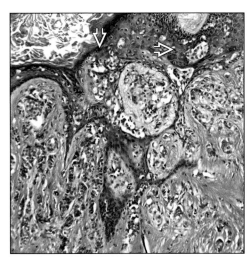
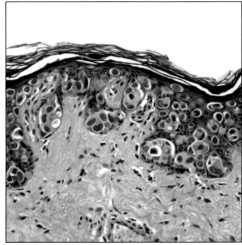

(Left) This central ulcerating carcinoma is associated with numerous satellite skin nodules ⇨. The satellite nodules are not in continuity with the main tumor and are a result of dermal lymph-vascular invasion (i.e., intramammary skin metastases). *(Right)* This is a focus of invasive carcinoma in the skin ⇨ and would be considered a satellite skin nodule if it were located away from the main tumor mass. To qualify for classification as T4b, the nodule must be clinically apparent.

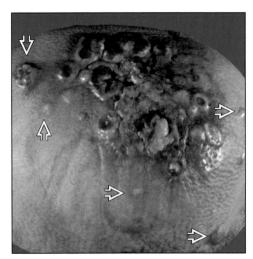
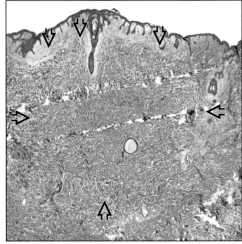

AJCC T4 CARCINOMAS (CHEST WALL OR SKIN INVOLVEMENT)

Carcinomas with Skin Involvement

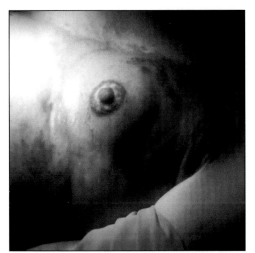

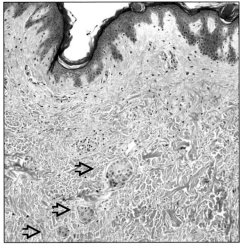

(Left) Inflammatory carcinoma is diagnosed based on erythema and edema of the skin involving 1/3 or more of the breast. Dermal lymph-vascular invasion in the absence of skin changes is insufficient for this diagnosis. (Right) The pathologic correlate of clinical inflammatory carcinoma is dermal lymph-vascular invasion ➢. The lymphatics are obstructed, resulting in a swollen erythematous breast. The prognosis is poor in most cases.

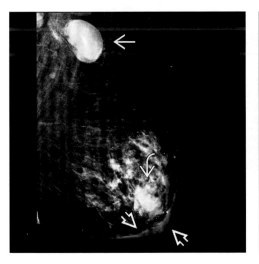

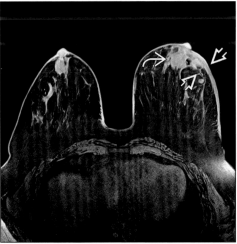

(Left) This subareolar carcinoma ➢ is associated with skin edema ➢. This clinical finding is included in the definition of T4b. However, edema cannot be determined with certainty grossly or microscopically in pathologic specimens. This patient also has metastatic carcinoma in a lymph node ➢. (Right) This patient was suspected to have inflammatory carcinoma due to marked skin edema and thickening ➢ associated with a mass ➢. She had a subareolar abscess.

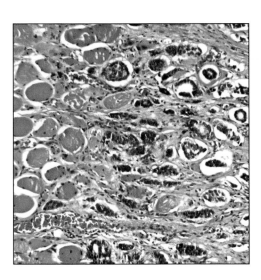

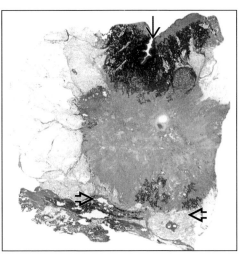

(Left) Skeletal muscle invasion can sometimes be seen at the deep aspect of a breast excision. The muscle is generally the pectoralis muscle, and this is not considered chest wall invasion. (Right) This carcinoma invades into the skin causing skin retraction ➢. However, the skin is not ulcerated, and there are no satellite nodules. The carcinoma does not invade into the chest wall ➢. Therefore, this carcinoma would be classified based on its size.

LYMPH NODE METASTASES

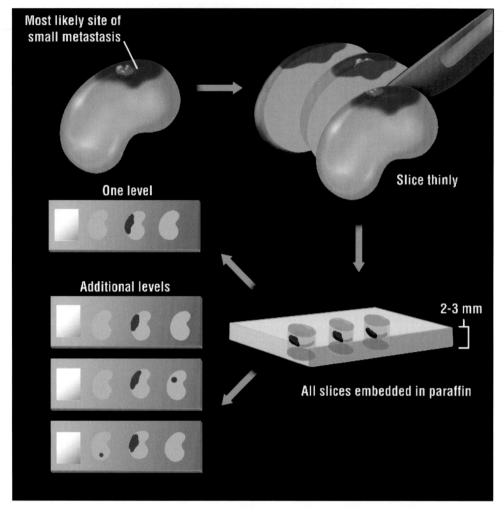

Radioactive tracer or blue dye can be used to identify the sentinel node, which is the node (or often 2 nodes) that first receives lymphatic drainage from the breast. Metastases are most frequent at the pole of the node stained by the dye. In order to find all macrometastases (> 2 mm), each node must be thinly sectioned (at 2-3 mm) and all slices embedded in paraffin for slide preparation. Macrometastases will be seen in > 98% of cases on 1 representative H&E section. Smaller metastases (micrometastases or ITCs) may or may not be seen if additional deeper levels through the block are prepared. To identify all tumor cells, the entire node, or ~ 500 slides, needs to be examined.

TERMINOLOGY

Abbreviations
- Individual tumor cells or individual tumor cell clusters (ITCs)

ETIOLOGY/PATHOGENESIS

Histogenesis
- Majority of breast cancers metastasize via lymphatics and likely also metastasize via blood vessels
  - A subgroup of cancers metastasize only via blood vessels and do not involve lymph nodes
    - Spindle cell carcinomas, high-grade phyllodes tumors, and sarcomas typically metastasize without involving regional nodes
- Major outflow of lymph from the breast is to 1 or 2 sentinel lymph nodes in the axilla

- Negative sentinel node is predictive of absence of metastases in remainder of axillary nodes in ~ 90% of patients
- Nonsentinel node metastases occur in up to 10% of patients with a negative sentinel node
  - Some cases are due to sentinel node being replaced by tumor, not allowing uptake of radioactive tracer or dye
  - Some cases may be due to aberrant drainage patterns in a few patients
  - Some cases are due to failure of mapping technique
- Rare cancers metastasize via lymphatics draining to other nodal basins, such as internal mammary nodes
- Intramammary nodes may be involved by carcinoma but are rarely, if ever, the sentinel node

CLINICAL IMPLICATIONS

Clinical Significance of Lymph Node Metastases

- Macrometastases (≥ 0.2 cm) are prognostically significant for overall and disease-free survival
  - 0.2 cm was originally chosen as size that could be measured with a ruler and did not require special measuring devices
  - 0.2 cm is also size that can be reliably detected by thinly slicing nodes and examining all slices with 1 H&E section
- Prognosis is diminished with each additional lymph node metastasis
  - Difference in survival between 0 positive nodes and 1 positive node is similar to difference for each additional node; there is no sharp drop-off in survival
  - Total number of involved lymph nodes should be counted and reported
    - Nodes with ITCs are not included in total node count
    - Axillary nodes and intramammary nodes are counted together
  - Number of uninvolved nodes and ratio of positive/negative nodes also has prognostic significance
    - Very important to always identify as many separate nodes as possible
    - When 1 sentinel node is involved, number of additional negative nodes may be used to determine need for additional node dissection
- Extranodal invasion is an adverse prognostic factor
  - Not extensively studied due to rarity of this finding
  - Extensive extranodal invasion correlates with clinical finding of matted axillary nodes
    - It may be necessary to estimate number of nodes present when extensive
  - May be used in decisions on benefit of axillary radiation
- Smaller metastases (micrometastases and ITCs) have a very small effect on prognosis
  - Survival is diminished by < 3% at 5-10 years as compared with node-negative women
  - No practical technique can detect all small metastases; hundreds of slides per lymph node would need to be examined
  - Clinical impact is too small to uniformly recommend studies to detect a subset of these metastases
    - No currently used clinically feasible protocols detect all ITCs that may be present in nodes
    - Effect on prognosis is so small that treatment recommendations should be based on their presence with caution
  - Cancers associated with small metastases often have other adverse prognostic factors that would be indications for systemic treatment
- Rare cancers drain to internal mammary nodes
  - These nodes lie below ribs and sternum and are difficult to approach surgically

- If radiologic findings are inconclusive as to whether these nodes are involved, fine needle aspiration (FNA) to establish positivity may be attempted
- Lymph node metastases after neoadjuvant treatment are an adverse prognostic finding
  - Indication of an incomplete response to therapy
  - Small residual metastases are as prognostically important as larger metastases
    - Although ITCs are classified as pN0(i+), this finding is not considered a pathologic complete response (pCR)
  - Response in nodal metastases has more prognostic significance than the response of cancer in the breast
  - Degree of response of metastases to treatment should be reported (e.g., presence and extent of fibrosis)
  - Some metastases can resolve completely after treatment without leaving a fibrous scar
    - Alternatively, some nodes not involved by metastasis can have small areas of fibrosis
    - Therefore, if nodes are free of carcinoma after treatment, it cannot be determined with certainty whether or not they were involved prior to treatment
    - pCR in nodes cannot be determined with certainty unless a metastasis has been documented before treatment by either fine needle aspiration or core needle biopsy
  - Sentinel node biopsy after neoadjuvant treatment is less accurate than in absence of treatment
    - Response to treatment is not uniform across all nodes
    - Metastasis in sentinel node may completely respond to treatment, but this does not ensure that all metastases to nonsentinel nodes will also have undergone a complete response
  - Documenting metastatic disease to lymph nodes is necessary to accurately classify patients for neoadjuvant trials and to derive the most information about treatment response
    - Palpable nodes may be sampled by FNA or core needle biopsy
    - Nonpalpable but enlarged nodes can be identified by ultrasound and sampled by needle biopsy
    - If no enlarged nodes are identified, sentinel node biopsy can be used to document a negative node; no additional nodal sampling is then necessary after treatment

MACROSCOPIC FINDINGS

General Features

- Gross appearance
  - Large metastases efface surface of lymph node and appear as firm white nodule(s)
    - Gross size of metastasis should be noted
    - Sampling may be limited to 1 section most likely to show extranodal invasion
  - Metastases < 1 cm may not be grossly evident
  - Number of nodes examined and number of positive nodes must be determined as accurately as possible

LYMPH NODE METASTASES

- Each node should be separately identified
- Nodes should be inked with different colors if slices from more than 1 node will be placed in same cassette
  - Size &/or shape of node is not reliable to identify different nodes when submitted together
- ○ If extensive extranodal invasion is present, it may be difficult to determine number of positive nodes
  - Attempt must be made to identify as many separate nodes as possible

Specimen Handling

- **Sentinel lymph nodes**
- Should be identified as "sentinel" by surgeon
  - ○ May be identified by blue dye, radioactive tracer, or both
    - Success rate for finding sentinel node is highest when both methods are used
  - ○ Majority of sentinel nodes will be both blue and hot (i.e., radioactive)
    - ~ 5% of sentinel nodes are blue but not hot; these are likely true sentinel nodes
    - ~ 10-40% of nodes may be hot but not blue; these nodes rarely contain metastases and are likely due to tracer being taken up by nonsentinel lymph nodes
  - ○ Number of sentinel nodes identified may determine need for completion axillary dissection
    - Therefore, each node must be separately identified and evaluated
- Small metastases are at pole of lymph node identified by dye in > 80% of cases
  - ○ Metastasis can be missed if a node is bisected and only 1/2 of node examined
    - 20-40% of macrometastases can be missed if only 1/2 of node examined
  - ○ Examination of entire node histologically is recommended in order to find all macrometastases
  - ○ Ancillary studies (additional levels, IHC) will detect additional micrometastases and ITCs
    - Smaller metastases have very minimal impact on survival
    - Additional studies beyond H&E evaluation are not currently required for AJCC staging
    - Ancillary studies are not currently recommended by the College of American Pathologists or the Association of Directors of Surgical Pathology
- **Nonsentinel lymph nodes**
  - ○ Each node should be sliced thinly
  - ○ All nodal tissue should be examined microscopically
  - ○ Ancillary studies are not required and are not recommended
- **Methods of finding nodes**
  - ○ "Squash" method
    - Fatty tissue is compressed and flattened by firmly pressing with finger or thumb
    - Lymph nodes are firm nodules that cannot be compressed by firmly pressing on tissue
    - This method can find nodes as small as 1-2 mm in size
  - ○ Clearing methods
    - Special solutions cause adipose tissue to become transparent

- Additional very small nodes may be found
- Solutions generally contain toxic chemicals and are time-consuming to use
- Clinical significance of very small nodes found after using clearing methods and careful gross examination is unclear
- ○ Bouin solution
  - Adipose tissue is dyed yellow, and nodes appear white when sectioned
  - Bouin adversely affects immunoreactivity for hormone receptors
  - Bouin fixative should not be used on any tissue for which hormone receptor studies might be required
  - Bouin also degrades DNA and should not be used for tissue that may be used for FISH or other DNA/RNA studies
  - After node is identified, it should be dissected out of tissue to avoid counting multiple slices as multiple nodes
- ○ If lymph nodes are not found, or very few are found, examination of remaining tissue should be considered
  - Nodes with extensive fatty replacement may be difficult to see grossly
  - Small nodes may be found near vessels

REPORTING CRITERIA

AJCC/UICC N Classification

- N classification is based solely on axillary lymph nodes in majority of breast cancers
  - ○ In rare cases in which other nodal groups are involved at presentation (e.g., internal mammary nodes, infraclavicular or level III nodes), additional N categories apply
  - ○ Intramammary nodes are included in total count with axillary nodes
  - ○ At least 1 metastasis must be a macrometastasis for classification as pN1a or higher
  - ○ Nodes with ITCs are not included in total count of positive nodes
- pN0: No metastases are detected in nodes
- pN0(i+): Isolated tumor cells are present
  - ○ Largest cohesive cluster measures ≤ 0.02 cm
  - ○ No more than 200 cells should be present on any single complete cross section of node
  - ○ pN0 (i-) is undefined term, as no technique completely eliminates possibility of ITCs
- pN0(mol+): Molecular test (generally RT-PCR) is positive, but no metastases are seen on H&E
  - ○ Size of metastasis cannot be determined with certainty
  - ○ Macrometastases can be missed depending on amount of tissue apportioned for assay
  - ○ False-positive results occur with RT-PCR in 5% or more of patients
- pN1mi: A micrometastasis is present
  - ○ Defined as > 0.02 cm or more than 200 cells but ≤ 0.2 cm
- PN1a: Metastases in 1-3 axillary lymph nodes
- PN2a: Metastases in 4-10 axillary lymph nodes

LYMPH NODE METASTASES

- PN3a: Metastases in > 10 axillary lymph nodes
- **(sn) Modifier**
  - Modifier "(sn)" was introduced in the AJCC 6th edition to indicate cases in which nodal classification was based only on sentinel nodes
  - In these cases, only 1 or 2 nodes may be examined, and actual nodal classification could be different if all axillary nodes were examined
    - In some cases, however, several sentinel nodes are removed such that the number is similar to a low axillary dissection
  - In the 7th edition, modifier (sn) allowed only if ≤ 5 sentinel and nonsentinel nodes are removed

ANCILLARY STUDIES

Use of Ancillary Studies
- Ancillary studies for lymph node evaluation are not required or recommended by AJCC, CAP, or ADASP
- Lymph nodes can be classified for staging using a representative H&E slide
- In selected cases, additional levels or IHC studies can be helpful to identify and classify cells that are not clearly metastatic carcinoma by histologic appearance

Multiple H&E Levels
- Recommended that nodes be thinly sliced at 0.2-0.3 cm and that all slices be examined microscopically
- This method will detect > 95% of macrometastases (> 0.2 cm)
  - Additional levels deeper through paraffin block detect micrometastases and ITCs
  - Routine "levels" are generally only 10-20 microns apart
  - Levels used to detect additional metastases must be equally spaced in block of tissue and typically must be hundreds of microns apart
    - Need for widely spaced levels must be specifically communicated to histotechnologist
- Number of levels and spacing of levels determine size of metastases that can be detected
  - 1 level: ≥ 0.2 cm metastases
  - 3 equally spaced levels: ≥ 0.1 cm metastases
  - 6 equally spaced levels: ≥ 0.05 cm metastases

Immunohistochemistry (IHC)
- IHC for keratin or other epithelial markers can be used to identify cells difficult to classify as epithelial cells on H&E
- Cells should have morphology of breast carcinoma before classifying them as cancer cells
  - Plasma cells may be positive for many IHC markers
  - Reticulin cells can be positive for keratin CAM5.2
    - Reticulin cells have spindly processes, encircle germinal centers, and do not have epithelial cell morphology
  - Keratin positive cells can be artifactually transferred to slides but are usually out of plane of section
  - Benign epithelial inclusions will be keratin positive but may also be associated with myoepithelial cells or markers positive in endosalpingiosis

- IHC for keratin can be helpful to determine presence and extent of metastasis from invasive lobular carcinoma
  - Tumor cells can closely resemble lymphocytes or histiocytes and can be difficult to detect by H&E
- If IHC is performed on nodes negative by H&E, usually only ITCs are detected
  - Slide used for IHC is also a level, and sometimes metastases are detected due to deeper level rather than IHC
  - Metastases should be classified by size and not by method of detection

RT-PCR
- Fresh or frozen tissue is used for extraction of mRNA
- Tissue can only be used for histological examination or for RT-PCR
  - Both tests cannot be performed on same tissue
  - This requires that nodes be divided for these studies
    - Method of dividing node and amount of tissue used for each study will greatly influence results
    - Because small metastases are usually found in 1 pole of the node, bisecting nodes will often lead to 1 sample containing cancer and the other not containing cancer
- Presence of transcripts typical of epithelial cells can be assayed using RT-PCR
  - More than 1 transcript may be assayed
  - Not all carcinomas may express genes used for the assay
  - Transcripts are not specific for tumor cells
- False-positive results are possible
  - Production of mRNA is not always faithful to cell type
  - Contamination of small amounts of extraneous tissue can give false results
  - Under best conditions, approximately 5% of results are considered false-positive
- False-negative results are possible
  - May be too few cells to detect by this method
    - Assay may be adjusted to attempt to detect only metastases of certain size
    - However, size of metastasis is never certain using only RT-PCR results
  - Node may have been divided in such a way that metastasis is not present in tissue used for RT-PCR
- Management of patients classified as pN0(mol+) is problematic
  - Depending on how assay is performed, this group can include patients with false-positive results, ITCs, micrometastases, or macrometastases

DIFFERENTIAL DIAGNOSIS

Benign Inclusions
- In rare cases, normal ducts with luminal and myoepithelial cell layers or cells resembling endosalpingiosis are present in axillary nodes
  - Thought to be a developmental anomaly
- Benign inclusions are often located in the outer sinus or capsule of nodes

- Cells are usually arranged in well-formed tubules with low-grade nuclei
  - Cells resembling endosalpingiosis may be ciliated
    - Cells will be positive for Pax-8 and WT1
    - Metastatic breast carcinoma should be negative for these markers
  - Some have a myoepithelial cell layer and may be associated with stroma
    - IHC is helpful to document a true myoepithelial cell layer
- For suspected cases of benign inclusions, it is important to compare morphology of cells in lymph node to primary carcinoma in the breast
  - Distinction between benign inclusions and true metastases is usually not possible with molecular (RT-PCR) tests

Displaced Epithelium

- Epithelial cells may be iatrogenically pushed into vascular spaces and transported to lymph nodes after biopsy
  - Can be benign or malignant
  - Most commonly seen in patients with intraductal papillomas and multiple core needle biopsies
- Cells are present as detached fragments, sometimes with a papillary configuration
  - Displaced epithelium is usually located only in subcapsular sinus of node
  - Presence of giant cells, histiocytes, and degenerating blood cells has been suggested as evidence of artifactual displacement
    - Reliability of these criteria to distinguish true metastases from artifact is uncertain
    - Clinical significance of displaced malignant cells vs. true metastasis is unknown
- Benign cells may not morphologically resemble breast cancer
  - Important to compare morphology of cells in lymph node to histology of primary breast cancer
  - Morphologic difference (e.g., low-grade cells in papillary fragments in patient with high-grade tumor) supports classification as artifactual displacement
- IHC can be helpful in some cases
  - Demonstration of both luminal and myoepithelial cells supports artifactual displacement of benign cells
  - Differences in ER, PR, and HER2 results for cells in node and patient's breast cancer support that the cells are benign

Lymphoma

- High-grade lymphomas can have epithelial appearance
- Obstruction of lymph nodes can cause swelling and erythema of the breast, thus mimicking inflammatory carcinoma
- IHC for lymphocyte and epithelial markers will identify cell type
  - Some lymphomas can be positive for epithelial membrane antigen
  - Thus, preferred marker to identify malignancies as carcinoma is keratin

Medullary-like Carcinomas

- Some carcinomas are typically well circumscribed and associated with prominent lymphocytic infiltrate
- If located in upper outer quadrant of the breast, it may be difficult to distinguish this type of carcinoma from metastasis to a lymph node
- True lymph nodes have an outer capsule with a sinus
- Carcinomas are more likely to have adjacent DCIS although the DCIS may be scant and consist of cancerization of lobules
- Germinal centers can be associated with either and are not a helpful finding

Nevus Cell Nests

- Nevus cells are melanocytic-type cells that may be present in capsule of lymph nodes
  - Occasionally they involve interlobar septae and can appear to be within the node
- Cells are spindle-shaped with low- to intermediate-grade nuclei and usually do not resemble the breast cancer
- IHC can be used to show that cells are negative for keratin and positive for S100

SELECTED REFERENCES

1. Cserni G et al: Distinction of isolated tumour cells and micrometastasis in lymph nodes of breast cancer patients according to the new Tumour Node Metastasis (TNM) definitions. Eur J Cancer. 47(6):887-94, 2011
2. Weaver DL et al: Effect of occult metastases on survival in node-negative breast cancer. N Engl J Med. 364(5):412-21, 2011
3. Brown AS et al: Histologic changes associated with false-negative sentinel lymph nodes after preoperative chemotherapy in patients with confirmed lymph node-positive breast cancer before treatment. Cancer. 116(12):2878-83, 2010
4. Corben AD et al: Endosalpingiosis in axillary lymph nodes: a possible pitfall in the staging of patients with breast carcinoma. Am J Surg Pathol. 34(8):1211-6, 2010
5. Ohsie SJ et al: Heterotopic breast tissue versus occult metastatic carcinoma in lymph node, a diagnostic dilemma. Ann Diagn Pathol. 14(4):260-3, 2010
6. Pugliese M et al: The clinical impact and outcomes of immunohistochemistry-only metastasis in breast cancer. Am J Surg. 200(3):368-73, 2010
7. Weaver DL: Pathology evaluation of sentinel lymph nodes in breast cancer: protocol recommendations and rationale. Mod Pathol. 23 Suppl 2:S26-32, 2010
8. Lester SC et al: Protocol for the examination of specimens from patients with invasive carcinoma of the breast. Arch Pathol Lab Med. 133(10):1515-38, 2009
9. Vinh-Hung V et al: Prognostic value of nodal ratios in node-positive breast cancer: a compiled update. Future Oncol. 5(10):1585-603, 2009
10. Zynger DL et al: Paracortical axillary sentinel lymph node ectopic breast tissue. Pathol Res Pract. 205(6):427-32, 2009
11. Norton LE et al: Benign glandular inclusions a rare cause of a false positive sentinel node. J Surg Oncol. 95(7):593-6, 2007
12. Bleiweiss IJ et al: Axillary sentinel lymph nodes can be falsely positive due to iatrogenic displacement and transport of benign epithelial cells in patients with breast carcinoma. J Clin Oncol. 24(13):2013-8, 2006

LYMPH NODE METASTASES

Classification of Nodal Metastases Based on Size

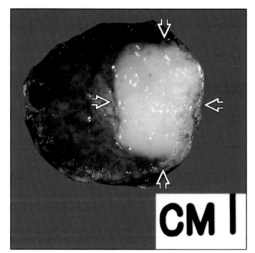

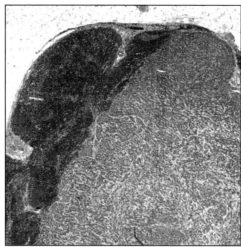

(Left) Lymph node metastases are the most important prognostic factor for breast carcinoma. Larger metastases can be seen grossly ➡. The size of the metastasis should be recorded and any areas of extracapsular invasion sampled and documented. (Right) All macrometastases (≥ 0.2 cm in size) can be detected by thinly slicing each node and examining all the slices microscopically on 1 representative H&E slide. Prognosis diminishes with each additional positive lymph node.

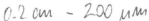

0.2 cm – 200 μm

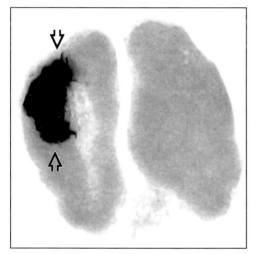

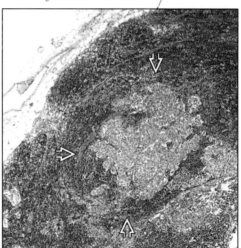

(Left) Small metastases are usually located at 1 pole of a lymph node. In this case, a macrometastasis is present only in 1 slice of a bisected node ➡. Examination of 1/2 a node or less will miss macrometastases in 20-40% of patients. (Right) This metastasis measures 0.2 cm ➡ and is at the upper limit to be classified as a micrometastasis. Metastases of this size have proliferated within the node, and small blood vessels will be associated with the nests of tumor cells.

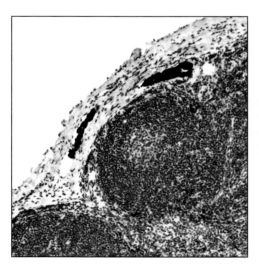

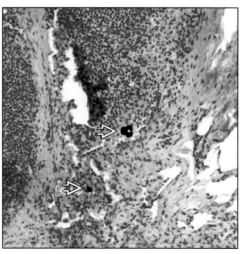

(Left) This metastasis approaches the upper size limit of ITCs. The 2 foci together would measure approximately 0.02 cm. However, as the foci are separate, neither fulfills the size requirement. Together, there are only about 50 tumor cells. (Right) When only a few keratin-positive cells ➡ are detected by IHC, it can be difficult to determine if the cells are more likely metastatic carcinoma, benign cells, or artifacts. True metastases should resemble the primary carcinoma.

Difficulties in Classification of Metastases

(Left) Metastatic carcinoma can completely destroy the underlying nodal architecture. Foci of invasive carcinoma within axillary adipose tissue are assumed to be the result of completely replaced lymph nodes and are counted as lymph node metastases. *(Right)* Extranodal invasion is included in measuring the overall size of a lymph node metastasis ⊵. It is also an additional poor prognostic factor and may be used as an indication for radiation therapy to the axilla.

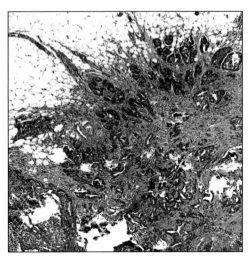
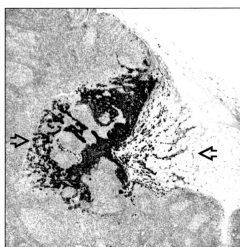

(Left) This metastasis is associated with a desmoplastic response. The entire involved area (tumor cells and stroma) ⊵ should be measured for classification, rather than the largest contiguous cluster ⊳. *(Right)* Metastases present as multiple clusters of tumor cells ⊵ are particularly difficult to classify. The N category may be based on the single largest contiguous focus of carcinoma, but the presence of multiple foci should be noted.

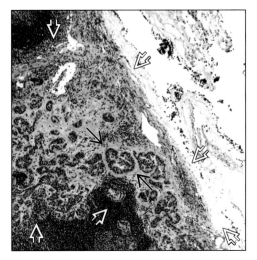
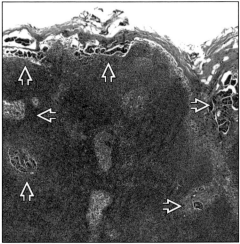

(Left) The lobular pattern of metastasis is difficult to quantify as the tumor cells are usually dispersed throughout the node. The largest area of contiguous cells can be used as the measurement, but judgment may be necessary to determine the best N category. *(Right)* Lymph nodes after neoadjuvant therapy are difficult to classify if there has been a marked response. Small metastases ⊳ represent an incomplete response to therapy. The number, size, and degree of response should be reported.

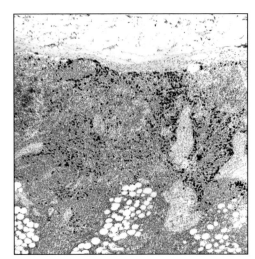
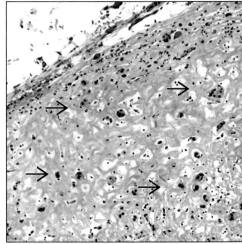

LYMPH NODE METASTASES

Difficulties in Classification of Metastases

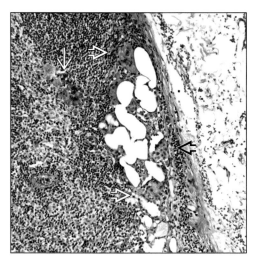

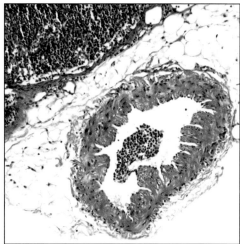

(Left) The presence of giant cells ➡ and hemosiderin-laden giant cells ➡ has been suggested as evidence that associated tumor cells ➡ are present due to artifactual displacement. **(Right)** Metastatic carcinoma is sometimes present only in lymphatics outside of the lymph node itself. Deeper levels frequently show the tumor actually extending into the node. If the only tumor present is in lymphatics, judgment should be used in determining the best classification.

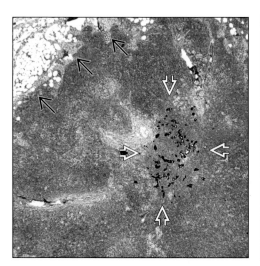

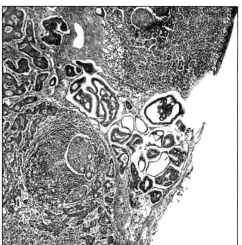

(Left) Metastases are usually located in the peripheral sinus ➡. However, on occasion, metastases are located within the central portion of the node ➡ and are more difficult to detect. **(Right)** Metastases should resemble the primary carcinoma. If they do not, alternative diagnoses or another primary should be considered. In this case, the breast carcinoma had a micropapillary pattern consisting of a hollow balls of cells. The metastasis shows the same histologic pattern.

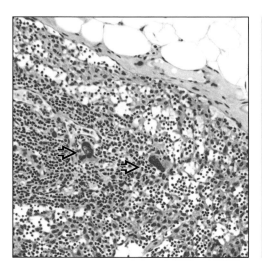

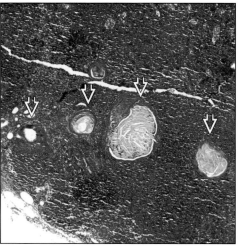

(Left) Megakaryocytes are large cells that can rarely be seen in lymph nodes. They usually have a single or multiple large, lobated nuclei with smudged chromatin ➡. If the identity of the cells is uncertain, they can be shown to be negative for keratins by IHC. **(Right)** This lymph node has multiple nests of keratin-producing squamous cells ➡. The breast carcinoma was an adenocarcinoma without squamous features. These are likely benign inclusions.

Difficulties in Lymph Node Classification

(Left) It may be difficult to prove that epithelial cells in lymph nodes are benign inclusions. In this case, IHC confirmed the presence of a myoepithelial cell layer ⮞ and a luminal cell layer ⮞. *(Right)* Benign inclusions can resemble endosalpingiosis. A single glandular structure is present in this axillary lymph node, and the cells are ciliated ⮞. The cells were strongly positive for Pax-8 and WT1 whereas the patient's breast cancer was negative for both of these markers.

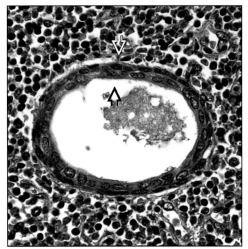 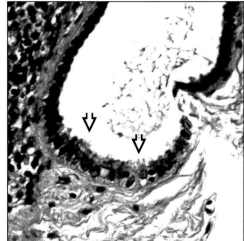

(Left) Normal plasma cells can be positive in many IHC studies due to the cytoplasmic presence of antibodies. They can also mimic ITCs. These cells are easily recognized by their eccentric nuclei with a clockface chromatin pattern. *(Right)* The cytokeratin antibody CAM5.2 can be positive in nonepithelial cell types. In this case, the reticular cells in this lymph node show cytoplasmic positivity but are recognizable due to their spindled shapes and arrangement around a germinal center.

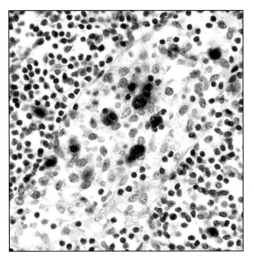 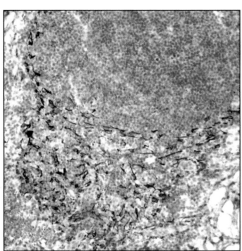

(Left) Nevus cell nests are typically present in the capsule of a lymph node ⮞. Less typically, they may be present in septae that appear to be outside the node ⮞ or within the node. In these locations, they are more likely to be confused with metastatic carcinoma. *(Right)* Nevus cells are spindled in shape and have low- to intermediate-grade nuclei. In general, they do not resemble breast carcinoma. IHC can demonstrate that the cells are keratin negative and S100 positive.

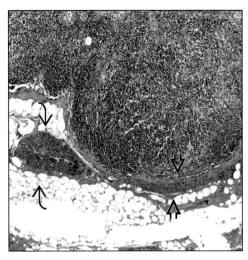 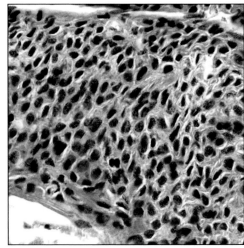

LYMPH NODE METASTASES

Lymph Node Anatomy

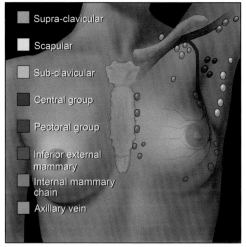

Supra-clavicular

Scapular

Sub-clavicular

Central group

Pectoral group

Inferior external mammary

Internal mammary chain

Axillary vein

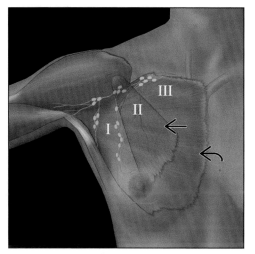

(Left) The majority of breast cancers metastasize first to the axillary nodes and only subsequently to other nodal basins. **(Right)** Regional lymph nodes are divided into levels I, II, and III according to their relationship to the pectoralis minor muscle ➡, which lies under the pectoralis major muscle ➡. Level II nodes lie below both muscles whereas Rotter nodes lie between the 2 muscles. These latter nodes may or may not be removed during an axillary dissection.

Sentinel nodes

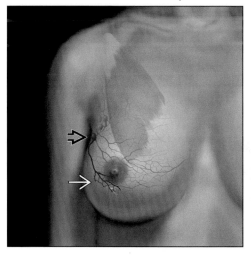

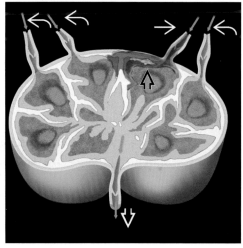

(Left) In the majority of women, lymphatic drainage is initially directed to 1 or 2 sentinel lymph nodes ➡. Sentinel nodes can be identified by using blue dye or radioactive tracer or both, injected around the carcinoma or adjacent to the nipple ➡. **(Right)** Lymphatic drainage enters by afferent lymphatics ➡ and exits via efferent lymphatics ➡. In this case, blue dye used for sentinel node mapping ➡ identifies the most likely location of a metastasis ➡.

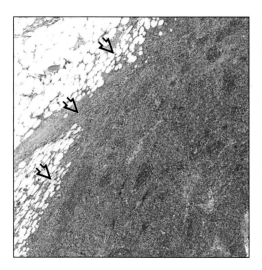

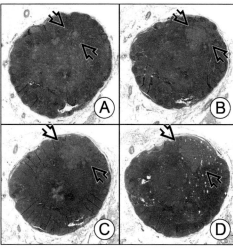

(Left) Occasionally, normal nodal anatomy is useful to distinguish a carcinoma arising in the upper outer quadrant from a nodal metastasis. This carcinoma is associated with numerous lymphocytes ➡, but unlike a metastasis, it lacks a nodal capsule. **(Right)** The size of small metastases can vary depending on the plane of section. In this case, a small micrometastasis ➡ (A) becomes a larger metastasis in deeper levels (B and C) and, finally, a macrometastasis (D).

HISTOLOGIC GRADE

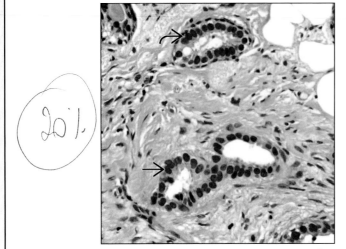

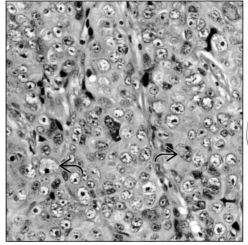

Approximately 20% of invasive carcinomas are low grade, characterized by well-formed glands, small uniform nuclei ➡ similar in appearance to benign luminal cells ➡, and rare or absent mitoses.

About 1/2 of breast cancers are high grade and are identified by their lack of gland formation, large, bizarre, pleomorphic nuclei that vary in size and shape ➡, and numerous mitotic figures.

TERMINOLOGY

Abbreviations
- Elston and Ellis modification of Scarff-Bloom-Richardson histologic grading (MSBR)

Synonyms
- Elston and Ellis grading
- Modified Bloom-Richardson grade
- Nottingham combined histologic grade

INTRODUCTION

Grade and Breast Cancer
- MSBR is most widely used system for breast tumor grading
  - Recommended by College of American Pathologists, American Joint Committee on Cancer, and European Commission Working Group on Breast Screening Pathology
- Grading divides breast cancers into groups that have different natural histories and biologic characteristics
  - MSBR grade describes features related to tumor differentiation and proliferation
  - Grade 1(well differentiated): 20% of cancers
    - Incidence higher in older &/or screened populations
  - Grade 2 (moderately differentiated): 30-35% of cancers
  - Grade 3 (poorly differentiated): 45-50% of cancers
    - Incidence higher in younger &/or unscreened populations
- Other grading systems have been described but have not been as widely used or validated with as many studies as MSBR

Prognosis and Grade
- Histologic grade is strongly correlated with breast cancer-specific survival and disease-free survival

- Many clinical studies have validated and confirmed important prognostic significance of tumor grade
  - Significant association between grade and survival holds true for different tumor subgroups
    - Tumor size (pT1a, pT1b, pT1c, and pT2)
    - Lymph node stages (pN0, pN1, and pN2)
  - Grade correlated with overall length of survival regardless of clinical stage

ETIOLOGY/PATHOGENESIS

Grade and Genomic Grade Index (GGI)
- GGI was developed using gene expression profiling
  - 97 genes were found to be differentially expressed between low and high histologic grade carcinomas
  - Majority of genes are associated with cell cycle regulation and proliferation
  - Low and high GGI strongly associated with disease-free and overall survival in ER-positive cancers
    - Low GGI found in luminal A cancers
    - High GGI found in luminal B, HER2, and basal-like cancers
  - Low and high GGI associated with histologic grade
    - Histologic grade 1: ~ 85% low GGI
    - Histologic grade 3: ~ 90% high GGI
- GGI reclassified histologic grade 2 carcinomas into 2 groups
  - Approximately 2/3 were low GGI and had outcomes similar to other low-grade cancers
  - Approximately 1/3 were high GGI and had outcomes similar to other high-grade cancers
  - GGI has challenged clinical relevance of grade 2 category
- GGI has helped validate histologic grade as important prognostic factor
  - Provides molecular basis underlying different grades of breast cancer
- Simplified index using 4 genes associated with cell cycle progression and proliferation is determined

using qRT-PCR ("PCR-GGI") and can be used to analyze formalin fixed tissue
- ○ Genes used are *MYBL2* (also used in Oncotype DX [Genomic Health; Redwood City, CA]), *KPNA2* (also used in Mammaprint [Agendia; Irvine, CA]), *CDC2*, and *CDC20*
- ○ Results are similar to 97 gene assay
- Histologic grade 2 carcinomas can also be subdivided by other measures of proliferation
  - ○ Ki-67 (MIB-1) is positive in all cycling cells (i.e., all cells not in G0)
    - ▪ Histologic grade 1: 1-15% positive cells (mean ~ 10%)
    - ▪ Histologic grade 2: 3-40% positive cells (mean ~ 10%)
    - ▪ Histologic grade 3: 8-85% positive cells (mean ~ 20%)
  - ○ Grade 2 cancers can be divided into 2 groups based on Ki-67 scores; generally, cut-off point of 15% is used

Grade and Changes in DNA
- Number and pattern of genomic copy number alterations differed significantly when stratified by grade
  - ○ Average number of chromosomal changes increases with increasing grade
  - ○ Low-grade carcinomas had fewer genomic alterations
- Close correlation between DNA copy number and mRNA expression levels has been reported
- Gene amplification may be common mechanism for increased gene expression in breast tumors
  - ○ May help explain GGI
  - ○ Genomic changes provide further validation for histologic grade as important prognostic factor

MICROSCOPIC FINDINGS

MSBR Grading
- 3 features are evaluated separately; given scores of 1-3
- Sum of scores determines final grade

MSBR (Sum of the Scores)
- MSBR grade 1 (sum of scores = 3-5)
  - ○ Well-differentiated breast cancer
- MSBR grade 2 (sum of scores = 6-7)
  - ○ Moderately differentiated breast cancer
- MSBR grade 3 (sum of scores = 8-9)
  - ○ Poorly differentiated breast cancer

Glandular (Acinar)/Tubular Differentiation Score
- Architecture of carcinoma is assessed over entire area of carcinoma
- Includes tubules, cell nests with lumens, papillae, as well as cribriform patterns
- Absence of tubule formation particularly unfavorable when combined with high nuclear grade
- "Micropapillary" structures in invasive micropapillary carcinomas are cellular spheroids and not indicative of gland formation

Nuclear Score (Nuclear Pleomorphism)
- Nuclei are scored at the periphery or in area of carcinoma with highest nuclear grade

Mitotic Score
- Count mitotic figures in 10 high-power fields (40x objective) in most mitotically active part of carcinoma
  - ○ Mitotic counts are usually highest at periphery
  - ○ If score is close to a cut-off point, additional fields should be counted
  - ○ Only fields that are representative of cellularity of carcinoma should be chosen
- Only clearly identifiable mitotic figures should be included
  - ○ Hyperchromatic, karyorrhectic, or apoptotic nuclei should not be counted
- Size of microscope field must be known in order to determine correct score
  - ○ Sizes of microscope fields can vary more than 6x
  - ○ Tables are available correlating mitotic counts with field sizes and scores for grading

Special Histologic Types and Grade
- All breast cancers should be graded
- Majority (70-80%) are of no special type ("ductal" cancers)
  - ○ Grading is effective method of subclassifying these cancers
- Some special histologic types of breast cancer are always associated with a specific grade
  - ○ Tubular carcinoma: Grade 1
  - ○ Medullary carcinoma: Grade 3
    - ▪ This is the 1 type of carcinoma for which grade is not good predictor of clinical outcome
- Other histologic types can be of any grade
  - ○ Lobular carcinoma: 15% grade 1, 75% grade 2, 10% grade 3
  - ○ Mucinous (colloid) carcinoma: Usually grade 1, can be grade 2, or rarely grade 3
  - ○ Micropapillary carcinoma: Usually grade 2 or 3 (hollow spheres are not true papillae or tubules)
  - ○ Papillary carcinoma: Usually grade 1 or 2, rarely grade 3
  - ○ Metaplastic carcinoma: Almost always grade 3

Grade on Needle Core Biopsies
- Accuracy of histologic grading in needle core biopsy is variable compared with excised tumor
  - ○ Dependent on quality of needle core biopsy sample
  - ○ Dependent on degree of heterogeneity in breast tumor
  - ○ Dependent on size of invasive carcinoma on core relative to size on excision
  - ○ Reported concordance rates between biopsy and excision range from 60-75%
- Grading of tumors on needle core biopsy should be considered provisional
  - ○ Grade on cores tends to be lower than grade on excision
  - ○ Important consideration for patients who are candidates for neoadjuvant chemotherapy

Elston and Ellis Modification of Scarff-Bloom-Richardson Score

Value	Glandular Score	Nuclear Score	Mitotic Score
1	≥ 75% of tumor area forming glandular/tubular structures	Nuclei small, regular, and uniform; similar to normal epithelial cells	≤ 3 mitoses per mm²
2	10-75% of tumor area forming glandular/tubular structures	Nuclei enlarged, somewhat variable in size; nucleoli present but not prominent	4-7 mitoses per mm²
3	< 10% of tumor area forming glandular/tubular structures	Nuclei significantly enlarged, vary in size and contour; nucleoli typically prominent	≥ 8 mitoses per mm²

The 3 values are added together to derive a final grade.

Final Grade

MSBR Grade	Sum of Scores	Description	Genomic Grade Index (GGI)
1	3, 4, or 5	Well differentiated	Low GGI
2	6 or 7	Moderately differentiated	Reclassified as low or high GGI
3	8 or 9	Poorly differentiated	High GGI

Interobserver Agreement and Grade
- Tissue handling, fixation, and specimen preparation should be optimized
  - Delayed fixation can reduce mitotic count
  - High-quality tissue sections necessary for morphologic assessment of histologic grade
  - Quality of histologic sections may have significant influence on accuracy and observer agreement
- Accuracy and interobserver agreement dependent on experience and application of strict criteria
  - Kappa values for tubule formation indicate substantial level of agreement
  - Lower levels of agreement reported for mitotic count and nuclear score
  - Accurate grading important for ensuring prognostic significance

Clinical/Pathologic Correlates and Grade
- **MSBR grade 1 carcinomas**
  - More common in older women
  - Frequently found by mammographic screening
    - Account for majority of excess invasive carcinomas detected in screened populations
  - Almost all ER &/or PR positive
  - Very rarely HER2 positive
  - Less likely to demonstrate axillary lymph node metastases at presentation
    - When present, metastases are usually small and few in number
  - Generally slow growing with recurrence occurring late in course (> 10 years after diagnosis)
    - Metastases are typically to bone
    - Patients can survive for long time periods (decades) after distant recurrence with hormonal therapy
  - Less likely to benefit from chemotherapy
- **MSBR grade 3 carcinomas**
  - Higher incidence in younger individuals
  - Most commonly present as palpable mass in younger women or as interval carcinoma in older women undergoing screening
  - About 1/2 ER &/or PR negative
  - About 1/3-1/2 HER2 positive
  - More likely to demonstrate axillary lymph node metastases at presentation
    - Metastases may be large and multiple
  - Recurrences usually early in course (3-5 years after diagnosis)
    - Metastases typically to brain and viscera
    - Long survival after distant recurrence is unusual
  - Subset (~ 15%) will have pathologic complete response to chemotherapy
    - Many of these patients have long-term survival and may be cured
- **MSBR grade 2 carcinomas**
  - Features of these tumors are intermediate between MSBR grade 1 and 2 carcinomas
    - May be due to intermingling of cancers that are actually grade 1 and grade 2
  - Genomic grading and separation by other measures of proliferation indicates that this may not be a true biologic category

SELECTED REFERENCES

1. Filho OM et al: Genomic Grade Index: An important tool for assessing breast cancer tumor grade and prognosis. Crit Rev Oncol Hematol. 77(1):20-9, 2011
2. Ellsworth RE et al: Molecular changes in primary breast tumors and the Nottingham Histologic Score. Pathol Oncol Res. 15(4):541-7, 2009
3. Liedtke C et al: Genomic grade index is associated with response to chemotherapy in patients with breast cancer. J Clin Oncol. 27(19):3185-91, 2009
4. Ignatiadis M et al: Understanding the molecular basis of histologic grade. Pathobiology. 75(2):104-11, 2008
5. Rakha EA et al: Prognostic significance of Nottingham histologic grade in invasive breast carcinoma. J Clin Oncol. 26(19):3153-8, 2008
6. Dalton LW et al: Histologic grading of breast cancer: linkage of patient outcome with level of pathologist agreement. Mod Pathol. 13(7):730-5, 2000

Carcinomas

HISTOLOGIC GRADE

Microscopic Features

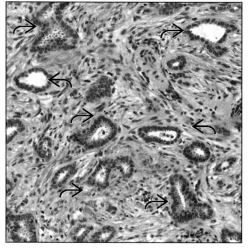

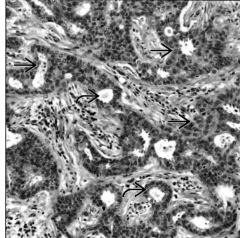

(Left) The glandular/tubular differentiation score is based on assessment of acinar formation by the tumor. This well-differentiated invasive ductal carcinoma shows good acinar formation ⇗ by tumor cells (> 75%) and would be given a score of 1. The small uniform nuclei would be given a nuclear score of 1. (Right) Tubule formation ⇗, as well as cribriform patterns ⇘, are included as glandular/tubular differentiation. The pattern is assessed over the entire area of the carcinoma.

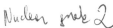

Nuclear grade 2   Nuclear grade 3

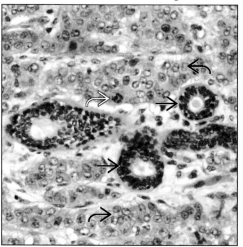

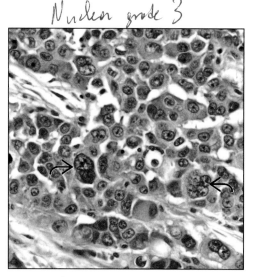

(Left) The nuclear score is based on assessment of nuclear pleomorphism. This invasive ductal carcinoma contains cells with enlarged nuclei (relative to normal ducts ⇗) that are somewhat variable in size and shape ⇗ and that have distinct nucleoli (nuclear grade of 2). A mitotic figure is present ⇗. (Right) This carcinoma shows significant nuclear enlargement ⇗, variability in size, irregular nuclear contours, and vesicular chromatin with prominent nucleoli (nuclear grade 3).

Mitosy   Apoptosis

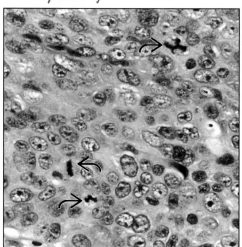

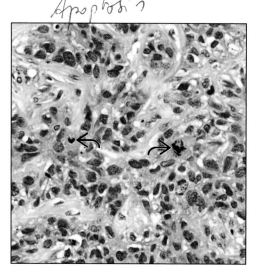

(Left) The mitotic score is based on careful assessment of mitotic activity. In the area with the highest proliferative rate, often at the periphery of the cancer, the average number of mitotic figures seen in 10 HPFs is determined. This high-grade tumor shows several mitotic figures in which individual chromosomes can be discerned ⇗. (Right) Only definite mitotic figures ⇗ are counted. Hyperchromatic cells and apoptotic cells should not be included.

LYMPH-VASCULAR INVASION

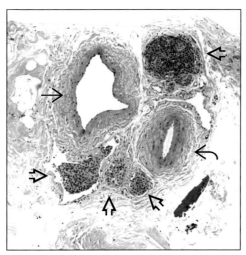

LVI is the presence of tumor emboli within lymphatic spaces ⮞ that are typically associated with small arterioles ⮞ and veins ⮞. The presence of LVI is associated with lymph node metastases and recurrence.

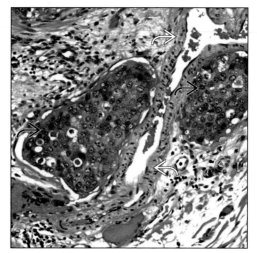

The diagnosis of LVI ⮞ is made easier by recognizing the normal microanatomy. Lymphatic spaces are typically present within the interlobular septae adjacent to small arterioles ⮞.

TERMINOLOGY

Abbreviations
- Lymph-vascular invasion (LVI)

Synonyms
- Lymphatic/vascular invasion
- Lymphovascular invasion
- Vascular invasion

Definitions
- Tumor emboli within peritumoral vascular channels (lymphatics and capillaries)

EPIDEMIOLOGY

Incidence
- Reported to be present in 10-90% of invasive breast carcinomas
- Incidence varies with patient population and diagnostic criteria

CLINICAL IMPLICATIONS

Clinical Risk Factors
- Pathologic factors and risk
  - Breast carcinomas metastasize via both lymphatics and blood vessels
  - Lymphatic channels are main route for metastasis (in approximately 2/3 of cancers)
    - LVI is associated with the presence of lymph node metastases
  - In a subset of breast carcinomas, metastasis is via blood vessels
    - Not associated with lymph node metastasis
    - Fewer vessels are involved, and tumor emboli are smaller than those in lymphatics
    - Approximately 20-30% of node-negative patients develop distant metastases, presumably due to blood vessel invasion
    - Spindle cell carcinomas, phyllodes tumors, and angiosarcomas are examples of tumors that rarely involve lymph nodes
    - May be specific molecular signatures associated with pattern of metastasis
  - Difficult to distinguish lymphatics from small capillaries
    - Immunoperoxidase markers cannot always identify type of vessel with confidence
    - Many patients have both lymphatic and blood vessel involvement
    - For practical purposes, no need to distinguish lymphatic from capillary to diagnose LVI
  - Peritumoral LVI has independent prognostic significance
    - Associated with increased risk of axillary lymph node metastasis as well as local and distant recurrence
  - Intratumoral LVI likely has little or no prognostic significance
    - Difficult to distinguish LVI within confines of invasive carcinoma from retraction artifact
    - Tumor in vascular channels that has not traveled beyond the tumor is less likely to be prognostically significant
    - Not associated with lymph node metastasis
    - Recommended that intratumoral LVI alone not be reported
  - LVI is more frequently associated with breast cancers demonstrating other aggressive features
    - High Ki-67 score
    - High histologic grade
    - Absence of hormone receptor expression
- Prognostic factors and risk
  - LVI is associated with significantly increased risk for tumor recurrence or death independent of axillary node status

- Recurrence for stage I (node-negative) invasive breast cancer increases from 22% without LVI to 38% with LVI
- Presence of LVI increases risk for metastases in additional nodes if sentinel node is positive
- LVI may be associated with resistance to chemotherapy

Therapeutic Implications

- LVI is useful in therapeutic decision making, particularly for node-negative patients with small cancers

MICROSCOPIC FINDINGS

General Features

- Strict criteria for LVI aid in making correct diagnosis
- LVI should be assessed at periphery, beyond advancing border of invasive carcinoma
  - Majority of LVI will be within 1-2 mm of edge of invasive carcinoma
  - If foci are only seen at greater distance, they are more likely to be artifactual
- Tumor emboli should be within vascular channels lined by a single layer of endothelial cells
  - Nuclei of endothelial cells are not always apparent in all spaces
  - Lymphatics and small capillaries are not surrounded by muscular layer or elastica
    - Red blood cells may be present in either structure
  - Large arteries or veins with muscular walls are rarely involved
    - Larger vessels can be identified with elastic stains
    - Elastin fibers are also present surrounding ducts and should not be mistaken for blood vessels
    - IHC for smooth muscle markers is also helpful for identifying larger vessels
- Tumor emboli usually do not completely conform to shape of space
  - If space is completely filled by tumor cells, it is difficult to recognize as LVI
  - Tumor cells within a larger space of different shape favors LVI
    - In retraction artifact, shape of tumor and space are usually identical
  - Spaces may be elongated and sinusoidal as lymphatic passes in and out of plane of section
  - Branch points (Y-shaped focus) are more likely to be due to LVI than invasive carcinoma
- Recognizing anatomic distribution of lymphatics aids in their identification
  - Lymphatics and small blood vessels usually run together between lobules
  - Lymphatics are often seen adjacent to small arteriole and vein
  - Lymphatics may cup around arteriole

Immunohistochemistry

- Can be used to identify endothelial cells
  - Clinical significance of LVI detected only by IHC and not seen after careful review of H&E sections remains unclear

- CD31 and CD34 are positive in endothelial cells
  - CD31 is predominantly positive in blood vessels
  - CD34 is positive in blood vessels and also in some lymphatics
  - CD34 is also positive in stromal cells, which limits its usefulness for distinguishing LVI from retraction artifact
- Podoplanin is a mucin-type transmembrane glycoprotein 1st described in lymphatic endothelial cells
  - Monoclonal antibody D2-40 (against podoplanin) selectively detects lymphatic vessels
    - Most sensitive and specific marker for lymphatic endothelial cells
    - Pattern should be strong and linear
    - Endothelial cells of arteries, veins, and capillaries should not be positive
    - Myoepithelial cells can be positive for D2-40; therefore, not very useful to distinguish DCIS from LVI
    - Pattern in myoepithelial cells is often weak, granular, and membranous
  - Use of D2-40 can increase number of foci of LVI detected by 20% over H&E sections alone
  - D2-40 may also be positive in basal-like carcinomas, squamous cell carcinomas, and angiosarcomas
    - Use of this marker to evaluate LVI in these tumor types may be more difficult

Positive Lymph Node in Absence of LVI

- Usually occurs when there is 1 or only a few positive lymph nodes
- Frequently occurs with discohesive (e.g., lobular) carcinomas
  - Cohesive carcinomas grow as contiguous plugs of tumor within lymphatics with adhesion to vessel wall
  - Discohesive carcinomas are present as dispersed cells, not adherent to wall, and may only be present transiently
- In some cases, extensive LVI can be mistaken for DCIS
- Diagnosis of LVI should not be made based only on presence of lymph node metastases

Negative Lymph Nodes in Presence of LVI

- LVI may be present although no metastases are present in lymph nodes
  - Reported in 5-10% of node-negative carcinomas
- Lymphatic drainage may be toward internal mammary nodes, particularly for medially located carcinomas
- Metastatic foci may not have reached axillary nodes or may not be able to establish viable growth in nodes

DIFFERENTIAL DIAGNOSIS

DCIS

- Both LIV and DCIS appear as circumscribed nests of tumor cells
  - Stromal reaction is usually absent surrounding LVI and may be absent or minimal surrounding DCIS

- Stromal reaction (e.g., lymphocytic infiltrate) favors DCIS
  - ○ Central necrosis may be present in either LVI or DCIS
- DCIS will be present in normal distribution of ducts and lobules
  - ○ LVI more typically present in sinusoidal-shaped spaces associated with blood vessels running between lobules that are often not involved by DCIS
  - ○ DCIS is typically present in a terminal duct lobular unit and involves multiple adjacent spaces
- DCIS will have myoepithelial cell layer, which can be identified by IHC
  - ○ Compressed cells at edges of LVI can mimic appearance of myoepithelial cells
  - ○ Both myoepithelial cells and lymphatic lining cells can be positive for podoplanin (D2-40)
  - ○ p63 is better than muscle-type markers to identify myoepithelial cells in this situation
- DCIS generally completely fills spaces whereas LVI should only partially fill space

Invasive Carcinoma

- Retraction artifact is most commonly seen around foci of invasive carcinoma in main tumor mass
  - ○ LVI should only be assessed outside borders of invasive carcinoma
- In retraction artifact, tumor cells are usually same shape as surrounding space
  - ○ In LVI, tumor cells may not completely conform to space or space may be larger than cell cluster
- Invasive carcinomas with retraction artifact are typically associated with stromal response
  - ○ LVI typically not associated with stromal response
- Spaces forming retraction artifacts should not be lined by endothelial cells
  - ○ True endothelial cells can be identified by vascular markers (CD31 or podoplanin)
  - ○ Fibroblasts and myofibroblasts can mimic lining endothelial cells in retraction artifact
- Some invasive carcinomas typically will show clear spaces around infiltrating tumor cells
  - ○ Invasive micropapillary carcinoma has invasive pattern of clusters of cells in cleared out spaces
    - Also associated with extensive LVI and an increased incidence of lymph node metastases at presentation
    - It may be difficult to distinguish between LVI and invasive micropapillary morphology
  - ○ Retraction or clear spaces around tumor cells in other cancer types has been associated with increased risk of lymph node metastases
    - This pattern is most commonly seen with poorly differentiated carcinomas
    - These cancers are frequently associated with true LVI

Artifactual Displacement of Epithelial Cells

- Both benign and malignant cells can be pushed into lymphatic spaces or artifactual clefts
  - ○ Phenomenon generally seen after biopsy and near prior biopsy site

- If cells appear benign and do not resemble the carcinoma, LVI should not be diagnosed
- LVI should not be diagnosed if tumor cells within spaces are only seen in the biopsy site and are not present elsewhere in the tissue

SELECTED REFERENCES

1. Hasebe T et al: Grading system for lymph vessel tumor emboli: significant outcome predictor for invasive ductal carcinoma of the breast. Hum Pathol. 41(5):706-15, 2010
2. Kanner WA et al: Podoplanin expression in basal and myoepithelial cells: utility and potential pitfalls. Appl Immunohistochem Mol Morphol. 18(3):226-30, 2010
3. Koo JS et al: Epithelial displacement into the lymphovascular space can be seen in breast core needle biopsy specimens. Am J Clin Pathol. 133(5):781-7, 2010
4. Ragage F et al: Is it useful to detect lymphovascular invasion in lymph node-positive patients with primary operable breast cancer? Cancer. 116(13):3093-101, 2010
5. Uematsu T et al: Is lymphovascular invasion degree one of the important factors to predict neoadjuvant chemotherapy efficacy in breast cancer? Breast Cancer. Epub ahead of print, 2010
6. Mohammed RA et al: Lymphatic and angiogenic characteristics in breast cancer: morphometric analysis and prognostic implications. Breast Cancer Res Treat. 113(2):261-73, 2009
7. Yang Z et al: Attenuated podoplanin staining in breast myoepithelial cells: a potential caveat in the diagnosis of lymphatic invasion. Appl Immunohistochem Mol Morphol. 17(5):425-30, 2009
8. Marinho VF et al: Lymph vascular invasion in invasive mammary carcinomas identified by the endothelial lymphatic marker D2-40 is associated with other indicators of poor prognosis. BMC Cancer. 8:64, 2008
9. Arnaout-Alkarain A et al: Significance of lymph vessel invasion identified by the endothelial lymphatic marker D2-40 in node negative breast cancer. Mod Pathol. 20(2):183-91, 2007
10. Mohammed RA et al: Improved methods of detection of lymphovascular invasion demonstrate that it is the predominant method of vascular invasion in breast cancer and has important clinical consequences. Am J Surg Pathol. 31(12):1825-33, 2007
11. Van den Eynden GG et al: Distinguishing blood and lymph vessel invasion in breast cancer: a prospective immunohistochemical study. Br J Cancer. 94(11):1643-9, 2006
12. Truong PT et al: Lymphovascular invasion is associated with reduced locoregional control and survival in women with node-negative breast cancer treated with mastectomy and systemic therapy. J Am Coll Surg. 200(6):912-21, 2005
13. Woo CS et al: Lymph node status combined with lymphovascular invasion creates a more powerful tool for predicting outcome in patients with invasive breast cancer. Am J Surg. 184(4):337-40, 2002
14. Rosen PP: Tumor emboli in intramammary lymphatics in breast carcinoma: pathologic criteria for diagnosis and clinical significance. Pathol Annu. 18 Pt 2:215-32, 1983

LYMPH-VASCULAR INVASION

Microscopic and Immunohistochemical Features

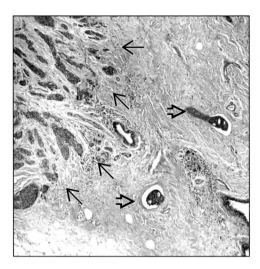

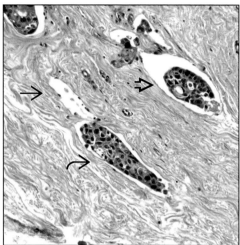

(Left) LVI should not be reported if only present within the confines of an invasive carcinoma. In this location, it is difficult to distinguish from retraction artifact. Peritumoral LVI ⊟ is most commonly seen 1-2 mm beyond the periphery of an invasive carcinoma ⊟. (Right) The tumor emboli may partially ⊟, almost completely ⊟, or completely fill the lymphatic space. Lymphatics are more easily identified in foci in which the space is larger than the embolus ⊟.

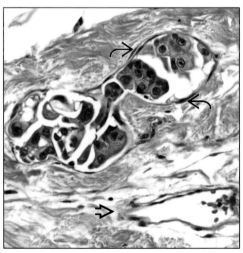

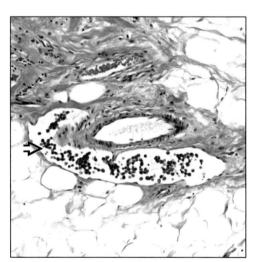

(Left) The presence of a vascular endothelial lining ⊟ around tumor cell emboli is very important for identifying LVI. Lymphatics are generally found adjacent to blood vessels ⊟. (Right) Lymphatics typically encircle or cup around blood vessels. This is an unusual case of lobular carcinoma involving lymphatics. LVI is rarely seen in this tumor type, likely due to the discohesion of the tumor cells ⊟ and the lack of adhesion to the vessel walls.

D2-40

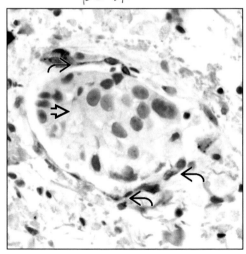

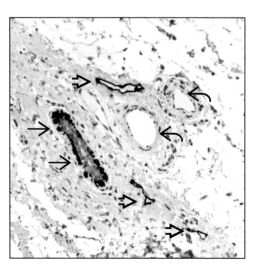

(Left) Podoplanin (D2-40) can be used to confirm that a tumor cell embolus ⊟ is in a space lined by lymphatic endothelial cells ⊟. However, not all lymphatic endothelial cells are positive for podoplanin. (Right) In addition to lymphatic endothelial cells ⊟, myoepithelial cells ⊟ can also be positive for podoplanin. Thus, DCIS with retraction artifact can mimic LVI. Some stromal cells may also be positive. Blood vessel endothelium is generally negative ⊟.

LYMPH-VASCULAR INVASION

Microscopic Features

(Left) LVI in the dermis signifies a poorer prognosis than LVI deeper in the breast. The plugging of dermal vessels by tumor ➔ gives rise to the clinical signs of inflammatory carcinoma such as breast enlargement, swelling, peau d'orange, and erythema. No true inflammation is present. Dermal LVI can also be seen in the absence of clinical skin changes. *(Right)* In this case of an edematous breast, the normal pattern of blood vessels and lymphatics running between lobules can be readily seen.

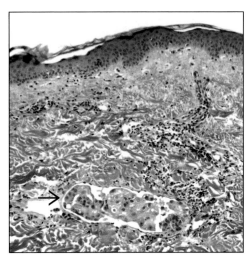
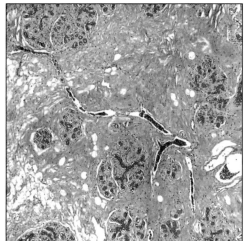

(Left) Although these foci completely fill spaces ➔, they can be recognized as LVI since they are elongated and run between the normal lobules ⇒. There is no stromal response. *(Right)* In most carcinomas, 1-3 foci of LVI are seen. Rarely, almost every lymphatic can appear to be involved, as in this case. The involved lymphatics traverse either side of normal lobules ⇨ or surround blood vessels ➔. Central necrosis may be present ⬈, causing confusion with DCIS.

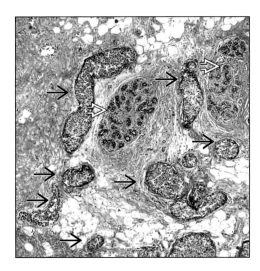
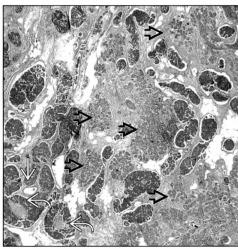

(Left) LVI completely filling the lumen ⇨ of the vascular space can mimics DCIS. The lack of a stromal response favors LVI. Podoplanin (D2-40) may be positive in both lymphatic endothelial cells and myoepithelial cells. Other myoepithelial markers may be more helpful. *(Right)* After neoadjuvant therapy, the majority of the residual carcinoma may be in lymphatics ➔. It is possible that tumor cells are less susceptible at this site. Although the volume of tumor may be low, this is a poor prognostic finding.

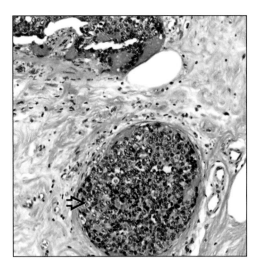
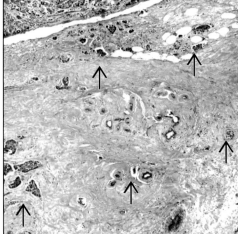

LYMPH-VASCULAR INVASION

Differential Diagnosis

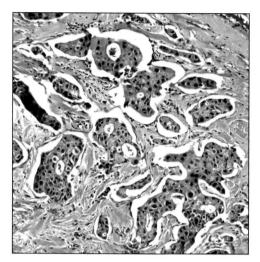

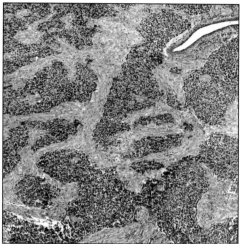

(Left) Retraction artifact around an invasive carcinoma can mimic LVI. The tumor cells generally conform exactly to the spaces. Lining cells are not present, but stromal fibroblasts can mimic their appearance. In general, LVI does not appear in clustered spaces and is more typically seen in a linear pattern. (Right) Some invasive carcinomas appear to grow in the clefts characteristic of pseudoangiomatous stromal hyperplasia. It is possible that these are prelymphatic channels.

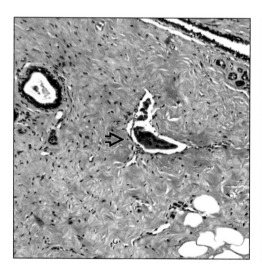

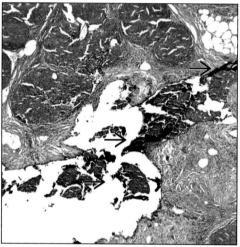

(Left) This cluster of apocrine-appearing cells ⊋ was found at a distance from a carcinoma that did not have apocrine features. They are most likely benign epithelial cells artifactually pushed into the space. (Right) Some cancers are friable and prone to be smeared into tissue sections. Artifactual pushing of tumor into stroma or vascular spaces can often be distinguished from true invasion or LVI. In this case, the presence of ink on tumor clusters ⊋ is a helpful sign.

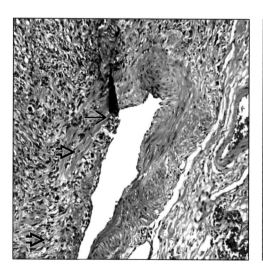

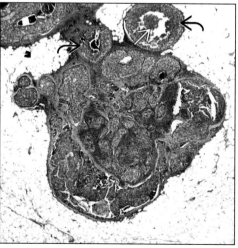

(Left) Invasion of large vessels with muscular walls is an unusual finding. In this case, the carcinoma ⊋ directly invades a large artery and extends into the lumen ⊋. (Right) LVI is sometimes difficult to distinguish from DCIS. In this case, the clustering of involved spaces ⊋, the presence of a fibrotic stromal response with a lymphocytic infiltrate, and foci of necrosis ⊋ would suggest that this represents a focus of DCIS. However, this is LVI in perinodal lymphatics in the axillary tail.

HORMONE RECEPTORS (ER/PR)

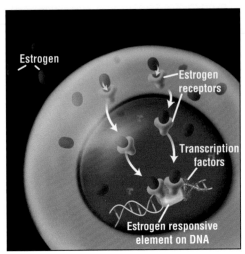

Estrogen receptor binds with its ligand estrogen and is transported to the nucleus of the cell where it acts as a transcription factor, regulating the expression of ER responsive genes.

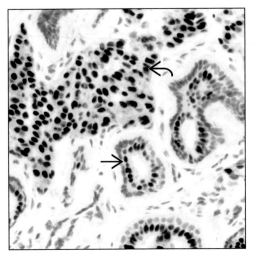

This invasive breast carcinoma has a high level of ER-α expression in the nuclei of the tumor cells ➡. Adjacent benign luminal cells also show strong positivity ➡.

TERMINOLOGY

Abbreviations
- Estrogen receptor (ER), progesterone receptor (PR)

Synonyms
- Estrogen receptor α

Definitions
- ER is activated by binding with hormone 17 β-estradiol (estrogen)
- ER is found in endometrium, breast, ovarian stroma
- 2 different forms of estrogen receptor exist: ER-α and ER-β
  - Each estrogen receptor is encoded by a separate gene: *ESR1* (ER-α) and *ESR2* (ER-β)
- ER-α is most important ER in breast cancer
  - After binding to its ligand, estrogen, ER is transported to nucleus of cell
  - In nucleus, ER functions as transcription factor
  - ER regulates expression of a number of genes important in breast cancer biology
- PR expression is regulated by ER
  - PR is expressed in majority of ER(+) breast carcinomas

EPIDEMIOLOGY

Incidence
- ER expression is present in 70-80% of breast cancers
  - ER(+)/PR(+) ~ 65%: Usually well- or moderately differentiated cancers
    - Includes almost all tubular carcinomas, well- or moderately differentiated lobular carcinomas, and mucinous carcinomas
    - If well-differentiated carcinoma is ER(-), assay may be faulty and should be repeated
  - ER(+)/PR(-) ~ 15%: Usually moderately or poorly differentiated; rarely well differentiated

- PR is downregulated by HER2; approximately 25% of PR(-) cancers will show HER2 amplification
    - More frequent in older women with larger cancers with higher rate of proliferation, when compared to ER(+)/PR(+) cancers
  - ER(-)/PR(+) ~ 5%: Reported to be more common in younger women with more advanced cancers
    - Some cases are due to technical problems with either ER assay or PR assay
    - Biologic basis of PR expression in absence of ER expression is not well understood
  - ER(-)/PR(-) ~ 15%: Usually poorly differentiated
    - About 1/3 of these cancers will show HER2 amplification
    - These cancers are more common in young women, African-American women, and Latino women

Diet
- Cruciferous vegetables (e.g., broccoli, Brussels sprouts) can decrease estrogen exposure
  - Indole-3-carbinol causes estrogen to be changed to inactive metabolite
- Excessive alcohol consumption can increase estrogen exposure
  - Decreased liver function increases estrogen levels

ETIOLOGY/PATHOGENESIS

Histogenesis
- Factors associated with prolonged increased exposure to estrogen are associated with elevated lifetime risk for developing ER(+) breast cancer
  - Female gender
  - Early menarche
  - Late menopause
  - Obesity after menopause (adipose tissue can be converted into estrogens)
  - Nulliparity

HORMONE RECEPTORS (ER/PR)

○ Hormone replacement therapy
- Factors associated with lower estrogen exposure are associated with decreased lifetime risk for developing ER(+) breast cancer
  ○ Late menarche
  ○ Early menopause
  ○ Obesity prior to menopause (menstrual cycles may be reduced or absent)
  ○ Child bearing (especially beginning at early age)
  ○ Breastfeeding
  ○ Oophorectomy
- Inappropriate, abnormal, &/or prolonged estrogen exposure stimulates proliferation of ER(+) breast epithelial cells
  ○ Increases number of epithelial cells and predisposes cells to mutations, increasing likelihood of ER-dependent breast cancers

CLINICAL IMPLICATIONS

Prognostic Implications

- ER expression by breast cancer cells is weak prognostic marker of clinical outcome in most studies
  ○ ER expression in breast cancer is highly predictive for clinical benefit from endocrine therapies
    ▪ Some patients with distant metastases survive for many years with hormonal treatment
  ○ In general, ER(+) and HER2(-) carcinomas do not respond well to chemotherapy
- *PR* gene is regulated by ER, and PR is usually detected in tumor cells with activated ER pathway
  ○ Recent data has demonstrated that PR status may be independently associated with outcome
    ▪ ER(+)/PR(+) cancers confer better prognosis than ER(+)/PR(-) cancers
    ▪ This may be related to different tumor biology for ER(+)/PR(-) subset of cancers
- Carcinomas negative for ER and PR have worse prognosis than hormone receptor positive cancers
  ○ However, a subset of these cancers (~ 20%) will have pathologic complete response after chemotherapy, and prognosis for this group is favorable
  ○ Patients who develop distant metastases after treatment rarely have prolonged survival

Treatment Implications

- **ER/PR expression in invasive breast cancer**
- Clinical benefit from endocrine therapy is only seen in carcinomas that test positive for ER &/or PR
- Clinically validated assays for ER and PR should be part of diagnostic work-up of every newly diagnosed invasive breast carcinoma
- Endocrine therapy for ER- or PR-positive breast cancer can be achieved using pharmaceuticals or surgery
  ○ Drugs
    ▪ Selective ER modulators (SERMs) act as ER antagonists in breast tissue (e.g., tamoxifen)
    ▪ Aromatase inhibitors block conversion of precursors to estrogen in peripheral tissue
    ▪ Gonadotropin-releasing factor can be blocked by antagonists or refractory agonists
  ○ Surgery: Ovarian ablation

▪ In patients with *BRCA1* or *BRCA2* mutations, surgery also reduces risk of ovarian or tubal carcinomas
- ER(+)/PR(-) cancers may be more resistant to endocrine therapy
  ○ Clinical trial data are unclear as to whether these patients should be treated differently compared to patients with ER(+)/PR(+) cancers
  ○ Some medical oncologists are more likely to include chemotherapy in addition to hormonal therapy for ER(+)/PR(-) cancers
- **ER/PR expression in ductal carcinoma in situ (DCIS)**
  ○ DCIS typically expresses ER and PR
    ▪ ER(+)/PR(+) ~ 85%; ER(-)/PR(-) ~ 15%; other combinations < 5%
    ▪ Immunoreactivity can be markedly heterogeneous with both positive and negative areas
    ▪ May be difficult to distinguish rare tumor cell positivity from residual normal epithelial cells
    ▪ In majority of cases, ER and PR expression is same for invasive carcinoma and its associated DCIS
    ▪ In rare cases, expression is discordant (typically DCIS positive and invasive carcinoma negative)
    ▪ This can lead to inaccurate results for methods that do not distinguish in situ from invasive carcinoma (e.g., some gene profiling assays, automated image analysis)
  ○ NSABP B24 DCIS trial had treatment arms with or without tamoxifen; retrospective analysis revealed
    ▪ Addition of tamoxifen to treatment for DCIS reduced likelihood of recurrence if DCIS was ER(+)
    ▪ Benefit was not seen for ER(-) DCIS
    ▪ However, there were too few cases of ER(-) DCIS to exclude possibility of small effect
  ○ ER testing of DCIS may be requested by some oncologists to guide treatment decisions

Clinical Assay to Assess ER and PR Status

- Currently, ER and PR assessment is performed using IHC techniques
- IHC has a number of advantages over ligand-binding assay methodologies
  ○ Lower cost
  ○ Morphologic confirmation of evaluation of tumor cells and not normal breast elements
    ▪ IHC detects nuclear hormone receptor proteins and excludes cases with cytoplasmic positivity
  ○ Rapid turn around time
  ○ Ability to assay smaller tissue samples, such as needle core biopsies

Specimen Handling

- ER, PR, and HER2 should be assessed in every newly diagnosed invasive breast carcinoma
- Ideally, breast specimens should be sectioned and placed in adequate volume of fixative within 1 hour of removal
- If gross tumor is identified during initial specimen evaluation
  ○ Sample of tumor and fibrous normal tissue can be placed together in same cassette and immediately placed in formalin

- Ensures good fixation of cancer as well as normal breast tissue for internal control for ER and PR

Breast Tissue Fixation
- Breast tissue samples must be fixed in 10% neutral buffered formalin
  - Fixation time: Recommended to be at least 6 hours and no more than 72 hours before processing
    - Under- or overfixation can lead to technical problems with IHC assay and may give false-negative results
    - Small biopsy samples require same amount of fixation time as larger resection samples

ER/PR Methodology: IHC
- ER/PR IHC assays should be performed following standardized methods using validated assay
- Antibodies for ER and PR IHC should have well-established specificity and sensitivity
  - Assays should be clinically validated, demonstrating good correlation with patient outcomes in published reports
  - Antibodies for ER meeting these criteria are 1D5, 6F11, and SP1
  - Antibodies for PR meeting these criteria are 1294, 1A6, and 312
    - Each of these antibodies is equivalent or superior to ligand-binding assays in correlation with outcome and benefit from endocrine therapy

ER/PR IHC Interpretation
- Goal for ER/PR analysis: Identification of patients most likely to benefit from endocrine therapy
- Interpretation should include % of positive tumor cell nuclei and average intensity of staining reaction
- Level of expression of ER in carcinomas demonstrates broad dynamic range that can vary by several hundred fold
  - ER expression levels may provide valuable information that could influence decision making for specific types of adjuvant therapy
  - IHC assay for ER and PR should be optimized so that staining captures broad dynamic range of expression in terms of both distribution and intensity of staining
- Threshold cut-off point for defining ER positivity should be clinically validated against patient outcome
  - Clinical studies have shown that patients with as few as 1% ER(+) cells derived benefit from endocrine treatment with tamoxifen
  - Magnitude of benefit appears to vary with different levels of ER expression
    - Greatest benefit from tamoxifen seen for those patients with high levels of ER expression
  - ASCO/CAP guidelines define 1% or greater immunoreactive cells as positive result
    - Patients with carcinomas showing this level of ER/PR expression should be considered for endocrine treatment
    - 0 or < 1% immunoreactive cells defined as negative result

- However, in Allred system, < 1% immunoreactive cells of moderate or strong intensity is considered a positive result

QA and QC for ER/PR Testing
- **Routine use of control materials**
  - Positive and negative controls should be included with every ER and PR IHC assay
  - Batch controls can be used to monitor assay performance and to detect loss of sensitivity or assay analytical drift
  - "On slide" controls can be used to help ensure that all reagents were properly dispensed onto slide
- Different tissues and cell types, including internal and external controls, can be used as well
- Best "on slide" positive controls are normal breast elements from patient's breast tissue
  - Normal breast elements usually show ER expression in about 5-10% of luminal epithelial cells
    - In some cases, number of ER(+) nonmalignant breast epithelial cells will be higher
    - Nonepithelial cells can also be ER(+): Myofibroblasts, smooth muscle of areola, rare lymphocytes
  - Tissue block selected for ER/PR testing should contain, if possible, adjacent normal breast elements
- Endometrial tissue shows a range of levels of ER and PR expression
  - Levels of expression vary over course of menstrual cycle
  - Small portion of endometrium can be used as "on slide" positive control tissue
- **Analytical validation**
  - Helps ensure accuracy, sensitivity, and specificity for assay performance
  - Assay validation should be against clinically validated method
- **Monitor daily testing results**
  - Review of batch controls and "on slide" controls to document accurate assay performance
    - Evaluate results for analytical drift and loss of assay sensitivity
- **Perform periodic trend analysis**
  - Percentage of ER- and PR-positive and negative cases should be within expected norm for breast cancer in similar population
- **Participate in ER/PR IHC proficiency program**
  - Must be high concordance between central laboratory analysis and individual laboratory results

SELECTED REFERENCES
1. Hammond ME et al: American Society of Clinical Oncology/College of American Pathologists guideline recommendations for immunohistochemical testing of estrogen and progesterone receptors in breast cancer (unabridged version). Arch Pathol Lab Med. 134(7):e48-72, 2010

Ancillary Techniques

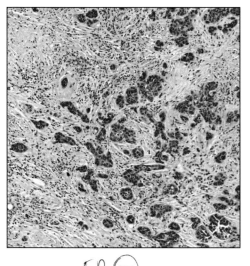

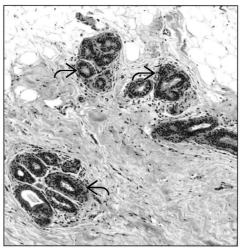

(Left) This poorly differentiated invasive ductal carcinoma was placed in formalin at the time of initial gross examination to help ensure good tissue fixation. (Right) This fibroglandular breast tissue with normal breast elements ⇨ was placed in the same cassette with a section of invasive carcinoma to provide an internal control that has been handled and fixed in the same manner. The ability to evaluate the patient's normal breast tissue optimizes breast marker analysis.

ER ⊖

ER ⊕

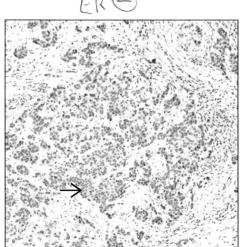

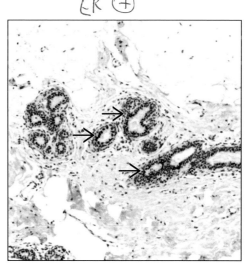

(Left) This poorly differentiated carcinoma is negative for ER expression ⇨. There are no normal adjacent breast epithelial cells to act as an internal control. The possibility of a false-negative result should be considered. (Right) This fibroglandular normal breast tissue placed in the same cassette with the carcinoma shows reactivity for ER in luminal cells ⇨. This ensures that the negative results in the carcinoma reflect a true lack of ER expression by the tumor cells.

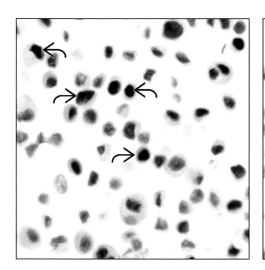

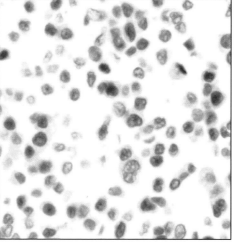

(Left) Commercially available FDA-approved ER/PR testing kits provide sections of formalin-fixed paraffin-embedded breast cancer cell lines that can be used as batch controls for monitoring performance and assess for assay drift of ER/PR IHC assays. This cell line (CAMA-1) shows moderate ER nuclear expression ⇨. PR shows a similar staining pattern. (Right) The commercially available HT-29 cell line is ER/PR negative as shown in this IHC study for ER.

HORMONE RECEPTORS (ER/PR)

Ancillary Techniques

(Left) This invasive carcinoma shows strong nuclear reactivity for ER ➡. Normal breast elements ➡ within the same tissue block serve as an internal positive control for the assay. *(Right)* The invasive carcinoma is negative for PR ➡, while the internal positive controls show strong reactivity ➡. ER(+)/PR(-) breast cancers usually have a poorer prognosis compared to PR(+) cancers. However, they may be more likely to respond to chemotherapy added to endocrine treatment.

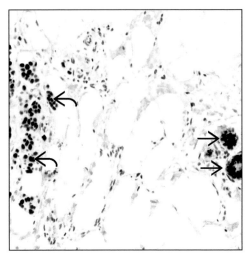 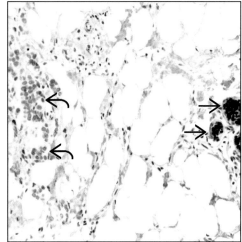

(Left) ER expression correlates with histologic grade. Well-differentiated breast cancers, such as this tubular carcinoma, should show high levels of ER and PR expression. *(Right)* The expected result for well-differentiated carcinomas is that the majority of tumor cells will show strong positivity, as seen in this invasive tubular carcinoma ➡. If negative results are obtained, the possibility of a false-negative result should be considered, and repeat studies may be indicated.

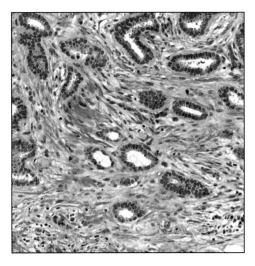 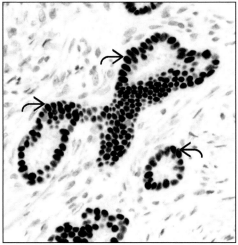

(Left) This is a poorly differentiated invasive ductal carcinoma with poor tubule formation ➡, pleomorphic nuclei ➡, and a high mitotic rate. *(Right)* The poorly differentiated invasive carcinoma shows scattered weak positivity for ER ➡, suggesting that the tumor demonstrates a low level of ER expression. The presence of intense ER reactivity within normal breast elements ➡ confirms that the assay is performing appropriately and that the ER results are valid.

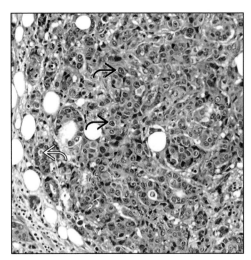 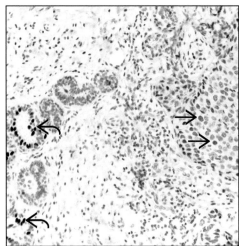

Difficult Cases

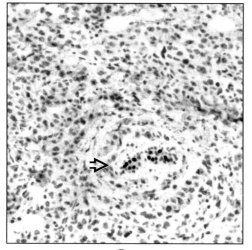

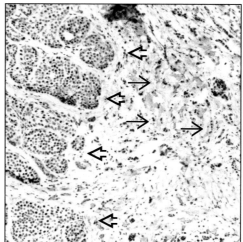

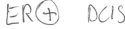
ER⊕ DCIS

ER⊕

(Left) False-positive results are very unusual for hormone receptor tests. One rare cause is the misinterpretation of entrapped normal ER(+) ducts ⊵ as tumor cells. (Right) In situ carcinoma and associated invasive carcinoma are concordant for ER in > 80% of cases. In this unusual case, LCIS is ER(+) ⊵ and invasive carcinoma is ER(-) ➡. This can cause discrepancies if results are compared to assays that do not distinguish in situ from invasive carcinoma.

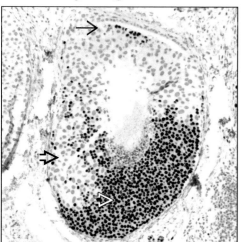

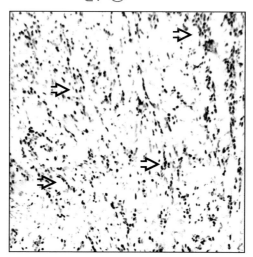

(Left) DCIS is ER(+) in 85% of cases but can show marked heterogeneity, as in this case with low-grade ER(+) areas ⊵ and high-grade ER(-) areas ⊵. Some residual normal epithelial cells are present on the periphery ➡. Such residual cells may be difficult to distinguish from tumor cells in some cases. (Right) Other cell types can also be ER(+), such as myofibroblasts in this myofibroblastoma ⊵, smooth muscle cells of the areola, and rare lymphocytes.

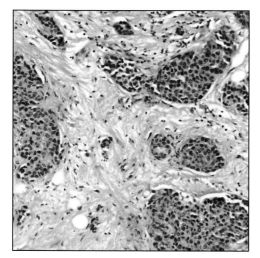

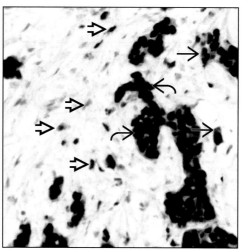

(Left) This is a moderately differentiated invasive ductal carcinoma diagnosed on core biopsy. The ER study was submitted for a 2nd opinion. (Right) This ER assay shows strong nuclear reactivity within tumor cells ➡. However, there is also atypical cytoplasmic staining ➡ and positivity in adjacent stromal nuclei ⊵ suggesting a technical problem with nonspecific immunoreactivity. Assay results such as this should be rejected as uninterpretable and repeated.

HER2

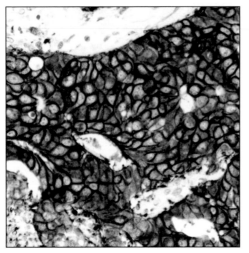

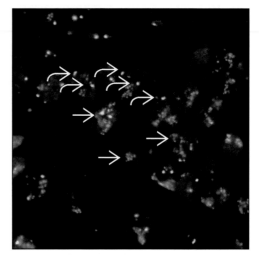

This is a typical HER2-positive invasive ductal carcinoma with high nuclear grade and intense circumferential membrane immunoreactivity ("chicken wire" pattern), which is uniform throughout the tumor.

An increased number of HER2 genes (red signals ➡), compared to 1 or 2 copies of chromosome 17 centromere sequences (green signals ➡), would be classified as marked HER2 gene amplification.

TERMINOLOGY

Abbreviations
- HER2-positive breast cancer (HER2+BC)
- Human epidermal growth factor receptor-2 (HER2)
- Chromosome 17 centromere enumeration probe (CEP17)

Synonyms
- HER2, HER2/neu, NEU, NGL, TKR1, c-erb, CD340, ERBB2

Definitions
- *HER2* is a proto-oncogene located on chromosome 17q12
  - Expressed normally in a number of glandular epithelia including breast
- Translated into a 185 kDa transmembrane growth factor receptor protein
  - HER2 transmits signals regulating normal cell growth, development, and survival
- In 15-20% of breast cancers, HER2 protein is overexpressed
  - In > 95% of HER2+BC, the mechanism of overexpression is due to increased numbers of *HER2* gene (gene amplification)
    - Amplification of the gene drives mRNA production and protein expression
    - Clinical assays evaluate DNA, mRNA, or protein
  - In ~ 5% of HER2+BC, there may be other mechanisms resulting in protein overexpression
    - These mechanisms have not been well studied
- HER2 is a member of HER-family of growth factor receptors
  - This family also includes HER1 (EGFR), HER3, and HER4
    - Regulate intracellular signaling through MAP-kinase and PI3-kinase pathways
    - Regulate normal cell proliferation and cell survival
  - Overexpression results in increased HER2 receptors on the surface of tumor cells

ETIOLOGY/PATHOGENESIS

Histogenesis
- HER2 alteration is thought to be early event in pathogenesis of HER2+BC
  - May play important role in carcinogenesis and tumor development
  - Higher proportions of DCIS overexpress HER2 compared to invasive carcinoma
- HER2 alteration is stable genetic change in tumor cells
  - HER2 overexpression is seen in primary tumor as well as metastases from HER2+BC
  - However, in some cases HER2 overexpression is lost in residual carcinoma after treatment or in metastases
    - Most likely due to initial tumor heterogeneity and the selective effects of targeted therapy

Molecular Pathology
- Binding of high affinity ligands to HER-receptors leads to conformational change in molecule
  - Conformational change promotes receptor activation through dimerization
    - HER-family members form homo-dimers and hetero-dimers
  - Receptor dimerization leads to activation of intracellular tyrosine kinase portion of molecule
    - Tyrosine kinase activation initiates receptor signaling through phosphorylation
- Overexpression of HER2 increases likelihood of receptor activation and signaling
  - Active HER2 pathway signaling
    - Promotes angiogenesis
    - Drives proliferation
    - Protects cells against apoptosis
    - Increases tumor cell motility and invasion

HER2

- Contributes to more aggressive biologic behavior and malignant phenotype

CLINICAL IMPLICATIONS

Prognostic Implications

- *HER2* gene amplification/overexpression plays a pivotal role in driving tumor biology
  - ○ Contributes to more aggressive clinical course for HER2+BC
    - ■ Significantly decreased disease-free and overall survival
    - ■ Higher incidence of local recurrence compared to luminal A cancers (ER positive and HER2 negative)
    - ■ Increased incidence of lymph node metastases
    - ■ More frequent metastases to brain, liver, and lung compared to luminal A cancers
    - ■ 40-50% of patients with brain metastases have HER2+BC
- HER2 overexpression significantly correlates with a number of unfavorable tumor characteristics
  - ○ Higher proliferative index
  - ○ Larger tumor size
  - ○ Higher tumor grade
- HER2 overexpression may predict response to certain adjuvant chemotherapy regimens and endocrine therapy

Treatment Implications

- HER2 overexpression in breast cancer represents ideal target for therapy
  - ○ Receptor located on surface of cell and is accessible
  - ○ Receptor plays a pivotal role in driving clinical course of disease
  - ○ Targeted therapy utilizes either a HER2 specific antibody or a HER2 small molecule inhibitor
- **Trastuzumab (Herceptin)**
  - ○ Humanized monoclonal antibody that targets the HER2 receptor
  - ○ Combines mouse recognition sequence of monoclonal antibody (4D5) with human IgG1
    - ■ Trastuzumab binds to extracellular epitope of HER2 receptor
- Trastuzumab demonstrates high affinity and specificity for HER2 receptor
  - ○ In preclinical studies, this drug inhibits growth of HER2 overexpressing breast cancer cells
  - ○ Trastuzumab binding blocks receptor signaling
    - ■ May stimulate immune-mediated tumor cell cytotoxicity
    - ■ May act synergistically with chemotherapy to induce tumor cell apoptosis
- In clinical trials, trastuzumab plus chemotherapy demonstrated remarkable efficacy against HER2+BC
  - ○ Efficacy has been demonstrated for metastatic, adjuvant, and neoadjuvant therapy
  - ○ Adjuvant trastuzumab plus chemotherapy can reduce relative risk of recurrence by 50% in early stage HER2+BC
    - ■ Data suggest that only HER2+BC are likely to benefit from this therapy

- ○ Safety considerations
  - ■ Cardiac dysfunction seen in 2-4% of patients treated with trastuzumab plus anthracycline-based chemotherapy
- ○ Data highlight the importance of accurate HER2 testing
  - ■ Important to identify only those patients who will be most suitable candidates for treatment
  - ■ Benefit from targeted therapy is not related to the degree of gene amplification
  - ■ Cancers with low levels of gene amplification respond as well as cancers with large numbers of genes
- **Lapatinib (Tykerb)**
  - ○ Dual tyrosine kinase inhibitor that interrupts the kinase activity of both HER2 and EGFR (HER1)
    - ■ Oral agent
  - ○ Used for initial therapy in combination with chemotherapy or after carcinomas have progressed after treatment with trastuzumab

Clinical Assays for HER2 Status

- Immunohistochemistry (IHC) detects HER2 protein overexpression
- In situ hybridization (FISH or CISH) detects *HER2* gene amplification
  - ○ Both IHC and FISH have been clinically validated to help predict response to HER2-targeted therapy
- Oncotype DX (Genomic Health; Redwood City, CA) assay detects *HER2* mRNA overexpression using quantitative RT-PCR
  - ○ Not currently used to make treatment decisions
  - ○ Requires tissue microdissection if DCIS shows stronger HER2 positivity or if little carcinoma in relation to stroma is present
  - ○ Will not detect heterogeneity of overexpression
- HER2 testing has become an essential part of clinical evaluation for breast cancer patients
  - ○ Treatment guidelines from ASCO and the NCCN recommend HER2 testing for all newly diagnosed breast cancer patients
- Decisions about HER2-targeted therapy include concerns about cost and potential toxicities
  - ○ HER2-targeted therapy should only be used in patients whose tumors have been evaluated by a validated HER2 assay

Specimen Handling

- Breast specimens should be sectioned and placed in adequate volume of fixative within 1 hour from removal
- If gross tumor is identified during initial specimen evaluation
  - ○ Sample of tumor and fibrous normal tissue can be placed together into same cassette
    - ■ Tissue is placed immediately into formalin; fixation start time should be recorded
    - ■ Helpful to initiate good and rapid fixation
    - ■ Helps ensure normal breast tissue is available as internal control for breast marker testing

Breast Tissue Fixation

- Breast tissue samples must be fixed in 10% neutral buffered formalin
  - Formalin fixation is part of FDA approval for test kits that evaluate HER2 by IHC and FISH
- Fixation time recommended to be no less than 6-8 hours and no more than 48 hours before processing
  - Underfixation can lead to technical problems with IHC assay
  - Only very long fixation times (weeks) have been demonstrated to alter results
  - Small biopsy samples require same amount of fixation time as larger resection samples
- Acid decalcification can interfere with evaluation of specimens by FISH due to DNA degradation
  - Specimens treated with very careful EDTA decalcification and daily monitoring by specimen radiography can be used for FISH and IHC
  - Negative results using other methods of decalcification should be interpreted with caution

HER2 Assay Methodologies: IHC

- Different antibodies have been used for evaluation of HER2 protein expression in formalin-fixed, paraffin-embedded samples
  - Antibody clones have varying sensitivities and specificities
    - 3B5 (mouse, monoclonal), predominantly used in older studies: C-terminus, preferentially recognizes unphosphorylated form
    - AO85 (rabbit, polyclonal), part of FDA-approved kit: Cytoplasmic portion
    - CB11 (mouse, monoclonal), part of FDA-approved kit: Internal portion of receptor
    - 4B5 (rabbit, monoclonal), part of FDA-approved kit
    - SP3 (rabbit, monoclonal): Extracellular domain

HER2 IHC Interpretation

- Scoring of HER2 results by IHC needs to be semi-quantitatively evaluated to be clinically relevant
  - Only areas of invasive carcinoma are scored
- HER2+BC (IHC scored as 3+) ~10-15% of cancers
  - Diffuse intense circumferential membrane "chicken wire" staining pattern in > 30% of invasive cancer
    - Score as HER2 IHC positive (3+)
    - In most cancers, the majority of the carcinoma is positive
    - If only focal positivity is present (e.g., strong positivity in 20% of the cancer), this should be described; these cases may correlate with genetic heterogeneity
  - Carcinomas with this staining pattern typically show good concordance with gene amplification by FISH (> 95%)
  - Patients with HER2 3+ carcinomas are candidates for treatment with HER2-targeted therapy
  - In rare cases, the associated DCIS overexpresses HER2 but the invasive carcinoma is HER2 negative
    - This finding should be documented to ensure this is taken into account during the evaluation of other assays

- HER2-BC (IHC scored as 0 or 1+) ~ 70-75% of cancers
  - Absent or weak incomplete membrane staining in invasive cancer
    - Score as HER2 IHC negative (0/1+)
  - Cancers with this staining pattern show a good concordance with absence of amplification by FISH (> 95%)
  - Breast cancer patients with HER2 IHC 0/1+ tumors are unlikely to benefit from targeted therapy
- HER2 equivocal breast cancer (IHC scored as 2+) ~ 15% of cancers
  - Weak, circumferential membrane staining &/or heterogeneity in staining distribution < 30% of invasive tumor
    - Score as HER2 IHC equivocal (2+)
  - In correlative studies, approximately 1/5-1/4 of 2+ cancers show HER2 gene amplification
  - Breast cancers with equivocal HER2 IHC result should be analyzed by FISH to assess for HER2 gene amplification
    - These cases are more likely to have low numbers of HER2 genes
  - If the studies are performed on a core needle biopsy, it is helpful to repeat on a larger area of carcinoma in the excision
  - Some cancers will have "equivocal" HER2 results by both IHC and FISH, reflecting that HER2 expression is continuous and not bimodal
- HER2 IHC inadequate for interpretation (rejection); in some cases scoring is not possible
  - Needle core biopsies with crush artifact are inadequate for interpretation
    - Should not be overinterpreted as positive
  - Staining of adjacent normal breast tissue suggests that the assay is too sensitive
    - Results for the assay should be considered inadequate for interpretation
    - May lead to false-positive interpretation
  - Prolonged period of ischemia prior to initiation of formalin fixation
    - Time from tissue collection to fixation > than 1-2 hours
    - HER2 assay result may not be accurate
    - May lead to false-negative interpretation
  - Samples fixed for < 6-8 hours in neutral buffered formalin
  - Samples fixed for > 48 hours in neutral buffered formalin
  - Samples fixed in fixatives other than formalin
    - Alternative fixatives must be rigorously validated by laboratory
  - Samples with no residual invasive carcinoma on deeper levels
  - Samples on unstained slides stored for > 6 weeks prior to testing
- Many laboratories utilize a HER2 testing algorithm in which tumor samples are initially screened by IHC
  - FISH testing is reflexively performed only on equivocal cases
  - Testing algorithm assumes that IHC assays are highly standardized

HER2

- Laboratories must exercise rigorous quality control and follow published guidelines
- Assay must be validated to show high degree of concordance with FISH results

HER2 Assay Methodologies: In Situ Hybridization (ISH)

- Morphology-based assay to evaluate gene copy number
  - Single probe methods evaluate the number of *HER2* genes
  - Dual probe methods evaluate the number of *HER2* genes and chromosome 17 centromere sequences (CEP17)
    - Results are reported as the ratio HER2:CEP17
- Multiple methods for ISH are available
  - FISH utilizes fluorescent labeled probes and fluorescence microscopy
  - Chromogenic/bright-field in situ hybridization (CISH, Duo-CISH) and silver-enhanced in situ hybridization (SISH) use light microscopy
    - Chromogen dye or silver deposition replaces fluorescent label for detection of gene copy number
    - Light microscopy facilitates correlation with histologic appearance
    - These methods correlate well with FISH
- With FISH, quantitative interpretation of results more straightforward than with IHC
  - Concordance rates between observers are higher with FISH than with IHC in some studies
  - However, heterogeneity of expression is easier to detect with IHC
- ISH and IHC assays are best viewed as complementary methodologies
  - Each assay examines a different aspect of HER2 biology
  - ISH assays can be used in conjunction with IHC or as primary methodology for HER2 testing
- **Chromosome 17 centromere sequences (CEP17)**
  - Probe to the centromeric region of chromosome 17 is utilized in dual probe methods to determine the number of chromosomes present
  - 10-50% of HER2+BC are reported to have increased CEP17 sequences
    - "Polysomy" is usually defined as ≥ 3 CEP17 signals per nucleus
    - However, true polysomy (duplication of the entire chromosome) is only present in 1-2% of cancers
    - In the majority of cancers, increased CEP17 is due to duplication of a segment of centromeric DNA
  - Carcinomas with 3-5 copies of the *HER2* gene and increased CEP17 generally do not show increased protein expression
  - Carcinomas with > 6 gene copies are usually associated with HER2 overexpression
    - > 90% of these cases will also have HER2:CEP17 ratios > 2.2, and the carcinoma is classified as HER2 amplified
    - In rare cases, the ratio is < 2.2 due to the increased CEP17 numbers, and the 2 methods for

determining *HER2* amplification have different interpretations
  - If not previously performed, an IHC assay should be performed
  - Carcinomas with 3+ scores by IHC are classified as HER2+BC
  - It is not yet clear if carcinomas with 2+ scores by IHC, > 6 gene copies, but ratios < 2.2 will benefit from targeted therapy
    - Monosomy for chromosome 17 occurs in < 5% of cancers
    - It is not clear if ratios > 2.2 in the presence of monosomy will predict benefit from targeted therapy

HER2 FISH Interpretation

- Guidelines for HER2 FISH interpretation were recommended by an ASCO/CAP task force
  - Different criteria for interpretation of CISH or SISH
- H&E slide corresponding to the block used for FISH should be examined
  - Areas of invasive carcinoma are identified and marked
  - Areas of DCIS should be noted in order to exclude them from the evaluation
    - In rare cases, DCIS will show amplification but not the associated invasive carcinoma
  - Review of the HER2 IHC slide is helpful to identify areas of heterogeneous protein expression that should be correlated with FISH results
- Slide prepared for FISH is examined using a fluorescence microscope
  - Entire slide is scanned to select the best areas for analysis and to evaluate genetic heterogeneity
    - At least 2, and up to 4, representative fields are analyzed
  - Fluorescent counterstains allow identification of areas of invasive cancer
  - Number of signals from randomly selected invasive tumor cell nuclei are counted
    - Cells should be nonoverlapping with distinct nuclear membranes, and at least 1 signal should be clearly visible
    - If 2 different probes are used, at least 1 signal from each probe should be seen in each cell counted
    - Good gene signals should be present in > 75% of tumor cells to help ensure adequate hybridization of probe
    - Sufficient numbers of nuclei are counted to ensure that the ratio is representative of the entire cancer
    - At least 40 cells, 20 in each of 2 fields, should be counted
    - In dual probe systems, both the HER2 count and the CEP17 count are determined in the same set of cells; the average number of signals are used to calculate the HER2:CEP17 ratio
    - If the result would be classified as "equivocal," additional cells should be counted &/or the assay should be repeated
- **HER2+BC (FISH amplified)**
  - HER2:CEP17 ratio is > 2.2 or HER2 count is > 6.0
    - Score as *HER2* gene amplified

- > 90% of tumors with gene amplification show HER2 protein overexpression by IHC (scored as 3+)
  - These 2 methods of scoring ISH are concordant in the majority of cases
  ○ Breast cancers with *HER2* gene amplification are candidates for treatment with HER2-targeted therapy
  ○ Nonconcordance between the 2 methods of scoring can occur in carcinomas with increased CEP17 signals (i.e., > 6 genes but ratio < 2.2)
    - Approximately 1/3 of these cases have IHC 3+, and the cancer would be classified as being HER2 positive
    - If the cancer shows equivocal 2+ expression, it is not yet clear if the patient would benefit from targeted therapy
- **HER2(-) breast cancer (FISH not amplified)**
  ○ Calculated HER2:CEP17 ratio is < 1.8 or HER2 count is < 4.0
    - Score as *HER2* gene not amplified
    - > 95% of tumors without gene amplification do not show HER2 protein overexpression (0/1+)
  ○ Breast cancer patients without *HER2* gene amplification are not candidates for treatment with HER2-targeted therapy
- **HER2 FISH equivocal breast cancer**
  ○ Calculated HER2:CEP17 ratio is 1.8-2.2 or HER2 count is 4.0-6.0
    - New category created by ASCO/CAP Task Force on HER2 guidelines; previously any ratio ≥ 2 was considered amplification
    - 3-5% of cases will have HER2:CEP17 ratio that falls very close to this cut-off point
    - Most appropriate HER2 status for HER2 FISH equivocal patients is unclear
  ○ Carcinomas with equivocal HER2 FISH result need additional analysis to resolve HER2 status
    - Count additional tumor nuclei by FISH
    - Reflex testing by IHC to assess for HER2 protein overexpression (if not previously done)
    - Additional testing on other specimens may be of value (e.g., an excisional specimen after a core needle biopsy)
    - Some carcinomas biologically have "borderline" expression after repeat testing; reflects that expression is continuous and not bimodal
- **HER2 FISH inadequate for interpretation**
  ○ Some assay results are inadequate for interpretation and must be repeated
    - Total of at least 40 nonoverlapping, intact tumor nuclei cannot be identified
    - Either positive or negative control results fall outside expected values
    - Hybridization signals are not uniform throughout areas of invasive tumor (> 75% of cells)
    - Background is too high or obscures gene signals
    - Enzymatic digestion is not optimized to produce scorable signals
    - Nuclear borders are indistinct or lost (overdigestion)

- Persistence of green autofluorescence that obscures signal (underdigestion)

HER2 Genetic Heterogeneity (GH)

- Some cancers show more than 1 population of tumor cells according to HER2 amplification
- Genetic heterogeneity is present when > 5% but < 50% of the tumor cells show amplification (ratio > 2.2 or > 6 genes)
  ○ If > 50% of the cells show amplification, the carcinoma is reported as HER2 positive without GH
- Classification of the cancer is based on the average results over the entire carcinoma
  ○ Significance of GH for determining benefit from HER2-targeted therapy is unknown
- The statement "*HER2* genetic heterogeneity is present (see comment)" should be included, and the comment should state the following
  ○ Percent of invasive carcinoma showing *HER2* amplification
  ○ Indication of whether the amplified cells are scattered or in a specific cluster
  ○ If a cluster of cells showing amplification is seen, the HER2/CEP17 results for the cluster should be provided and it should be stated if these cells have a histologically distinct appearance
- If GH is detected on a core needle biopsy
  ○ Report should state that the findings might not be representative of the entire carcinoma
  ○ Additional testing on the excisional specimen may be of value

QA and QC for HER2 Testing

- **Analytical validation requirements**
- Initial test validation with 25-100 samples fixed in formalin using standardized operating procedures
  ○ Samples are tested in parallel by alternative validated method (FISH if validating IHC)
    - Tests can be performed in either the same or another laboratory
  ○ Must achieve > 95% concordance for positive and negative results
  ○ Validation is ASCO/CAP guideline requirement before HER2 test can be offered clinically
- **Routine use of control materials**
  ○ Positive and negative controls should be run with every assay to help ensure proper assay performance
    - Batch control using HER2(+) cell lines helps ensure appropriate assay sensitivity
    - Batch controls can be used to monitor assay performance and to detect loss of sensitivity or assay analytical drift
    - Known HER2(+) sample on the same slide as test sample helps to ensure that all reagents were dispensed appropriately
- **Monitor daily testing results**
  ○ Review of batch controls and "on slide controls" to ensure accurate assay performance
    - Evaluate results for analytical drift and loss of assay sensitivity
- **Perform periodic trend analysis**
  ○ Helps ensure that percentage of HER2(+) cases are within expected norm for breast cancer population

HER2

HER2 Immunohistochemistry Scoring Criteria

HER2 Status	Tumor Cell Membrane Staining
Positive = 3+	Intense circumferential membrane staining pattern ("chicken wire") > 30% invasive tumor
Negative = 0 or 1+	Absent (0) or weak partial membrane staining, > 10% invasive tumor (1+)
Equivocal = 2+; reflex FISH test required	Weak complete membrane staining, nonuniform or stronger staining in < 30% invasive tumor

HER2 FISH Scoring Criteria

Probes	Nonamplified	Equivocal	Amplified
Dual probes (HER2 and CEP17)	HER2/CEP17 < 1.8	HER2/CEP17 = 1.8-2.2	HER2/CEP17 > 2.2
Single probe (HER2)	HER < 4	HER2 = 4-6	HER2 > 6

- **Participate in HER2 testing proficiency program**
  - Helps ensure high concordance and accuracy of individual laboratory results

Critical Evaluation of HER2 Assays

- Make sure tissue handling and fixation parameters comply with guidelines
- Make sure controls demonstrate expected results
- Question tissue antigenicity if everything is negative by IHC
- Make sure HER2 test results fit histologic appearance and clinical history (e.g., concordant with prior assays on the same or other specimens)
- IHC and ISH testing are complementary methods
  - Examine different aspects of HER2 biology
  - Technical validation is critical
- Continuous monitoring of QA/QC and assay performance is essential

CORE NEEDLE BIOPSIES

Evaluation of HER2

- Both IHC and ISH can be performed on core needle biopsies
- This testing may be required to identify patients eligible for neoadjuvant therapy
- Concordance between core needle biopsies and subsequent excisions is 85-90%
- Discordant results can result from tumor heterogeneity (i.e., only a small portion of a large carcinoma may be sampled in a needle biopsy) or differences in fixation
- If the results on the core needle biopsy do not show amplification, repeat studies on the subsequent excision should be considered in the following situations
  - Amount of carcinoma in the needle biopsy is small (~ < 0.5 cm), especially if the primary carcinoma is large
  - Carcinoma is poorly differentiated
  - Multiple foci of invasion are present
  - Equivocal results are obtained on the needle biopsy
  - Patient has received neoadjuvant therapy and residual carcinoma is present

SELECTED REFERENCES

1. Vranic S et al: Assessment of HER2 gene status in breast carcinomas with polysomy of chromosome 17. Cancer. 117(1):48-53, 2011
2. Babic A et al: The impact of pre-analytical processing on staining quality for H&E, dual hapten, dual color in situ hybridization and fluorescent in situ hybridization assays. Methods. 52(4):287-300, 2010
3. Ibarra JA et al: Fixation time does not affect expression of HER2/neu: a pilot study. Am J Clin Pathol. 134(4):594-6, 2010
4. Moelans CB et al: Absence of chromosome 17 polysomy in breast cancer: analysis by CEP17 chromogenic in situ hybridization and multiplex ligation-dependent probe amplification. Breast Cancer Res Treat. 120(1):1-7, 2010
5. Chibon F et al: Prediction of HER2 gene status in Her2 2+ invasive breast cancer: a study of 108 cases comparing ASCO/CAP and FDA recommendations. Mod Pathol. 22(3):403-9, 2009
6. Krishnamurti U et al: Poor prognostic significance of unamplified chromosome 17 polysomy in invasive breast carcinoma. Mod Pathol. 22(8):1044-8, 2009
7. Marchiò C et al: Does chromosome 17 centromere copy number predict polysomy in breast cancer? A fluorescence in situ hybridization and microarray-based CGH analysis. J Pathol. 219(1):16-24, 2009
8. Shah SS et al: Effect of high copy number of HER2 associated with polysomy 17 on HER2 protein expression in invasive breast carcinoma. Diagn Mol Pathol. 18(1):30-3, 2009
9. Vance GH et al: Genetic heterogeneity in HER2 testing in breast cancer: panel summary and guidelines. Arch Pathol Lab Med. 133(4):611-2, 2009
10. Hicks DG et al: HER2+ breast cancer: review of biologic relevance and optimal use of diagnostic tools. Am J Clin Pathol. 129(2):263-73, 2008
11. Hicks DG et al: Trastuzumab as adjuvant therapy for early breast cancer: the importance of accurate human epidermal growth factor receptor 2 testing. Arch Pathol Lab Med. 132(6):1008-15, 2008
12. Wolff AC et al: American Society of Clinical Oncology/College of American Pathologists guideline recommendations for human epidermal growth factor receptor 2 testing in breast cancer. Arch Pathol Lab Med. 131(1):18-43, 2007

HER2

Immunohistochemical Assay

(Left) Low-grade infiltrating ductal carcinomas show good tubule formation ➔. Breast tumors with these morphologic features would be unlikely to show HER2 gene amplification or protein overexpression. *(Right)* Well-differentiated carcinomas are expected to show absent or partial weak membrane HER2 staining. This result ➔ would be scored as a negative (1+ staining). The majority of tumors with this staining pattern do not show evidence for HER2 gene amplification by FISH.

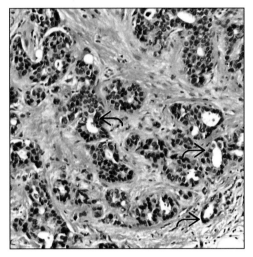
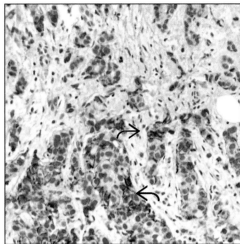

(Left) Moderately differentiated invasive ductal carcinomas show partial tubule formation ➔ and higher grade nuclei. *(Right)* There is complete membrane staining ➔ that is weak and nonuniform ➔ throughout the tumor. This would be scored as an equivocal result for HER2 overexpression (2+ staining). Tumors with this staining pattern are inconclusive for HER2 overexpression and should be sent for reflex HER2 FISH testing. About 1/5-1/4 will show low levels of amplification.

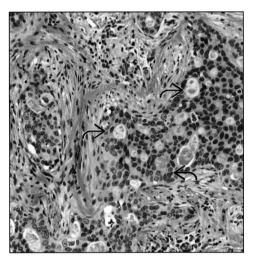
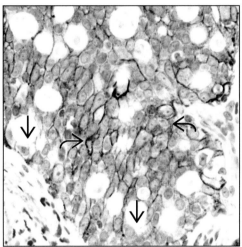

(Left) Poorly differentiated invasive ductal carcinomas show high-grade nuclei ➔ as well as numerous mitotic figures ➔. Tumors with these features are more likely to show HER2 overexpression. *(Right)* The IHC for HER2 shows complete, uniformly distributed membrane staining ➔ ("chicken wire" pattern) and would be scored as a positive result for HER2 overexpression (3+ staining). Tumors with this staining pattern show gene amplification by FISH in over 90% of cases.

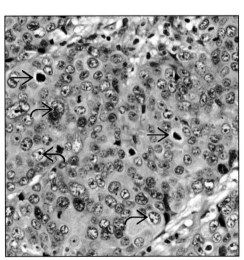
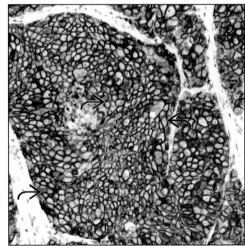

Controls and QA for HER2 Evaluation by IHC

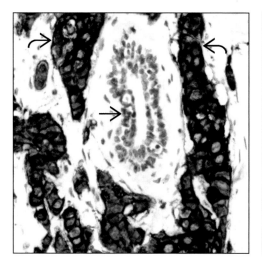

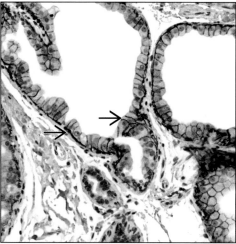

(Left) This invasive carcinoma has the classic "chicken wire" membrane positive staining pattern for HER2+BC ➡. Normal breast elements should be HER2 negative ➡ if the assay is performing properly. *(Right)* In an optimized HER2 assay, normal breast elements should be completely negative for HER2. One exception is apocrine metaplasia, which typically shows basal-lateral HER2 membrane staining ➡. If other normal elements are HER2 positive, the assay should be repeated.

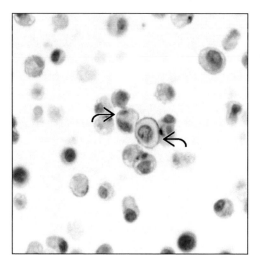

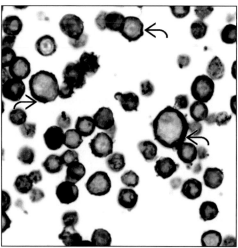

(Left) The cell line MDA-175, when formalin fixed and paraffin embedded, shows partial weak membrane staining for HER2 ➡. Use of cell lines as "batch" controls helps ensure proper assay performance, sensitivity, and dynamic range for each staining run. *(Right)* The cell line SK-BR3, when formalin fixed and paraffin embedded, shows a high level of HER2 expression with the expected intense circumferential membrane staining ➡. This cell line can be used as a positive control.

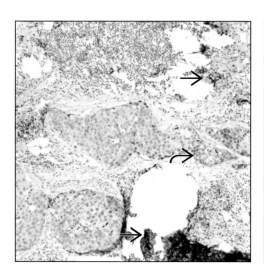

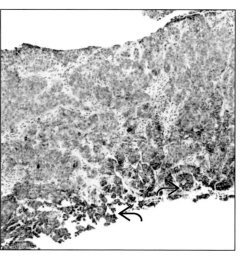

(Left) This invasive ductal carcinoma was fixed for only 2 hours in formalin prior to processing. Accurate HER2 results depend on proper tissue fixation. Tumor cells show partial weak membrane staining ➡. The presence of tissue folding ➡ also suggests that there is a technical problem with the assay and the results should be rejected. *(Right)* This HER2-negative invasive carcinoma shows edge artifact ➡. Membrane staining is concentrated at the periphery of tissue.

HER2

HER2 Genotyping (FISH, CISH)

(Left) This FISH assay shows > 6 HER2 signals (red ➡) and 0-2 CEP17 signals (green ➡). Therefore, this carcinoma would be classified as showing HER2 gene amplification by either using the number of genes or the ratio (HER2:CEP17 > 2.2). *(Right)* The relative number of HER2 signals ➡ and CEP17 signals ➡ is similar and therefore the HER2/CEP17 ratio is < 1.8. There are also fewer than 6 HER2 signals, and thus the carcinoma would be classified as not showing amplification.

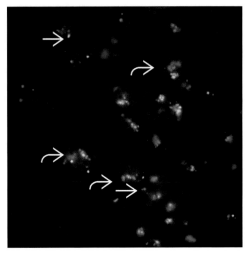 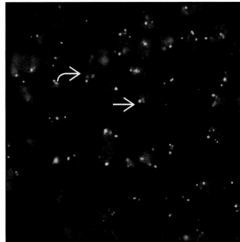

(Left) The number of HER2 signals ➡ and CEP17 signals ➡ are both increased, giving a HER2/CEP17 ratio of < 1.8. In most cases the centromeric sequences are amplified, and in only rare cancers is there true polysomy. Some of these cases show protein overexpression. *(Right)* This FISH assay shows poor hybridization. The tumor cells appear faint, some are fragmented ➡, and many lack hybridization signals. The assay is technically inadequate and should be rejected.

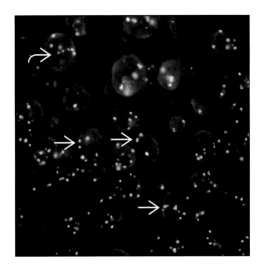 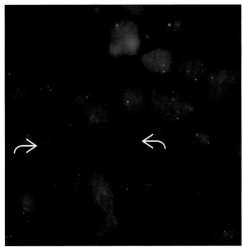

(Left) HER2 CISH allows for chromogenic detection of HER2 signals (red ➡) and CEP17 signals (blue ➡) and interpretation by light microscopy. This carcinoma shows a similar number of HER2 and CEP17 signals and is not amplified (HER2/CEP17 < 1.8). *(Right)* In this CISH assay, the number of HER2 signals ➡ is markedly increased, and the carcinoma would be considered as having HER2 gene amplification. A normal duct shows the normal number of HER2 and CEP17 signals ➡.

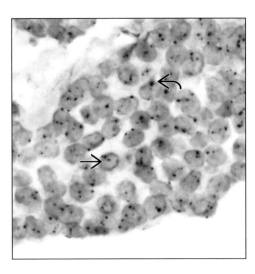 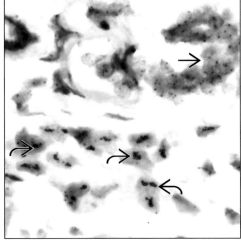

HER2

Difficult Cases for HER2 Evaluation

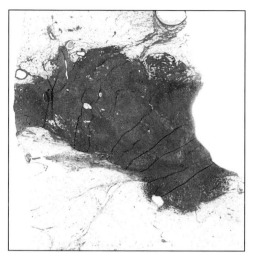

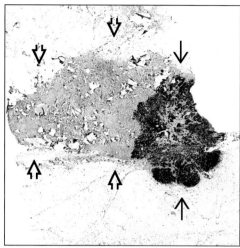

(Left) This is a 1.1 cm moderately differentiated carcinoma that was positive for both ER and PR throughout the carcinoma. *(Right)* The carcinoma shows genetic heterogeneity for HER2. Approximately 2/3 of the carcinoma is completely negative ⊡, but 1/3 is strongly positive by immunohistochemistry ➔ and was amplified by FISH. There was no morphologic correlate for the different areas with or without HER2 expression. A lymph node metastasis was negative for HER2.

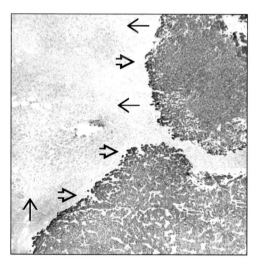

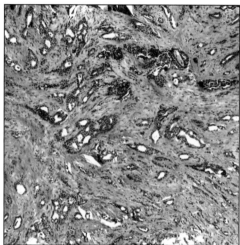

(Left) This patient with carcinoma had marked heterogeneity for HER2 expression. Lymph node metastasis also shows strongly HER2 positive ⊡ & negative ➔ areas. *(Right)* This well-differentiated invasive ductal carcinoma showed weak (1+) immunoreactivity for HER2. FISH showed marked amplification with 20 copies of HER2 & a ratio of 10. Repeat FISH gave the same results. Cases like this will not be detected by IHC alone. Response to HER2-based therapy is unknown.

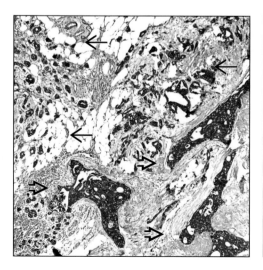

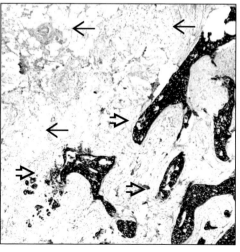

(Left) This carcinoma consists of areas of invasive carcinoma positive for cytokeratin AE1/AE3 ➔, as well as adjacent areas of DCIS positive for cytokeratin and with myoepithelial cells positive for p63 ⊡. *(Right)* The DCIS is strongly positive for HER2 ⊡, but the invasive carcinoma is completely negative ➔. Only invasive carcinoma is scored for IHC and FISH. Microdissection would be necessary to test such an invasive carcinoma by multigene assays such as Oncotype DX.

Difficulties in HER2 Evaluation

*(**Left**) This carcinoma has 2 HER2 signals* 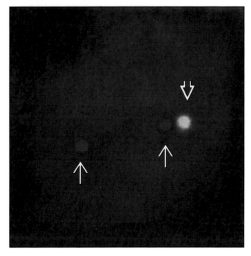 *and 1 CEP17 signal* . *The ratio is 2.0, and the patient would be eligible for HER2-targeted therapy. Such cancers are unlikely to show protein overexpression, and response to targeted therapy is unclear. (**Right**) This carcinoma has 8 CEP17 signals and 8 HER2 signals. It would be considered amplified according to the number of genes but not according to the ratio. The best method to predict response to HER2-targeted therapy is unclear.*

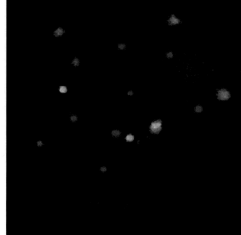

*(**Left**) Cytoplasmic HER2 immunoreactivity is sometimes present but is not scored as a positive result. This pattern can make membrane positivity difficult to evaluate. FISH studies can be helpful in some cases. (**Right**) Well- and moderately differentiated breast cancers such as tubular, papillary, lobular, and mucinous carcinomas rarely, if ever, overexpress HER2. Positive results, such as in this mucinous carcinoma, are often best confirmed by FISH.*

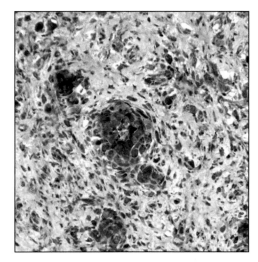

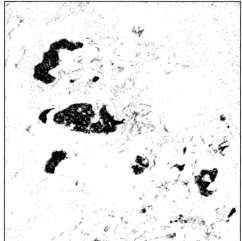

*(**Left**) Well- and moderately differentiated invasive lobular carcinomas rarely overexpress HER2. However, due to the discohesion of the cells, edge enhancement can occur* . *This should not be overinterpreted as positivity. (**Right**) Invasive lobular carcinoma and LCIS can show edge enhancement for HER2 because the cells are not attached to adjacent cells or stroma. In this case of LCIS, the chromogen appears to be in the cracks between the cells* .

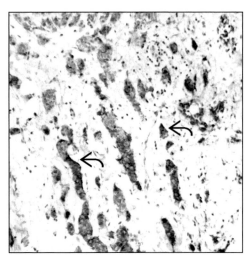

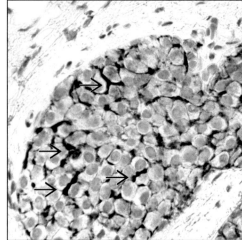

HER2 and Histologic Types of Breast Carcinomas

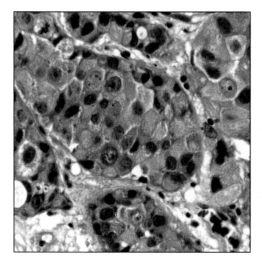

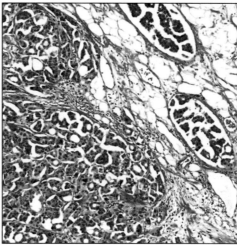

(Left) Apocrine carcinomas are more likely than other subtypes of carcinoma to overexpress HER2. Approximately 50% of cases are positive by IHC or are amplified by FISH. These carcinomas are also frequently positive for androgen receptor and GCDFP-15. (Right) In addition to apocrine carcinoma, invasive micropapillary carcinoma (pictured) and inflammatory carcinoma have a higher rate of HER2 overexpression compared to carcinomas of no special type.

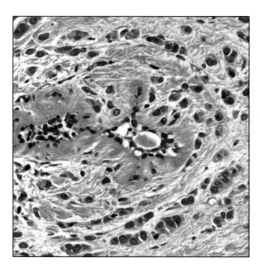

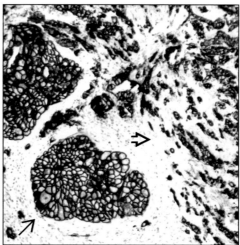

(Left) Well- and moderately differentiated carcinomas including tubular carcinoma, papillary carcinoma, mucinous carcinoma, and low-grade lobular carcinoma (pictured) very rarely overexpress HER2. If the HER2 findings are not typical for a histologic type, repeat studies or additional studies (e.g., both IHC and FISH) should be considered. (Right) This is an unusual case of an E-cadherin(-) poorly differentiated invasive lobular carcinoma ➡ & LCIS ➡ that overexpress HER2.

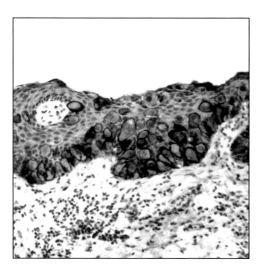

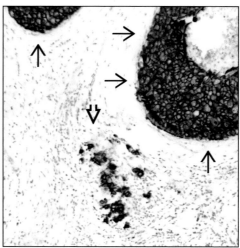

(Left) Approximately 80% of cases of DCIS in nipple skin (Paget disease of the nipple) are positive for HER2. These specimens can be useful controls for HER2 assays. (Right) DCIS ➡ is more commonly positive for HER2 (40-50% of cases, higher in cases with high grade nuclei) than is invasive carcinoma (approximately 20% of cases). In this case, an area of microinvasion is also HER2 positive ➡. However, associated invasive carcinomas can be negative for HER2.

DNA ANALYSIS

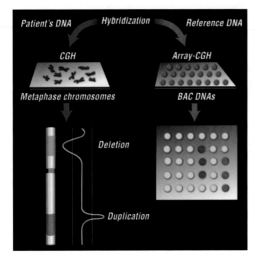

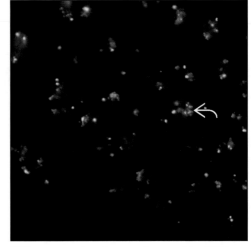

Labeled DNA from a tumor is hybridized to either metaphase chromosomes (CGH) or a DNA microarray (array-CGH). Deletions or duplications of DNA are detected by comparison with reference normal DNA.

DNA copy number changes discovered by CGH can be validated by FISH. Amplification of the HER2 gene (red signals) ⇒ is the prototype for genomic changes associated with high-grade breast cancers.

TERMINOLOGY

Abbreviations
- Conventional cytogenetics (CC)
- Comparative genomic hybridization (CGH)
- Loss of heterozygosity (LOH)
- Copy number alterations (CNA)

Definitions
- Completion of human genome project will expand knowledge of human DNA sequences
- Development of new genomic technologies provide new tools to study human disease
  - CC: Visualizes all chromosomes; detects large translocations and chromosomal duplication or loss
  - CGH: Detects gains or losses of short DNA segments throughout genome
  - LOH: Detects loss of 1 of 2 alleles of specific genes
  - FISH: Uses specific probes to visualize increased copies of genes or to identify gene translocations
- These genomic technologies can be applied to clinical breast cancer samples
- Possible to study complex genomic aberrations and recurrent genomic imbalances characterizing tumors
  - CGH allows genome-wide investigation of CNA
  - Has resulted in major advances in understanding of breast carcinogenesis and tumor progression

ETIOLOGY/PATHOGENESIS

Histogenesis
- Breast cancers are characterized by complex genomic changes and CNA
  - Common and specific recurrent genomic changes described in breast tumors
    - Most common recurrent chromosomal genomic gains: 1q, 8q, 17q, 20q, and 11q
    - Most common recurrent chromosomal genomic losses: 8p, 11q, 13q, 16q, and 18q

- Many of these changes occur in regions that harbor known proto-oncogenes and tumor suppressor genes
  - May cause gene overexpression or loss of function

CLINICAL IMPLICATIONS

Genomic Changes and Tumor Grade
- Genomic aberrations and CNA are correlated with traditional clinicopathologic factors in breast cancer
  - Number and pattern of genomic aberrations differ most significantly when stratified by tumor grade
    - Average number of chromosomal changes increase with increasing tumor grade
    - Patterns of genomic alterations (genomic signatures) differ significantly when stratified by grade
- Prototype for significant changes in DNA copy number is amplification of HER2 gene on long arm of chromosome 17 (17q12)
  - Increased number of genes leads to higher levels of mRNA and increase in protein expression
  - This genomic change is significantly and independently correlated with high-grade carcinomas
    - < 1% of low-grade carcinomas show evidence of HER2 gene amplification

Low-Grade Invasive Ductal Carcinoma
- Tend to have fewer chromosomal alterations compared with high-grade carcinomas
  - HER2 nonamplified
  - Diploid
  - Low proliferative index
- Most frequent genomic changes
  - Losses on chromosome 16q and gains on 1q
  - Other reported changes include chromosomal gains on 8q, 11q, 16p, and 17q and losses on 1p, 8p, 11q, 13q, and 22q

DNA ANALYSIS

Genomic Alterations in Breast Cancer

Tumor Grade	Chromosomal Gains (Amplifications)	Chromosomal Losses (Deletions)
Low grade	Gains on 1q, 8q, 11q, 16p, and 17q	Losses on 16q, 1p, 8p, 11q, 13q, and 22q
High grade	Gains on 8q, 17q, and 20q	Losses on 17p, 1p, 19p, and 19q

- ○ Similar genomic changes have been described in low-grade DCIS, LCIS, and non-high-grade invasive lobular carcinoma
- ○ Genomic changes found in low-grade invasive carcinomas are shared with low-grade DCIS (precursor lesions)
  - ▪ Changes likely occur early in course of disease and play a role in pathogenesis
  - ▪ Low-grade ductal and lobular carcinomas may share common molecular origin

High-Grade Invasive Ductal Carcinoma

- Tend to have more frequent, extensive, and complex chromosomal alterations
  - ○ Overexpress *C-MYC* and *HER2* by gene amplification
  - ○ Demonstrate frequent loss of p53 function
  - ○ Aneuploid
  - ○ High proliferative index
- Most frequent genomic changes
  - ○ Losses on chromosome 17p, 1p, 19p, and 19q; infrequent losses on 16q
  - ○ Genomic chromosomal gains on 8q, 17q, and 20q
- Similar genomic changes have been described in high-grade DCIS
  - ○ Changes likely occur early in course of development of disease and likely play a role in pathogenesis

Molecular Pathogenesis

- Cancer development and progression is due to accumulation of recurrent genomic alterations
  - ○ Genomic changes can alter gene expression inducing growth advantage and clonal expansion
- Genomic studies suggest separate molecular pathways lead to development of low- and high-grade breast carcinomas
  - ○ Tumorigenesis is associated with unique patterns of genomic alterations for low- and high-grade carcinomas

- ▪ Gene expression profiling studies also show distinctive patterns of mRNA expression for low- and high-grade carcinomas
- ○ Differential changes found in low- and high-grade invasive carcinomas are also shared with low- and high-grade DCIS
  - ▪ Molecular heterogeneity of breast cancer already exists in in situ lesions
  - ▪ Thus, genomic changes occur early in course of development of cancer
  - ▪ Likely play a role in disease pathogenesis, initiation of tumor formation, and tumor progression
- Studies comparing CNA by CGH and gene expression analysis
  - ○ Close correlation between DNA copy number and mRNA expression levels has been reported
  - ○ Suggests gene amplification is common mechanism for increased gene expression in breast tumors

SELECTED REFERENCES

1. Andre F et al: Molecular characterization of breast cancer with high-resolution oligonucleotide comparative genomic hybridization array. Clin Cancer Res. 15(2):441-51, 2009
2. Vincent-Salomon A et al: Integrated genomic and transcriptomic analysis of ductal carcinoma in situ of the breast. Clin Cancer Res. 14(7):1956-65, 2008
3. Climent J et al: Characterization of breast cancer by array comparative genomic hybridization. Biochem Cell Biol. 85(4):497-508, 2007

IMAGE GALLERY

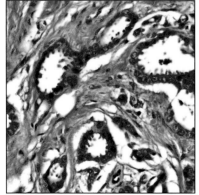 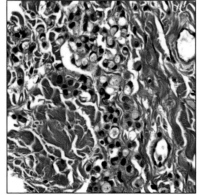 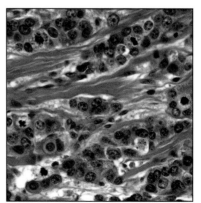

(Left) H&E shows well-differentiated tubular carcinoma of the breast. *(Center)* Invasive lobular carcinoma with signet ring cells is shown. *(Right)* Poorly differentiated invasive ductal carcinoma is depicted. Low-grade carcinomas show fewer genomic alterations compared with high-grade carcinomas. Low-grade ductal and lobular carcinomas show similar patterns and types of genomic changes and may share a common molecular origin, which is distinct and different from that of high-grade tumors.

EXPRESSION PROFILING, mRNA

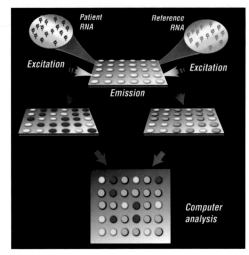

GEP is performed by mixing labeled tumor RNA with reference RNA and hybridizing to complementary sequences. Relative RNA expression may be increased (red), decreased (green), or unchanged (yellow).

GEP data are analyzed to find biologically meaningful patterns based on similar patterns of gene expression. This approach was used to develop the intrinsic molecular classification of breast cancers.

TERMINOLOGY

Abbreviations
- Gene expression profiling (GEP)

Definitions
- Methods that measure relative amounts of mRNA in cancers; overall pattern is referred to as the gene profile or signature

GENE EXPRESSION PROFILING

Introduction
- GEP uses cDNA microarrays or quantitative RT-PCR on clinical samples of breast tumor tissue to detect mRNA levels
  - Simultaneous examination of global changes in patterns of gene expression
  - Ability to molecularly profile breast tumors at the level of the expression of 20,000-25,000 genes
- GEP has added greatly to our understanding of biologic diversity of breast cancer
  - Provides important insights into breast tumor biology
  - Provides clinically meaningful molecular tumor classification
  - Identifies good and poor prognostic groups
  - Defines cancers more susceptible to specific types of therapy
- GEP has potential to provide value beyond traditional clinical/pathologic prognostic and predictive factors

GEP, Unsupervised "Cluster" Analysis
- Requires fresh or snap-frozen tissue samples from cohort of breast cancer patients with outcome data
  - RNA isolated from tumor tissue
  - Analyzed using cDNA microarrays
    - Determines level of mRNA gene expression relative to reference RNA

- Data on expression levels for thousands of genes collected for analysis
- Computer and statistical analysis needed to look for biologically meaningful patterns
- Unsupervised cluster analysis (class discovery approach)
  - Sorts tumors into related clusters based on similarities in gene expression profiles
  - "Dendrograms" used to illustrate degree of relatedness between different tumors
  - Sorts tumors into different groups of imputed biologic significance
- This approach used to develop intrinsic molecular classification of breast cancer

CLINICAL IMPLICATIONS

GEP Identifies Four Major Types of Cancer
- Microarrays and unsupervised analysis group breast cancers into distinctive subsets using patterns of mRNA levels
- Reproducible differences in gene expression patterns help define distinct subtypes of breast cancer
  - Likely represent different distinct tumor types
    - Reflect underlying differences in biology
    - Influence clinical course, likelihood of recurrence, and overall survival
    - Influence response to therapy
- Results of GEP support that groups of cancers defined by ER, PR, HER2, and proliferation also share a much broader range of gene expression patterns

Luminal Subtype A
- Gene expression pattern (~ 55% of breast cancers)
  - High levels of ER
    - Genes regulated by ER (including PR) and genes associated with ER activation
  - Luminal cytokeratins (e.g., cytokeratins 8/18)
  - Does not overexpress HER2

○ Lower expression of proliferation-related genes
- Clinical features
  - ○ Indolent clinical course of disease
  - ○ Better prognosis compared with luminal B cancers or other subtypes
  - ○ Metastatic pattern is to bone, often after a long disease-free interval

Luminal Subtype B

- Gene expression pattern (~ 15% of breast cancers)
  - ○ Generally lower level of expression of ER and ER-related genes
  - ○ Often negative for PR or low-level expression
  - ○ HER2 overexpressed in 30-50% of cases
  - ○ May overexpress EGFR (HER1)
  - ○ Higher expression of proliferation-related genes
    - ▪ Ki-67 proliferation index may be useful to help separate luminal B from luminal A tumors
- Clinical features
  - ○ More aggressive clinical course, worse prognosis

HER2 Subtype

- Gene expression pattern (15-20% of breast cancers)
  - ○ HER2 overexpressed
    - ▪ Also overexpresses adjacent genes on HER2 amplicon; number of genes varies in different cancers
    - ▪ May include TOP2-α (associated with sensitivity to anthracyclines) and GRB7
  - ○ Does not express ER or PR
  - ○ Higher expression of proliferation-related genes
- Clinical features
  - ○ More likely to have multiple involved lymph nodes
  - ○ More aggressive clinical course; poor prognosis but modified by HER2-targeted therapy
- Identification of HER2 subtype by GEP confirmed that these cancers represent a clinically distinct subset
  - ○ HER2(+) tumors defined by GEP do not completely overlap with HER2(+) tumors defined by IHC &/or FISH

Basal Subtype

- Gene expression pattern (~ 10% of breast cancers)
  - ○ Does not express ER or PR
  - ○ Does not overexpress HER2
  - ○ High expression of proliferation-related genes
  - ○ Strong expression of basal cytokeratins 5, 14, and 17
  - ○ May show gene amplification and overexpression of EGFR (HER1)
- Clinical features
  - ○ Typically younger patients
    - ▪ May have positive breast cancer family history
    - ▪ May benefit from genetic testing
  - ○ Poor prognosis and aggressive clinical course for majority of basal cancers
  - ○ Increased likelihood of early local or systemic recurrence within 3-5 years
  - ○ Visceral recurrence and brain metastases more likely than in other subtypes
  - ○ Some cancers that fall within this group have a favorable prognosis (e.g., adenoid cystic carcinoma, low-grade adenosquamous carcinoma, medullary carcinoma)

- Triple negative phenotype (ER, PR, HER2 negative) commonly used as surrogate for basal subtype
  - ○ Triple negative and basal subtype only overlap by 70-80%
  - ○ ~ 10% of basal subtype are ER positive, and ~ 10% overexpress HER2

EXPRESSION PROFILING ASSAYS

Oncotype DX®

- Marketed by Genomic Health, Inc.; Redwood City, CA, USA
- 21 gene RT-PCR assay
  - ○ 16 genes are cancer related
  - ○ Includes ER, PR, and HER2; individual values provided for each
  - ○ Includes proliferation-related genes including Ki-67
- Test results
  - ○ Recurrence score (RS) with values from 0-100
    - ▪ Low risk: RS < 18 (~ 51% of patients)
    - ▪ Intermediate risk: RS > 18 but < 30 (~ 22% of patients)
    - ▪ High risk: RS > 30 (~ 27% of patients)
  - ○ RS provides risk of distant recurrence at 10 years for node-negative women treated with tamoxifen
    - ▪ Low risk, ~ 7%; intermediate risk, ~ 14%; high risk, ~ 31%
  - ○ RS correlated with magnitude of benefit of chemotherapy
    - ▪ Greatest benefit for high-risk women; benefit under investigation for intermediate-risk women; no apparent benefit for low-risk women
- Cost: $3,978 (USA, current as of March 17, 2011)

MammaPrint®

- Marketed by Agendia BV; Amsterdam, the Netherlands
- 70 gene microarray assay (Amsterdam signature)
  - ○ Includes only 1 gene used for Oncotype DX
- Test results
  - ○ Correlation coefficient > 0.4: Good prognosis
  - ○ Correlation coefficient ≤ 0.4: Poor prognosis
- Prognosis score correlated with distant disease-free survival at 5 years for patients not receiving treatment
  - ○ Good prognosis: 85% disease-free and 95% survival
  - ○ Poor prognosis: 51% disease-free and 55% survival
- Cost: $4,200 (USA, current as of March 17, 2011)

Theros H/I® (H:I Ratio)

- Marketed by bioTheranostics; San Diego, CA, USA
- 6 gene RT-PCR assay
  - ○ 2 genes are cancer related: *HOXB13* and *IL17BR*
- Test results
  - ○ Ratio of H:I, normalized to expression of other genes
- High ratio is predictive of decreased disease-free survival
- Cost: $1,400 (USA, current as of March 17, 2011)

MapQuant Dx™ (Genomic Grade Index [GGI])

- Marketed by Ipsogen SA; Marseille, France
- 97 gene microarray assay

Commercially Available GEP Assays

Name	Assay	Tissue Required	Patient Population	Results
Oncotype DX (Genomic Health, Inc.)	RT-PCR for 21 genes (16 cancer related) including ER, PR, HER2	Formalin-fixed paraffin-embedded tissue	Stage I or II; ER positive	Distant recurrence at 10 years for node-negative patients if treated with tamoxifen; relative benefit of chemotherapy; values of ER, PR, HER2
MammaPrint (Agendia BV)	Microarray for 70 genes	Fresh-frozen tissue or saved in RNA preservative with at least 30% tumor cells	Age < 61 years; stage I or II; ≤ 5 cm; node negative	Good or poor prognosis signatures; distant recurrence at 5 years (Amsterdam signature)
Theros H:I Expression Ratio (bioTheranostics)	RT-PCR assay for 6 genes (2 cancer related)	Formalin-fixed paraffin-embedded tissue	ER-positive cancer; node negative	Low- or high-risk groups: Disease-free survival at 5 years
MapQuant Dx Genomic Grade Index (Ipsogen)	Microarray for 97 genes or RT-PCR for 8 genes	Fresh-frozen, tissue- or formalin-fixed, paraffin-embedded tissue	ER-positive cancer	Low or high GGI: Correlates with disease-free and overall survival

- Modified quantitative RT-PCR assay using 4 genes has been developed
  - *MYBL2* (also used in Oncotype DX), *KPNA2* (also used in MammaPrint), *CDC2*, and *CDC20*
- Test results
  - High or low GGI
- Correlates with disease-free and overall survival
- Associated with histologic grade
  - Grade 1: ~ 85% low GGI
  - Grade 3: ~ 90% high GGI
  - Grade 2: Cancers are split into low and high categories

Second Generation GEP Assays

- Designed for defined subsets of cancers and to address specific clinical questions rather than overall prognosis
  - Prediction of response to types of therapy
  - Wound response indicator: May predict survival
  - Invasive gene signature: 186 gene profile

Limitations of Current GEP Assays

- Identify largely overlapping good and poor prognostic groups
  - Choice of different gene sets for each assay is likely due to basing selection on relatively small numbers of cancers expressing thousands of different genes
  - Consistent assignment by different assays to same molecular group is only modest for luminal A, B, and HER2 types
- Information is complementary to traditional prognostic factors
  - Tumor size and lymph node status add important independent information
  - Few cancers < 1 cm in size are included in tumor banks used for development of assays
- Prediction is limited to ER positive and HER2 negative cancers
  - ER negative and HER2 positive cancers are generally placed in high-risk category; better predictors are needed for these cancers
  - PR negative and cancers with high proliferative rates are also generally intermediate to high risk and additional information may not be provided by GEP assay

- Predictive power is largely driven by genes related to proliferation and cell cycle
  - Other measures of proliferation such as mitotic count or Ki-67 might yield similar information if combined into weighted score
- Predict short-term but not long-term relapse
  - Many breast cancers have long natural history
- Reproducibility
  - Assays can only be performed by a single laboratory; reproducibility and accuracy cannot be independently evaluated
- Cost
  - High cost will limit use of these tests for patient care in some settings
    - Reduced use of chemotherapy for low-risk patients may offset cost of testing
  - High cost makes it difficult for independent researchers to study these assays

SELECTED REFERENCES

1. Fumagalli D et al: Treatment of pT1N0 breast cancer: multigene predictors to assess risk of relapse. Ann Oncol. 21 Suppl 7:vii103-vii106, 2010
2. Nielsen TO et al: A comparison of PAM50 intrinsic subtyping with immunohistochemistry and clinical prognostic factors in tamoxifen-treated estrogen receptor-positive breast cancer. Clin Cancer Res. 16(21):5222-32, 2010
3. Weigelt B et al: The contribution of gene expression profiling to breast cancer classification, prognostication and prediction: a retrospective of the last decade. J Pathol. 220(2):263-80, 2010
4. Cheang MC et al: Ki67 index, HER2 status, and prognosis of patients with luminal B breast cancer. J Natl Cancer Inst. 101(10):736-50, 2009
5. Dunn L et al: Genomic predictors of outcome and treatment response in breast cancer. Mol Diagn Ther. 13(2):73-90, 2009
6. Sørlie T et al: Gene expression patterns of breast carcinomas distinguish tumor subclasses with clinical implications. Proc Natl Acad Sci U S A. 98(19):10869-74, 2001
7. Perou CM et al: Molecular portraits of human breast tumours. Nature. 406(6797):747-52, 2000

Molecular Classification of Breast Cancer Subtypes

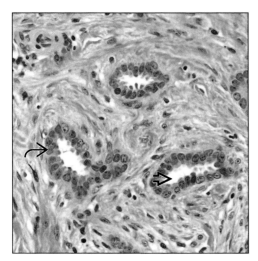
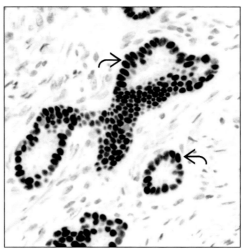

(Left) Luminal subtypes of breast cancer are defined by expression of ER and dozens of genes regulated by ER. Luminal A cancers typically have a low nuclear grade ➡ and have a pattern of well-formed tubules ➡. (Right) Luminal A cancers typically show strong ER positivity in almost all tumor cells ➡ as well as strong PR positivity. Luminal B cancers may have low levels of ER expression, and PR may be absent or only focally expressed. Some luminal B cancers overexpress HER2.

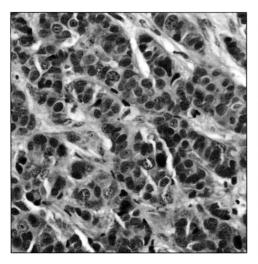
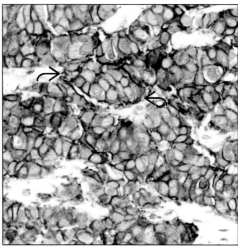

(Left) The HER2 subtype as defined by GEP overexpresses HER2, other genes on the same amplicon, and proliferation-related genes, but it does not express ER. These tumors typically are high grade with a high mitotic rate. (Right) HER2 gene amplification (detected by FISH) results in increased mRNA (detected by GEP) and increased protein in the membranes of tumor cells ➡ (detected by IHC). HER2 is unusual in that overexpression almost always occurs via gene amplification.

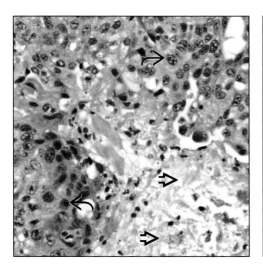
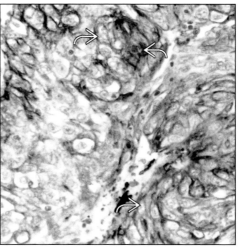

(Left) This poorly differentiated carcinoma shows pleomorphic cells arranged in syncytial-like sheets ➡ and no evidence of tubule formation. The central portion of the tumor shows geographic necrosis ➡, a feature frequently associated with basal-like carcinomas. (Right) Basal-like breast cancers are most often negative for ER, PR, and HER2 but frequently show strong expression for basal cytokeratins such as CK5 ➡, EGFR, or other "basal" markers.

EXPRESSION PROFILING, PROTEIN

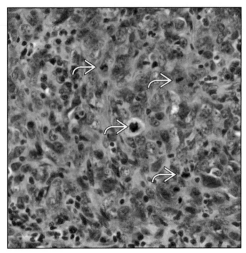

This grade 3 invasive carcinoma has a high mitotic rate ➡. Additional information is provided by the use of IHC markers to determine prognosis and guide selection of the most effective therapy.

IHC SURROGATES FOR MOLECULAR CLASSIFICATION OF BREAST CANCER

Invasive Breast Cancer
(Classified by Immunophenotype)
ER
+
HER2
+
KI-67

ER(+)			ER(-)		
HER2(-)		HER2(+)	HER2(+)	HER2(-)	
				CK5/6 + EGFR	
ER(+)/HER2(-) Ki-67 low	ER(+)/HER2(-) Ki-67 high	ER(+)/HER2(+)	ER(-)/HER2(+)	ER(-) HER2(-) CK5/6+ &/or EGFR(+)	ER(-) HER2(-) CK5/6- and EGFR(-)
Luminal A	Luminal B	Luminal HER2	HER2 Classic	Basal Phenotype	Non-Basal Normal-Breast Phenotype

IHC markers classify breast cancers into distinct cancer subsets that demonstrate differences in patient characteristics, prognosis, patterns of recurrence, and response to types of treatments.

TERMINOLOGY

Definitions
- Protein expression profiling is identification of patterns of expression that identify clinically significant subtypes of breast cancer
- Breast cancer encompasses a group of very heterogeneous malignancies
  - Carcinomas show distinct differences in natural history, pathologic features, and biologic behavior
  - Multiple treatment options are available, including use of targeted therapies
    - Increasingly, clinical decisions on utility of treatment options and targeted therapy require assessment of underlying tumor biology
  - Need for clinically useful breast cancer classification scheme to help assess prognosis and aid treatment decisions

Breast Cancer Biology and Classification
- Technical advances have made it possible to study underlying biology of breast cancer samples
  - Tumor tissue can be analyzed for changes at level of genome
    - DNA copy number changes; genomic gains and losses
    - Global changes in gene expression (mRNA)
    - Global changes in protein expression
- Each of these approaches can be used to classify breast cancers into different biologic subsets
  - Biologic classification has potential to provide additional prognostic and predictive information
    - Potential aid to clinical decision making
  - Each approach has different specimen requirements
    - Some of these methodologies require fresh or snap frozen tumor samples
    - Other methodologies can be used to study formalin-fixed paraffin-embedded breast tumors

CLINICAL IMPLICATIONS

Clinically Relevant Tumor Classification
- Classification should help distinguish different prognostic groups among patients with similar features
  - Classification should help predict response to different therapies
    - Endocrine therapies and type of endocrine therapy (e.g., tamoxifen or aromatase inhibitors)
    - Chemotherapy: Many types, doses, and combinations available
    - Biologic/targeted therapies: HER2-targeted treatment has been very successful for cancers overexpressing the protein
- Clinically useful breast cancer classification will aid in optimal patient management

Gene Expression Profiling (GEP), mRNA
- 4 major groups of "molecular subtypes" of cancers identified
  - 2 subgroups of ER(-) cancers
    - HER2(+) tumors with low or absent expression of ER-related genes
    - HER2(-) tumors with increased expression of basal cytokeratins
  - 2 subgroups of ER(+) cancers
    - Luminal A: High ER expression, low levels of proliferation-related gene expression
    - Luminal B: Lower levels of ER expression, high levels of proliferation-related gene expression, 1/3-1/2 overexpress HER2
- These molecular subtypes have been confirmed as reproducible and statistically robust in independent data sets
  - Significantly correlated with prognosis, independent of traditional prognostic factors
  - Associated with different patterns of metastatic recurrence

○ May help predict likelihood of response to chemotherapy
- Limitations of GEP
  ○ Clinical applicability of gene expression profiling limited
  ○ Requires fresh or frozen tissue
    ▪ Only applicable for larger carcinomas for which diagnosis is known prior to surgery
    ▪ Not suitable for small carcinomas < 1 cm
    ▪ If tissue is harvested for this assay, reduces tumor available for histologic evaluation or other types of assays
  ○ Technical complexity and technical feasibility in routine practice setting
  ○ Reproducibility
    ▪ Consistency of results across different laboratories or on repeat specimens has not been extensively examined
  ○ Cost

IHC Profiling: Single Antibodies

- IHC evaluation of single protein markers has demonstrated clinical utility
  ○ ER, PR, HER2, Ki-67 (MIB-1)
  ○ Clinically validated as useful for risk stratification and decision for specific adjuvant therapies
    ▪ ER and PR: Response to tamoxifen, aromatase inhibitors
    ▪ HER2: Response to trastuzumab, lapatinib, other HER2-directed therapy
    ▪ Ki-67: High proliferative rate may predict increased benefit from chemotherapy
- Selected IHC antibody panels can be used to profile breast tumors
  ○ Able to identify breast cancer subsets with differing outcomes
  ○ Analytical techniques developed for GEP can be applied to IHC
- Examination of multiple prognostic markers by IHC in well-defined cohort using unsupervised hierarchical clustering
  ○ Demonstrated ability to identify prognostic relevant groups of breast cancer patients
  ○ Determined optimal panel of IHC markers necessary to define these groups
- Numerous investigators have attempted to "translate" gene expression data into IHC panels for clinical application in breast cancer
  ○ Studies suggest that application of selected antibody panels using IHC can identify breast cancer subsets with differing outcomes
    ▪ May help predict response to specific therapies

IHC Profiling: Cytokeratin (CK) Classification

- Breast cancers can be classified based on differential patterns of expression of cytokeratins by IHC
  ○ Basal subtype
    ▪ Expression of high molecular weight "basal" cytokeratins CK5/6, CK14, CK17
    ▪ Also frequently expresses luminal cytokeratins
  ○ Luminal subtype
    ▪ Expression of low molecular weight "luminal" cytokeratins CK8, CK18

▪ Usually do not express basal cytokeratins
- Expression of basal cytokeratins in breast cancer shows a number of clinical correlations
  ○ Absence of ER expression
  ○ Aggressive clinical course with poor prognosis and increased incidence of early recurrence
    ▪ Increased incidence of metastases to lungs and brain
  ○ High histological and nuclear grade with pushing borders and marked increase in proliferation
  ○ *BRCA1*-associated tumors and familial breast cancer
  ○ Poor responses to standard adjuvant chemotherapy
    ▪ May be more sensitive to anthracycline-based chemotherapy compared with luminal subtype
  ○ Tends to occur in patients under age of 40
    ▪ More common in premenopausal African-American and Hispanic women

IHC Profiling: Surrogates for Molecular Classification by GEP

- Limited panel of IHC markers can identify clinically relevant groups
  ○ Panel includes ER, HER2, HER1 (EGFR), Ki-67, and basal cytokeratins (e.g., CK5/6)
  ○ Stratify breast cancer samples into subsets similar to molecular subtypes defined by expression profiling
  ○ Can be used as surrogate for intrinsic molecular classification of breast cancer
    ▪ IHC surrogates for molecular subsets demonstrate similar prognostic significance compared with expression profiling
    ▪ May be predictive for patterns of metastatic recurrence
- **Luminal A subtype**
  ○ ER(+), HER2(-), Ki-67 low; usually PR(+)
  ○ Usually grade 1 or 2
  ○ Approximately 70% of all breast cancers
  ○ Metastasizes most commonly to bone; least likely subtype to metastasize to brain, liver, or lung
  ○ In general, shows little benefit from addition of chemotherapy to hormonal therapy
- **Luminal B subtype: HER2(-)**
  ○ ER(+), HER2(-), Ki-67 high; may be PR(-)
  ○ Usually grade 2 or 3
  ○ Approximately 10% of all breast cancers
  ○ Most commonly metastasizes to bone, followed by liver and lung
  ○ In general, benefits from chemotherapy and hormonal therapy
- **Luminal B subtype: HER2(+)**
  ○ ER(+), HER2(+), Ki-67 high; may be PR(-)
  ○ Usually grade 3
  ○ Approximately 10% of all breast cancers
  ○ Metastasizes most commonly to bone, brain, liver, and lung
  ○ More likely to have multicentric disease, multiple positive nodes, and higher risk of local recurrence
  ○ In general, benefit from chemotherapy, HER2-targeted therapy, and hormonal therapy
- **HER2 subtype**
  ○ ER(-), HER2(+), Ki-67 high; usually PR(-)
  ○ Usually grade 3

- o Approximately 10% of all breast cancers
- o More likely to have multicentric disease, multiple positive nodes, and higher risk of local recurrence
- o Metastasizes most commonly to bone, brain, liver, and lung
- o In general, benefits from chemotherapy and HER2-targeted therapy but not hormonal therapy
- o Patients are younger compared to women with luminal A cancers
- **Basal subtype**
  - o ER(-), HER2(-), basal cytokeratin(+), EGFR(+), PR(-)
    - Identifies basal-like carcinomas defined by gene expression with 76% sensitivity, 100% specificity
    - Other IHC panels have also been used to define this group
    - Does not identify ~ 10% that are ER positive or ~ 10% that overexpress HER2
  - o Usually poorly differentiated
  - o Approximately 15% of all breast cancers
  - o Less likely to have involved nodes but higher risk for local recurrence
  - o Metastasizes most commonly to brain, lung, and distant nodes
  - o May respond to specific types of chemotherapy
  - o Patients are younger compared to women with luminal A cancers

IHC Profiling: Mammostrat® Assay

- Alternative approach to profiling breast cancer patients for prognosis and treatment response utilizing IHC
  - o Developed by Applied Genomics, Inc. (Huntsville, AL) in collaboration with researchers at Stanford University
    - Attempted to translate diversity revealed by gene expression studies into new IHC tests with potential clinical utility
  - o Utilized gene expression data sets to select hundreds of novel targets for production of new antibodies
    - Antibodies screened across several thousand formalin-fixed paraffin-embedded (FFPE) tumor samples to identify quality IHC reagents
    - Most robust IHC markers further investigated for their ability to identify clinically significant subsets of solid tumors
- Panel developed for determining prognosis of early-stage ER(+) and node(-) breast cancer
  - o Step 1: Panel of antibodies was used to score well-characterized breast cancer cohort
  - o Step 2: Identified antibodies with univariate association with breast cancer recurrence
  - o Step 3: Generated Cox Proportional Hazard models using stage I/II cohort data "fit" to predict recurrence
- 5 antibodies identified as minimal panel for prediction of recurrence
  - o SLC7A5: Amino acid transport (may help sustain tumor cell growth)
    - Positive: > 10% membrane positivity
    - 31.4% of score
  - o P53: Tumor suppressor gene (involved in cell cycle control)
    - Positive: > 10% nuclear positivity

- 22.9% of score
  - o NDRG1: Stress/hypoxia response protein
    - Positive: Confluent uniform cytoplasmic or membrane positivity
    - 20.9% of score
  - o *HTF9C*: Methyl transferase gene family homology
    - Positive: > 10% cytoplasmic positivity
    - 14.5% of score
  - o CEACAM5: Embryonic expressed protein
    - Positive: > 10% cytoplasmic or membrane positivity
    - 10.3% of score
- Biologic assessment independent of proliferation, HER2, and hormone receptors
- Results are scored as positive or negative and used in an algorithm to calculate a risk index (RI)
  - o Clinically validated on 3 independent institutional cohorts of patients
  - o Clinically validated on archival tissue samples from NSABP B14 and B20 clinical trials
  - o Results similar to Oncotype DX on same patient samples
- RI classifies ER(+) and node(-) patients into 3 groups with different risks of recurrence at 10 years
  - o Low risk: 7.6%
  - o Moderate risk: 16.3%
  - o High risk: 20.9%
- Patients with high RI appear to derive greatest benefit from adjuvant chemotherapy

IHC Profiling: Use of Image Analysis

- IHC stains are analogous to ELISA tests performed in clinical laboratories
  - o Protein detection chemistry in ELISA test is similar to what is performed for IHC
    - ELISA tests are recognized as being quantitative
    - IHC stained slides have potential to be quantified
    - Strict standardization and quality assurance for all pre-analytical and analytical variables are important for meaningful quantitation
- Several computerized image analysis applications for IHC quantification have been developed
  - o Image analysis systems are commercially available for clinical and research applications
    - Some commercially available systems have received clearance from the FDA for quantitative assessment of ER, PR, and HER2
  - o Computer algorithms can measure IHC staining localized to nuclear, membrane, and cytoplasmic cellular compartments
    - Reporting tools integrate picture, graphics, and multiple assay results into clinical reports
- Computerized image analysis has been shown to provide more accurate and objective ER, PR, and HER2 IHC interpretation relative to manual microscopy
  - o Assistance of digital microscopy improves inter-pathologist reproducibility in numerous reports
    - May be helpful in defining clinically relevant thresholds of staining that cannot be accurately detected by eye
- Not yet shown to provide clinically relevant information beyond standard manual interpretation

EXPRESSION PROFILING, PROTEIN

Biologic Profiling of Clinical Breast Cancer Samples

Features	DNA	mRNA	Protein
Technology platforms	Traditional cytogenetic, array-based comparative genomic hybridization; FISH	Array-based gene expression profiling, quantitative RT-PCR	Protein expression arrays; immunohistochemistry
Sample requirements	Fresh tissue (CGH), FFPE tissue (FISH)	Fresh tissue (cDNA microarrays), FFPE tissue (QRTPCR)	Fresh tissue (protein arrays), FFPE tissue IHC
Assay target	Genomic DNA (copy number changes)	mRNA gene transcripts	Expressed proteins
Quantitative analysis	++ (DNA copy number changes: CGH), (average number of gene signals/cell: FISH)	+++ (QRTPCR, broad dynamic range, less so with cDNA expression arrays)	+/- (IHC qualitative assessment), image analysis and immunofluorescence may improve quantitative aspects of analysis
Feasibility	CGH: Technically demanding; FISH: Adaptable to most laboratory settings	QRTPCR: Technically demanding, availability limited to reference laboratories	IHC: Broadly applicable technology, currently available in most laboratory settings

IHC Profiling: Use of Automated Quantitative Immunofluorescence Analysis (AQUA)

- Fluorescence-based method that provides objective and continuous protein expression scores in tissue
  - Method utilizes automated fluorescence microscopy and advanced image analysis algorithms
    - Molecular identification of compartments is used to quantify biomarker expression as function of pixel intensity in specific tissues or subcellular compartments
    - Measured AQUA scores are directly proportional to molecules per unit area or protein concentration
  - Assessment of HER2 by AQUA analysis has significant linear relationship with FISH
    - HER2 expression as determined by AQUA analysis predicts response to trastuzumab
  - Quantitative assessment of ER as continuous variable may be clinically useful
- Clinical utility will require that additional information acquired by this technique is useful for patient management

FOXA1 Expression in Breast Cancer

- FOXA1: Forkhead family transcription factor
  - Protein essential for optimum expression of many estrogen-responsive genes
  - Expression segregates with genes that characterize luminal subtypes by expression analysis
    - May represent independent prognostic factor for ER(+) breast cancer
- In large clinical cohorts, FOXA1 expression correlates with luminal subtype A breast cancer
  - Expression of FOXA1 was significant predictor of improved cancer-specific survival in patients with ER(+) tumors
  - Prognostic ability of FOXA1 in these low-risk breast cancers may prove to be useful in clinical treatment decisions

PREDICTIVE CANCER TESTING SUMMARY

General Issues

- Standard IHC antibody panels are used in routine pathologic evaluation of newly diagnosed breast cancers
  - Wide availability, lower cost, fast turnaround time
  - Readily adaptable to most pathology practices
  - Morphologic confirmation of tissue assayed
- Expanded IHC panels have potential to provide additional information to help guide clinical decisions on adjuvant therapies
  - Need to establish optimal panels correlated with patient outcome or response to treatment
  - Need to standardize tissue handling and fixation protocols
  - Need to standardize assay procedures, positive and negative controls, criteria for interpretation

SELECTED REFERENCES

1. Harigopal M et al: Multiplexed assessment of the Southwest Oncology Group-directed Intergroup Breast Cancer Trial S9313 by AQUA shows that both high and low levels of HER2 are associated with poor outcome. Am J Pathol. 176(4):1639-47, 2010
2. Weigelt B et al: Molecular profiling currently offers no more than tumour morphology and basic immunohistochemistry. Breast Cancer Res. 12 Suppl 4:S5, 2010
3. Yerushalmi R et al: Ki67 in breast cancer: prognostic and predictive potential. Lancet Oncol. 11(2):174-83, 2010
4. Cheang MC et al: Ki67 index, HER2 status, and prognosis of patients with luminal B breast cancer. J Natl Cancer Inst. 101(10):736-50, 2009
5. Gustavson MD et al: Standardization of HER2 immunohistochemistry in breast cancer by automated quantitative analysis. Arch Pathol Lab Med. 133(9):1413-9, 2009
6. Ross DT et al: Chemosensitivity and stratification by a five monoclonal antibody immunohistochemistry test in the NSABP B14 and B20 trials. Clin Cancer Res. 14(20):6602-9, 2008
7. Badve S et al: FOXA1 expression in breast cancer--correlation with luminal subtype A and survival. Clin Cancer Res. 13(15 Pt 1):4415-21, 2007
8. Livasy CA et al: Phenotypic evaluation of the basal-like subtype of invasive breast carcinoma. Mod Pathol. 19(2):264-71, 2006

Immunohistochemical Profiles

(Left) *This patient presented with a poorly differentiated invasive ductal carcinoma with axillary lymph node metastases. Selection of the most appropriate therapy will be guided by the immunophenotype of the tumor cells. (Right) This poorly differentiated breast cancer is weakly ER(+) ⊡ and also has a high rate of proliferation, consistent with a luminal B breast cancer. Patients with this type of cancer likely benefit from both chemotherapy and endocrine therapy.*

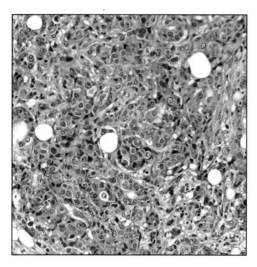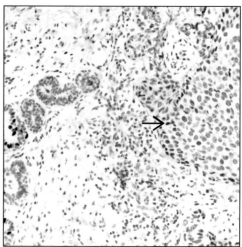

(Left) *This young patient presented with a poorly differentiated invasive ductal carcinoma. IHC profiling can help assess the biology of the tumor and aid in the selection of appropriate adjuvant therapy. (Right) This high-grade cancer is ER(-) and shows strong circumferential membrane expression for HER2 ⊡, consistent with a HER2-positive breast cancer. Patients with HER2 positive cancers benefit from HER2-targeted therapy in addition to chemotherapy.*

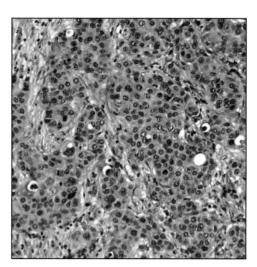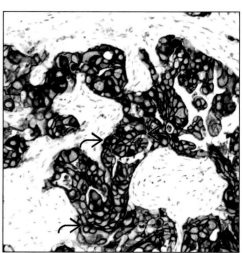

(Left) *This poorly differentiated invasive ductal carcinoma is ER and PR negative and shows foci of geographic tumor necrosis ⊡. On further work-up, the tumor was negative for HER2 and would be classified as a triple negative breast cancer. (Right) Triple negative breast cancers that express basal cytokeratin 5 ⊡ correlate well with basal-like carcinomas by gene expression profiling. IHC markers do not predict the response to a specific type of treatment in this group.*

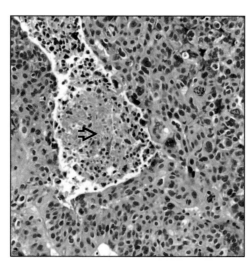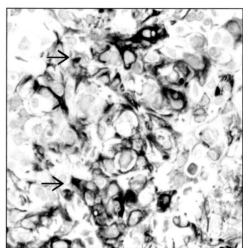

EXPRESSION PROFILING, PROTEIN

Mammostrat® Assay for ER-Positive Breast Cancer

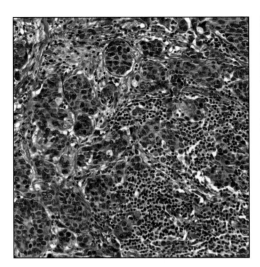

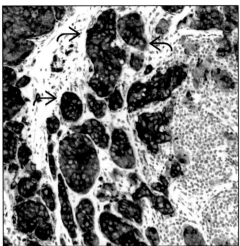

(Left) The Mammostrat assay is a 5-antibody IHC panel used to help predict prognosis and appropriate therapy for patients with ER(+) and node(-) cancers. The staining results from the 5 markers are used in an algorithm to calculate a risk index (RI). (Right) CEACAM5 is one of the antibodies used in Mammostrat and is strongly positive in this cancer ⊿. A positive result is > 10% of the carcinoma showing cytoplasmic or membrane immunoreactivity.

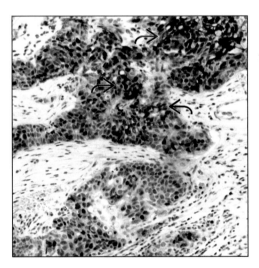

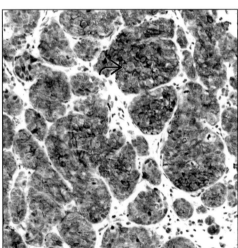

(Left) Another Mammostrat antibody is HTF9C. A positive result is defined by > 10% of the cells showing positivity. This cancer shows strong cytoplasmic positivity throughout the tumor ⊿. (Right) NDRG1 is another Mammostrat antibody, is expressed under conditions of hypoxia and other stresses, and may function to improve tumor cell survival within the microenvironment of the cancer. This carcinoma shows positive cytoplasmic immunoreactivity ⊿.

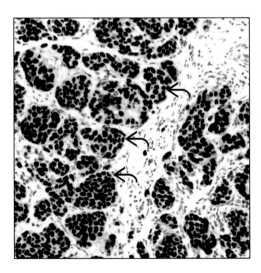

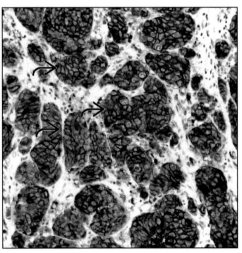

(Left) Mammostrat also incorporates p53. Having more than 10% of cells with nuclear immunoreactivity is considered a positive result. This carcinoma shows strong diffuse nuclear positivity ⊿. (Right) SLC7A5 is scored as positive if > 10% of tumor cells are immunoreactive and is part of the Mammostrat panel. This carcinoma shows strong membrane positivity ⊿. The scores for the 5 markers are used to generate an RI of 4.081, identifying this patient as being at high risk for recurrence.

Mammostrat® Assay for ER-Positive Breast Cancer

(Left) This invasive ductal carcinoma is ER positive. Many patients with such carcinomas gain little or no benefit from chemotherapy and may do equally well with endocrine therapy alone. Mammostrat is one of many assays to help select the subset of patients most likely to benefit from chemotherapy. *(Right)* This carcinoma shows strong diffuse positivity for CEACAM5 ➘. This protein is normally expressed in embryonic tissues and aberrantly expressed in some carcinomas.

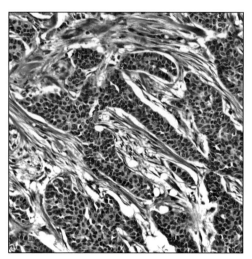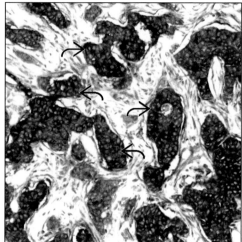

(Left) HTF9C is coexpressed with proteins involved in DNA replication and likely plays a role in both DNA replication and cell cycle control. This carcinoma does not show any immunoreactivity for this protein. *(Right)* NDRG1 is expressed under conditions of hypoxia and other stressors and likely increases the ability of tumor cells to survive in a hostile tumor microenvironment. There is no expression of NDRG1 in this carcinoma.

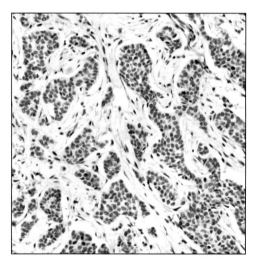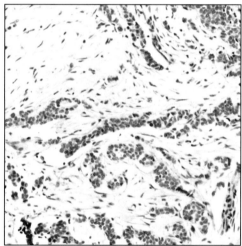

(Left) The oncoprotein p53 plays a central role in cell cycle regulation, DNA repair, and the maintenance of genomic integrity. This carcinoma shows no immunoreactivity. *(Right)* SLC7A5 is involved in nutrient transport and is not expressed by this cancer. The calculated RI score for this patient is -0.359, placing her in the low-risk group. Patients in this group have a 7% probability of distant recurrence at 10 years.

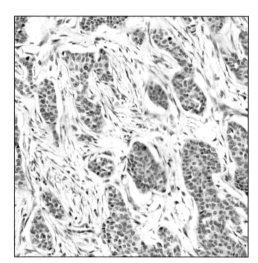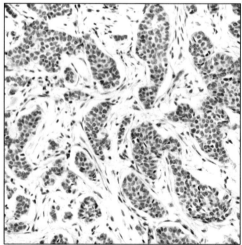

Ki-67 Proliferation Index

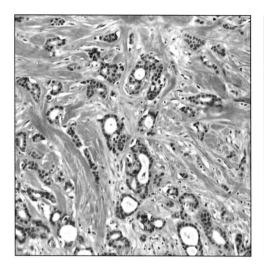
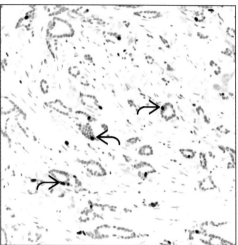

(Left) Most ER(-) cancers are high grade and have high proliferative rates. In contrast, ER(+) cancers show a wide range of grade and proliferation. Proliferation has been used to identify the subset of ER(+) cancers most likely to benefit from chemotherapy. This grade 1 cancer is expected to have a low rate of proliferation. (Right) This well-differentiated carcinoma shows only rare Ki-67 positive cells ➔, consistent with the grade and mitotic rate.

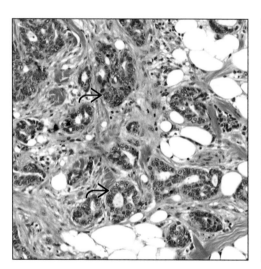
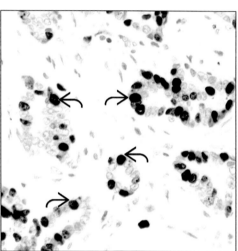

(Left) Grade 2 and 3 ER(+) cancers ➔ often have decreased or absent PR expression and are associated with a higher mitotic index and increased expression of Ki-67. (Right) Ki-67 is a nuclear protein ➔ that plays a role in cell division and is expressed in all cell cycle phases except G0. A high Ki-67 proliferation index (> 15-20% positive cells) is associated with decreased disease-free survival and may also be helpful as a predictor of a better response to chemotherapy.

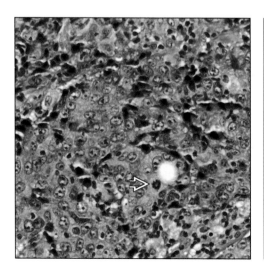
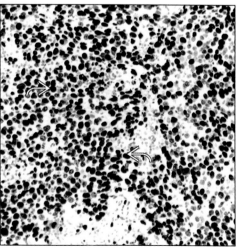

(Left) The prognostic groups identified by gene expression profiling are largely driven by expression of proliferation-related proteins. The increased number of cells in mitosis ➔ in high-grade breast cancers can be identified morphologically, or proliferation-related proteins can be identified in larger populations of cycling cells by IHC. (Right) Almost every cell in this poorly differentiated cancer shows nuclear positivity for Ki-67 ➔. The mitotic rate is also very high.

EXPRESSION PROFILING, ONCOTYPE DX ASSAY

TERMINOLOGY

Abbreviations
- Quantitative reverse transcriptase polymerase chain reaction (QRT-PCR)
- 21 gene RT-PCR breast cancer gene profiling assay (Oncotype Dx [Genomic Health; Redwood City, CA])
- Recurrence score (RS)
- National Surgical Adjuvant Breast and Bowel Project (NSABP)

Types of Tests
- Gene expression profiling studies of breast cancer have demonstrated potential clinical applications
  - Provide clinically relevant biologic classification of breast cancer patients
  - Assessment of prognosis and potential for recurrence that is significant and independent of other pathologic factors
  - Help predict response to adjuvant and neoadjuvant therapies
    - Endocrine therapy
    - Chemotherapy
    - Targeted therapies
- Significant technical limitations of expression profiling studies for clinical samples in routine practice
  - Current technology requires fresh or snap frozen tissue, which contain high quality RNA that has not degraded
    - Limited dynamic range for gene assays, difficult to control
- Alternative approach to molecular profiling of breast cancer
  - Application of QRT-PCR to formalin-fixed paraffin-embedded clinical samples
    - Used to quantify expression of potentially clinically important, tumor-related gene transcripts in multigene approach
- QRT-PCR assay for genes utilizes forward primer, reverse primer, and probe
  - Probes and primers are specific sequences that are complementary and bind to specific RNA transcript to be assayed
  - Ends of gene probe are capped with fluorescence label on 1 end and fluorescence quencher on other
    - Used to measure amount of RNA present and level of gene expression
  - During PCR, DNA polymerase displaces and cleaves probe, releasing fluorescent label
    - Rate of rise of fluorescence as label is released depends on amount of starting RNA present
    - Rate of rise of fluorescence can be used to quantitatively measure level of gene expression
  - QRT-PCR has wide dynamic range
    - High sensitivity and specificity for results
    - Results are highly reproducible

Definitions
- Validated 21-gene RT-PCR assay (Oncotype Dx) was developed for use in routine paraffin-embedded breast cancer samples

- Developed through collaborations between Genomic Health Incorporated (Redwood City, CA) and NSABP
  - Helps predict likelihood of recurrence and the magnitude of benefit from adjuvant chemotherapy
- Oncotype Dx assay utilizes TaqMan® (Invitrogen; Carlsbad, CA) quantitative PCR
  - Measures quantitatively a selected panel of 21 gene transcripts
    - 16 cancer-related genes and 5 reference genes
    - Algorithm based on level of gene expression used to calculate recurrence score
    - Assay validated for patients with ER positive, node-negative breast cancers treated with tamoxifen
  - Reference genes are used to normalize level of expression of cancer-related genes
    - Helps to control for RNA fragmentation, which occurs in formalin-fixed tissue

Target Gene or Antigen
- 16 cancer-related genes are used to calculate RS
  - Selected genes weigh most heavily tumor proliferation, hormone receptor status, and HER2 expression
  - Used to help predict likelihood of disease recurrence at 10 years
- Calculated RS in ER(+) node(-) breast cancer ranges from 0-100
  - Divides patents into 3 categories in terms of their 10-year distant recurrence-free survival
    - Low RS: < 18
    - Intermediate RS: 18-31
    - High RS: > 31

CLINICAL ISSUES

Epidemiology
- Prevalence
  - 60-70% of breast tumors will express estrogen receptors
    - Patients likely to benefit from hormonal therapy with tamoxifen or aromatase inhibitors
  - Established consensus that adjuvant chemotherapy improves survival in breast cancer patients
    - Chemotherapy is included in treatment regimen for many women with breast cancer at time of diagnosis
    - Not all patients receiving chemotherapy will benefit and may be unnecessarily exposed to potentially significant toxicity
  - Many ER(+) patients are adequately treated with surgery/radiation and adjuvant hormonal treatment
    - Clinically challenging to define which ER(+) patients could potentially avoid chemotherapy
  - Oncotype Dx assay developed to help independently predict likelihood of recurrence for ER(+) tumors
    - Help assess magnitude of benefit from adjuvant chemotherapy in ER(+) node(-) breast cancer patients

EXPRESSION PROFILING, ONCOTYPE DX ASSAY

RT-PCR Gene Sets Used to Calculate Recurrence Score

Proliferation	ER	HER2	Invasion	Unrelated Genes	Reference Genes
Ki-67	ER	HER2	MMP11	GSTM1	β-actin
STK15	PR	GRB7	CTSL2 (cathepsin L2)	CD68	GAPDH
Survivin	BCL2			BAG1	RPLPO
CCNB1 (cyclin-B1)	SCUBE2				GUS
MYBL2					TFRC

RS = level of gene expression for each group x weighted coefficient (scale 0-100). Divides patients into 3 groups: Low (< 18), intermediate (18-31), and high (> 31) risk for disease recurrence.

Prognostic Value

- RS has been shown to be highly significant and independent predictor of disease recurrence in several studies
- Clinical validation study of RS performed on paraffin blocks from patients treated on NSABP B-14 clinical trial
  - B-14 trial demonstrated benefit from tamoxifen treatment in ER(+) node(-) breast cancer patients
    - Paraffin blocks from 668 ER-positive patients from the tamoxifen-treated arm were used for validation of assay
  - RS was independent and highly significant predictors of 10-year recurrence-free survival
    - Low RS (< 18): 6.8% risk for recurrence
    - Intermediate RS (18-30): 14.3% risk for recurrence
    - High RS (> 31): 30.5% risk for recurrence
  - In multivariate analysis, only tumor grade and RS were independent predictors of outcome
    - Tumor grade showed a higher hazard ratio than RS for predicting disease recurrence
  - Approximately 50% of ER(+) node(-) breast cancer patients fell within low RS category in B-14 patient cohort
- RS is also prognostic in untreated patients

Treatment Implications

- Predictive Value
  - Chemotherapy benefit for ER(+) node(-) breast cancer
    - RS has been examined in clinical samples from NSABP clinical trial B-20
    - B-20 examined benefit of adding chemotherapy to tamoxifen for ER(+) node(-) breast cancer patients
  - RS was predictive of response to chemotherapy
    - Patients with high RS appeared to receive greatest benefit from adding chemotherapy to their endocrine treatment
    - Patients with low RS appeared not to receive any additional benefit from adding chemotherapy to their adjuvant treatment regimen
  - RS appears to be predictive for tamoxifen efficacy
    - Patients with low RS appear to receive greatest benefit from tamoxifen
    - Patients with low RS may be able to be spared potential toxicity of chemotherapy
  - RS should be correlated with other pathologic risk factors in making treatment decisions
  - RS should be considered as adjunct to pathologic phenotyping as indication for potential benefit from chemotherapy

Quality Control and Quality Assurance

- Formalin-fixed paraffin-embedded tissue blocks selected for Oncotype assay should contain invasive tumor
  - Blocks with extensive amount of ductal carcinoma in situ, normal tissue, and inflammation should be avoided if possible
  - Some tissue samples will need to be macro-dissected to enrich for invasive tumor prior to performing assay
    - These non-tumor tissues may affect RS assay results

SELECTED REFERENCES

1. Asad J et al: Does oncotype DX recurrence score affect the management of patients with early-stage breast cancer? Am J Surg. 196(4):527-9, 2008
2. Badve SS et al: Estrogen- and progesterone-receptor status in ECOG 2197: comparison of immunohistochemistry by local and central laboratories and quantitative reverse transcription polymerase chain reaction by central laboratory. J Clin Oncol. 2008 May 20;26(15):2473-81. Erratum in: J Clin Oncol. 26(20):3472, 2008
3. Flanagan MB et al: Histopathologic variables predict Oncotype DX recurrence score. Mod Pathol. 21(10):1255-61, 2008
4. Habel LA et al: A population-based study of tumor gene expression and risk of breast cancer death among lymph node-negative patients. Breast Cancer Res. 8(3):R25, 2006
5. Paik S et al: Gene expression and benefit of chemotherapy in women with node-negative, estrogen receptor-positive breast cancer. J Clin Oncol. 24(23):3726-34, 2006
6. Esteva FJ et al: Prognostic role of a multigene reverse transcriptase-PCR assay in patients with node-negative breast cancer not receiving adjuvant systemic therapy. Clin Cancer Res. 11(9):3315-9, 2005
7. Cronin M et al: Measurement of gene expression in archival paraffin-embedded tissues: development and performance of a 92-gene reverse transcriptase-polymerase chain reaction assay. Am J Pathol. 164(1):35-42, 2004
8. Paik S et al: A multigene assay to predict recurrence of tamoxifen-treated, node-negative breast cancer. N Engl J Med. 351(27):2817-26, 2004

TERMINOLOGY

Abbreviations
- MammaPrint breast cancer assay (MPA)

Definitions
- Gene expression profiling (GEP) studies have added greatly to our understanding of biologic diversity of breast cancer
  - Expression array studies allow simultaneous examination of global changes in gene expression from clinical breast cancer samples

Target Gene or Antigen
- GEP studies allow simultaneous examination of thousands of genes without need to define function or relationship among genes
  - Application to breast cancer has potential to provide important insights into tumor biology and clinically meaningful tumor subtypes
    - Large data sets generated by these studies require computer and statistical analysis to look for biologically meaningful patterns
- Statistical and computer analysis need to identify groups of genes (gene signatures) that correlate with clinical outcome

Types of Tests
- GEP of clinical breast cancer samples using cDNA microarray
  - Requires fresh or snap frozen tissue samples from a cohort of breast cancer patients with outcome data
    - RNA isolated from tumor tissue for GEP analysis

Supervised Analysis of GEP
- Goal of supervised classification of breast cancer using GEP data
  - Detect gene expression patterns that are predictive of outcome in clinically well-defined patient cohorts
- Initial step: Separate breast cancer patients in the large patient cohort into clinically defined subsets or groups
  - Different patient groups usually defined by clinical outcome
    - Disease recurrence = poor outcome
    - No disease recurrence = good outcome
  - Mathematical models and statistics used to identify gene sets or "genomic classifiers"
    - Should predict which outcome group each patient belongs to ("class prediction")
  - Validation of gene sets for classification of outcome must be done in additional patient cohorts to help establish clinical utility
    - Validation of assay results in additional patients important to help exclude "false discovery"
    - GEP studies are associated with high "false discovery" due to larger number of genes evaluated in limited number of patients
    - Numbers of genes tested is quite large compared with number of clinical samples used to create these models
    - Potential for high "false discovery" rate for genes that appear to be correlated with outcome

MammaPrint (70 Gene Prognostic Panel)
- MPA developed by investigators from the Netherlands Cancer Institute
- MPA: Test development
  - 1st cohort used frozen tumor tissue from 98 patients with node-negative invasive breast cancer
  - RNA from individual cases was hybridized to 25,000 gene microarray
  - Preliminary unsupervised statistical clustering analysis
    - 5,000 genes showed significant variation between different breast cancer cases
  - Tumor samples could be separated into 2 general classes of tumor
    - 1 class correlated with mostly ER(+) tumors
    - 1 class correlated with mostly ER(-) tumors
  - Statistical methods that incorporated clinical outcome data were then applied
    - Patients separated into 2 groups based on outcome
      - Relapse within 5 years (34 patients) and disease free at 5 years or more (44 patients)
    - Identified 231 genes whose expression was correlated with outcome
    - Further statistical methods identified 70 genes as optimal number to use to develop GEP prognostic classifier
  - Final 70 gene set for determining good and bad prognosis in breast cancer patients
    - Included genes involved in cell cycle and proliferation
    - Genes involved in invasion and metastasis
    - Genes involved in angiogenesis
    - Genes involved in signal transduction
  - Some genes commonly thought to be associated with prognosis in breast cancer were not part of panel
    - ER, UPA, PAI-1, HER2
- 70 genes classifier was independently correlated with poor prognosis
  - Able to stratify patients into different prognostic group and predict outcome

CLINICAL ISSUES

MPA: Test Validation
- Validation study included 295 consecutive breast cancers with available banked fresh-frozen tissue from the Netherlands Cancer Institute
  - Cohort included node(-) and node(+) patients
  - Included some ER(-) patients and some patients who had received chemotherapy
- Study showed strikingly different outcomes for patients with good vs. poor genetic signatures
  - Good prognosis genetic signature
    - 14.8% 10-year distant recurrence (confidence interval [CI] ± 4.3)
  - Poor prognosis genetic signature
    - 50% 10-year distant recurrence (CI ± 4.5)
  - Multivariate analysis

Comparison of MammaPrint and Oncotype Assays in Breast Cancer

Feature	MammaPrint	Oncotype
Starting material	Fresh frozen breast tumor	Formalin-fixed paraffin-embedded breast tumor
Technology platform	Gene expression microarray	RT-PCR
Number of genes assayed	70 gene signature	21 genes (16 cancer related and 5 reference genes used for normalization of gene expression)
Assay results	Poor vs. good prognostic signature (binary results)	Low, intermediate, and high recurrence score (continuous variable)
Validation cohort	ER(+), ER(-) and node(+), node(-) patients	ER(+) node(-) patients
Adjuvant treatment validation cohort	Some received chemo and hormonal treatment	Tamoxifen
Outcome good prognostic group	14.8% 10-year distant recurrence (CI ± 4.3)	6.8% 10-year distant recurrence (CI 4.0-9.6)
Outcome poor prognostic group	50% 10-year distant recurrence (CI ± 4.5)	30.5% 10-year distant recurrence (CI 23.6 - 37.4)
Gene sets included in assay	Cell cycle, invasion and metastasis, angiogenesis, signal transduction	Proliferation, *HER2*, invasion, *ER*
Multivariate analysis for assay	Strong independent factor in predicting disease outcome	Strong independent factor in predicting disease outcome
Predicts response to adjuvant therapy	Yes	Yes
Clinical trial utilizing assay	MINDACT trial: Microarray in node(-) disease may avoid chemotherapy	PACCT-1 or TAILORx: Trial assigning individualized options for treatment

- MPA was statistically independent predictor of disease outcome
- Test added to predictive power of classic pathologic parameters
- Estimated hazard ratio for distant metastases in poor prognosis vs. good prognosis signature = 5.1 (CI 2.9-9.0; p < 0.001)

Epidemiology

- Poor prognostic signature was found in 180 patients (61%) in reported validation cohort
  - Poor prognostic signature correlated with traditional high-risk pathologic tumor features
    - Increased tumor size
    - Higher histologic grade
    - Estrogen receptor negativity
- Age Range
  - Poor prognostic signature for MPA is correlated with younger patient age
- MPA test is now commercially available
  - Agendia: http://agendia.com or Molecular Profiling Institute Inc: http://www.molecularprofiling.com/products/mammaprint.cfm
  - Test requires unfixed frozen breast tumor tissue

Prognostic Value

- MPA test has been demonstrated to be statistically significant independent predictor of disease outcome
  - Prognostic power of MPA is independent of patient age and lymph node status

Treatment Implications

- Predictive Value
  - Recent studies suggest that poor prognostic signature is predictive for pathologic response to neoadjuvant chemotherapy
- MINDACT clinical trial in breast cancer
  - Encouraging results with MPA have led to initiation of large clinical trial in Europe utilizing gene profiling

- MINDACT trial: Microarray in node-negative disease may avoid chemotherapy
- All enrolled patients will have MPA performed on their breast tumor tissue
- Trial design compares traditional clinical/pathologic prognostic factors with MPA for selection of adjuvant therapy
  - Patients with good prognostic factors and good prognostic GEP will receive hormonal therapy
  - Patients with poor prognostic factors and poor prognostic GEP will receive chemotherapy + hormonal therapy
- For discordant expression profiles (MPA) and traditional pathologic factors
  - Patients randomized to receive hormonal therapy alone vs. chemotherapy + hormonal therapy
- This prospective randomized trial employing molecular triage should help answer questions on clinical utility of MPA testing

SELECTED REFERENCES

1. Mook S et al: The 70-gene prognosis-signature predicts disease outcome in breast cancer patients with 1-3 positive lymph nodes in an independent validation study. Breast Cancer Res Treat. 116(2):295-302, 2009
2. Wittner BS et al: Analysis of the MammaPrint breast cancer assay in a predominantly postmenopausal cohort. Clin Cancer Res. 14(10):2988-93, 2008
3. Mook S et al: Individualization of therapy using Mammaprint: from development to the MINDACT Trial. Cancer Genomics Proteomics. 4(3):147-55, 2007
4. Buyse M et al: Validation and clinical utility of a 70-gene prognostic signature for women with node-negative breast cancer. J Natl Cancer Inst. 98(17):1183-92, 2006
5. Weigelt B et al: Molecular portraits and 70-gene prognosis signature are preserved throughout the metastatic process of breast cancer. Cancer Res. 65(20):9155-8, 2005
6. van 't Veer LJ et al: Gene expression profiling predicts clinical outcome of breast cancer. Nature. 415(6871):530-6, 2002

CIRCULATING TUMOR CELLS

TERMINOLOGY

Abbreviations
- Circulating tumor cell (CTC)

Definitions
- Pathologic staging of breast cancer is clinically useful in determining course of disease
  - Identification of tumor cells in lymph nodes and bone marrow indicates increased risk for recurrence/ metastasis
    - Indication for systemic treatment as part of therapeutic regimen
- Significant number of early stage breast cancers will recur following theoretically curative surgical excision
  - Suggests that current clinical staging is inadequate for some patients
    - More sensitive methods for determining tumor cell dissemination and risk for metastasis needed
    - Tumor cells spread to distant sites through venous and lymphatic circulation before development of clinically detectable disease
  - Number of investigators have attempted to look for circulating tumor cells in peripheral blood as surrogate for early dissemination
    - Detection of CTCs may reflect aggressiveness of breast tumor
    - May assist in therapeutic decisions in patients with breast cancer
    - CTCs may have role as surrogate markers to monitor treatment response
  - Recent technical advances have made reliable detection of CTCs possible

Target Gene or Antigen
- CTCs are rare findings within blood stream requiring specific and sensitive methodologies for detection
  - Strategies for detection have attempted to exploit differences between epithelial cells and blood or between benign and malignant cells
  - Most technical methods for detecting CTCs rely on combination of cell enrichment and detection step
    - Immunomagnetic bead coated with antibodies can be used to tag and separate epithelial cells from whole blood
    - These isolated cells are then characterized as CTC based on detection of some biologic marker
    - In breast cancer, RT-PCR for cytokeratin, MUC1, CEA, mammaglobin, and HER2 have been used to identify punitive CTC
    - IHC and immunofluorescence for epithelial markers have also been used to identify CTCs

Types of Tests
- Blood represents convenient clinical sample, is easily obtained, and has been the most extensively studied for CTCs
  - Some studies have suggested that assessment of bone marrow for tumor cells may yield better predictor of disease outcome
- Current methods are limited to the ability to identify and count CTCs

- Newer methods under development are seeking to capture viable tumor cells from the circulation
  - Isolated viable CTCs may be able to be grown in tissue culture
  - Viable CTCs can undergo further molecular analysis
    - May provide clinically useful information

CLINICAL ISSUES

CTC Technology
- Detection of circulating tumor cells may represent early indication of micrometastasis
  - May be useful in identification of aggressive tumors, which are able to shed cells into bloodstream
    - Current data are unclear on how this information can be used in breast cancer management
- Commercially available CTC detection methodology (Cell Search assay [Veridex; Raritan, NJ])
  - Assay utilizes immunomagnetic selection to enrich for CTC
    - Immunomagnetic selection followed by immunofluorescent detection of CTCs
    - Epithelial markers such as cytokeratin and HER2 used to identify tumor cells
    - Nuclear staining with 4'-6-diamidino-2-phenylindole used to help identify intact cells
    - Fluorescent staining with CD45 used to highlight contaminating leukocytes that are eliminated from analysis
  - Assay cleared by FDA for use as prognostic test in patients with metastatic cancers of breast, prostate, and colon
- Sample type, volume, and collection can influence results of CTC assays
  - Rapid processing of samples to avoid detection target degradation is recommended
    - RT-PCR detected transcript may decline or increase over time

Epidemiology
- Prevalence
  - CTCs demonstrated in peripheral blood in up to 40% of patients with newly diagnosed breast cancer
    - Incidence of CTC is higher for methods that use RT-PCR compared with immunologic methods
    - 20-30% of stage I or II breast cancer patients will have CTC detected by RT-PCR for *CK19* mRNA
  - CTCs can be found in 50-75% of patients with metastatic breast cancer

Prognostic Value
- Newly diagnosed breast cancer patients may demonstrate CTCs in peripheral blood
  - Detection of CTCs associated with worse prognosis
    - Prognostic association of CTC is independent of nodal status or whether patient receives adjuvant chemotherapy
- Metastatic breast cancer patients with CTCs have worse prognosis than those without elevated CTCs
  - In 1 study, patients who were negative for CTCs showed median overall survival of 28.3 months

CIRCULATING TUMOR CELLS

Detection Methodologies for Circulating Tumor Cells

Features	Immunologic Detection	RT-PCR Detection
Detection methodology	Immunohistochemistry or immunofluorescence	PCR for RNA transcripts
Detection targets	Epithelial antigens, cytokeratin (may use cocktails), HER2	Cytokeratin, MUC1, mammaglobin, CEA, HER2 transcripts
Sensitivity	Less sensitive	More sensitive
Specificity	More specific (ability to view captured cells)	Less specific (no ability to visualize captured cells)
Detection limits	Approximately 1 tumor cell per 1 million non-tumor cells	Approximately 1 tumor cell per 10^7 cells
Expense	More expensive (requires image analysis equipment)	Less expensive
Quantitative results	Yes (yields results in terms of number of tumor cells)	Yes (yields results in terms of measured number of gene transcripts, may vary widely between cells and between tumors)

- ○ Metastatic breast cancer patients with elevated CTCs had median overall survival of only 12.8 months

Treatment Implications

- Predictive Value
  - ○ **CTC and adjuvant therapy**
    - ■ *CK19* mRNA has been used to detect CTC in clinical studies for adjuvant treatment
    - ■ Peripheral blood samples can be used to assess for CTC before and after adjuvant chemotherapy
  - ○ Detection of *CK19* mRNA-positive CTCs post chemotherapy demonstrates a number of clinical associations
    - ■ Involvement of > 3 axillary lymph nodes
    - ■ Increased incidence of clinical relapse and disease-related deaths
    - ■ Significant reduction in disease-free and overall survival
  - ○ In multivariate analysis, detection of *CK19* mRNA-positive CTCs before and after adjuvant chemotherapy
    - ■ Independent factor associated with reduced disease-free survival
  - ○ Detection of *CK19* mRNA-positive CTCs in blood after adjuvant chemotherapy
    - ■ Independent risk factor indicating presence of chemotherapy-resistant residual disease
  - ○ **CTCs and metastatic therapy**
    - ■ Prospective randomized clinical trial was conducted that looked at CTCs
    - ■ Eligible patients had measurable metastatic disease and were started on new therapeutic regimen
    - ■ Elevated CTCs at any time point was associated with high likelihood of short time to disease progression
    - ■ At 1st follow-up visit, patients with elevated CTC had worse prognosis than patients who did not
    - ■ Elevated CTCs at later time point also associated with rapid subsequent disease progression
    - ■ It remains unclear whether changing therapy when elevated CTCs are found will impact ultimate clinical outcome
    - ■ Prospective clinical trials are currently underway to address this question

Future Directions for CTC

- Studies of secondary phenotyping and genotyping of immunomagnetically detected CTCs have been reported
  - ○ Potential to provide additional important information on tumor biology
    - ■ May prove useful for clinical decision making
  - ○ Incorporation of CTC assays into well-designed clinical trials will help define clinical utility of this technology

SELECTED REFERENCES

1. Hayes DF et al: Is there a role for circulating tumor cells in the management of breast cancer? Clin Cancer Res. 14(12):3646-50, 2008
2. Ignatiadis M et al: Prognostic value of the molecular detection of circulating tumor cells using a multimarker reverse transcription-PCR assay for cytokeratin 19, mammaglobin A, and HER2 in early breast cancer. Clin Cancer Res. 14(9):2593-600, 2008
3. Pierga JY et al: Circulating tumor cell detection predicts early metastatic relapse after neoadjuvant chemotherapy in large operable and locally advanced breast cancer in a phase II randomized trial. Clin Cancer Res. 14(21):7004-10, 2008
4. Müller V et al: Recent translational research: circulating tumor cells in breast cancer patients. Breast Cancer Res. 8(5):110, 2006
5. Cristofanilli M et al: Circulating tumor cells, disease progression, and survival in metastatic breast cancer. N Engl J Med. 351(8):781-91, 2004
6. Pierga JY et al: Clinical significance of immunocytochemical detection of tumor cells using digital microscopy in peripheral blood and bone marrow of breast cancer patients. Clin Cancer Res. 10(4):1392-400, 2004
7. Pantel K et al: Detection and clinical implications of early systemic tumor cell dissemination in breast cancer. Clin Cancer Res. 9(17):6326-34, 2003
8. Smith BM et al: Response of circulating tumor cells to systemic therapy in patients with metastatic breast cancer: comparison of quantitative polymerase chain reaction and immunocytochemical techniques. J Clin Oncol. 18(7):1432-9, 2000
9. Tondini C et al: Circulating tumor markers in breast cancer. Hematol Oncol Clin North Am. 3(4):653-74, 1989

NEOADJUVANT THERAPY

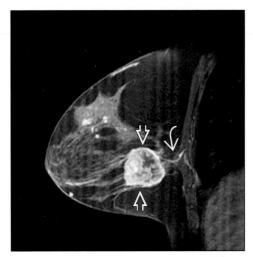

This MR study shows a large enhancing mass ⇒ with tethering to the chest wall ➚. A core needle biopsy confirmed a poorly differentiated carcinoma that was negative for ER, PR, and HER2.

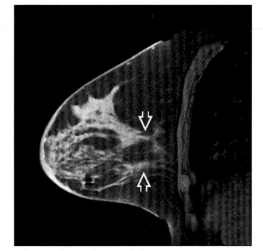

After neoadjuvant therapy, the large invasive carcinoma is no longer seen ⇒. Pathologic examination of the tumor bed confirmed a complete response. The patient has an excellent prognosis.

TERMINOLOGY

Abbreviations
- Neoadjuvant therapy (NAT)

Synonyms
- Preoperative therapy
- Presurgical therapy

Definitions
- NAT is treatment of patients with chemotherapy &/ or hormonal therapy prior to surgical removal of carcinoma
  - Diagnosis of primary carcinoma is generally made by core needle biopsy; histologic type, grade, and tumor markers are determined on this specimen
  - Size and extent of primary carcinoma (i.e., multicentricity, involvement of skin or chest wall) is determined by imaging studies
  - Lymph nodes must be evaluated prior to treatment in order to gain maximum amount of information about tumor response
    - Palpable or enlarged nodes on ultrasound should be sampled by fine needle aspiration
    - If no nodes suitable for fine needle aspiration can be identified, sentinel node biopsy may be performed
    - However, if the only positive node is excised, response to treatment in lymph nodes cannot be determined

CLINICAL IMPLICATIONS

Response to NAT
- Degree of response to NAT provides additional information
  - Individual patients: Prognostic information can be used to guide further treatment and help determine benefit of prophylactic surgery
  - Clinical trials: Response to NAT is short-term endpoint that can be used to compare different treatments using fewer patients over shorter period of time
  - Research: Paired samples of cancers pre- and post-treatment are valuable resource for research
    - Can be used to investigate types of carcinomas that respond to specific treatments
    - Can be used to investigate how carcinomas respond and how to predict which carcinomas will respond
- Clinical/radiologic evaluation of response may be inaccurate
  - Residual palpable masses and radiologic densities may be due to tumor bed without viable tumor
  - Carcinomas undergoing partial response typically become softer, show less uptake by MR, and break up into multiple small tumor foci
    - Considerable residual carcinoma can be present even if no palpable mass remains and imaging findings resolve after treatment
- Pathologic evaluation of response to NAT
  - All prognostic factors prior to treatment are also prognostic after NAT
  - Additional prognostic factors after NAT have been used in multiple different systems for evaluating response
    - Change in tumor size
    - Change in tumor cellularity: Most carcinomas become less cellular
    - Response in lymph nodes: Response of metastatic carcinoma has greater prognostic value than response in breast
    - Pathologic complete response (pCR) is associated with exceptionally good outcome for majority of patients

Clinical Value of NAT
- NAT does not improve survival over adjuvant therapy (treatment after surgical removal of cancer)

NEOADJUVANT THERAPY

- In some patients, decrease in size of large cancer will make them eligible for breast conservation
  - However, there is small increased risk of local recurrence
- Primary value of NAT is prognostic and scientific information gained from degree of response of cancer to treatment

Predicting Response to NAT

- Likelihood of response to therapy can be predicted by features of pre-treatment carcinoma
- Response to endocrine therapy
  - ER status: ER/PR-positive carcinomas respond more than ER-negative carcinomas or PR-negative carcinomas
- Response to chemotherapy
  - Grade 3 (poorly differentiated) carcinomas: More likely to respond
  - High mitotic rate: More likely to respond
  - Tumor necrosis: More likely to respond
  - ER negative: More likely to respond
  - HER2 overexpression: More likely to respond to HER2-based therapy
  - Lobular type: Less likely to respond
- Future predictors
  - NAT trials are designed to develop new methods (such as RNA profiling) that will provide better indicators of response to enable more individualized treatment for patients

MACROSCOPIC FINDINGS

Specimen Radiographs

- Clip should be placed prior to treatment to identify tumor bed
  - If there is complete or near complete response, there may not be alternative method to identify site of carcinoma
- Calcifications associated with carcinoma generally remain after treatment
  - Not all carcinomas are associated with calcifications, and this finding should not be relied upon to identify tumor site

Specimen Handling

- Tissue adjacent to clip(s) must be identified grossly
- If grossly evident invasive carcinoma is present, size, number of cancers, and relationship of cancers to each other should be described
  - Typical partial response to treatment is seen as multiple foci of invasion scattered over tumor bed
- Extent of sampling adjacent to clip(s) if gross carcinoma is not present depends on extent of carcinoma prior to treatment
  - If practical, entire tumor bed should be sampled if patient may have had a pCR
  - If tumor bed is quite large, at least 1 block of tissue per cm of tumor bed is suggested
    - Additional tissue sampling can be determined after examination of initial sampling
- Gross presence of tumor bed at margins should be noted

- All margins should be sampled with perpendicular sections
- Lymph nodes should be carefully searched for and completely submitted for microscopic examination
  - Nodes may be smaller and fewer in number after treatment

MICROSCOPIC FINDINGS

General Features

- Tumor bed must be identified microscopically
  - Typical findings are dense fibrosis, histiocytes, lymphocytes, occasional giant cells, and hemosiderin-laden macrophages
  - Tumor bed will not look like normal breast tissue
    - If only normal breast tissue is present, additional gross sampling is indicated
- Residual invasive carcinoma usually resembles pre-treatment carcinoma but is often less cellular
  - In rare cases, the carcinoma may appear to be more poorly differentiated or very rarely more well differentiated
- Residual DCIS may be present
  - In some cases, there can be pCR for invasive carcinoma but with residual DCIS
  - DCIS may be similar in appearance or may have higher nuclear grade
  - Presence of DCIS can be helpful in identifying the location of tumor bed
- Normal breast tissue may undergo treatment-related changes
  - Ducts and lobules may appear atrophic with thickened basement membranes
  - Scattered cells with nuclear pleomorphism may be seen
  - In some cases, it may be difficult to distinguish treatment-related changes from residual DCIS

REPORTING CONSIDERATIONS

Reporting Residual Invasive Carcinoma

- Histologic type, grade, lymph-vascular invasion, and size should be reported
  - Size may be difficult to determine if there are multiple scattered foci over tumor bed
    - Reporting options are size of largest contiguous focus, number of foci, and number of blocks
- Tumor cellularity and change in cellularity is prognostic factor and is used in some systems of reporting response to therapy
  - For very paucicellular carcinomas, cytokeratin studies may be helpful to identify location and extent of residual carcinoma
- ER, PR, and HER2 should be repeated if residual invasive carcinoma is present
  - Markers negative before treatment may be positive after treatment due to limited pre-treatment sampling, selection of tumor subclones by treatment, or (less likely) treatment effect on tumor cells

NEOADJUVANT THERAPY

Systems for Evaluating the Response to Neoadjuvant Therapy

Name of System	Reference	Features Evaluated	Categories of Response	Comments
Miller-Payne	Ogston, 2003	Change in tumor cellularity comparing pre- and post-treatment carcinoma	5 grades from 1 (no change in cellularity) to 5 (pathologic complete response in breast)	Does not include lymph node metastases; requires review of pre-treatment core needle biopsy for cellularity
Residual Cancer Burden (RCB)	Symmans, 2007	Average cellularity over size of tumor bed (in 2 dimensions), number of lymph node metastases, size of largest metastasis	Continuous variable divided into 4 categories from 0 (pathologic complete response) to RCB-3 (generally little or no response)	Categories correlate with response if pre-treatment cancer would have been RCB-3; a web-based calculator is available at www.mdanderson.org/breastcancer_RCB
AJCC	7th edition, 2010	Size and extent of carcinoma, number of lymph node metastases	Change in T or N category, 4 post-treatment stages	Prognostic power is enhanced if both pre- and post-treatment AJCC staging is used in combination
Rodenhuis	Rodenhuis, 2009	Point system based on change in AJCC T category and change in N category divided by total possible points	0 (no response or progression) to 1 (pathologic complete response in breast and nodes)	Requires clinical and imaging information to determine pre-treatment T and N categories

Reporting Residual DCIS

- Report type and extent
- In only DCIS is present, this is considered pCR in most systems
- IHC should be used, if necessary, to distinguish DCIS from residual invasive carcinoma

Reporting Margins

- Margins should be evaluated for presence of invasive carcinoma, DCIS, and tumor bed
- In general, size of tumor bed is size of carcinoma prior to treatment
  - Entire tumor bed should be removed as carcinoma can be present as multiple foci throughout tumor bed if there has been partial response
  - If tumor bed is present at margin, there may be increased likelihood of residual carcinoma in breast

Reporting Lymph Node Status

- Lymph nodes should be evaluated for metastatic carcinoma and response to treatment
  - If metastatic carcinoma is present, associated features suggesting treatment response (e.g., scarring fibrosis) should be noted
    - In selected cases with fibrosis and scattered atypical cells, cytokeratin studies may be helpful to document presence of residual carcinoma
  - Small lymph node metastases (< 2 mm) have same prognostic significance as larger metastases without treatment
    - Small metastases after NAT are indicative of partial response
    - Any tumor cells in nodes (including isolated tumor cells) excludes pCR
  - In nodes without carcinoma, presence of features suggesting prior involvement (e.g., scarring fibrosis) should be noted
    - However, metastatic carcinoma in nodes can undergo a pCR without leaving histologic evidence in node

- Pathologic evaluation of nodes only after treatment is not reliable to determine nodal status prior to treatment

Reporting Response to NAT

- More than 8 systems have been developed to classify response of breast carcinomas to treatment
- In general, NAT trials have the following results
  - Up to 20% of patients have pCR
  - Up to 20% of patients do not respond or progress
  - Up to 60% of patients have partial response
    - These are most difficult cases to evaluate and classify consistently
- Category of pCR is easiest to define
  - In most systems, pCR can include residual DCIS, but invasive carcinoma in breast or metastatic carcinoma in nodes must be absent
- Some systems compare carcinomas before and after treatment (e.g., Miller-Payne, Rodenhuis), whereas other systems quantify amount of residual carcinoma after treatment (e.g., RCB, AJCC)
- Extent of tumor prior to treatment is also important prognostic factor
  - For example, > 90% of all patients with pCR will not recur; however, 50% of patients with pre-treatment inflammatory carcinoma and pCR do recur

SELECTED REFERENCES

1. Rodenhuis S et al: A simple system for grading the response of breast cancer to neoadjuvant chemotherapy. Ann Oncol. 21(3):481-7, 2010
2. Sahoo S et al: Pathology of breast carcinomas after neoadjuvant chemotherapy: an overview with recommendations on specimen processing and reporting. Arch Pathol Lab Med. 133(4):633-42, 2009
3. Symmans WF et al: Measurement of residual breast cancer burden to predict survival after neoadjuvant chemotherapy. J Clin Oncol. 25(28):4414-22, 2007
4. Ogston KN et al: A new histological grading system to assess response of breast cancers to primary chemotherapy: prognostic significance and survival. Breast. 12(5):320-7, 2003

NEOADJUVANT THERAPY

Imaging and Gross Features and Core Needle Biopsy

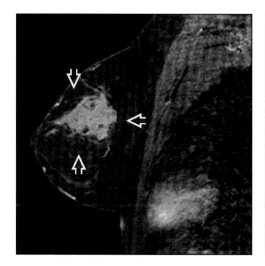
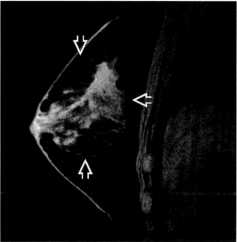

(Left) This patient presented with a large palpable mass that correlated with an area of enhancement by MR ➡. A moderately differentiated invasive carcinoma positive for ER and PR and negative for HER2 was confirmed by core needle biopsy. *(Right)* After treatment, the mass is still present, but the enhancement is diminished ➡. Pathologic examination confirmed residual invasive carcinoma within the tumor bed. ER positive carcinomas typically respond less well to chemotherapy.

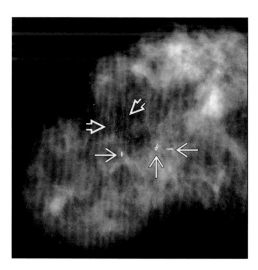
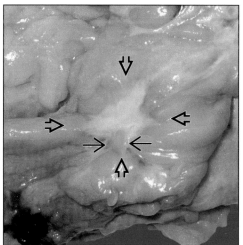

(Left) Clips must be placed during the diagnostic biopsy or at the time of subsequent biopsies taken for research in order to identify the tumor bed. In this case, 3 clips are seen ➡. Calcifications present prior to treatment are usually present after treatment, as in this case ➡. However, carcinomas are not always associated with calcifications. *(Right)* After NAT, a fibrotic tumor bed is present ➡ with a 0.8 cm focus of residual invasive carcinoma ➡.

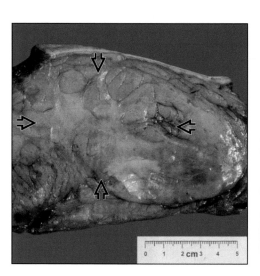
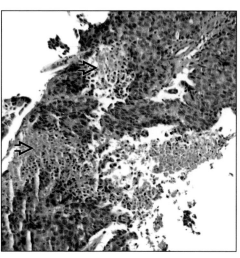

(Left) This patient had an 8 cm palpable HER2 positive carcinoma. After NAT, a large fibrotic tumor bed is present ➡, which could only be identified by radiographing the specimen and finding clips. *(Right)* The initial core needle biopsy is essential to guide treatment. The predictors of a good response to chemotherapy are high nuclear grade, increased proliferative rate, extensive necrosis ➡, absence of lobular morphology, absence of ER, and presence of HER2.

NEOADJUVANT THERAPY

Microscopic Features

(Left) Tumor beds consist of areas of dense fibrosis. They do not look like typical normal breast tissue but can be difficult to distinguish from breast tissue with dense interlobular stroma. In this case, the tumor bed consists of dense collagenized tissue lacking normal ducts and lobules ➲. *(Right)* A tumor bed can also consist of a dense infiltrate of histiocytes and lymphocytes. An IHC study for cytokeratin confirmed that no residual carcinoma was present.

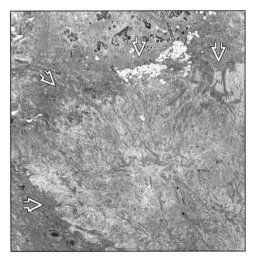 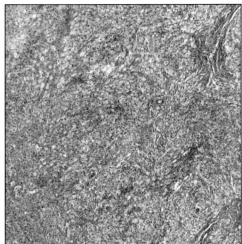

(Left) A giant cell reaction ➲ or hemosiderin-laden macrophages ➲ may also identify the location of a treated carcinoma &/or the prior core needle biopsy site. *(Right)* Normal breast tissue may appear atrophic after treatment, and basement membranes may be thickened ➲. Sporadic cells may show marked nuclear atypia ➲. In some cases, it may be difficult to distinguish such atypia from residual carcinoma in situ. Atypical cells due to treatment should not proliferate.

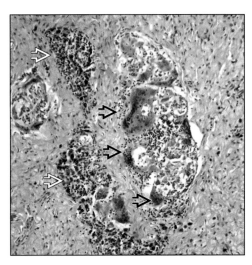 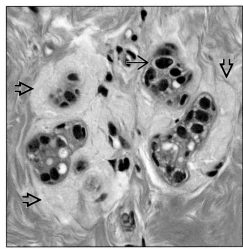

(Left) This untreated invasive carcinoma is highly cellular and shows moderate nuclear pleomorphism. *(Right)* This carcinoma had a partial response to chemotherapy as a single large carcinoma was reduced to multiple small foci of cancer scattered over the tumor bed. However, the residual foci of carcinoma are similar in appearance to the pre-treatment carcinoma, and there has been no change in cellularity. In general, treatment does not change the cytologic appearance of carcinomas.

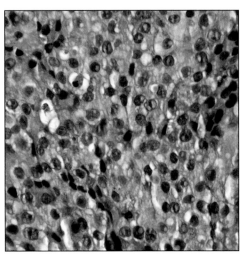 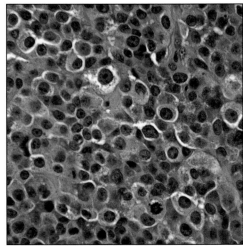

NEOADJUVANT THERAPY

Microscopic Features

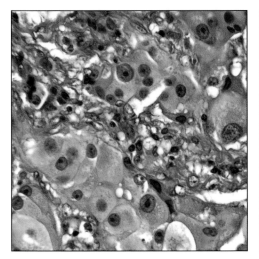

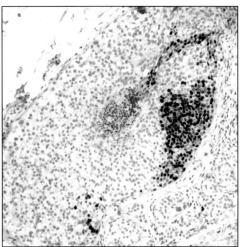

(Left) This carcinoma has an altered appearance after NAT, consisting of abundant granular cytoplasm and large pleomorphic nuclei. However, such changes cannot be attributed to treatment unless the pre-treatment carcinoma is available for comparison. *(Right)* This carcinoma shows marked heterogeneity for estrogen receptor (ER), which might not be detected by core needle biopsy. The carcinoma after treatment may consist predominantly of therapy-resistant ER positive tumor cells.

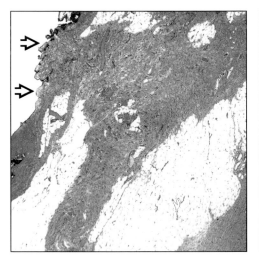

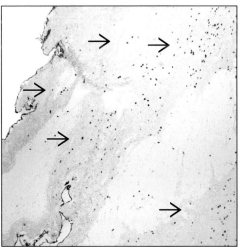

(Left) Margins can be difficult to evaluate after treatment when there are scattered foci of carcinoma in the tumor bed and the tumor bed appears to extend to the margin. In this case, the fibrotic tumor bed appears to have been transected ⊟. *(Right)* A cytokeratin study demonstrates the presence of scattered residual tumor cells ⇒. Although the cells are not touching ink, it is possible that the tumor bed has been transected and that there is residual carcinoma in the patient.

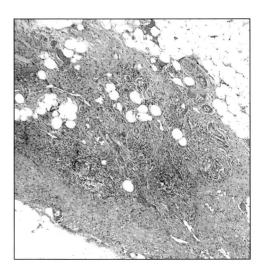

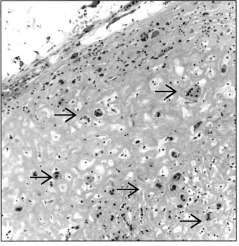

(Left) Lymph nodes after treatment are often fibrotic with few lymphocytes. However, it is difficult to determine with certainty whether or not a lymph node was involved by carcinoma prior to treatment. In some cases, a metastasis can respond completely, and the node will appear normal. *(Right)* If there has been a marked response in the lymph nodes, there may be scattered tumor cells in a fibrous scar ⇒, as seen in this case, indicating an incomplete response to treatment.

Stromal Lesions

FIBROADENOMA

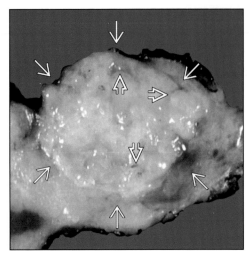

Fibroadenomas are benign proliferations of intralobular stroma. They form circumscribed masses ➡ that bulge out from the adjacent fatty tissue. Clefts ⬌ correspond to epithelial-lined spaces.

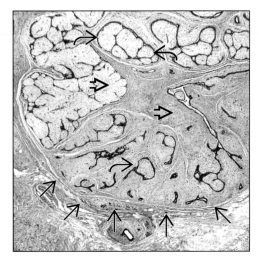

Fibroadenomas are formed by a proliferation of stromal cells ⬌ that usually push and distort the associated epithelium ⬌. These lesions are well circumscribed with pushing borders ⬌.

TERMINOLOGY

Abbreviations
- Fibroadenoma (FA)

Synonyms
- Adenofibroma

Definitions
- Biphasic fibroepithelial tumor consisting of intralobular stromal cells and associated epithelial cells

ETIOLOGY/PATHOGENESIS

Abnormal Growth of Intralobular Stromal Cells
- **Normal breast development**
  - During embryological development, stroma differentiates 1st and induces downgrowth of cells from epidermis to form ductal system
    - This synergistic relationship between epithelial and stromal cells persists in duct/lobular unit
    - Increased growth of stromal cells is accompanied by corresponding hyperplasia of epithelial cells
  - Several possible etiologies for abnormal growth of intralobular stromal cells
- **Hormonal stimulation**
  - Most FAs are polyclonal hyperplasias of lobular stroma
    - Some stromal cells have estrogen receptor β &/or progesterone receptors
  - FAs occur most commonly in young premenopausal women
  - FAs can grow during pregnancy
    - If rapid growth occurs, lesion may infarct
    - May be mistaken for malignancy
- **Iatrogenic**
  - Cyclosporine in kidney transplant recipients is associated with increase in FAs

- Attributed to possible similarity to prolactin
- Can regress when patient is switched to different medication
- **Genetic/hereditary**
  - More common in African-American women
  - Myxoid FAs occur in Carney complex
    - Myxomas (cardiac, cutaneous, breast), primary pigmented nodular adrenocortical disease, large cell calcifying Sertoli cell tumors, multiple thyroid lesions, growth hormone-producing pituitary adenoma, other tumors
    - Pigmented skin lesions (lentigos, blue nevi, café au lait spots), typically involving vermillion border of lip and intercanthal portion of eye
    - Type 1 (CNC1): *PRKAR1A* (17q23-24)
    - Type 2 (CNC2): Locus at 2p16
    - 30% of patients do not have an identified germline mutation
- **Neoplastic**
  - Some FAs are monoclonal stromal tumors
    - Clonal genetic changes may be present in stromal cells
    - Associated epithelial cells are usually polyclonal
  - In general, FAs have few genetic changes
    - Some have gain of 1q similar to phyllodes tumors
  - As stromal proliferation becomes more pronounced and autonomous, spectrum of changes seen in FAs overlaps with low-grade phyllodes tumors
    - Some phyllodes tumors likely arise from FAs

CLINICAL ISSUES

Epidemiology
- Incidence
  - Most common solid benign breast lesion
- Age
  - Typically occur in younger patients (20-35 years)

FIBROADENOMA

Key Facts

Terminology
- Fibroadenoma (FA)
  - Most common benign solid breast neoplasm
  - Well-circumscribed lesion
  - Proliferation of epithelial and stromal elements

Etiology/Pathogenesis
- FAs are due to proliferation of lobular stroma and may be polyclonal or monoclonal

Clinical Issues
- Typically occur in younger patients between ages 20-35
- Painless, slowly growing, mobile, well-defined mass
- Most FAs can be diagnosed by core needle biopsy and followed radiographically

Image Findings
- Circumscribed or lobulated mass
- Calcifications may be present, particularly in older women

Microscopic Pathology
- Admixed glands and stromal elements

Top Differential Diagnoses
- Phyllodes tumor
- Hamartoma (fibroadenolipoma)
- Fibroadenomatoid changes
- Fibrous tumor
- Pseudoangiomatous stromal hyperplasia
- Tubular adenoma

  - In older women, associated with continued elevated hormone levels either due to replacement therapy or obesity

Presentation
- Most commonly presents as painless, slowly growing, mobile, well-defined, palpable nodule in a young woman
- In older women, may be detected as mammographic circumscribed density or calcifications

Natural History
- May regress in size with age
- Stroma typically undergoes hyalinization, which can serve as substrate for calcifications

Treatment
- Surgical approaches
  - Most FAs can be diagnosed by core needle biopsy and followed radiographically
  - Surgery to remove a FA may be indicated for large lesions, if patient requests removal, or for rare lesions that continue to grow in size

Prognosis
- FAs are benign
  - Only clinical importance is in distinguishing FAs from malignancies
  - For some women, FAs may be excised due to cosmetic issues if lesion is large
- FAs are classified as proliferative breast disease without atypia
  - Relative risk increased 1.5-2x; absolute lifetime risk of breast cancer is 5-7%
  - Risk is to both breasts
  - In 1 study, only women with complex FAs had increased risk

Core Needle Biopsy
- Diagnosis of FA can usually be made on core biopsy
  - Targeted lesion is usually a circumscribed mass or cluster of calcifications

  - Diagnosis of FA does not correlate well with an irregular mass
- Some fibroepithelial lesions on core needle biopsy are difficult to classify as FA or phyllodes tumor
  - Stroma may show increased cellularity
  - Mitoses may be present
    - Mitoses > 2 per 10 HPFs favors phyllodes tumor; lower scores do not discriminate between these lesions
    - Ki-67 > 5% favors phyllodes tumor; lower scores do not discriminate between these lesions
    - Because FAs can grow during pregnancy, increased proliferation may be present at this time
  - Focal stromal overgrowth may be seen
  - Infiltration of adjacent stroma may be difficult to evaluate due to fragmentation of cores
- Certain clinical features increase likelihood that lesion is a phyllodes tumor
  - Large size
  - Increase in size
  - History of prior phyllodes tumor
- If a definitive diagnosis cannot be made, lesion should be classified as a "fibroepithelial tumor"
  - This type of lesion is best classified after complete surgical excision

IMAGE FINDINGS

Mammographic Findings
- Circumscribed or lobulated mass
  - May be ill defined if obscured by dense stroma or if fibroadenomatoid changes are present
- Calcifications may be present, particularly in older women, and will appear as a cluster
  - Calcifications may be coarse (large "popcorn" calcifications) or numerous and small
  - May mimic calcifications seen in DCIS due to clustering

Ultrasonographic Findings
- Circumscribed or lobulated mass

FIBROADENOMA

MR Findings

- Smooth bordered mass; may have nonenhancing internal septations
- Enhancement is generally slower than that seen with carcinomas

MACROSCOPIC FEATURES

General Features

- Circumscribed, white, firm but not hard (rubbery), palpable mass
  - Mass usually bulges above normal breast tissue; slit-like spaces may be present
    - Carcinomas usually do not bulge; typically have flat surface
  - Large FAs may have a leaf-like appearance due to areas of stromal growth separated by epithelial-lined clefts
- Multiple synchronous FAs can be present

Size

- Majority < 3 cm but can be very large

MICROSCOPIC PATHOLOGY

Histologic Features

- **Biphasic growth pattern**
  - Admixed glandular and stromal elements
    - Variable morphologic appearance, depends on relative amount and configuration of each element
    - Regular and symmetric distribution of epithelial and fibrous elements should be present
  - FAs typically have well-circumscribed pushing borders and do not infiltrate adjacent parenchyma
    - Can be difficult to distinguish infiltration of stroma from fibroadenomatoid changes in adjacent stroma
  - Infarction can occur during pregnancy
    - Resulting necrosis should not be interpreted as indicating malignancy
- **Stromal component**
  - Typically loose and may have myxoid appearance
    - Myxoid stroma is more typical in younger individuals
    - Dense hyalinized stroma is more common in older individuals
  - Stroma typically shows low cellularity and lacks mitotic activity, and spindle cells are cytologically bland
    - Stromal spindle cells concentrically cuff glandular structures or array themselves perpendicular to basement membrane
    - Stromal spindle cells are predominantly CD34-positive specialized fibroblasts
    - CD34-positive spindle cells are seen in perilobular and to a lesser extent interlobular stroma of normal breasts
  - Pseudoangiomatous stromal hyperplasia can be present

- Benign heterologous elements including adipose tissue, smooth muscle, or bone are rare findings
- In rare cases, atypical bizarre multinucleated giant cells may be present
  - These should not be used to classify a tumor as a phyllodes tumor
- **Glandular component**
  - Epithelial component of FA is composed of cuboidal or columnar cells with uniform nuclei
    - Glandular structures are surrounded by a supportive myoepithelial layer
  - Glandular elements may be elongated and compressed with beaded appearance (intracanalicular pattern)
    - Some FAs have glandular elements arranged as small open and round acinar structures (pericanalicular pattern)
    - Many FAs have both patterns
  - Sclerosing adenosis, apocrine cysts, and epithelial hyperplasia may be present
    - Some tumors appear to be hybrid lesions with areas of both epithelial predominance and stromal predominance
  - Squamous metaplasia may be present
  - Although rare, ALH, LCIS, ADH, and DCIS may involve FAs
    - LCIS and DCIS can be found entirely within confines of FA or may involve surrounding breast tissues
- **Calcifications**
  - Some are associated with epithelial component; probably form on glandular secretions
  - Calcifications also form directly on regularly repeating collagenized stroma
    - This is the only type of breast stroma that frequently calcifies
    - Small calcifications can appear as minute blue bubbles in stroma
- **Variants**
  - Complex FA: FAs that include cysts > 3 mm, sclerosing adenosis, epithelial calcifications, or papillary apocrine change
    - 1 study provided evidence that only FAs with these features increase the risk of subsequent breast carcinoma
    - Not yet confirmed by other studies
  - Cellular FA: FA with a hypercellular stroma
  - Juvenile FA: This term has been used for several different types of lesions and, therefore, should only be used if lesion type is defined
    - FA with ADH: Does not necessarily present in young women
    - FA in a young woman: May show greater stromal cellularity and epithelial hyperplasia
    - Cellular FA
    - Large rapidly growing FA, usually in a young woman
  - Giant FA: FA of large size
    - Can have leaf-like ("phyllodes") architecture
  - Myxoid FA: FA with prominent myxoid changes in stromal component
    - Stromal changes can resemble mucin

ANCILLARY TESTS

Immunohistochemistry

- Ki-67
  - Typically very low (< 5%)
  - Some phyllodes tumors can also have low Ki-67 scores
  - Not typically used for diagnosis

DIFFERENTIAL DIAGNOSIS

Phyllodes Tumor

- Uncommon fibroepithelial neoplasm accounting for < 1% of primary mammary tumors
  - Typically occurs in older patients compared with FA (median age at diagnosis is 45)
- Appearance of stromal component is main diagnostic feature used to distinguish FA and phyllodes tumor
  - Increased stromal cellularity: Cells often form fascicles
  - Stroma proliferates to the extent that there are areas of cellular stroma without epithelial elements (stromal overgrowth)
  - Stromal cells may have nuclear atypia
  - Mitoses are usually present and may be numerous
    - Mitoses are typically absent or rare in FAs; they could possibly be increased during pregnancy
  - Tumor may invade into surrounding breast parenchyma
  - Heterologous malignant stromal elements are rarely present; most commonly liposarcoma or rhabdomyosarcoma
  - Necrosis may be present in high-grade lesions
- Some tumors are difficult to classify as either FA or phyllodes tumor as there is a continuum of histologic findings
  - Both FAs and low-grade phyllodes tumors have risk of local recurrence and essentially no risk of distant metastasis

Fibroadenomatoid Changes

- Same features as FA but do not form a discrete mass
  - Most likely represents hyperplastic stromal changes and not a neoplastic proliferation
- Typically presents as ill-defined palpable mass or mammographic density
- In rare cases, stromal invasion by phyllodes tumor can be mistaken for fibroadenomatoid changes

Hamartoma (Fibroadenolipoma)

- Well-circumscribed lesion composed of overgrowth of epithelial and stromal cells
- Considerable morphologic overlap between FA and hamartoma
  - Epithelial component is more disorganized and irregularly dispersed
  - Stromal predominance is not characteristic
  - Adipose tissue is usually found in hamartoma but very unusual for FA

Fibrous Tumor

- May present as palpable mass or mammographic circumscribed density
- Most common in premenopausal women or older women using hormone replacement therapy
- Appear to be proliferations of interlobular stromal cells
  - Tumor cells blend into surrounding tissue on microscopic examination
  - Correlation with clinical findings &/or imaging generally necessary to make diagnosis
- Findings on core needle biopsy are nonspecific
  - At least 0.4 cm span of fibrous tissue without adipose tissue is consistent with fibrous tumor
  - Radiologist must confirm that targeted lesion was sampled

Pseudoangiomatous Stromal Hyperplasia (PASH)

- Proliferation of interlobular myofibroblasts
  - Associated with a characteristic clefting of stroma
- Epithelial elements are surrounded rather than distorted by stromal proliferation
- Can form a circumscribed or ill-defined mass
  - Also common as an incidental finding
- Can be present within the stroma of a FA

Tubular Adenoma

- Circumscribed lesion consisting of small round acinar spaces surrounded by scant loosely cellular stroma
- Less common than FA
  - Also occurs in young women
- May be brown on gross examination
  - FAs are usually white
- Some lesions appear to consist of both tubular adenoma and FA
  - Probably hyperplasias with differing relative predominance of stromal and epithelial elements
  - Tubular adenoma is sometimes classified as a variant of FA

SELECTED REFERENCES

1. Iaria G et al: Prospective study of switch from cyclosporine to tacrolimus for fibroadenomas of the breast in kidney transplantation. Transplant Proc. 42(4):1169-70, 2010
2. Resetkova E et al: Clinical and radiologic data and core needle biopsy findings should dictate management of cellular fibroepithelial tumors of the breast. Breast J. 16(6):573-80, 2010
3. Sapino A et al: Estrogen receptor-beta is expressed in stromal cells of fibroadenoma and phyllodes tumors of the breast. Mod Pathol. 19(4):599-606, 2006
4. Carter BA et al: No elevation in long-term breast carcinoma risk for women with fibroadenomas that contain atypical hyperplasia. Cancer. 92(1):30-6, 2001
5. Dupont WD et al: Long-term risk of breast cancer in women with fibroadenoma. N Engl J Med. 331(1):10-5, 1994
6. Carney JA et al: Myxoid fibroadenoma and allied conditions (myxomatosis) of the breast. A heritable disorder with special associations including cardiac and cutaneous myxomas. Am J Surg Pathol. 15(8):713-21, 1991

FIBROADENOMA

Imaging and Microscopic Features

(Left) FAs are detected as circumscribed masses ⇒ by mammography. The appearance is not specific. The differential diagnosis also includes circumscribed carcinomas such as mucinous, medullary, and triple negative types. *(Right)* Some FAs are associated with radiographic calcifications, which are typically coarse and clustered ⇒ but may be pleomorphic and mimic ductal carcinoma in situ on imaging. The calcifications may form on secretions within the epithelium or directly on the dense stroma.

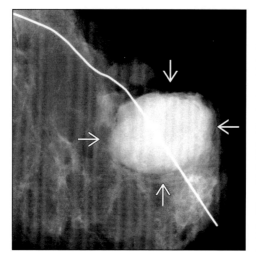 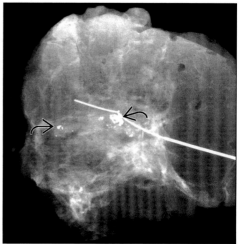

(Left) This FA has circumscribed borders and consists predominantly of stroma ⇒, but it also contains areas of sclerosing adenosis ⇒. This type of lesion is more likely to be hyperplastic than neoplastic. *(Right)* Fibroadenomas are often associated with large calcifications ⇒, which are not typically associated with malignancy. However, numerous smaller stromal calcifications ⇒ can appear very suspicious if they are clustered in the vicinity of the fibroadenoma.

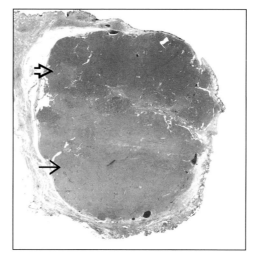 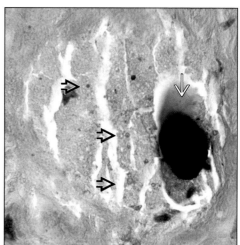

(Left) The epithelium of FA can be involved by florid epithelial hyperplasia ⇒. The pushing and distortion within the lesion can sometimes make classification difficult. *(Right)* FAs may be involved by DCIS ⇒, LCIS, ADH, or ALH. The clinical significance of these lesions when limited to a FA is unknown. Evidence of these lesions should be sought in the surrounding breast tissue.

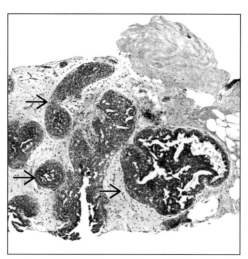 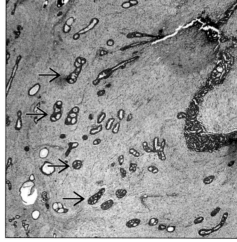

FIBROADENOMA

Microscopic and Immunohistochemical Features

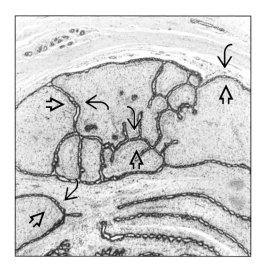

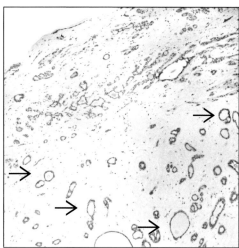

(Left) The most common growth pattern of FA is intracanicular. The stromal cells ⮞ push and distort the epithelium ➡. This pattern gives rise to the leaf-like pattern seen in large FAs and phyllodes tumors. (Right) In the pericanalicular pattern of FA, the stromal cells surround the epithelium but do not distort the shape ➡. When this pattern is present in phyllodes tumors, the leaf-like architecture is not present. These tumors have been called periductal stromal sarcomas.

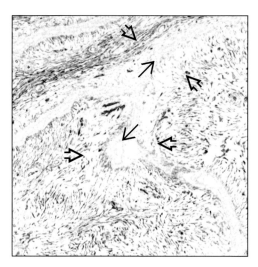

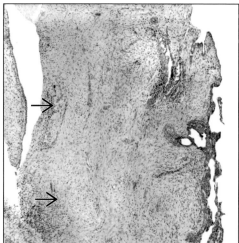

(Left) The stromal cells of a FA are predominantly CD34-positive fibroblasts ⮞, which concentrically cuff glandular structures ➡. The majority of breast fibroblasts are CD34 positive. The only stromal lesions commonly negative for this marker are fibromatosis and nodular fasciitis. (Right) FAs can be difficult to distinguish from phyllodes tumors on core needle biopsy. The presence of stromal mitoses &/or stromal overgrowth ➡ raises the possibility of a phyllodes tumor.

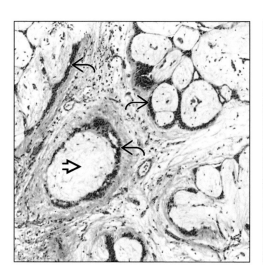

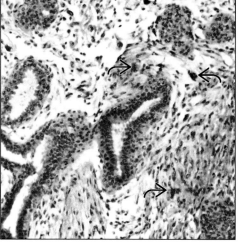

(Left) Myxoid changes ⮞ in a fibroadenoma can be prominent and are more typically seen in younger patients. The glandular elements are elongated and compressed ➡, showing an intracanalicular pattern. If prominent, these stromal changes can mimic a mucinous carcinoma. (Right) FA can have scattered atypical giant cells ➡. These cells are often multinucleated and are likely degenerative in nature. They should not be used as evidence of nuclear atypia in a phyllodes tumor.

FIBROADENOMA

Differential Diagnosis

(Left) *Fibroadenomatoid changes are most likely hyperplastic rather than neoplastic changes and involve multiple lobules. These changes can be associated with ill-defined masses but usually not circumscribed masses.* *(Right)* *Like FAs, fibrous nodules form circumscribed palpable masses or mammographic densities ➡. They appear to be benign proliferations of interlobular fibroblasts. If myofibroblasts are involved, the lesion may be classified as pseudoangiomatous stromal hyperplasia.*

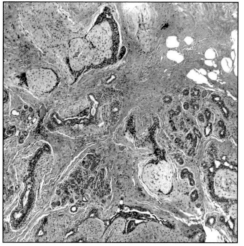
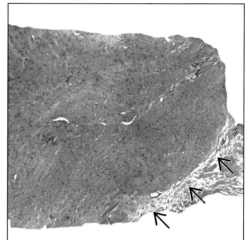

(Left) *Pseudoangiomatous stromal hyperplasia is a proliferative lesion of interlobular myofibroblasts. There can be characteristic stromal clefts or a fascicular pattern ➡. The cells often surround epithelial elements ➡ but do not push or distort them.* *(Right)* *Hamartomas, like FAs, also consist of epithelium and stroma. However, hamartomas contain adipose tissue ➡, which would be unusual for FA. In this case, the stroma has a smooth muscle appearance ("myoid hamartoma").*

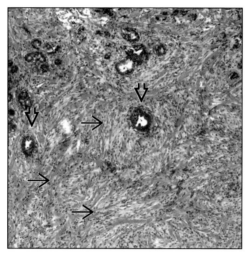
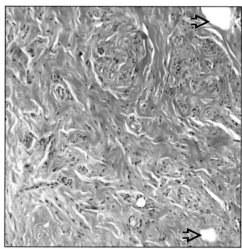

(Left) *Phyllodes tumors may form circumscribed masses ➡. The leaf-like pattern is formed by large areas of stroma surrounded by clefts lined by epithelial cells ➡.* *(Right)* *Like FAs, phyllodes tumors are also biphasic lesions that arise from intralobular stromal cells. Clefts are formed because the epithelial lined spaces ➡ are distorted by the large areas of neoplastic stromal cells ➡. Phyllodes tumors are typically larger, more cellular, and have a higher mitotic rate than FAs.*

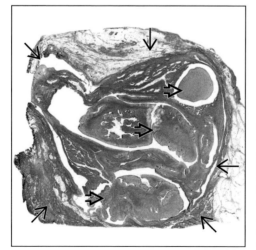
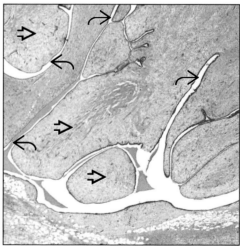

FIBROADENOMA

Fibroadenoma vs. Phyllodes Tumor

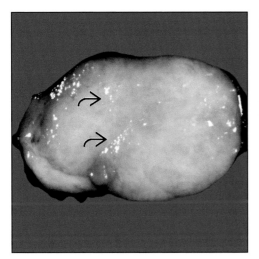 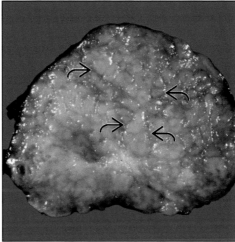

(Left) FAs are well-circumscribed rubbery lesions that are easily separated from surrounding breast tissue. The cut surface typically bulges and may appear glistening ➔ due to myxoid stromal changes. *(Right)* Phyllodes tumors typically have more stromal overgrowth compared to FAs. This feature can be seen grossly by areas of nodularity separated by slit-like spaces ➔ that are lined by benign epithelium. When more pronounced, larger leaf-like protuberances are formed.

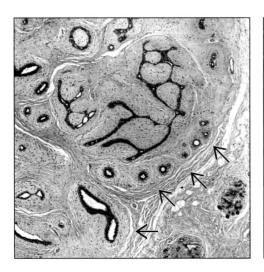 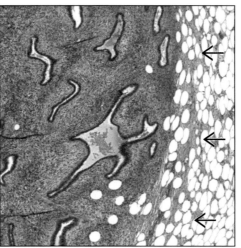

(Left) FAs have an even balance of epithelial and stromal components, which are usually pauci- or mildly cellular. The border is well circumscribed ➔. *(Right)* The stroma of phyllodes tumors is often highly cellular and often forms a fascicular pattern. Stromal overgrowth is typical. Extensive invasion into the surrounding breast tissue may be present ➔ and would not be seen in a fibroadenoma.

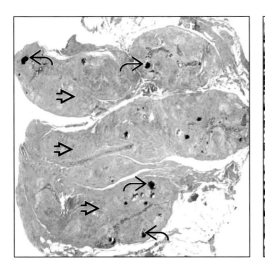 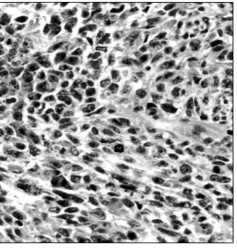

(Left) FAs, particularly those in older women, may undergo hyalinization ➔. The loss of epithelium in these areas should not be interpreted as stromal overgrowth. Calcifications may form directly on the regularly repeating collagen ➔. *(Right)* In high-grade phyllodes tumors, the benign epithelial component may be lost, the cells may show nuclear pleomorphism, and numerous mitotic figures may be present. In these tumors, the differential diagnosis includes a primary sarcoma.

PHYLLODES TUMOR

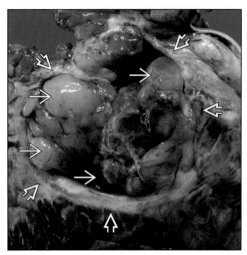

Phyllodes tumors were named after their leaf-like architecture characterized by protruding tumor nodules ➡ within a cystic cavity ⮑. These tumors can resemble complex cysts on breast imaging.

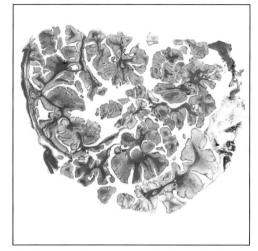

The tumor nodules are lined by benign epithelial cells. The characteristic clefts are formed as the stroma becomes more prominent and the spaces separating the epithelial surfaces widen.

TERMINOLOGY

Abbreviations
- Phyllodes tumor (PT)

Synonyms
- Cystosarcoma phyllodes
- Periductal stromal sarcoma

Definitions
- Biphasic tumor consisting of neoplastic intralobular-type stromal cells and benign epithelial cells

ETIOLOGY/PATHOGENESIS

Cell of Origin
- During development of embryo, 1st breast cells to differentiate are stromal cells
  - Stroma induces downgrowth of overlying epithelium to form primitive ducts
  - This molecular cross-talk continues throughout development
- Neoplastic stromal cells of PT arise from fibroblasts of specialized intralobular stroma
  - Fibroadenomas (FAs) are closely related tumors that also arise from same cells
  - Some FAs are hyperplasias and some neoplasias
  - FA and low-grade PT are on a spectrum of increasing autonomous growth of stromal cells
    - Some PT may arise from a preexisting FA
- Associated epithelial cells are benign
  - Epithelial cells are stimulated to proliferate by stromal cells
    - In some PTs, epithelial cells have some of the same genetic changes as stromal cells
    - May reflect fact that lobules are derived from a clone of cells
    - In other cases, epithelial cells are polyclonal

- With very rare exceptions, only stromal cells progress to malignancy
  - With increasing autonomy and growth, stromal cells outgrow epithelial cells
    - High-grade PT may consist almost entirely of stromal cells
  - Only stromal cells are present in distant metastases

DNA Changes
- Number of chromosomal changes increases with grade of PT
- Most common changes are gain of 1q and loss of 13, 7p12, 3p24, 10p12, and 9p21
  - Changes are very variable from tumor to tumor
  - Changes are also very variable within tumors
    - Suggests that many subclones with different genetic changes arise during progression
- Loss of heterozygosity (LOH) is very low in FAs, more common in low- and intermediate-grade PT, and most common in high-grade PT
- Recurrent PT often gains genetic changes
  - Correlates with increase in histologic grade in ~ 1/3 of cases

Gene Expression Profiling
- Patterns of expression vary by PT grade
  - Supports separation into 3 groups
- Major categories of changes are in genes related to proliferation and stromal/epithelial interactions

CLINICAL ISSUES

Epidemiology
- Incidence
  - Uncommon: < 1% of all breast tumors
- Age
  - Peak age range for occurrence is 35-55
    - Can occur at any age
- Ethnicity

PHYLLODES TUMOR

Key Facts

Terminology
- Derived from the Greek word "phyllos" meaning "leaf"
- Biphasic tumor consisting of epithelial-lined clefts separating areas of cellular stroma, creating leaf-like fronds

Clinical Issues
- Uncommon: < 1% of all breast tumors
- Peak age range is 35 -55
- More common in Asian populations (~ 7% of breast tumors)
- > 90% of PTs follow benign clinical course and are adequately treated by surgical resection
- In rare cases (< 5%), distant metastases occur and usually result in death of patient

Microscopic Pathology
- Evaluation of stroma is used to classify PT into 3 grades
- Margins can be difficult to evaluate, particularly in reexcision specimens
- Recurrent PT can progress to a higher grade and acquire additional genetic changes
- Metastases consist only of the stromal component
  - Bone and lung are most common sites

Top Differential Diagnoses
- Fibroadenoma with cellular stroma
- Spindle cell carcinoma
- Primary sarcoma of breast
- Fibromatosis
- Metastatic spindle cell carcinoma

  - More common in Asian populations (~ 7% of breast tumors)

Presentation
- Most common presentation is as palpable painless mass
- Less commonly detected as a density on mammographic screening

Treatment
- Surgical approaches
  - Complete excision of all PTs recommended
    - Incomplete excision increases risk for local recurrence
    - Recurrence rates increase from low-grade to high-grade PT; majority occur in 1st 2 years
  - Lower rates of recurrence after mastectomy
- Adjuvant therapy
  - Chemotherapy has not been shown to be effective
- Radiation
  - May reduce local recurrence rate
  - Not generally used for initial treatment

Prognosis
- Difficult to predict
  - Rare and difficult to study
  - Large series from referral centers may not be representative of prognosis in general
  - Treatment is not standardized
- Outcome can be predicted to some extent by grade of tumor
  - **Low-grade PT** (also termed "benign") ~ 60% of PT
    - Features overlap with cellular FA
    - ~ 4-10% risk of local recurrence; lower with more extensive surgery
    - < 1% risk of distant metastasis; reported to occur in large series, but these cases have never been described in detail
    - PT can recur at a higher grade; this may explain rare cases with metastasis
  - **Intermediate-grade PT** (also termed "borderline") ~ 10-20% of PT

- ~ 20% risk of local recurrence; lower with more extensive surgery
- < 10% risk of distant metastasis
  - **High-grade PT** (also termed "malignant") ~ 10-20% of PT
    - ~ 20% risk of local recurrence; lower with more extensive surgery
    - ~ 30% risk of distant metastasis

Core Needle Biopsy
- It can be difficult to distinguish PT from FA on core needle biopsies
  - PT can be heterogeneous with some areas having appearance of FA
  - History of recent increase in size favors PT unless patient is pregnant
- Features favoring PT on core needle biopsy
  - Markedly cellular stroma
  - Invasive border
  - Stromal overgrowth
  - Mitotic rate > 2 per 10 HPF I
    - If 0 or 1, not helpful for distinction
  - Ki-67 > 5%
    - If < 5%, not helpful for distinction
- If diagnosis is uncertain, best to diagnose "fibroepithelial lesion" and suggest classification after excision

IMAGE FINDINGS

General Features
- Circumscribed mass
  - May have history of slow or rapid growth
  - Calcifications not usually present

Mammographic Findings
- Circumscribed mass
- Partially indistinct margins may be indicative of infiltrative border

Ultrasonographic Findings
- Usually a hypoechoic mass

PHYLLODES TUMOR

- o Internal hyperechoic striations correlate with histologic clefts
- o May have intramural cystic spaces

MACROSCOPIC FEATURES

General Features
- Typically well-defined lobulated masses with bosselated borders
  - o Higher grade PT may show tongues of tumor protruding into adjacent breast parenchyma
- May show cleft-like cystic spaces

Size
- Most often 4-8 cm (range: 1-40 cm)

Sections to Be Submitted
- PT can be very heterogeneous
  - o High-grade features or malignant heterologous elements may be focal
  - o Epithelial component may be focal in high-grade lesions
- Tumors should be sampled with at least 1 section per cm of greatest size
  - o Preferable to completely sample PT when possible
- Margins should be extensively sampled if undergoing breast-conserving therapy

MICROSCOPIC PATHOLOGY

Histologic Features
- Diagnosis of PT requires presence of both spindle stromal cells and benign epithelium
- Characteristics of stromal cells are used to distinguish PT from FA and for classification
  - o Cellularity can vary from paucicellular to highly cellular areas
    - In very cellular areas, cells are organized in parallel arrays (fascicles)
    - Condensation (increased cellularity) is often found adjacent to epithelium ("cambium" layer)
  - o Stromal overgrowth
    - Areas of stroma that lack a benign epithelial component (at least 1 HPF)
    - Does not include paucicellular hyalinized areas
    - More common in higher grade tumors; uncommon or absent in FAs
  - o Nuclear pleomorphism
    - Usually mild or moderate
    - Markedly pleomorphic nuclei are only seen in high-grade PT
    - Does not include scattered multinucleated cells that may be degenerative in nature
  - o Mitotic rate
    - Majority of PT will have at least some mitoses
    - Mitoses in epithelial component are not used for classification
  - o Infiltrative border
    - Higher grade PT can invade into surrounding breast tissue, creating an irregular border
    - FA and low-grade PT have pushing circumscribed borders

- Must be distinguished from fibroadenomatoid changes in adjacent tissue
- Adipose tissue within a PT is usually an indication of invasion; liposarcoma must also be considered
- o Heterologous elements
  - Liposarcoma, chondrosarcoma, osteosarcoma, and rhabdomyosarcoma can occur in PT
  - More common as part of PT than as primary sarcomas
  - Extensive sampling may be necessary to identify benign epithelium diagnostic of PT
- o Growth pattern
  - Intracanicular growth pattern: Stromal cells push and distort epithelium; creates cleft-like spaces lined by epithelium that form leaf-like structures
  - Pericanalicular growth pattern: Stromal cells surround epithelium; results in a solid pattern without leaf-like structures
  - Many PTs show mixtures of these 2 growth patterns
- PT can be classified into low- ("benign"), intermediate- ("borderline"), and high-grade ("malignant") categories based on combination of stromal features
- Epithelial component must be present but is not used for classification
  - o Usually shows little or no nuclear atypia
  - o Epithelial hyperplasia may be present
    - Most common in low-grade PT; usually absent in high-grade PT
  - o Normal myoepithelial layer is present
  - o In rare cases, ALH, ADH, LCIS, DCIS, or invasive carcinoma may involve a PT
- **Margin evaluation**
  - o Residual PT at margin is a predictor of higher likelihood of recurrence
  - o Margins can be difficult to evaluate for low-grade PT if stroma is not very cellular
  - o Margin reexcisions are very difficult to evaluate if biopsy site changes are present at margin
    - Reactive fibroblasts present due to surgery may be impossible to distinguish from tumor cells
    - IHC studies are generally not helpful
- **Recurrent PT**
  - o May recur as multiple nodules surrounding tumor bed
  - o Grade may be higher than original tumor
    - ~ 25% recur as higher grade lesion
    - Additional genetic changes are often acquired
- **Metastatic PT**
  - o Only stromal component metastasizes
  - o Lymph node metastases very rare
  - o Distant metastases most common to lung and bone

ANCILLARY TESTS

Immunohistochemistry
- Ki-67
  - o More Ki-67-positive cells are found in PT as compared to FA
    - Low-grade PT ~ 1-5%
    - Intermediate-grade PT ~ 6-25%
    - High-grade PT ~ 10-50%

PHYLLODES TUMOR

Classification of Phyllodes Tumors and Fibroadenoma

Feature	Fibroadenoma	Low-Grade PT ("Benign")	Intermediate-Grade PT ("Borderline")	High-Grade PT ("Malignant")
Incidence	100x more common than PT	60-80% of PT	10-20% of PT	10-20% of PT
Tumor borders	Pushing/circumscribed	Pushing/circumscribed	May be invasive; usually focal	Usually invasive
Stromal cellularity	Low to intermediate	Low to intermediate	Intermediate	High
Mitotic figures (per 10 HPF)	Absent or rare	< 5	Usually 5-10	Often > 10
Stromal pleomorphism	Absent	Mild	Moderate	Usually marked
Stromal overgrowth	Absent	Usually focal	Present; may be focal	Usually extensive
Malignant heterologous elements	Absent	Absent	Absent	May be present
Local recurrence	Metachronous tumors may develop	~ 10%	~ 10-20%	~ 30% but low after mastectomy
Incidence of metastases	Absent	< 1%	< 10%	10-30%

- o Does not provide additional prediction for recurrence or metastases beyond morphology
  - Not routinely used in clinical practice
- CD34
  - o Majority of PT are CD34 positive as are most breast stromal cells
  - o Degree of positivity for CD34 decreases with grade and may be absent in high-grade PT
- p53
  - o More common in high-grade PT; rare or absent in FA and low-grade PT
  - o Not correlated with recurrence or death
- β-catenin
  - o Nuclear positivity is often present in PT
    - More common in lower grade tumors and FA and in zone adjacent to epithelium

DIFFERENTIAL DIAGNOSIS

Fibroadenoma (FA) with Cellular Stroma

- FAs are typically smaller than PTs, but there is a broad overlap in sizes
- FA has uniform distribution of glandular and stromal elements with no stromal overgrowth
  - o Areas of low cellularity and hyalinization are not considered stromal overgrowth
- Cytologic atypia is minimal and mitotic figures absent or rare
  - o FA can grow during pregnancy and could possibly have more mitoses in this setting
- Histologic features of some cellular FAs overlap with low-grade PT

Spindle Cell Carcinoma

- Can be difficult to distinguish from sarcomas and high-grade PT
  - o Carcinomas may invade around normal structures
  - o Neoplastic epithelioid nests of cells merging with spindle cell elements often seen
- Immunoperoxidase studies are often necessary
  - o Cytokeratins, especially basal keratins 14 and 17, identify the majority of carcinomas

- o p63 is positive in about 1/3 of carcinomas

Primary Sarcoma

- Extremely rare breast malignancy
  - o More common to see heterologous elements in PT
- Diagnosis should be made only after through sampling of lesion

Metastatic Spindle Cell Tumors

- Usually prior history of spindle cell malignancy
  - o Need to exclude metastatic spindle cell carcinoma, melanoma, or sarcoma in some cases
- Metastatic tumors do not have an epithelial component

Periductal Stromal Sarcoma

- PT with a pericanalicular pattern of growth
- This pattern confers a solid appearance in contrast to leaf-like appearance of intracanicular growth pattern

Fibromatosis

- Both fibromatosis and PT are tumors of stromal cells
- Fibromatosis does not have an epithelial component
- CD34 is typically negative in fibromatosis and positive in PT but may be negative in high-grade lesions
- Both fibromatosis and PT commonly have nuclear β-catenin; therefore, this marker is not useful to distinguish these entities

SELECTED REFERENCES

1. Guillot E et al: Management of phyllodes breast tumors. Breast J. 17(2):129-37, 2011
2. Korcheva VB et al: Immunohistochemical and molecular markers in breast phyllodes tumors. Appl Immunohistochem Mol Morphol. 19(2):119-25, 2011
3. Noronha Y et al: CD34, CD117, and Ki-67 Expression in Phyllodes Tumor of the Breast: An Immunohistochemical Study of 33 Cases. Int J Surg Pathol. 19(2):152-8, 2011

PHYLLODES TUMOR

Imaging, Gross, and Microscopic Features

(Left) The typical imaging finding associated with PT is a circumscribed or lobulated mass ➡. The radiographic appearance may overlap with FA and other benign lesions. An indistinct border may correlate with areas of stromal invasion. *(Right)* PT typically appears circumscribed, although microscopically there may be areas of stromal invasion. The surface is tan and fleshy. The numerous small cleft-like slits ➡ correspond to areas of stromal overgrowth lined by epithelium.

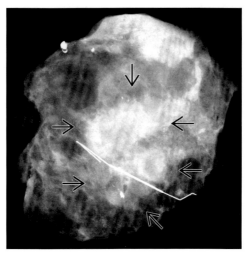
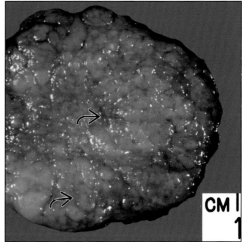

(Left) The most common growth pattern for PT is intracanicular. The epithelial cells are pushed and distorted by the stromal cells. The resulting clefts ➡ form the characteristic leaf-like appearance. *(Right)* A less common growth pattern in PT is pericanalicular. The epithelial component ➡ is surrounded, rather than distorted, by the tumor cells. This results in a solid pattern without leaf-like areas. This type of PT has been referred to as periductal stromal sarcoma.

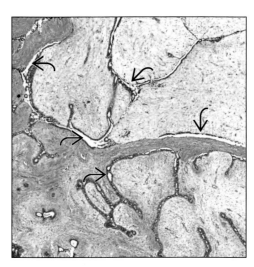
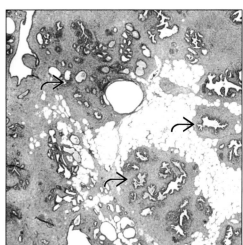

(Left) The region of greatest stromal cellularity is usually adjacent to the epithelium (a cambium layer) ➡. Mitoses are most likely to be present in this area ➡. This may reflect the biologic cross-talk between stromal and epithelial cells. *(Right)* Stromal mitoses ➡ are usually found in PT but are rare in FA. They are most commonly seen close to the epithelium ➡ in a cambium layer, as is the expression of some oncogenes such as p53 and C-Kit.

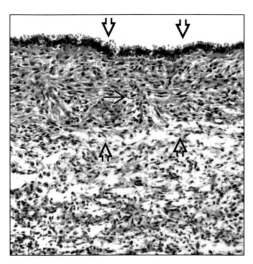
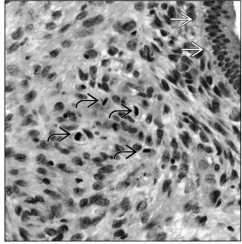

PHYLLODES TUMOR

Microscopic Features

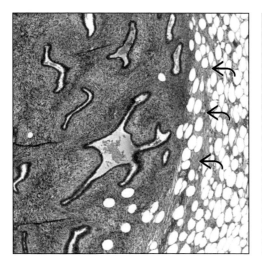

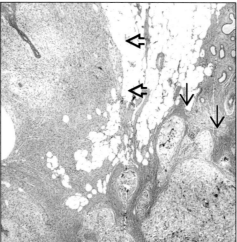

(Left) Unlike FA, PT can invade into the surrounding stroma ⤻. Stromal invasion is more frequent and more extensive in higher grade tumors. Stromal invasion must be distinguished from adjacent fibroadenomatoid changes. (Right) A prior excisional site ➡ is adjacent to a recurrent PT ⤹, which is now of intermediate grade. Progression to a higher grade occurs in about 1/3 of such cases and is frequently associated with acquisition of additional genetic changes.

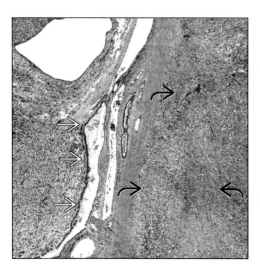

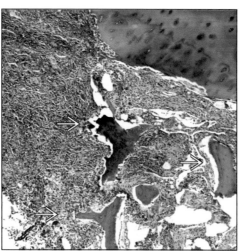

(Left) Stromal overgrowth ⤻ with loss of the benign epithelial component is typical for high-grade PT. The monophasic portion of the tumor can have the appearance of a fibrosarcoma. Extensive sampling may be necessary to find diagnostic areas of benign epithelium ➡. (Right) Only the stromal component of PT metastasizes, supporting that the epithelial cells are not malignant. The most common sites of metastases are to bone ➡ and lung. Nodal metastases are rare.

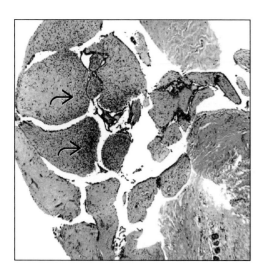

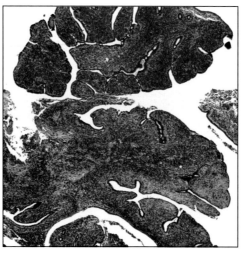

(Left) Distinguishing cellular FA and PT on core needle biopsies may be difficult due to the limited sampling. For lesions with increased stromal cellularity ⤻, atypia, or mitotic activity that cannot be categorized with certainty, a diagnosis of "fibroepithelial lesion" can be rendered and classification made after excision. (Right) Some cases of PT can be diagnosed on core needle biopsy if there is sufficient stromal overgrowth, nuclear atypia, &/or a high mitotic rate.

PHYLLODES TUMOR

Heterologous Elements

(Left) This 15 cm PT ➡ has a tan-white bosselated surface. In the center of the tumor is a discrete homogeneous yellow nodule ⮞. This area corresponds to liposarcoma arising within this PT. *(Right)* PT with malignant heterologous elements is considered high grade. This PT has areas of stromal overgrowth ➡ and benign epithelial elements ➡. In the central zone is an area of liposarcoma ⮞. This finding can be misinterpreted as invasion into benign adipose tissue.

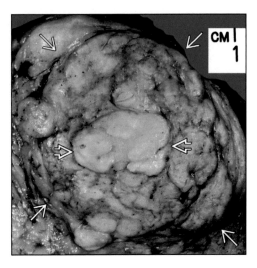
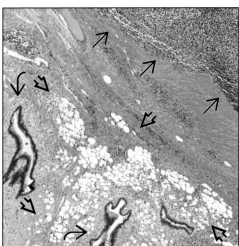

(Left) Adipose tissue within a PT is usually due to invasion into the surrounding breast tissues. These areas must be examined closely as nuclear pleomorphism ➡, abundant vacuolated cytoplasm ⮞, and lipoblasts are diagnostic of liposarcoma. These cases of PT are considered high grade. *(Right)* High-grade PT with marked nuclear pleomorphism ⮞, frequent mitoses ➡, and stromal overgrowth can be difficult to distinguish from primary sarcomas and poorly differentiated carcinomas.

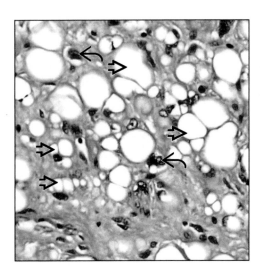
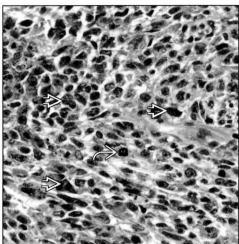

(Left) Malignant heterologous differentiation can consist of liposarcoma, osteosarcoma, chondrosarcoma, or rhabdomyosarcoma. In this example, the stromal overgrowth ➡ is forming a cartilage matrix ⮞, diagnostic of chondrosarcoma. *(Right)* This PT shows malignant osteoid production ➡ adjacent to a hypercellular stroma ⮞. Osteosarcoma in PT is much more common than primary osteosarcoma of the breast. Extensive sampling is often necessary for correct classification.

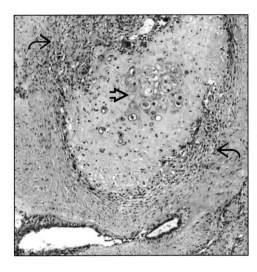
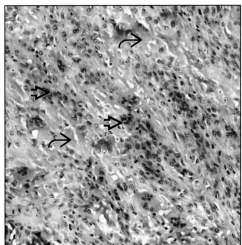

6

PHYLLODES TUMOR

Differential Diagnosis

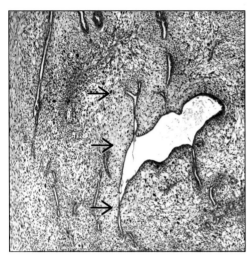

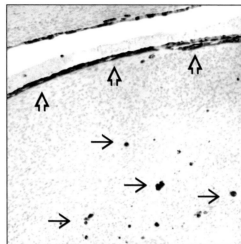

(Left) This spindle cell carcinoma has an unusual pattern surrounding distorted benign epithelial structures ➡. The pattern is very similar to that of a PT. (Right) Only rare cells are keratin positive ➡ in this spindle cell carcinoma that closely resembles a PT. The carcinoma surrounds normal-appearing ducts, which are also keratin positive ➢. Because of the differences in treatment, carcinoma should always be excluded when making a diagnosis of high-grade PT.

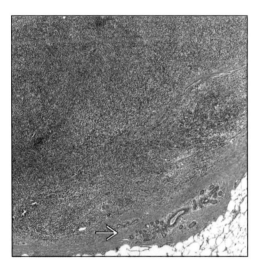

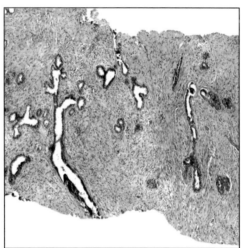

(Left) Primary sarcomas of the breast are extremely rare. They may resemble high-grade PT with stromal overgrowth. Extensive sampling may be necessary to exclude an epithelial component. This is an unusual rhabdomyosarcoma invading into normal breast stroma ➡. (Right) Cellular FAs and phyllodes tumors have overlapping histologic features and may be difficult to distinguish on the limited sampling on core needle biopsies. Mitoses and stromal overgrowth favor a phyllodes tumor.

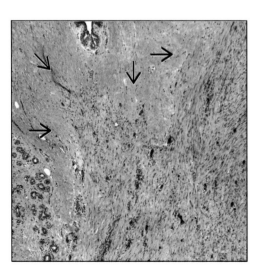

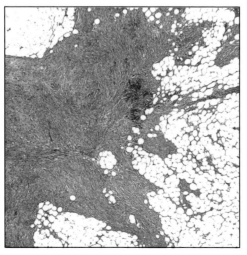

(Left) Reactive stromal changes around a biopsy site ➡ can be difficult to distinguish from small areas of residual PT as both consist of fibroblastic cells. If these areas are present at the margin, it may be impossible to know for sure if the tumor has been completely resected. (Right) Fibromatosis does not have the benign epithelial component of PT. High-grade PTs without a stromal component are generally more cellular and have more nuclear pleomorphism than fibromatosis.

PSEUDOANGIOMATOUS STROMAL HYPERPLASIA

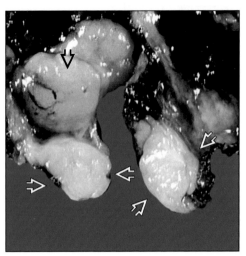

Some cases of PASH form firm rubbery circumscribed masses. This lesion has been bisected to show the white whorled surface of the tumor ➡ within an area of yellow adipose tissue ➡.

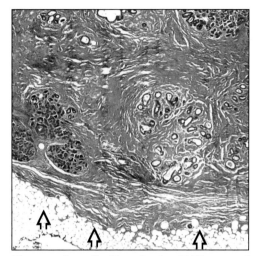

The stromal myofibroblasts forming PASH surround normal ducts and lobules and are associated with characteristic clefts. In this case, there is a discrete mass with a circumscribed border ➡.

TERMINOLOGY

Abbreviations
- Pseudoangiomatous stromal hyperplasia (PASH)

Synonyms
- Pseudoangiomatous hyperplasia of mammary stroma
- Nodular myofibroblastic stromal hyperplasia
- Nodular or tumorous PASH

Definitions
- Proliferation of myofibroblasts associated with stromal clefts that resemble vascular spaces

ETIOLOGY/PATHOGENESIS

Possible Relation to Hormonal Milieu
- Occurs most frequently in women of childbearing age
- Postmenopausal women receiving hormonal therapy may also be affected
- Similar stromal changes are often present in gynecomastia and juvenile hyperplasia
  - Thus, stromal proliferation of myofibroblasts is likely due to hormonal stimulation or hormonal imbalance
- It has been suggested that the clefts are prelymphatic channels that drain into true lymphatics
  - Some carcinomas invade with pattern suggesting that they involve clefts seen in PASH

CLINICAL ISSUES

Presentation
- May be incidental finding in approximately 23% of biopsies
- Also forms palpable masses or radiographic densities (nodular or tumorous PASH)
  - Masses are circumscribed or ill defined
- PASH frequently grows in size
  - Rapid growth can occur during pregnancy and may be associated with peau d'orange and skin necrosis

Treatment
- Mass-forming PASH should be biopsied to exclude malignancy
  - After malignancy is excluded, no other treatment is necessary
- Symptomatic mass-forming PASH may be surgically excised

Prognosis
- PASH is benign lesion
  - Rarely, mass-forming PASH may recur after surgical excision
  - Recurrent lesions are more likely in younger patients

Core Needle Biopsy
- Histologic findings are not specific for mass-forming lesion on core needle biopsy because stromal changes can also be an incidental finding
  - Radiologic correlation is necessary for final diagnosis

IMAGE FINDINGS

Mammographic Findings
- Circumscribed or ill-defined mass
- Calcifications are not characteristic

Ultrasonographic Findings
- Borders may be well defined, or ill-defined mass may be present

MR Findings
- Smooth-bordered mass with slow enhancement is characteristic
  - In some cases, there may be clumped enhancement or irregular mass

PSEUDOANGIOMATOUS STROMAL HYPERPLASIA

Key Facts

Terminology
- Pseudoangiomatous stromal hyperplasia (PASH)
- Proliferation of stromal myofibroblasts forming clefts that resemble vascular spaces

Etiology/Pathogenesis
- Majority of affected persons are women of childbearing age
  - Postmenopausal women taking hormonal therapy may also be affected
- Similar stromal changes are seen in gynecomastia and juvenile hyperplasia

Clinical Issues
- May be incidental finding in approximately 23% of biopsies

- PASH can also form palpable masses or radiographic densities
- Masses are circumscribed or ill defined
- Frequently grow in size

Microscopic Pathology
- Prominent slit-like stromal clefts are present
- Immunoperoxidase studies will confirm that cells are myofibroblasts

Top Differential Diagnoses
- Angiosarcoma
- Myofibroblastoma
- Fibrous tumors

Diagnostic Checklist
- Most important lesion in differential diagnosis is angiosarcoma

MACROSCOPIC FEATURES

General Features
- Nodular PASH can appear as firm, rubbery, circumscribed, white nodule
  - Size ranges from 1-10 cm
- Large clefts seen grossly in some fibroadenomas are not present

MICROSCOPIC PATHOLOGY

Histologic Features
- Prominent slit-like stromal clefts are present
  - Clefts are lined by bland stromal myofibroblasts
  - Clefts can involve both inter- and intralobular stroma and appear to invade into lobules
- Spaces are empty or contain only rare red blood cells
- Immunoperoxidase studies will confirm that cells lining clefts are myofibroblasts

ANCILLARY TESTS

Immunohistochemistry
- Stromal cells are positive for CD34, actin, and vimentin and may be positive for PR
- Stromal cells are negative for CD31, factor VIII, and other vascular markers

DIFFERENTIAL DIAGNOSIS

Angiosarcoma
- Angiosarcomas have nuclear pleomorphism, mitoses, and solid areas or tufting
- True vascular spaces are filled with blood
  - Pseudoangiomatous clefts of PASH can involve lobules and mimic invasive pattern of an angiosarcoma
- Angiosarcomas are usually large irregular masses; unlikely to present as circumscribed mass

- Immunoperoxidase studies distinguish endothelial cells of vascular lesions from myofibroblasts of PASH

Myofibroblastoma
- Also lesions of myofibroblasts
- However, these tumors form solid masses of spindle cells and do not proliferate around ducts and lobules
- Generally more cellular than PASH
  - Fascicular PASH can mimic myofibroblastoma, particularly on core needle biopsy

Fibrous Tumors
- Proliferations of interlobular fibroblasts that surround ducts and lobules
- Unlike PASH, characteristic stromal clefting is not seen
- Epithelial elements are usually scant and atrophic in appearance

SELECTED REFERENCES

1. Virk RK et al: Pseudoangiomatous stromal hyperplasia: an overview. Arch Pathol Lab Med. 134(7):1070-4, 2010
2. Asioli S et al: The pre-lymphatic pathway, the rooths of the lymphatic system in breast tissue: a 3D study. Virchows Arch. 453(4):401-6, 2008
3. Ferreira M et al: Pseudoangiomatous stromal hyperplasia tumor: a clinical, radiologic and pathologic study of 26 cases. Mod Pathol. 21(2):201-7, 2008
4. Hargaden GC et al: Analysis of the mammographic and sonographic features of pseudoangiomatous stromal hyperplasia. AJR Am J Roentgenol. 191(2):359-63, 2008
5. Damiani S et al: Malignant neoplasms infiltrating pseudoangiomatous' stromal hyperplasia of the breast: an unrecognized pathway of tumour spread. Histopathology. 41(3):208-15, 2002
6. Powell CM et al: Pseudoangiomatous stromal hyperplasia (PASH). A mammary stromal tumor with myofibroblastic differentiation. Am J Surg Pathol. 19(3):270-7, 1995
7. Anderson C et al: Immunocytochemical analysis of estrogen and progesterone receptors in benign stromal lesions of the breast. Evidence for hormonal etiology in pseudoangiomatous hyperplasia of mammary stroma. Am J Surg Pathol. 15(2):145-9, 1991

PSEUDOANGIOMATOUS STROMAL HYPERPLASIA

Imaging and Microscopic Features

(Left) PASH can form a circumscribed or lobulated mammographic density ⇨. Calcifications are generally not present and would be unusual. Some lesions have ill-defined borders due to the nature of the proliferation or because the lesion is present in an area of dense breast tissue. *(Right)* On MR, PASH may present as a slowly enhancing circumscribed mass ⇨, similar in appearance to other benign lesions such as fibroadenomas.

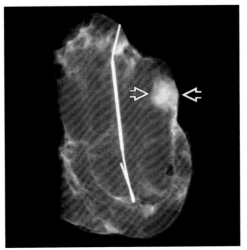
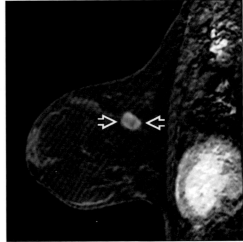

(Left) PASH is characterized by increased stromal cellularity with prominent stromal clefts. The stromal proliferation is evident around lobules and ducts. In this lesion, the clefting is very prominent ⇨. *(Right)* The cells lining the clefts have small bland nuclei. No nuclear pleomorphism is present, and mitoses are absent. The stroma between the clefts is collagenized and paucicellular.

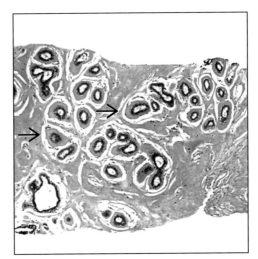
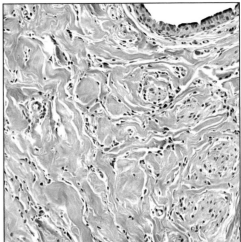

(Left) The stromal clefting is present in both interlobular and intralobular stroma. The clefts are empty or contain only rare red blood cells. *(Right)* Fascicular PASH is a variant in which the stromal myofibroblasts are more abundant and present in loose bundles in the stroma. The appearance may be very similar to that of a myofibroblastoma. However, PASH surrounds ducts and lobules, whereas myofibroblastomas consist solely of stromal cells.

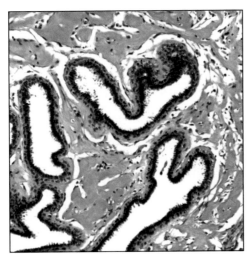
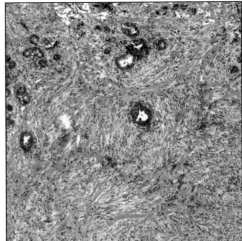

PSEUDOANGIOMATOUS STROMAL HYPERPLASIA

Ancillary Studies and Differential Diagnosis

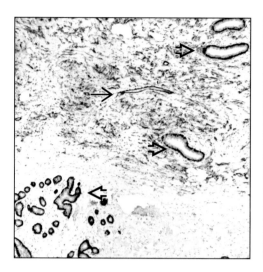

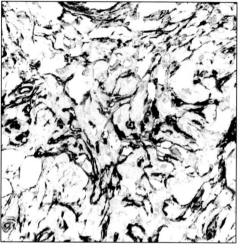

(Left) The myofibroblasts forming PASH are immunoreactive for smooth muscle myosin heavy chain and are more abundant in the area of PASH (top) than in normal stroma (bottom). Myoepithelial cells ⊡ and endothelial cells ⊡ are also positive for this marker. *(Right)* The myofibroblasts of PASH are positive for CD34, as are almost all stromal lesions of the breast. The 2 exceptions are fibromatosis and nodular fasciitis.

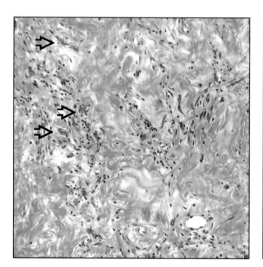

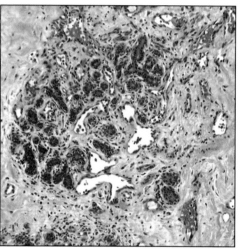

(Left) PASH can mimic the appearance of a low-grade angiosarcoma due to the clefting that simulates anastomosing blood vessels. However, as shown here, angiosarcomas have red blood cells in the lumens of the vessels ⊡. In other areas, nuclear pleomorphism was more apparent. *(Right)* Angiosarcomas invade into lobules, as shown here. The stromal clefting of PASH may also involve intralobular stroma. However, the other diagnostic features of angiosarcoma will not be present.

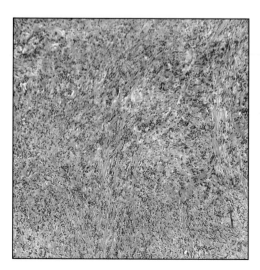

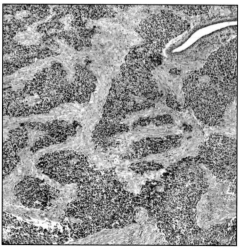

(Left) Myofibroblastomas consist of solid proliferations of myofibroblasts. Epithelial elements will not be present within the lesion. Fascicular PASH has a similar appearance but surrounds ducts and lobules. *(Right)* It is possible that the clefts of PASH are prelymphatic spaces. Some carcinomas, such as this one, appear to involve similar anastomosing spaces in the stroma. The stromal clefts may also be the path of least resistance for stromal invasion by lobular carcinomas.

MYOFIBROBLASTOMA

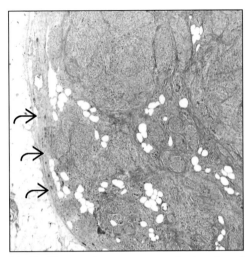

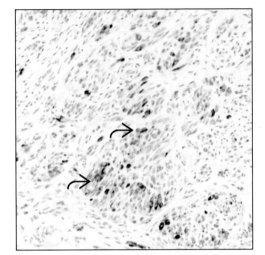

Myofibroblastoma is an uncommon benign stromal spindle cell tumor of the breast. The typical lesion is circumscribed ⮕ and composed of fascicles of spindle cells in a collagenized stroma.

The spindle cells of myofibroblastoma typically demonstrate myofibroblastic features by ultrastructure and immunohistochemistry, including immunoreactivity for desmin as seen here ⮕.

TERMINOLOGY

Abbreviations
- Myofibroblastoma (MFB)

Definitions
- Benign spindle cell mammary tumor
  - Original description: "Cells having features of both fibroblasts and smooth muscle"
- Derived from mammary myofibroblasts
  - Cells demonstrate ultrastructural and IHC similarities to myofibroblasts from other sites
- Morphologic, structural, and IHC overlap between MFB, spindle cell lipoma, and solitary fibrous tumor of breast
  - Some authors suggest that these entities represent a spectrum of lesions derived from myofibroblasts

ETIOLOGY/PATHOGENESIS

Hormone Receptors
- MFB characteristically express androgen, estrogen, and progesterone receptors
  - Possible role for sex hormones in pathogenesis of this tumor
  - MFB may be associated with androgen deprivation in treatment of some prostate cancers
  - MFB may be associated with gynecomastia or pseudoangiomatous stromal hyperplasia (PASH)
    - These conditions are also thought to share hormonal etiology

Cytogenetic Abnormalities
- Chromosome 13 rearrangements associated with loss of 13q14, partial loss of 16q
  - These chromosomal alterations are typically also observed in spindle cell lipoma

CLINICAL ISSUES

Epidemiology
- Incidence
  - Uncommon mammary neoplasm; < 1% of mammary tumors
- Age
  - Typically seen in older patient population; peak incidence: 50-75 years
- Gender
  - Initial reports suggested majority of cases of MFB occurred in male patients
    - Similar lesions have been reported in females
    - Majority of reported cases of MFB have occurred in male patients; however, overall incidence is likely equal in males and females
    - Coincidental gynecomastia may be seen in males

Presentation
- Palpable painless mass
  - Mobile
  - Slow growing
  - Can be solitary unilateral, bilateral, or multicentric
- Lesions with similar appearance can occur in extramammary locations

Treatment
- Surgical approaches
  - Complete surgical excision is recommended for lesions diagnosed on needle core biopsy

Prognosis
- Benign stromal tumor
- No recurrences have been reported to date in follow-up studies

IMAGE FINDINGS

Mammographic Findings
- Well-demarcated lobulated mass lesion

MYOFIBROBLASTOMA

Key Facts

Terminology
- Myofibroblastoma (MFB)
- Benign spindle cell mammary tumor, thought to be derived from mammary stromal myofibroblasts

Clinical Issues
- Uncommon mammary neoplasm
- Typically seen in older patient population
- Majority of reported cases of MFB have occurred in male patients; however, overall incidence is likely equal in males and females
- Presentation: Painless mass
- Complete surgical excision recommended for lesions diagnosed on needle core biopsy
- No recurrences have been reported to date

Image Findings
- Well-demarcated lobulated mass lesion

Macroscopic Features
- Typical lesion about 2 cm in diameter

Microscopic Pathology
- Uniform spindle cell proliferation
  - Spindle cells closely apposed and arranged in discrete intersecting bundles
- Hyalinized bands of collagen separate cells into groups or clusters
- Varying degrees of fat cells seen in some lesions

Ancillary Tests
- Lesional cells show immunophenotype typical of myofibroblasts

---

- Absence of microcalcifications

Ultrasonographic Findings
- Circumscribed or lobulated mass
  - Features similar to those seen in fibroadenoma

MR Findings
- Uniform enhancement with internal septation

MACROSCOPIC FEATURES

General Features
- Well circumscribed, lobulated, firm or rubbery consistency
- Cut surface has pink-tan, homogeneous whorled or nodular appearance

Size
- Typical lesion is about 2 cm; most are < 4 cm
  - MFB up to 10 cm in diameter have been reported

MICROSCOPIC PATHOLOGY

Histologic Features
- Uniform spindle cell proliferation
  - Slender, bipolar or fusiform-shaped spindle cells
  - Ovoid nuclei, pale cytoplasm
  - Mitotic figures rare/undetectable
  - Spindle cells closely apposed and arranged in discrete intersecting bundles and clusters
- Well-circumscribed borders
  - Pushing borders tend to compress normal breast parenchyma at periphery
  - Circumscribed with no true capsule
  - Usually no entrapment of ducts &/or lobules
- Hyalinized bands of collagen
  - Distributed throughout lesion
  - Collagen bands separate spindle cells into groups or clusters
- Varying degrees of fat cells seen in some lesions
  - Rarely, abundant fat suggests lipomatous element or component

- Term "lipomatous myofibroblastoma" describes lesions with abundant fatty component
- Morphologic and molecular overlap between lipomatous myofibroblastoma and spindle cell lipoma
- MFB rarely shows evidence of myoid and cartilaginous differentiation
- Rare variant forms of MFB may be encountered
  - Collagenized or fibrous variant
  - Epithelioid variant
    - Can mimic invasive lobular carcinoma, particularly if ER and PR positive on core needle biopsy
  - Infiltrating variant
  - Atypical variant
  - Immunohistochemistry helpful in identifying myofibroblastic origin for variant forms

ANCILLARY TESTS

Immunohistochemistry
- Lesional cells show immunophenotype typical of myofibroblasts
- Lesional cells also express hormone receptors
  - Estrogen, progesterone, and androgen receptors
- Cell of origin is likely hormonally responsive mammary stromal cell

Cytogenetics
- Cytogenetic relationship to spindle cell lipoma and solitary fibrous tumor
- Loss of 13q and 16q
  - Reported in MFB, spindle cell lipoma, and solitary fibrous tumor

DIFFERENTIAL DIAGNOSIS

Spindle Cell Sarcoma
- Stellate and invasive tumor with infiltrating borders
- Typically more cellular, with cytologic atypia
- More frequent mitotic figures

MYOFIBROBLASTOMA

Immunohistochemistry

Antibody	Reactivity	Staining Pattern	Comment
CD34	Positive	Cell membrane & cytoplasm	Diffuse staining throughout lesion
Bcl-2	Positive	Cell membrane & cytoplasm	Diffuse staining throughout lesion
Desmin	Positive	Cytoplasmic	Focal staining
Actin-sm	Positive	Cytoplasmic	Focal staining
Vimentin	Positive	Cytoplasmic	Diffuse staining throughout lesion
PR	Positive	Nuclear	Suggests hormone responsive stromal cell
Androgen receptor	Positive	Nuclear	Suggests hormone responsive stromal cell
ER	Positive	Nuclear	Suggests hormone responsive stromal cell
AE1/AE3	Negative	Cytoplasmic	Multiple keratin antibodies may be necessary to exclude spindle cell cancers that may only be positive for "basal" keratins

Spindle Cell Metaplastic Carcinoma
- Stellate and invasive tumor with infiltrating borders
- May show nests and clusters of plump epithelioid cells demonstrating epithelial differentiation
- May be associated with areas of DCIS
- Typically demonstrates cytokeratin expression by IHC; however, these carcinomas may only be positive for basal-type keratins

Nodular Fasciitis
- Infiltrative borders
- Stellate and plump myofibroblastic cells
- Extravasated RBCs and inflammatory reaction seen at periphery of lesion
- Negative for CD34

Fibromatosis
- Highly infiltrative lesions
- Abundant collagenous matrix
- Spindle cells arranged in broad sweeping fascicles
- CD34 negative

Spindle Cell Lipoma
- More abundant adipose tissue compared to MFB
- Some authors consider MFB, spindle cell lipoma, and solitary fibrous tumors to represent a spectrum of benign myofibroblastic lesions
  - Other experts feel that these lesions should be classified separately

Solitary Fibrous Tumor
- Clinical and morphologic overlap with MFB
- Typical solitary fibrous tumor does not show expression of actin or desmin by IHC
- Some authors consider MFB, spindle cell lipoma, and solitary fibrous tumors to represent a spectrum of benign myofibroblastic lesions
  - Other experts feel that these lesions should be classified separately

Fascicular Pseudoangiomatous Stromal Hyperplasia
- Myofibroblastic proliferation in dense collagenous stroma
- Slit-like clefts in tissue resemble vascular spaces
- Most commonly an incidental finding in premenopausal women
- May demonstrate fascicles of myofibroblastic cells; extreme examples show growth pattern similar to MFB

DIAGNOSTIC CHECKLIST

Clinically Relevant Pathologic Features
- Age distribution
  - Lesion typically seen in older population
  - Occurs at equal frequency in males and females
- Imaging
  - Circumscribed or lobulated, uniformly enhancing lesion
  - Internal septations on MR
- Gross appearance
  - Typically well circumscribed with pushing borders

Pathologic Interpretation Pearls
- Look for short intersecting fascicular clusters of uniform spindle cells
- Look for bands of hyalinized collagen separating spindle cells into clusters
- Necrosis and hemorrhage should not be present unless associated with previous biopsy site
- Immunohistochemistry is helpful to confirm diagnosis
  - IHC may be especially helpful to confirm variant forms of MFB

SELECTED REFERENCES

1. Magro G: Mammary myofibroblastoma: a tumor with a wide morphologic spectrum. Arch Pathol Lab Med. 132(11):1813-20, 2008
2. Meguerditchian AN et al: Solitary fibrous tumor of the breast and mammary myofibroblastoma: the same lesion? Breast J. 14(3):287-92, 2008
3. Lichten JB et al: Myofibroblastoma of the breast. Breast J. 10(4):370-1, 2004
4. Magro G et al: Spindle cell lipoma-like tumor, solitary fibrous tumor and myofibroblastoma of the breast: a clinico-pathological analysis of 13 cases in favor of a unifying histogenetic concept. Virchows Arch. 440(3):249-60, 2002
5. McMenamin ME et al: Mammary-type myofibroblastoma of soft tissue: a tumor closely related to spindle cell lipoma. Am J Surg Pathol. 25(8):1022-9, 2001
6. Salomão DR et al: Myofibroblastoma and solitary fibrous tumour of the breast: histopathologic and immunohistochemical studies. Breast. 10(1):49-54, 2001

MYOFIBROBLASTOMA

Imaging and Microscopic Features

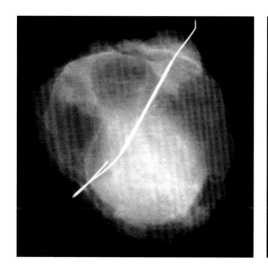 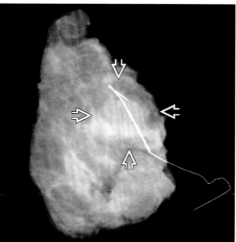

(Left) The characteristic imaging appearance of a myofibroblastoma is a circumscribed mass, as shown in this specimen radiograph. Myofibroblastoma with a component of adipose tissue could closely mimic hamartomas on mammography. *(Right)* This specimen radiograph shows a myofibroblastoma within an area of dense breast tissue ➡. The margins of the lesion are circumscribed, which is not readily appreciated due to surrounding tissue.

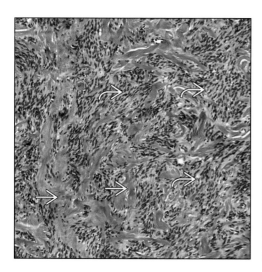 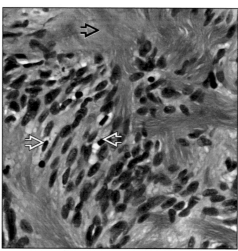

(Left) MFB has a typical low-power appearance. The lesion is devoid of mammary duct and lobular elements. Characteristic short intersecting bundles of uniform spindle cells ➡ are separated by broad bands of hyalinized collagen ➡. *(Right)* A higher power view shows spindle cells of similar size and shape arranged in short fascicles ➡ in a hyalinized stroma ➡. The nuclei are round to oval with dispersed chromatin and may contain distinct small nucleoli. Mitoses are infrequent.

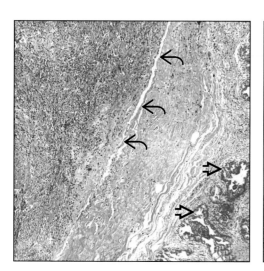 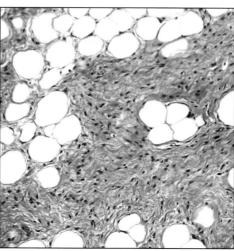

(Left) The borders of myofibroblastoma are well circumscribed and pushing ➡; they do not surround and entrap adjacent mammary ducts and glandular tissue ➡. *(Right)* Myofibroblastoma can infiltrate into stroma and into adipose tissue. Some lesions closely resemble spindle cell lipoma. These may be morphologic variants of the same lesion.

Ancillary Techniques

(Left) This MFB with an epithelioid pattern closely mimics an invasive lobular carcinoma histologically. The cells of MFB are also often ER and PR positive. However, spindle-shaped cells, which would be unusual for invasive lobular carcinoma, are usually also present. *(Right)* This is an invasive lobular carcinoma. These cells are keratin positive, and this finding will distinguish them from MFB. In addition, LCIS will often be present.

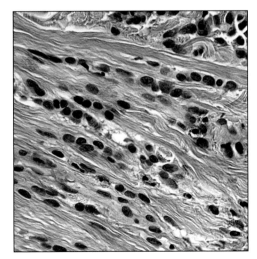
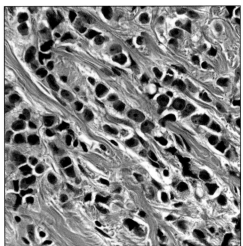

(Left) This MFB is composed of a homogeneous population of spindle cells with oval nuclei and pale cytoplasm arranged in intersecting bundles and fascicles. *(Right)* Desmin expression by these spindle cells ➔ is consistent with a myofibroblastic orgin for this tumor and is helpful in confirming the diagnosis of myofibroblastoma.

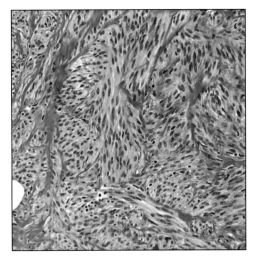
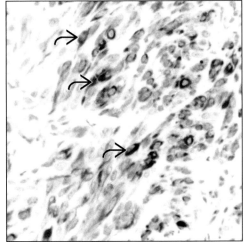

(Left) The cells of MFB typically show expression of CD34, as seen here ➔. These tumors most likely arise from CD34-positive mammary stromal cells, which can be seen throughout the breast parenchyma. *(Right)* Immunoreactivity for Bcl-2, as seen here ➔, is frequently encountered in MFB. Staining for CD34 and Bcl-2 can be extremely helpful in confirming the diagnosis of myofibroblastoma, particularly in unusual morphologic variants of this lesion.

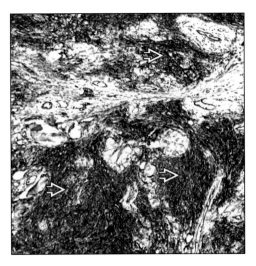
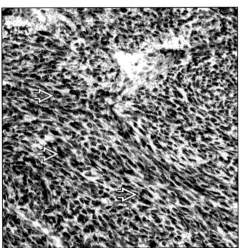

MYOFIBROBLASTOMA

Ancillary Techniques

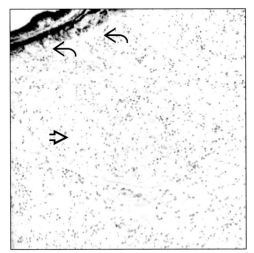

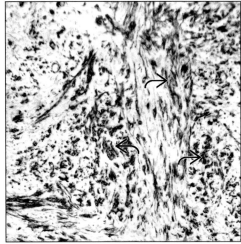

(Left) MFB is negative for keratins ⊳. This feature is helpful to distinguish MFB from spindle cell carcinoma or invasive lobular carcinoma. An adjacent duct is keratin positive ⊳. *(Right)* Myofibroblastoma is positive for smooth muscle actin ⊳. Positivity can also be seen in stromal cells of normal stroma, fibroadenomas, phyllodes tumors, PASH, spindle cell lipomas, and solitary fibrous tumors. The stromal cells of fibromatosis are usually negative.

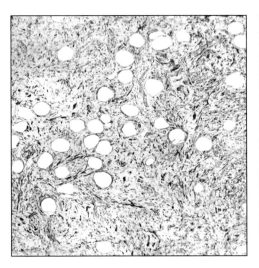

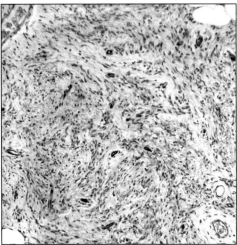

(Left) MFB is positive for desmin. Fibromatosis and the rare leiomyoma of the nipple will also be positive. *(Right)* MFB is positive for CD34. The stromal cells of the normal breast, fibroadenomas, phyllodes tumors, PASH, solitary fibrous tumors, and spindle cell lipomas are also positive for this marker. The stromal cells of fibromatosis are negative.

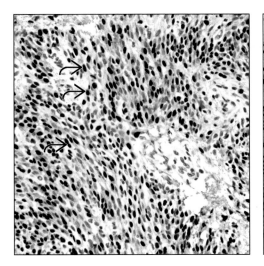

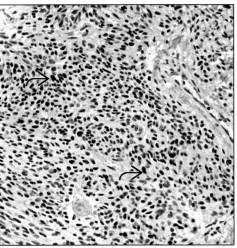

(Left) Most MFBs show expression of hormone receptors including estrogen, progesterone, and androgen receptor (seen here ⊳). Although the factors giving rise to these lesions are yet to be established, expression of sex steroid receptors suggests a hormonal etiology. *(Right)* ER expression, as seen here ⊳, is also a frequent finding in myofibroblastoma in both males and females. Other stromal lesions like gynecomastia can also express these receptors.

LIPOMA AND ANGIOLIPOMA

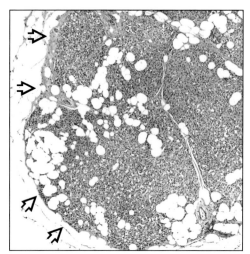

Angiolipomas consist of a mixture of small blood vessels and adipose tissue. The borders are well circumscribed ⮕. These lesions may present as a palpable mass or as a mammographic density.

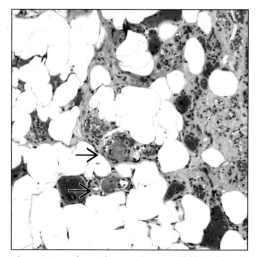

The majority of angiolipomas have small fibrin thrombi ⮕, which are an important diagnostic feature. Unlike dermal angiolipomas that may present with pain, breast lesions are usually asymptomatic.

TERMINOLOGY

Definitions
- Benign neoplasms consisting of mature adipose cells and blood vessels

CLINICAL ISSUES

Epidemiology
- Age
  - Most lipomas become clinically apparent in patients 40-60 years old

Presentation
- Lipomas and angiolipomas form soft palpable circumscribed masses
  - Typically present as slowly growing solitary lesions
- Also detected at screening mammography

Treatment
- Surgical approaches
  - Lesions are benign, and no treatment is necessary
  - Palpable masses, or those that are clinically apparent, may be excised for cosmetic reasons or due to patient preference
  - Superficial or subcutaneous lesions are more likely to be clinically apparent and undergo excision

Prognosis
- Benign lesions without risk of local recurrence

Core Needle Biopsies
- Histologic features of lipoma on core needle biopsy are nondiagnostic
  - Radiologic correlation is necessary for a final diagnosis
  - Lipomas are rarely biopsied as imaging findings are usually diagnostic
- Angiolipomas can be diagnosed on core needle biopsies
  - More commonly biopsied than lipomas due to dense appearance that can mimic carcinomas

IMAGE FINDINGS

Mammographic Findings
- Lipomas and angiolipomas form oval, round, or lobulated masses
- Lipomas consist entirely of adipose tissue and are radiolucent with thin capsule
  - Masses with typical appearance of lipoma need not be biopsied
- Angiolipomas form dense masses
  - Biopsies are often performed for definitive diagnosis

Ultrasonographic Findings
- Lipomas and angiolipomas form oval, round, or lobulated masses
- Masses are isoechoic or hyperechoic compared to subcutaneous adipose tissue

MACROSCOPIC FEATURES

General Features
- Rarely completely excised
- If excised, it is often as multiple fragments, without surrounding tissue
- In complete excisions, there will be an ovoid mass consisting of adipose tissue, separated from surrounding tissue by a thin capsule

MICROSCOPIC PATHOLOGY

Histologic Features
- Lipomas consist of mature adipose tissue without epithelial elements

LIPOMA AND ANGIOLIPOMA

Key Facts

Terminology
- Benign neoplasms consisting of mature adipose cells and blood vessels

Clinical Issues
- Lipomas and angiolipomas form soft palpable circumscribed masses
- Lesions are benign, and no treatment is necessary

Image Findings
- Lipomas consist entirely of adipose tissue and are radiolucent with a thin capsule
  - Do not require biopsy
- Angiolipomas form dense masses
  - Generally require biopsy for definitive diagnosis

Microscopic Pathology
- Mature adipose tissue without epithelial elements

- Adipose cells are uniform in size throughout lesion
- After trauma, may show varying degrees of fibrosis, myxoid change, and calcification

Top Differential Diagnoses
- Myofibroblastoma/spindle cell lipoma
- Hamartoma
- Hibernoma
- Liposarcoma or angiosarcoma

Reporting Considerations
- Histologic findings on fine needle aspiration, core needle biopsy, or in fragmented specimens are nonspecific for lipomas
  - Clinical, radiologic, and pathologic correlation is often necessary for diagnosis

---

  - Completely excised lesion is well circumscribed and encapsulated and may push adjacent fibroglandular breast elements
- Appearance of lipoma may be altered secondary to trauma or impaired blood supply
  - After trauma, lesions may show varying degrees of fibrosis, myxoid change, lipogranulomas, and calcification
- Angiolipomas consist of mature adipose tissue and small round blood vessels
  - Branching networks of small vessels are typically more prevalent in subcapsular region
  - Fibrin thrombi are typically present within vascular spaces
- Nuclei of adipocytes are small, uniform, and located at periphery of cell

DIFFERENTIAL DIAGNOSIS

Myofibroblastoma/Spindle Cell Lipoma
- Myofibroblastoma, spindle cell lipoma, and solitary fibrous tumor of breast are very similar, if not identical, tumors
- Consist of admixtures of mature fat, collagen-forming spindle cells, and varying degrees of myxoid changes
  - Spindle cells are CD34, CD10, and vimentin positive
  - Variably, α-smooth muscle actin or desmin positivity may be seen
- Myofibroblastoma and spindle cell lipoma both have rearrangements of 13q and 16q

Hamartoma
- Usually presents as mammographic circumscribed masses containing adipose tissue
- Consist of normal-appearing ducts and lobules in addition to minor component of fat

Liposarcoma
- Extremely rare in breast
- Variation in size of adipocytes, atypia, lipoblasts, and fibrous septae are good diagnostic clues for malignancy

- High-grade phyllodes tumors may have liposarcoma as a heterologous element
- Usually present as large palpable mass with irregular or ill-defined borders
  - Highly unlikely to present as mammographic finding or small circumscribed mass
  - Form dense masses on mammography

Hibernoma
- Lesion consisting of brown fat found most commonly in upper outer quadrant or axilla
- Hibernoma can occur in adults, potentially at any site where brown fat persists
- Most cases are asymptomatic and present as slow-growing mass lesions
- Microscopically, lesion is composed of coarsely multivacuolated fat cells that lack atypia

Angiosarcoma
- Malignant blood vessels are irregular in shape and dissect into surrounding tissue
- Nuclear pleomorphism, tufting, solid areas, and blood lakes are common
- Typical presentation is as large palpable mass with irregular or ill-defined borders
  - It would be highly unusual for angiosarcoma to present as small circumscribed mass

SELECTED REFERENCES

1. Kryvenko ON et al: Angiolipoma of the female breast: clinicomorphological correlation of 52 cases. Int J Surg Pathol. 19(1):35-43, 2011
2. Schmidt J et al: Giant lipoma of the breast. Breast J. 15(1):107-8, 2009
3. Magro G et al: CD10 is expressed by mammary myofibroblastoma and spindle cell lipoma of soft tissue: an additional evidence of their histogenetic linking. Virchows Arch. 450(6):727-8, 2007
4. Colville J et al: Mammary hibernoma. Breast J. 12(6):563-5, 2006
5. Kahng HC et al: Cellular angiolipoma of the breast: immunohistochemical study and review of the literature. Breast J. 8(1):47-9, 2002

LIPOMA AND ANGIOLIPOMA

Imaging, Gross, and Microscopic Features

(Left) Unlike radiolucent lipomas, angiolipomas form dense masses ⮊ due to the presence of blood vessels. Because carcinomas can also form circumscribed dense masses, most angiolipomas undergo biopsy or excision. *(Right)* This 5 cm radiolucent mass ➡ was not palpable. A core needle biopsy showed adipose tissue, consistent with lipoma. Lipomas are often in subcutaneous tissue, rather than arising deep in the breast. Biopsy is unnecessary if the imaging findings are diagnostic.

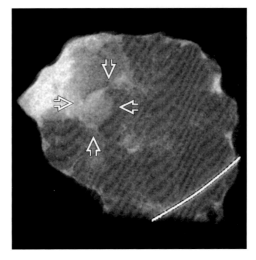
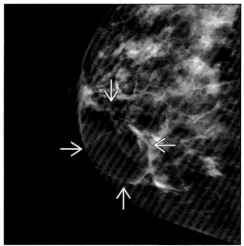

(Left) The majority of breast masses are hypoechoic on ultrasound in comparison to the surrounding breast tissue. Angiolipomas form circumscribed hyperechoic masses ⮊ due to the combination of adipose and angiomatous components in these lesions. *(Right)* Lipomas consist of mature fat without epithelial elements. The findings are nonspecific unless the entire lesion is excised with margins. Radiologic and clinical correlation are generally required for a final diagnosis of lipoma.

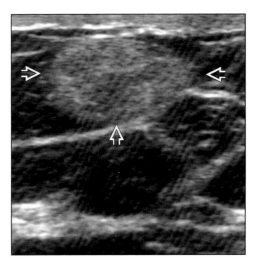
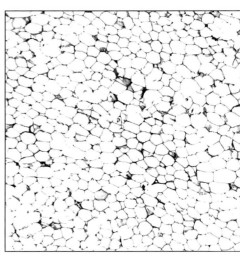

(Left) This angiolipoma ⮊ was an incidental finding in a mastectomy specimen for breast cancer. The lesion is well circumscribed with pushing borders and has a distinct homogeneous tan appearance as compared to the surrounding yellow adipose tissue. *(Right)* Compared to lipomas, angiolipomas have a prominent component of small, well-formed, round blood vessels. Fibrin thrombi may be present but are not as frequently seen as in angiolipomas of other sites.

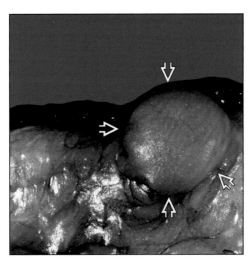
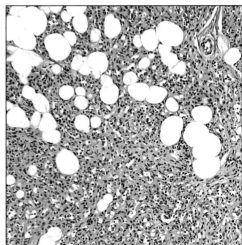

LIPOMA AND ANGIOLIPOMA

Differential Diagnosis

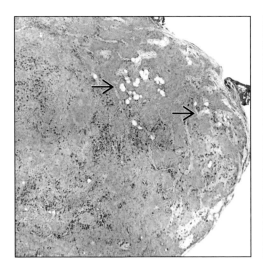

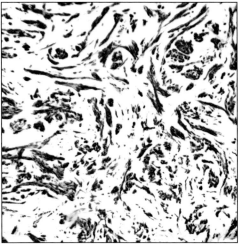

(Left) Hamartomas present as dense circumscribed masses and, unlike most other mammographically dense lesions, characteristically have a small component of adipose tissue ➡. However, hamartomas mostly consist of fibrous tissue as well as ducts and lobules. (Right) The stroma of hamartomas can be fibrous tissue or show muscle differentiation. This myoid hamartoma shows strong immunoreactivity in the stromal cells for desmin. Adipose tissue is also usually present.

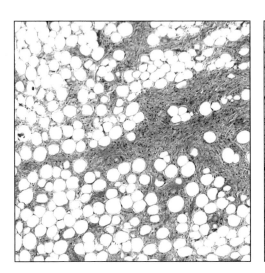

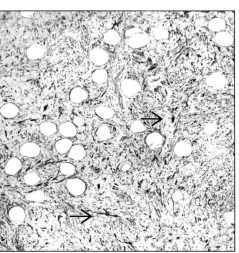

(Left) Myofibroblastomas and spindle cell lipomas are similar, if not identical, lesions. This myofibroblastoma has a prominent component of adipose tissue intermingled with areas of myofibroblasts. (Right) The myofibroblasts in this myofibroblastoma demonstrate immunoreactivity for desmin ➡. Although this finding has been used to differentiate these lesions from spindle cell lipomas, they both share the same cytogenetic changes.

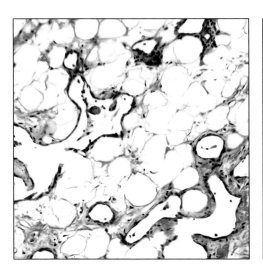

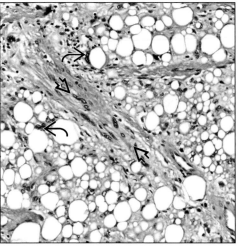

(Left) Angiosarcomas have irregular anastomosing vascular channels, nuclear atypia, and tufting of endothelial cells. Although they can invade into fat, they should not be mistaken for an angiolipoma. (Right) Liposarcomas of the breast are very rare. Unlike lipomas, they form a dense mass on mammography. Variation in the size of adipocytes, lipoblasts, atypia ➡, and fibrous septae ➤ are helpful diagnostic features to recognize the lesion as a sarcoma.

DIABETIC MASTOPATHY/LYMPHOCYTIC MASTOPATHY

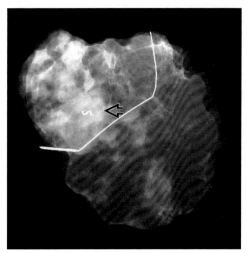

Diabetic mastopathy forms breast masses that may be palpable or present as circumscribed or ill-defined mammographic densities. In this case, a clip ⊵ from a prior core needle biopsy is present within the mass.

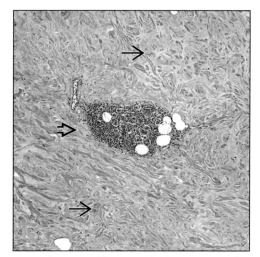

DM is characterized by extremely dense stroma with a glassy appearance to the collagen ⊵. Ducts, lobules ⊵, and blood vessels are surrounded by a dense lymphocytic infiltrate.

TERMINOLOGY

Abbreviations
- Diabetic mastopathy (DM)

Synonyms
- Diabetic fibrous mastopathy
- Lymphocytic mastopathy
- Sclerosing lymphocytic lobulitis

Definitions
- Periductal, perilobular, and perivascular lymphocytic infiltrate accompanied by proliferation of fibroblasts and myofibroblasts, occurring primarily in women with diabetes mellitus or other autoimmune diseases

ETIOLOGY/PATHOGENESIS

Etiology
- Majority of patients have longstanding insulin-dependent diabetes
  - Fewer patients have autoimmune thyroid disease
- Stromal changes may be due to abnormal glucose deposition on collagen
- However, some patients do not have autoimmune disease; it is unknown if DM is risk factor for developing these diseases

CLINICAL ISSUES

Presentation
- Very hard palpable mass, well circumscribed or ill defined
- May be multiple and bilateral
- Occurs in both men and women at any age
- Imaging findings may mimic carcinoma or be nonspecific
  - MR may be helpful as there is characteristic slow gradual enhancement

Treatment
- Unnecessary once carcinoma is excluded

Prognosis
- Lesion is benign, but new masses may form

IMAGE FINDINGS

Mammographic Findings
- Usually appears as circumscribed or ill-defined mass or may not be seen
- Calcifications would be unusual

MACROSCOPIC FEATURES

Gross Appearance
- Dense white masses, circumscribed or ill defined
- Masses can be 1 to > 6 cm in size

MICROSCOPIC PATHOLOGY

Histologic Features
- Dense lymphocytic infiltrates surround lobules, ducts, and blood vessels
- Basement membranes of ducts and lobules may be markedly thickened
- Lobules are small in size and sparse in number
- Stroma is very dense and paucicellular, often glassy in appearance
- In some cases, fibroblasts may have enlarged nuclei and appear epithelioid in shape
- Stromal cells are positive for fibroblast and myofibroblast markers (CD34, smooth muscle actin, desmin, CD10)
- Lymphocytes are predominantly B cells intermingled with smaller population of T cells

DIABETIC MASTOPATHY/LYMPHOCYTIC MASTOPATHY

Key Facts

Terminology
- Chronic inflammation and stromal changes occurring primarily in women with diabetes mellitus or other autoimmune diseases

Etiology/Pathogenesis
- Majority of patients have longstanding insulin-dependent diabetes
  - Fewer patients have autoimmune thyroid disease
- Some patients do not have autoimmune disease; it is unknown if DM is risk factor for developing these diseases

Clinical Issues
- Very hard palpable mass, well circumscribed or ill defined
- May be multiple and bilateral

- Treatment is unnecessary once carcinoma is excluded
- Imaging findings may mimic carcinoma or be nonspecific

Microscopic Pathology
- Dense lymphocytic infiltrates surround lobules, ducts, and blood vessels
- Lymphocytes are predominantly B cells intermingled with smaller population of T cells

Top Differential Diagnoses
- Pseudoangiomatous stromal hyperplasia (PASH)
- Fibrous nodule
- Lymphoma
- IgG4-related sclerosing mastitis
- Lymphocytic lobulitis associated with carcinomas

DIFFERENTIAL DIAGNOSIS

Pseudoangiomatous Stromal Hyperplasia (PASH)
- Lacks lymphocytic infiltrates of DM
- PASH has characteristic clefts within stroma that are not typical of DM

Fibrous Nodule
- Lacks lymphocytic infiltrates of DM
- Stroma is generally more cellular than stroma of DM

Lymphoma
- Lymphomas form masses composed of malignant cells; stromal proliferation is not prominent
- Findings similar to DM can be seen at edges of low-grade lymphomas occurring in breast

Inflammatory Pseudotumor (or Plasma Cell Granuloma) and IgG4-related Sclerosing Mastitis
- Patients present with palpable masses that may be multiple &/or bilateral
- Not associated with diabetes mellitus or connective tissue disease
- Lesion consists of dense lymphoplasmacytic infiltrate with germinal centers
- Unlike DM, lymphocytes are not centered around ducts, lobules, or blood vessels
- Stroma is sclerotic; ducts and lobules are absent or only present at periphery
  - Unlike DM, stroma is minor component of lesion
- Lymphocytes consist of mixture of B cells and T cells
- In IgG4-related sclerosing mastitis, plasma cells are predominantly IgG4(+) (40-85% of all IgG[+] cells)

Lymphocytic Lobulitis Associated with Carcinomas
- Lymphocytic infiltrates associated with carcinomas are predominantly T cells

- T-cell lymphocytic lobulitis has been described as finding in prophylactic mastectomies of high-risk women
  - Majority of these women are BRCA1 carriers
  - Have not been associated with mass-forming lesions

DIAGNOSTIC CHECKLIST

Pathologic Interpretation Pearls
- Fine needle aspiration or core needle biopsy may be difficult to perform due to density of lesion
  - Lesions are typically harder than invasive carcinomas
  - Needles may not penetrate easily or may not adequately sample the lesion for diagnosis
- Findings on core needle biopsy may suggest the diagnosis but not be definitive
- Excision may be necessary for final evaluation

SELECTED REFERENCES

1. Cheuk W et al: IgG4-related sclerosing mastitis: description of a new member of the IgG4-related sclerosing diseases. Am J Surg Pathol. 33(7):1058-64, 2009
2. Oba M et al: A case of lymphocytic mastopathy requiring differential diagnosis from primary breast lymphoma. Breast Cancer. 16(2):141-6, 2009
3. Guo X et al: Tumor infiltrating lymphocytes differ in invasive micropapillary carcinoma and medullary carcinoma of breast. Mod Pathol. 21(9):1101-7, 2008
4. Thorncroft K et al: The diagnosis and management of diabetic mastopathy. Breast J. 13(6):607-13, 2007
5. Douglas-Jones AG: Lymphocytic lobulitis in breast core biopsy: a peritumoral phenomenon. Histopathology. 48(2):209-12, 2006
6. Hermsen BB et al: Lobulitis is a frequent finding in prophylactically removed breast tissue from women at hereditary high risk of breast cancer. J Pathol. 206(2):220-3, 2005

DIABETIC MASTOPATHY/LYMPHOCYTIC MASTOPATHY

Microscopic Features

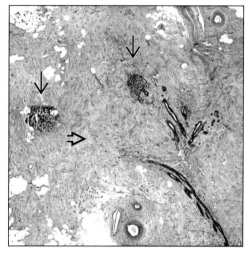
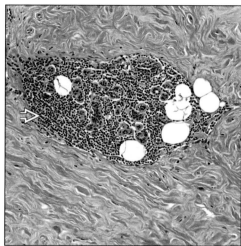

(Left) The predominant component of DM is very dense stroma ⊡. The hardness of the lesion can make it difficult to sample with needle biopsies. Epithelial elements are sparse, and lobules are generally small and atrophic ⊡. *(Right)* Lobules are sparse and small in size ⊡. The inflammatory infiltrate consists almost exclusively of small lymphocytes and surrounds epithelium and blood vessels. The lymphocytic infiltrate can be so dense as to obscure the epithelium.

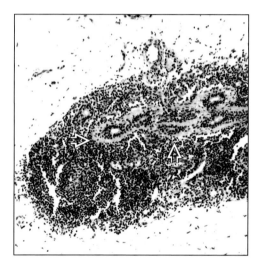
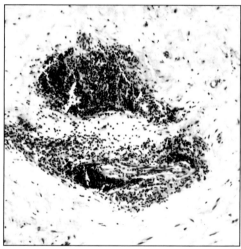

(Left) The lobules are characteristically atrophic in appearance, and the basement membranes are typically markedly thickened ⊡. A possible association with abnormal glucose deposition has been suggested for the abnormal stromal changes. *(Right)* In addition to the lymphocytic infiltrates associated with ducts and lobules, lymphocytic infiltrates also surround small blood vessels.

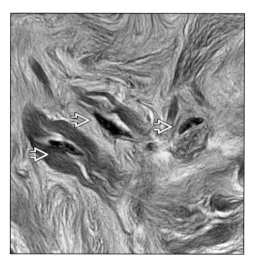
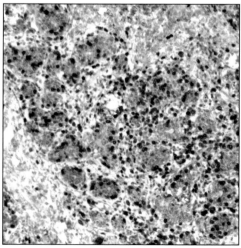

(Left) The stromal cells can have enlarged nuclei, and the cells may appear epithelioid ⊡. In rare cases, these cells can raise concern for a diffusely infiltrating carcinoma. However, these cells are fibroblasts and are immunoreactive for CD34 and negative for cytokeratins. *(Right)* The lymphocytes of DM are predominantly small B cells, as shown in this immunohistochemical study for CD20. B cells also predominate in other reactive inflammatory lesions of the breast.

DIABETIC MASTOPATHY/LYMPHOCYTIC MASTOPATHY

Differential Diagnosis

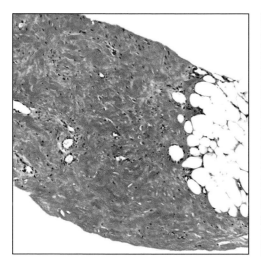

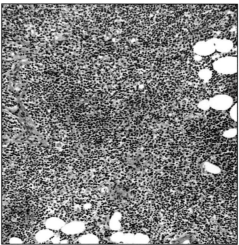

(Left) Fibrous nodules also consist of dense collagenized stromal tissue. Epithelial elements may be absent or scant and atrophic in appearance. However, a lymphocytic infiltrate is not present, and there is no association with diabetes. *(Right)* Lymphomas of the breast consist of a dense infiltrate of atypical cells forming a solid mass. The infiltrate is not centered on lobules and blood vessels as in DM. However, findings at the periphery of lymphomas can mimic DM.

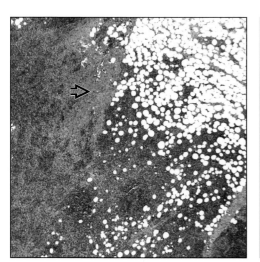

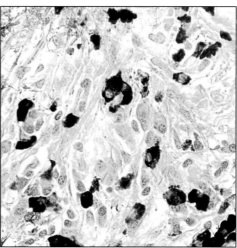

(Left) Inflammatory pseudotumors (also termed "plasma cell granulomas") consist of a lymphoplasmacytic infiltrate involving fibroadipose tissue. Unlike DM, breast elements are absent or only focally present at periphery of mass ⊵. Inflammatory cells, not stroma as in DM, form the bulk of the lesion. *(Right)* IgG4-related sclerosing mastopathy has identical histologic features as inflammatory pseudotumor but is characterized by numerous IgG4(+) plasma cells.

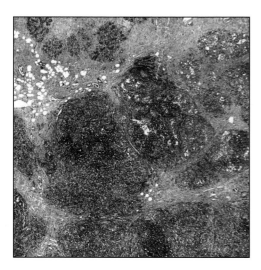

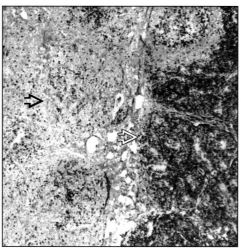

(Left) Lymphocytic lobulitis is described as a lesion found in prophylactic mastectomies from women at risk for breast cancer. A dense infiltrate of lymphocytes surrounds lobules. A milder lymphocytic infiltrate surrounds adjacent lobules. The lobules do not appear atrophic. *(Right)* Lymphocytic lobulitis in BRCA1 carriers consists of CD4(+) T cells ⊳ in the main lesion and in adjacent lobules ⊵. Lymphocytes associated with some types of carcinomas are also T cells.

GRANULAR CELL TUMOR

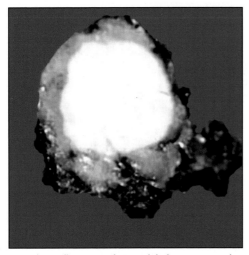

Granular cell tumors form solid firm masses that can be circumscribed or irregular. This tumor has a homogeneous white surface and pushing border in contrast to the surrounding yellow adipose tissue.

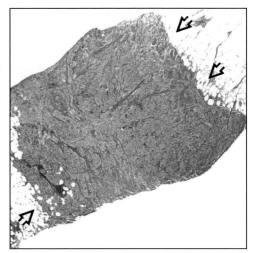

This core needle biopsy shows a granular cell tumor consisting of cells with abundant foamy eosinophilic cytoplasm infiltrating in a collagenous stroma. The borders are slightly irregular ⊡.

TERMINOLOGY

Abbreviations
• Granular cell tumor (GCT)

Synonyms
• Granular cell myoblastoma

Definitions
• Tumor thought to arise from Schwann cells, consisting of granular cells (cells with abundant eosinophilic bubbly cytoplasm)

CLINICAL ISSUES

Epidemiology
• Incidence
  ○ Rare breast lesion: Only 1 GCT occurs for every 100-200 cases of carcinoma
• Age
  ○ Occurs most commonly during childbearing years (range: 17-74 years of age)
• Gender
  ○ Similar to other breast lesions, majority occur in women with only 10% in men
• Ethnicity
  ○ African-American women are affected more commonly than Caucasian women

Presentation
• Majority of patients present with solitary palpable mass that may be firm or hard
  ○ Most common in upper inner breast (carcinomas are most common in upper outer breast)
  ○ Rarely, multiple masses are present (5-10%)
  ○ Mass may retract skin or be adherent to chest wall
• Smaller tumors may be detected as a density on mammographic screening

Natural History
• Benign and slow growing
• Rare reports of local recurrence
• Very rare reports of malignant GCT with metastases to lymph nodes or lung

Treatment
• Most tumors are completely excised by surgery

IMAGE FINDINGS

Mammographic Findings
• Mass with irregular, circumscribed, or lobulated borders
• Multiple masses are present in 5-10% of cases
• Calcifications are not typical

Ultrasonographic Findings
• Hypoechoic mass with irregular margins
• Marked posterior shadowing may be present

MACROSCOPIC FEATURES

General Features
• Gross palpable, white to yellow, firm to hard mass; closely resembles invasive carcinoma
• Borders may be circumscribed, ill defined, or irregular
• Usually 1-3 cm; rare reports of tumors up to 6 cm

MICROSCOPIC PATHOLOGY

Histologic Features
• Solid proliferation of tumor cells
  ○ Cells can also infiltrate as single cells or small nests
• Cells are rounded or spindle-shaped
• Cytoplasm is abundant and contains eosinophilic granules; in some cases, cytoplasm may appear clear
  ○ Granules are PAS positive and diastase resistant

GRANULAR CELL TUMOR

Key Facts

Terminology

- Previously termed "granular cell myoblastoma"
- Tumor thought to arise from Schwann cells, consisting of granular cells (cells with abundant eosinophilic bubbly cytoplasm)

Clinical Issues

- Rare; only 1 case per 100-200 cases of carcinoma
- Presents as firm to hard palpable mass or as a density on screening mammography
  - Some tumors can retract skin or be adherent to chest wall
- Majority of tumors are benign and cured by surgical excision
- Rare reports of local recurrence
- Very rare reports of malignant tumors with metastases to lymph nodes or lung

Image Findings

- Most common in upper inner breast (carcinomas are most common in upper outer breast)

Ancillary Tests

- Immunohistochemical studies are useful to distinguish granular cells from other types of cells
- Granules seen by light microscopy correspond to numerous lysosomes by electron microscopy
- Myelin figures are also present, supporting neural origin

Top Differential Diagnoses

- Benign inflammatory lesions containing histiocytes
- Invasive carcinoma (histiocytoid, secretory)
- Metastatic tumors (renal cell carcinoma, melanoma)
- Alveolar soft part sarcoma

- Nuclei are small and oval with minimal pleomorphism; nucleoli may be inconspicuous or prominent
  - Focal areas of nuclear pleomorphism or occasional mitoses should not be interpreted as evidence of malignancy

ANCILLARY TESTS

Immunohistochemistry

- Useful to distinguish granular cells from other types of cells
  - Tumor cells are positive for S100, calretinin, inhibin-α, neuron specific enolase, β-catenin, and vimentin
  - Tumor cells may be positive for CD68 or CEA
  - Tumor cells are negative for cytokeratin, myoglobin, estrogen receptor, and progesterone receptor

Electron Microscopy

- Granules seen by light microscopy correspond to numerous lysosomes
- Myelin figures are present, supporting neural origin

DIFFERENTIAL DIAGNOSIS

Benign Inflammatory Lesions

- Histiocytes and granular cells can be similar in appearance
- Cause of histiocytic infiltrate is usually apparent, most commonly ruptured cysts or fat necrosis

Invasive Carcinoma

- Carcinomas with apocrine or histiocytoid features can resemble GCT
- Nuclear pleomorphism and mitotic figures are usually present
- DCIS is usually present
- Carcinomas are positive for cytokeratin

Metastatic Tumors

- Melanomas are most common type of metastasis to breast
  - S100 is positive in melanoma and in GCT
  - Other melanoma markers should be negative in GCT
- Renal cell carcinoma may also have granular cytoplasm
  - Blood lakes are common due to delicate vasculature
  - Renal cell carcinoma is positive for cytokeratin

Alveolar Soft Part Sarcoma (ASPS)

- Originally named "malignant granular cell myoblastoma," as it was thought to be malignant counterpart to GCT
  - These tumors have specific translocation: der(17)t(X;17)(p11;q25)
  - Translocation fuses transcription factor 3 (TFE3) gene to novel gene named ASPL creating an ASPL-TFE3 fusion protein
  - Nuclear immunoreactivity for TFE3 product is present in ASPS, pediatric renal carcinomas with TFE3 fusion proteins, and some GCT (25%)
    - Translocation and TFE3 fusion proteins have not been reported in GCT
- Rare type of sarcoma that would be highly unusual in breast
- Cells are discohesive in clustered pseudoalveolar pattern and have distinct PAS-positive granules in cytoplasm
- ASPS is negative for cytokeratin, HMB-45, and S100 in majority of cases
- Desmin and other skeletal muscle markers are positive in about 1/2 of cases

SELECTED REFERENCES

1. Rekhi B et al: Morphologic spectrum, immunohistochemical analysis, and clinical features of a series of granular cell tumors of soft tissues: a study from a tertiary referral cancer center. Ann Diagn Pathol. 14(3):162-7, 2010

GRANULAR CELL TUMOR

Microscopic Features and Ancillary Techniques

(Left) GCT is characterized by solid sheets of cells in stroma divided by prominent fibrous septae. In this tumor, the cells infiltrate irregularly into the surrounding adipose tissue ⇨ giving the lesion an irregular border by imaging. *(Right)* This GCT has a more diffusely infiltrative pattern. Single cells and small clusters of cells are dispersed in fibrous stroma and adipose tissue.

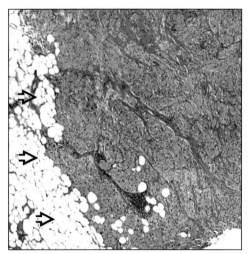
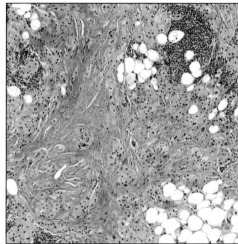

(Left) The tumor cells have small round nuclei with homogeneous chromatin and inconspicuous nucleoli. There is abundant amphophilic granular cytoplasm. Nuclear pleomorphism and mitoses are not characteristic. *(Right)* GCT can resemble invasive carcinomas with a histiocytoid or clear cell appearance. Immunohistochemical studies for broad spectrum cytokeratins confirm that tumor cells are negative ⇨, whereas adjacent benign epithelial cells are positive →.

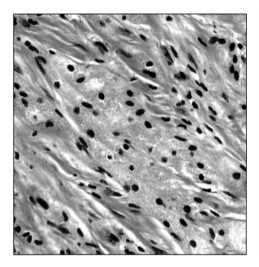
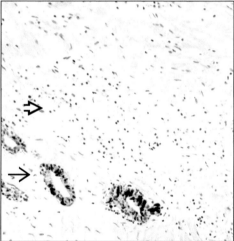

(Left) GCT is strongly positive for cytoplasmic and nuclear S100 protein. However, some invasive carcinomas and the majority of melanomas are also positive for S100. A panel of immunohistochemical markers should be employed to make a specific diagnosis. *(Right)* GCT is variably positive for CD68 as seen in this case. True histiocytes will also be positive for CD68 as well as S100. Histiocytes are more variable in appearance and associated with other types of inflammatory cells.

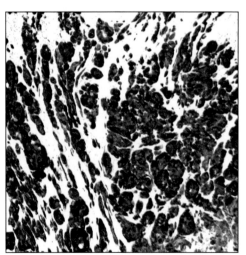
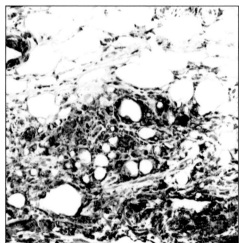

GRANULAR CELL TUMOR

Differential Diagnosis

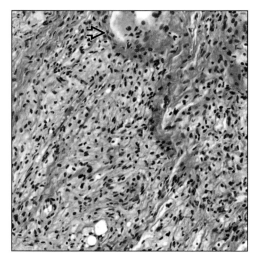

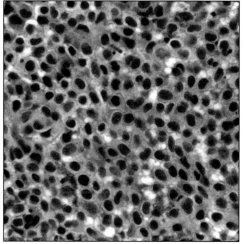

(Left) Histiocytes, such as in this case of fat necrosis, also may have abundant foamy cytoplasm. The nuclei tend to be more variable in shape and may be spindled. Other inflammatory cells, such as giant cells ⊵, are typically present. (Right) Metastatic melanoma can also consist of cells with abundant foamy cytoplasm. These tumors will be strongly S100 positive and cytokeratin negative, like GCT. Other melanoma markers, such as HMB-45, may be necessary to make a specific diagnosis.

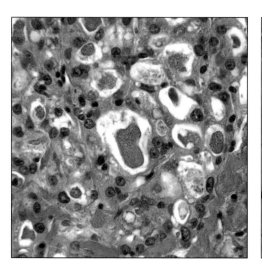

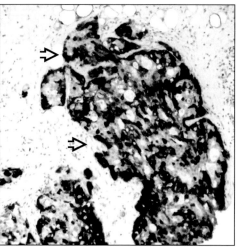

(Left) This secretory carcinoma has abundant amphophilic cytoplasm, similar to GCT. However, the tumor cells also form tubules containing secretory material. In difficult cases, carcinomas can be identified by immunoreactivity for cytokeratins. (Right) Secretory carcinoma ⊵ and GCT are both strongly positive for S100, as are some other breast carcinomas. However, immunoreactivity for cytokeratins will be present in carcinomas and absent within GCT.

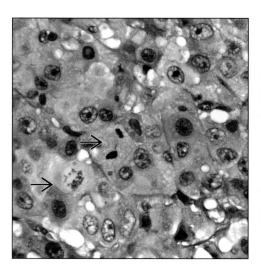

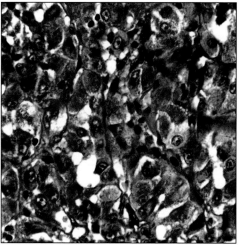

(Left) Some apocrine carcinomas have abundant eosinophilic cytoplasm, as seen here. The marked nuclear pleomorphism and the presence of mitotic figures ⇥ would not be seen in a typical GCT. In addition, areas of DCIS will usually be present in the adjacent breast tissue. (Right) Alveolar soft part sarcomas are also characterized by cells with abundant granular cytoplasm and PAS-positive, diastase-resistant crystals. About 1/2 will be positive for muscle markers such as desmin.

NODULAR FASCIITIS

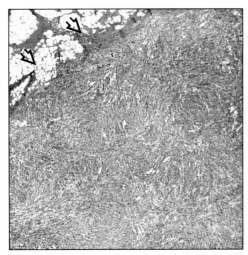

The stromal proliferation in nodular fasciitis generally forms a relatively circumscribed mass ⊵, although tumor cells can focally extend into adjacent stroma.

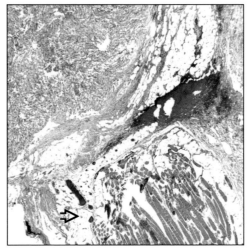

Nodular fasciitis is generally located in subcutaneous tissue or deep tissue close to the chest wall and skeletal muscle ⊵. Breast ducts and lobules are not present within the lesion.

TERMINOLOGY

Abbreviations
- Nodular fasciitis (NF)

Definitions
- Benign self-limited proliferation of fibroblasts and myofibroblasts

CLINICAL ISSUES

Presentation
- Presents as rapidly growing painful or tender mass
- Occurrence within breast is very rare
  - Location may be in subcutaneous tissue, muscle fascia, or within breast parenchyma

Treatment
- No treatment is necessary
  - In most cases, lesion will be excised to exclude other neoplasms

Prognosis
- Tumors spontaneously regress within a few months

IMAGE FINDINGS

Mammographic Findings
- Lesions present as mammographic densities with irregular margins

Ultrasonographic Findings
- Many lesions have irregular margins

MICROSCOPIC PATHOLOGY

Histologic Features
- Nodular fasciitis is composed of short spindle-shaped cells
  - Cells loosely arranged and are not organized in specific patterns
    - Tumor has a "tissue culture" appearance
  - Short fascicles or small whorls may be present
- Nuclei are small and uniform
  - Prominent nucleoli may be present
- Mitoses are typically frequent
- Cells form solid masses and do not infiltrate around ducts and lobules
- Thick bands of collagen are typical
- Chronic inflammation may be present; cells are distributed throughout and not restricted to periphery
- Red cell extravasation is common
- Borders are generally circumscribed
  - However, cells may focally infiltrate into surrounding stroma
- Large myoid type cells or multinucleated cells may be present
  - These cells must not be mistaken for epithelial cells in spindle cell carcinoma
  - This type of cell can be frequent in related lesion proliferative fasciitis

ANCILLARY TESTS

Immunohistochemistry
- Negative for CD34
- Cells may be positive for muscle markers (smooth muscle α-actin, calponin, desmin, etc.)
- Negative for cytokeratins
  - It is important to exclude spindle cell carcinoma, especially in limited biopsies such as core needle biopsies
- Negative for nuclear β-catenin
  - Cytoplasmic β-catenin may be present

NODULAR FASCIITIS

Key Facts

Terminology
- Benign self-limited proliferation of fibroblasts and myofibroblasts

Clinical Issues
- Presents as rapidly growing painful or tender mass
- Without treatment, tumors will spontaneously regress within a few months
- Location may be in subcutaneous tissue, muscle fascia, or within breast parenchyma

Image Findings
- There are no specific imaging findings that would identify a lesion as NF
- Many lesions have irregular margins and can closely resemble invasive carcinoma

Microscopic Pathology
- Mitoses are typically frequent
- Large myoid-type cells or multinucleated cells may be present
- Nodular fasciitis is composed of short spindle-shaped cells
- Cells are loosely organized and do not have specific pattern
  ○ Described as "tissue culture" appearance

Top Differential Diagnoses
- Fibromatosis
- Spindle cell carcinoma
- Myofibroblastoma
- Proliferative fasciitis and proliferative myositis
- Sarcoma

DIFFERENTIAL DIAGNOSIS

Fibromatosis
- Locally aggressive with frequent recurrence and must be distinguished from NF
- Tumor cells are arranged in long fascicles that infiltrate into adjacent breast tissue and possibly into muscle
- Mitoses are infrequent
- Chronic inflammatory cells are characteristically located at periphery
- Immunohistochemical studies may be helpful in distinguishing fibromatosis from NF
  ○ Both tumors have the same pattern of positivity for muscle markers present in myofibroblasts
  ○ Both tumors lack CD34 positivity, unlike other stromal lesions of the breast
  ○ Majority of cases of fibromatosis have nuclear positivity for β-catenin
    ▪ Nuclear β-catenin is absent in NF
    ▪ Some cases of fibromatosis are also negative for nuclear β-catenin

Spindle Cell Carcinoma
- Can have deceptively bland appearance
- Broad spectrum cytokeratins, including basal-type keratins, may be necessary to demonstrate keratin immunoreactivity
  ○ p63 may also be positive in about 1/3 of spindle cell carcinomas
- Nuclear pleomorphism and prominent nucleoli may be present
- Carcinomas typically invade in and around normal ducts and lobules and have irregular borders

Myofibroblastoma
- Cells are usually organized into short fascicles
- Chronic inflammation within lesion is not typical
- Extravasated red blood cells are not typical
- Cells are immunoreactive for CD34

Proliferative Fasciitis and Proliferative Myositis
- Do not usually occur in breast
  ○ Lesions on anterior chest wall can be mistaken for breast lesions
- Lesions usually grow rapidly within a few weeks, similar to NF
- Histologic appearance is similar to NF
  ○ Cells can entrap adipose tissue and skeletal muscle
  ○ Ganglion-like cells with abundant cytoplasm and 1 to several nuclei with prominent nucleoli may be frequent
    ▪ These cells can be mistaken for epithelioid cells in spindle cell carcinoma
    ▪ Cells may be positive for muscle specific actin, smooth muscle specific actin, and CD68
    ▪ Cells will be negative for cytokeratins

Sarcoma
- NF can mimic sarcoma due to high cellularity, focal infiltrative pattern, and numerous mitoses
- Most sarcomas are larger in size (> 4 cm), have greater nuclear pleomorphism, and may have abnormal mitoses
- Some sarcomas will be positive for CD34 or other markers specific for the type of sarcoma
  ○ In most cases, immunohistochemical studies will not be helpful for this differential diagnosis

SELECTED REFERENCES

1. Grobmyer SR et al: Nodular fasciitis: differential considerations and current management strategies. Am Surg. 75(7):610-4, 2009
2. Iwatani T et al: Nodular fasciitis of the breast. Breast Cancer. Epub ahead of print, 2009
3. Carlson JW et al: Immunohistochemistry for beta-catenin in the differential diagnosis of spindle cell lesions: analysis of a series and review of the literature. Histopathology. 51(4):509-14, 2007
4. Hayashi H et al: Nodular fasciitis of the breast. Breast Cancer. 14(3):337-9, 2007

NODULAR FASCIITIS

Microscopic and Immunohistochemical Features

(Left) The cells are loosely arranged without a specific pattern (a "tissue culture" appearance). Focal whorls or storiform formations can be present. Areas of keloid-like collagen are frequently seen ⊳. *(Right)* There is usually a clinical history of rapid tumor growth, correlating with the presence of frequent mitotic figures ⊳. The frequent mitoses can raise concern for a malignant tumor.

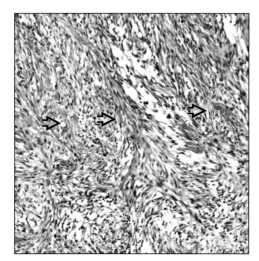
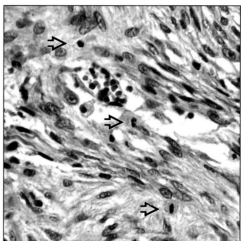

(Left) Extravasation of red blood cells is a common finding. *(Right)* Multinucleated giant cells or myoid cells may be present. These cells should not be mistaken for epithelioid cells in a spindle cell carcinoma. This type of cell may be more common in proliferative fasciitis and proliferative myositis.

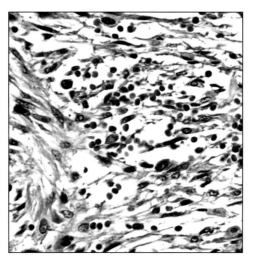
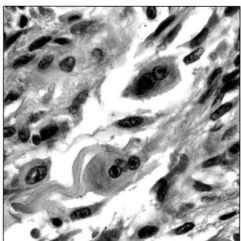

(Left) The lesional cells have features of myofibroblasts and are commonly immunoreactive for muscle markers such as calponin, as seen in this photomicrograph. A similar pattern would be seen for smooth muscle actin. *(Right)* The lesional cells of nodular fasciitis are negative for CD34 ⊳ as are the cells of fibromatosis. The majority of other stromal breast lesions are CD34 positive. Normal breast stroma ↗ and endothelial cells ➔ are positive for CD34.

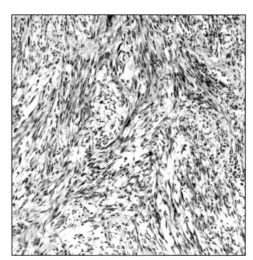
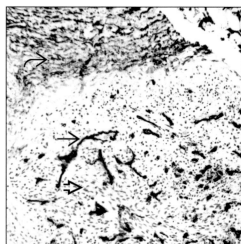

NODULAR FASCIITIS

Differential Diagnosis

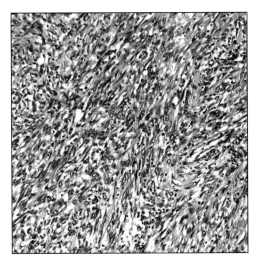

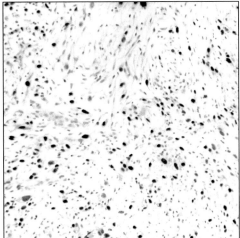

(Left) Spindle cell carcinomas generally have marked nuclear pleomorphism and may have atypical mitoses. The cells will be immunoreactive for cytokeratins. However, it may be necessary to use antibodies that detect basal-type keratins (CK14 and CK17). (Right) About 1/3 of spindle cell carcinomas will also be immunoreactive for nuclear p63. Squamous cell carcinomas are also positive for nuclear p63.

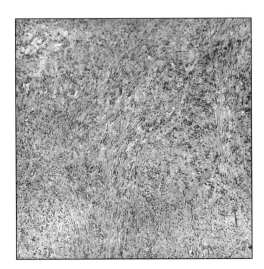

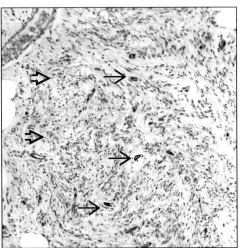

(Left) Myofibroblastomas consist of short spindle cells organized into fascicles. The cells are immunoreactive for CD34. Mitoses are absent or rare. (Right) The stromal cells of myofibroblastomas are immunoreactive for CD34 ▷ as are the endothelial cells of small blood vessels →.

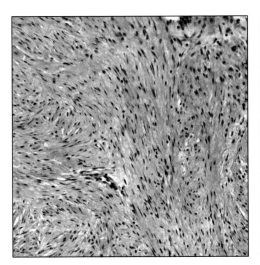

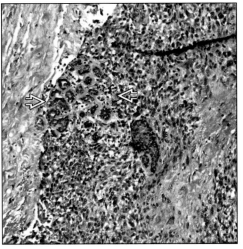

(Left) The cells of fibromatosis are organized into long sweeping fascicles. Fibromatosis and NF are the only breast stromal lesions that are typically CD34 negative. Unlike NF, fibromatosis may recur locally. (Right) Sarcomas of the breast are rare. These tumors usually invade into the breast stroma and around normal ducts and lobules ▷. Nuclear pleomorphism generally distinguishes these tumors from NF. Many sarcomas are immunoreactive for CD34, but some will be negative.

FIBROMATOSIS

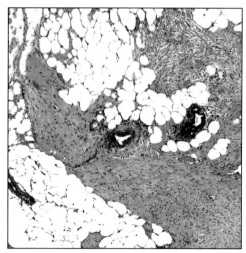

Fibromatosis is characterized by a proliferation of bland spindle cells organized in long fascicles that surround normal ducts and lobules and infiltrate into adipose tissue and skeletal muscle.

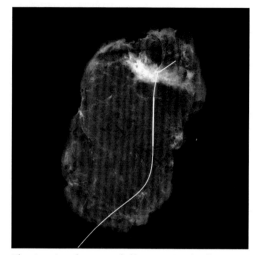

The imaging features of fibromatosis closely mimic those of invasive carcinomas. Most tumors appear as mammographic densities with irregular margins. Calcifications are not a feature.

TERMINOLOGY

Synonyms
- Mammary fibromatosis, aggressive fibromatosis
- Desmoid tumor, desmoid-type fibromatosis, extraabdominal desmoid tumor

Definitions
- Neoplastic proliferation of fibroblasts and myofibroblasts that is locally infiltrative but does not metastasize

ETIOLOGY/PATHOGENESIS

Genetic Causes
- Germline mutations
  - Familial adenomatous polyposis (FAP; includes Gardner syndrome and Turcot syndrome) is due to germline mutation in adenomatous polyposis coli (*APC*) gene
    - *APC* gene regulates β-catenin
  - Fibromatosis may occur in breast in patients with FAP, but fibromatosis is more common at other body sites
    - Abnormal regulation of β-catenin can result in accumulation of protein in nucleus, in addition to normal location in cytoplasm
    - Fibromatosis at any site associated with FAP shows nuclear β-catenin positivity in 67% of cases
- Somatic mutations
  - In sporadic cases, mutations in *APC* gene are present in 20% of tumors
    - Mutations in β-catenin gene in 50% of sporadic tumors
    - 80% of sporadic cases of fibromatosis are positive for nuclear β-catenin

Other Causes
- Trauma or prior surgery

  - In minority of cases, fibromatosis occurs in area of prior trauma or surgery (e.g., within capsule of breast implant)

CLINICAL ISSUES

Epidemiology
- Incidence
  - Rare; only 0.2% of breast tumors
- Age
  - Most patients are women in their 40s; however, any age can be affected

Presentation
- Most patients present with palpable mass or radiologic findings that closely mimic invasive carcinoma
  - Tumor can be fixed to pectoralis muscle or retract skin
  - Almost 1/2 of patients have prior history of breast surgery
  - Masses are usually painless
  - Tumors are irregular in shape

Treatment
- Tumor should be completely excised with an attempt at uninvolved margins
  - However, margin status does not accurately predict risk of local recurrence
- Radiation has been used for some patients; however, effectiveness of this treatment is uncertain
- Adjuvant treatment with cytotoxic therapy or hormonal therapy has been used
  - Too few cases reported to determine effectiveness of these treatments

Prognosis
- Local recurrence is common within 1st 3 years (20-30%), even with uninvolved margins
  - Younger patients with larger tumors are at increased risk for local recurrence

FIBROMATOSIS

Key Facts

Terminology
- Neoplastic proliferation of fibroblasts that is locally infiltrative but which does not metastasize

Etiology/Pathogenesis
- Some cases are associated with familial adenomatous polyposis (including Gardner and Turcot syndromes) and germline mutations in *APC* gene
- Sporadic cases are also associated with mutations in *APC* gene (20% of tumors) or β-catenin gene (50% of tumors)
- Minority of cases are associated with prior trauma or surgery

Clinical Issues
- Rare; only 0.2% of breast tumors

- Most patients present with palpable mass or radiologic findings that closely mimic invasive carcinoma
- Local recurrence is common within 1st 3 years (20-30%), even with uninvolved margins

Microscopic Pathology
- Long fascicles of spindle cells that infiltrate around normal ducts and lobules and may infiltrate into muscle

Ancillary Tests
- Fibromatosis characteristically shows aberrant nuclear β-catenin positivity and absence of CD34

- Not all patients with positive margins recur; therefore, careful observation with resection at time of recurrence is possible approach
- Histologic features do not identify tumors most likely to recur

IMAGE FINDINGS

Mammographic Findings
- Irregular dense mass; calcifications are not typical
  - Most typical location is close to, or arising from, pectoralis muscle fascia
  - If lesion is very large, breast can appear retracted and reduced in size

Ultrasonographic Findings
- Irregular mass with thick echogenic rim

MR Findings
- Mass-forming lesion with irregular margins
- Variable enhancement kinetics
  - Some reports of benign gradual enhancement pattern
  - Other enhancement patterns mimic malignancy

MACROSCOPIC FEATURES

General Features
- Firm to rubbery white mass
- Borders can appear circumscribed or irregular, or mass can be ill defined
- Size can range from 1 cm to > 10 cm

MICROSCOPIC PATHOLOGY

Histologic Features
- Long fascicles of spindle cells infiltrate around normal ducts and lobules and may infiltrate into muscle
- Cells are bland with minimal nuclear pleomorphism
- Mitoses are rare

- Lymphocytic aggregates are typically at periphery of tumor
- Stromal collagen bundles may be prominent
- Spindle cells consist of fibroblasts and myofibroblasts
- Diagnosis is often difficult to make on core needle biopsy

ANCILLARY TESTS

Immunohistochemistry
- Majority of tumors have aberrant nuclear β-catenin positivity, as well as typical cytoplasmic positivity
  - Not specific for fibromatosis and may be seen in other benign and malignant tumors
- Tumors frequently have subpopulation of cells positive for muscle markers: Desmin, actin, calponin
- Cells are negative for CD34; only other breast stromal tumor negative for CD34 is nodular fasciitis
- Spindle cell carcinoma should be excluded by use of broad spectrum keratins, including basal-like keratins
- Cells are negative for estrogen and progesterone receptors

DIFFERENTIAL DIAGNOSIS

Spindle Cell Carcinoma (Including Fibromatosis-like Metaplastic Carcinoma)
- Carcinomas generally have greater degree of cellular pleomorphism and more frequent mitoses
  - Fibromatosis-like metaplastic carcinomas can closely resemble fibromatosis
- Carcinomas will be immunoreactive for cytokeratins; it may be necessary to use basal keratins 14 and 17
  - Some spindle cell carcinomas will also be positive for p63

Reactive Changes Due to Prior Surgery or Trauma
- Prior history of surgery or trauma is helpful

FIBROMATOSIS

Fibromatosis and Other Spindle Cell Tumors of Breast

Name	Nuclear β-Catenin	SMA	Desmin	CD34	Keratin	ER
Fibromatosis	Positive (65-80%)	Positive (80%)	Positive (45%)	Negative	Negative	Negative
Nodular fasciitis	Negative	Positive (95%)	Rare (4%)	Negative	Negative	Unknown
Spindle cell carcinoma	May be positive	Positive (50%)	Positive (30%)	Negative	Positive	Negative
Spindle cell sarcoma	Positive (30%)	Positive (variable)	Positive (variable)	May be positive	Negative	Negative
Reactive stromal change	Negative	Positive (few cells)	Negative	Positive	Negative	Negative
Myofibroblastoma	Negative	Positive (75%)	Positive (90%)	Positive (90%)	Negative	Positive

- Inflammatory cells within mass, hemosiderin-laden macrophages, giant cells, and foreign material all favor reactive process to trauma or surgery
- Evaluation of prior excisions of fibromatosis for residual tumor may be difficult

Nodular Fasciitis

- Clinical history should be of rapidly growing painful mass
  - These tumors regress spontaneously within weeks to months
- Typically located in subcutaneous tissue
- Stroma is generally looser (myxoid) and lesion less cellular than fibromatosis
- Also negative for CD34 and can be positive for muscle markers; it should be negative for nuclear β-catenin
- Mitoses are usually present and are often frequent
- Tumor cells are usually haphazardly arranged and not in long fascicles
- Red cell extravasation is characteristic
- Tumor cells generally do not surround normal ducts and lobules
- Inflammatory cells are usually intermingled within tumor, rather than predominantly at periphery as in fibromatosis
- Margins are usually more circumscribed and less infiltrative than fibromatosis

Sarcomas of Breast

- Generally have markedly pleomorphic nuclei
- Mitoses are usually present and may be atypical
- Histologic features of specific sarcoma types may be present (e.g., liposarcoma, rhabdomyosarcoma, osteosarcoma)
- Most sarcomas are highly cellular
- Immunohistochemistry is not definitive, as some sarcomas show nuclear β-catenin positivity

Myofibroblastoma

- Most tumors are circumscribed
- Tumor forms solid mass and does not surround normal ducts and lobules
- Tumor cells are positive for CD34, muscle markers, as well as estrogen and progesterone receptors

Phyllodes Tumors

- Tumors with stromal overgrowth and infiltration into surrounding breast tissue can closely resemble fibromatosis
- Nuclear pleomorphism and mitoses are usually present

- Lesional cells are positive for CD34

DIAGNOSTIC CHECKLIST

Clinically Relevant Pathologic Features

- Local recurrence of fibromatosis after excision is common (20-30%)
  - Even with negative margins of resection
  - Careful observation and close clinical follow-up are warranted

Pathologic Interpretation Pearls

- Diagnosis can be difficult to make on core needle biopsy
  - Excision is usually necessary for definitive diagnosis and for treatment

SELECTED REFERENCES

1. Lee AH: Recent developments in the histological diagnosis of spindle cell carcinoma, fibromatosis and phyllodes tumour of the breast. Histopathology. 52(1):45-57, 2008
2. Neuman HB et al: Desmoid tumors (fibromatoses) of the breast: a 25-year experience. Ann Surg Oncol. 15(1):274-80, 2008
3. Schwarz GS et al: Fibromatosis of the breast: case report and current concepts in the management of an uncommon lesion. Breast J. 12(1):66-71, 2006
4. Brogi E: Benign and malignant spindle cell lesions of the breast. Semin Diagn Pathol. 21(1):57-64, 2004
5. Dunne B et al: An immunohistochemical study of metaplastic spindle cell carcinoma, phyllodes tumor and fibromatosis of the breast. Hum Pathol. 34(10):1009-15, 2003
6. Abraham SC et al: Fibromatosis of the breast and mutations involving the APC/beta-catenin pathway. Hum Pathol. 33(1):39-46, 2002
7. Devouassoux-Shisheboran M et al: Fibromatosis of the breast: age-correlated morphofunctional features of 33 cases. Arch Pathol Lab Med. 124(2):276-80, 2000

FIBROMATOSIS

Gross and Microscopic Features

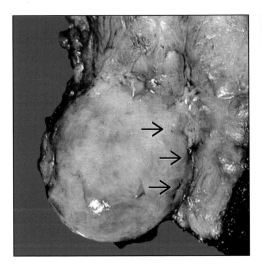

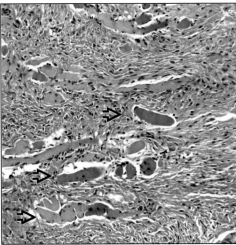

(Left) This case of fibromatosis arose near the chest wall in a young woman who had undergone previous breast reduction surgery. Sutures from the prior procedure are embedded at the periphery ➡. The tumor forms a firm tan mass with lobulated margins and focal infiltration into the adjacent tissue. (Right) Fibromatosis characteristically arises deep within the breast near the chest wall. The tumor cells are seen surrounding muscle fibers of the pectoralis ➡.

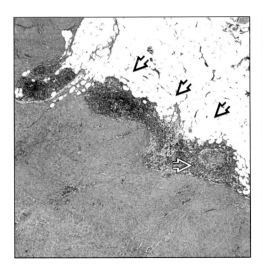

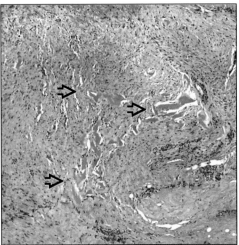

(Left) The edges of fibromatosis can be lobulated or irregular. Dense lymphocytic aggregates are commonly seen at the periphery of the tumor ➡. Germinal centers may be present ➡. Lymphocytic infiltrates within the tumor are not typical of fibromatosis. (Right) Thick bands of collagen may be present within the tumor ➡ and are characteristic. These bands should be distinguished from skeletal muscle.

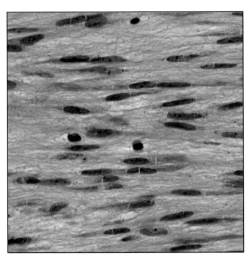

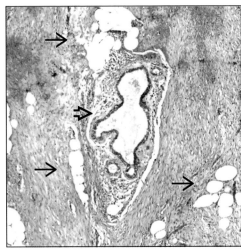

(Left) Minimal nuclear pleomorphism is typical for fibromatosis. Nuclei are usually elongated with rounded ends and small nucleoli. Significant nuclear atypia is more typical of carcinomas, sarcomas, or phyllodes tumors. Mitoses are absent or rare. A high mitotic rate would be more typical of malignant tumors or nodular fasciitis. (Right) Tumor cells surround normal ducts and lobules ➡ and infiltrate into adipose tissue ➡, which may result in formation of an irregular mass.

Ancillary Techniques and Differential Diagnosis

(Left) The majority of cases of fibromatosis show aberrant β-catenin nuclear immunoreactivity ➡ in addition to cytoplasmic immunoreactivity ⮕. However, other spindle cell tumors may also have this pattern. *(Right)* Unlike other stromal lesions of the breast, only fibromatosis and nodular fasciitis are characteristically negative for CD34. In this case, normal blood vessels within the fibromatosis are appropriately positive ➡.

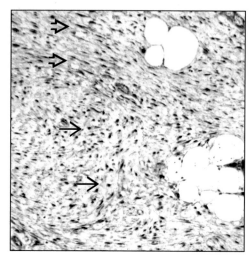 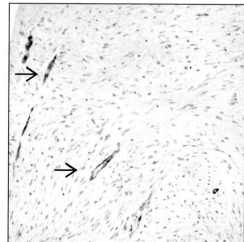

(Left) The cells of fibromatosis typically express muscle markers typical of myofibroblasts, such as actin and myosin. About 1/2 of cases will be immunoreactive for desmin, as in the illustrated case. *(Right)* It is important to confirm that the cells are not immunoreactive for cytokeratins to exclude a spindle cell carcinoma. Multiple cytokeratins, including the basal cytokeratins CK14 and CK17, should be used. An adjacent normal duct is positive for cytokeratin ⮕.

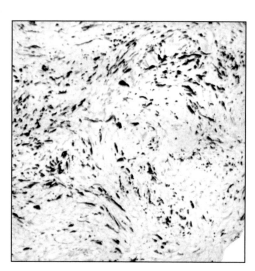 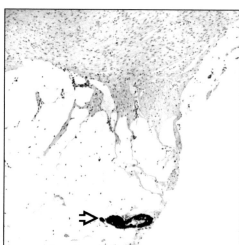

(Left) Spindle cell carcinomas can sometimes appear bland in appearance and resemble fibromatosis, as in this case. Almost all of the spindle cells in this image are carcinoma. *(Right)* This tumor is identified as a spindle cell carcinoma because it is immunoreactive for cytokeratin 14. Myoepithelial cells in an adjacent normal lobule are also positive ➡. Carcinomas are often positive for cytoplasmic β-catenin and 30% are positive for nuclear β-catenin.

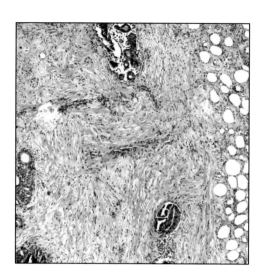 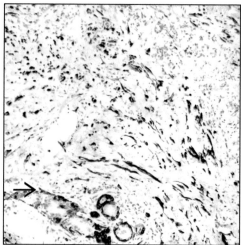

FIBROMATOSIS

Differential Diagnosis

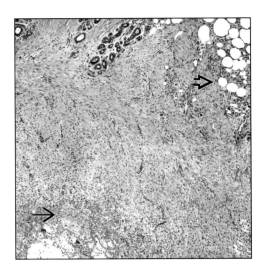

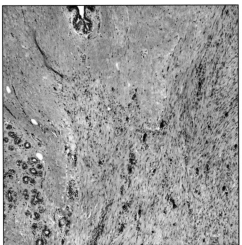

(Left) A clinical history of a prior biopsy is helpful to distinguish biopsy site changes from possible fibromatosis. Usually there is evidence of a biopsy cavity ⇒ and areas of fat necrosis ⊳. Suture material and other foreign material are also diagnostic clues. (Right) In this area of prior surgery, reactive fibroblasts appear to invade into the surrounding normal stroma. The granulation tissue type appearance and hemosiderin-laden macrophages are typical of scar tissue.

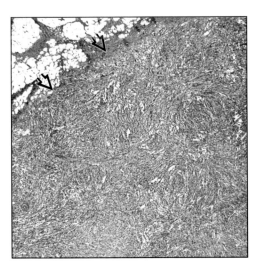

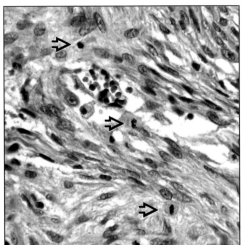

(Left) Nodular fasciitis, like fibromatosis, is also composed of myofibroblast-like cells that are negative for CD34. However, unlike fibromatosis, the cells are usually arranged loosely and not organized into long fascicles. The tumors are also usually more circumscribed ⊳ and not as irregular in shape. (Right) In this case of nodular fasciitis, mitotic figures ⊳ are frequent as is characteristic for this diagnosis. Mitoses are not typically seen in fibromatosis.

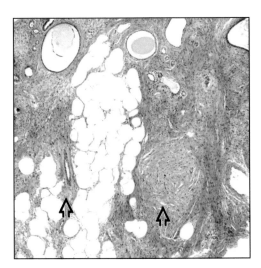

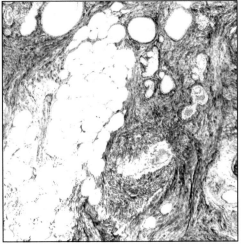

(Left) The infiltrating edge of a phyllodes tumor can resemble fibromatosis as the lesional cells surround normal ducts and lobules ⊳. In some phyllodes tumors, the stromal component is predominant with the epithelial component only present focally. (Right) The majority of stromal lesions of the breast are CD34(+). For example, this phyllodes tumor shows strong CD34 positivity. The exceptions are fibromatosis and nodular fasciitis, both of which are negative for CD34.

HEMANGIOMAS

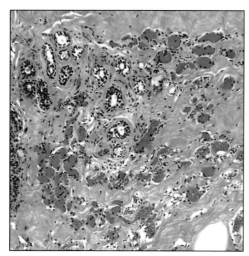

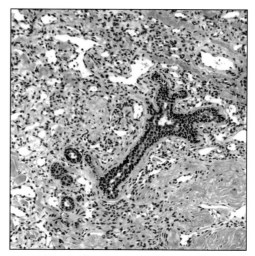

Perilobular hemangiomas are the most common type of vascular lesion in the breast and are usually incidental findings. The small round vessels are clustered in a lobulated mass next to a lobule.

Some benign hemangiomas have an infiltrative pattern with many small anastomosing vessels. Unlike angiosarcomas, however, nuclear pleomorphism, cellular tufting, and solid areas are not present.

TERMINOLOGY

Definitions
- Benign lesions of vascular origin occurring in or near breast parenchyma

ETIOLOGY/PATHOGENESIS

Estrogen
- Possible role for estrogen in development of hemangiomas
  - Hemangiomas are more common in women than in men
  - Hemangiomas at sites other than breast have been reported to
    - Occur after exogenous estrogen treatment
    - Increase in size during pregnancy
  - In a single case, a subcutaneous hemangioma of the breast was diagnosed after initiation of hormone replacement therapy
    - Partial involution was observed after discontinuation of hormone replacement

Hereditary Causes
- Hemangiomas occur as part of several genetic syndromes
  - Kasabach-Merritt syndrome
    - Most common in extremities but can involve any anatomic site, including breast
    - Breast hemangiomas and angiosarcoma have been reported
  - Poland syndrome
    - Unilateral defect of pectoral muscle and ipsilateral syndactyly
    - Breast may be absent or hypoplastic
    - Rarely, congenital hemangiomas may be present
- Tumors typically occur in infancy
- Breast involvement is very rare

CLINICAL ISSUES

Epidemiology
- Incidence
  - Uncommon: ~ 1% of mastectomies or ~ 5% of breast biopsies
    - May be found incidentally on microscopy of biopsy material for other indications
- Age
  - Wide range: 18 months to 82 years
- Gender
  - Males and females affected

Presentation
- Majority are incidental findings in biopsies for other lesions
- Larger hemangiomas can present as palpable mass
  - Some may be seen as red to purple skin lesion
- May also be detected as circumscribed masses on screening mammography

Natural History
- Some lesions may undergo involution or resolve spontaneously

Prognosis
- Hemangiomas are benign
  - Recurrence after incomplete excision has not been reported

Core Needle Biopsy
- Majority of vascular lesions diagnosed on core needle biopsy should undergo excision due to concern for undersampling an angiosarcoma
  - Vessels at periphery of an angiosarcoma can appear deceptively benign
- Majority of image-detected hemangiomas are small circumscribed masses
  - Angiosarcomas are typically larger and have irregular borders

HEMANGIOMAS

Key Facts

Clinical Issues
- Benign vascular lesions that occur in breast parenchyma and skin
- May be detected as palpable masses, circumscribed masses on imaging, or incidental findings
- Recurrence even after incomplete excision has not been reported
- Uncommon: ~ 1% of mastectomies or ~ 5% of breast biopsies
- Majority of vascular lesions diagnosed on core needle biopsy should undergo excision due to concern for undersampling an angiosarcoma

Microscopic Pathology
- Several types of hemangioma
  - Perilobular hemangioma
  - Cavernous hemangioma
  - Capillary hemangioma
  - Complex hemangioma
  - Venous hemangioma
  - Atypical hemangiomas
- Hemangiomas also occur in dermis of breast skin (nonparenchymal)
  - Cutaneous lesions are usually benign capillary hemangiomas
  - Must be distinguished from atypical vascular lesions occurring in skin after radiation treatment

Top Differential Diagnoses
- Low-grade angiosarcoma
- Pseudoangiomatous stromal hyperplasia
- Angiolipoma
- Papillary endothelial hyperplasia

- Changes caused by needle biopsy should not be mistaken for malignancy in excisional specimen
  - Hemorrhage simulating blood lakes
  - Thrombosis and papillary endothelial hyperplasia simulating anastomosing infiltrative vasculature
  - Infarction and necrosis

IMAGE FINDINGS

Mammographic Findings
- Oval or lobulated mass
- Punctate microcalcifications may be present
  - Calcifications likely related to thrombosis and phlebolith formation (coarse or eggshell-like calcifications)

Ultrasonographic Findings
- Oval mass with circumscribed margins

MACROSCOPIC FEATURES

General Features
- Hemangiomas are well-circumscribed, soft, spongy masses
- Rarely palpable
- Reddish brown color

Size
- Typically small (0.5-2 cm)
  - Lesions > 2 cm are more likely to be angiosarcomas

MICROSCOPIC PATHOLOGY

Histologic Features
- **Perilobular hemangioma**
  - Most common vascular breast lesion (1-5% of breast biopsies)
  - Typically, small incidental microscopic finding
  - Often intimately intermingled with lobular and terminal duct epithelial structures but can be located anywhere in breast tissue
  - Vascular spaces are lined by flattened endothelium
  - Vessels are small and rounded with little or no muscular coat
  - Atypical perilobular hemangiomas have hyperchromatic nuclei and may have anastomosing vascular channels
- **Cavernous hemangioma**
  - Composed of large cavernous vascular channels
  - Dilated thin-walled vessels are lined by flattened endothelium, congested with blood
  - Vessels appear separate; anastomosing pattern would be unusual
  - Smaller vessels may be present focally or at periphery
  - Thrombosis may be present with papillary endothelial hyperplasia (Masson lesion)
  - Dystrophic calcification may be found in organizing thrombi
  - Extramedullary hematopoiesis may be present
- **Capillary hemangioma**
  - Composed of capillary-sized well-formed blood vessels
  - Usually form circumscribed or lobulated mass; however, some have irregular margins
  - Cells may have hyperchromatic nuclei
- **Complex hemangioma**
  - Composed of variably sized small blood vessels, sometimes forming irregular anastomosing channels
  - No nuclear pleomorphism or atypia
  - Lesions are usually small (< 1 cm) with circumscribed borders
- **Venous hemangioma**
  - Composed largely of venous channels
  - Disorderly vascular proliferation with smooth muscle walls of varying thickness
  - Vascular spaces may be filled with blood or appear to be empty
- **Atypical hemangiomas**
  - Lesions with features not typical for benign hemangiomas may be classified as atypical
    - Complex anastomosing vessels
    - Central infarction

- Thrombosis with papillary endothelial hyperplasia; can simulate more complex architecture
- Pseudopapillary areas
- Focal endothelial hyperplasia; sometimes in association with thrombosis
- Hemangiomas also occur in dermis of breast skin (nonparenchymal)
  - Cutaneous lesions are usually benign capillary hemangiomas
  - Must be distinguished from atypical vascular lesions occurring in skin after radiation treatment

ANCILLARY TESTS

Immunohistochemistry
- Vascular markers
  - Endothelial cells express CD31, CD34, and factor VIII
- Supporting cell markers
  - Smooth muscle actin can be used to identify muscle coat
- Ki-67
  - Proliferation may be useful to help distinguish between benign and malignant vascular lesions
  - Hemangiomas typically have 4-8% positive endothelial cells
    - May be higher in areas of prior biopsy or thrombosis
  - Angiosarcomas typically have 30-45% positive cells
  - Some overlap in proliferation between benign and malignant lesions
    - Proliferation should not be used alone in making this distinction

DIFFERENTIAL DIAGNOSIS

Low-Grade Angiosarcoma (AS)
- Malignant vascular tumor with anastomosing growth pattern
  - Morphologic spectrum from scattered vessels with bland nuclei to solid sheets of poorly differentiated spindle or epithelioid cells
  - Typically have hyperchromatic endothelial cells, papillary endothelial proliferation, and mitoses
- Usually presents as clinically apparent palpable mass with irregular border
  - Diffuse infiltrative growth pattern invading into breast epithelium
  - Hemangiomas are generally well circumscribed
- Usually > 2 cm and may be many cm in size
  - Hemangiomas are usually small (< 2 cm)
- Ki-67 positivity is higher on average in AS as compared to hemangiomas

Pseudoangiomatous Stromal Hyperplasia (PASH)
- May mimic vascular lesions due to anastomosing slit-like spaces

- Pseudovascular spaces in PASH are not lined by true endothelial cells
  - Spaces do not contain intraluminal red blood cells
  - Lining cells are CD34(+) specialized fibroblasts and not endothelial cells
  - CD31 (endothelial marker) is negative in lining cells

Angiolipoma
- Benign lesion consisting of adipose tissue and small round blood vessels; can be considered a type of hemangioma
- Tumors are circumscribed and appear dense on mammography
  - However, pattern may appear infiltrative in small biopsies
- Presence of hyaline thrombi within vessels is good clue to correct diagnosis

Papillary Endothelial Hyperplasia (PEH)
- Organizing thrombi can closely resemble vascular lesions
- May develop within large vessel or within another vascular lesion such as cavernous hemangioma
  - Margins are circumscribed
  - May be surrounded by smooth muscle or elastic fibers
- May cause difficulty in histological interpretation due to its architectural complexity
  - Peripheral papillary endothelial proliferations surrounding central sclerosis &/or anastomosing vessels
  - Low mitotic activity, with < 1 mitosis per 10 HPF
  - Rarely, areas of necrosis may be identified and should not be misinterpreted as related to malignancy

Angiomatosis
- Very rare vascular lesion consisting of both blood and lymphatic vessels
- Presents as large palpable mass, typically > 9 cm
- Vessels are large throughout lesion and lined by bland endothelial cells
  - Some contain blood, and others appear empty
- Normal breast epithelium is surrounded, but not invaded, by vessels

SELECTED REFERENCES

1. Brodie C et al: Vascular proliferations of the breast. Histopathology. 52(1):30-44, 2008
2. Shin SJ et al: Hemangiomas and angiosarcomas of the breast: diagnostic utility of cell cycle markers with emphasis on Ki-67. Arch Pathol Lab Med. 131(4):538-44, 2007
3. Adwani A et al: Hemangioma of the breast: clinical, mammographic, and ultrasound features. Breast J. 12(3):271, 2006

HEMANGIOMAS

Types of Vascular Lesions

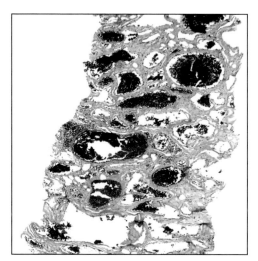 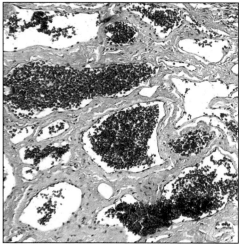

(Left) Cavernous hemangiomas consist of large, dilated, thin-walled vessels within stroma. Thrombosis and dystrophic calcifications may occur in some cases. In complex hemangiomas, vessels of both small and large size are present. *(Right)* The vessels of a cavernous hemangioma are large and dilated. The endothelial cells are present as a single flattened layer. There is no nuclear pleomorphism, tufting, or solid areas. Extramedullary hematopoiesis is sometimes present.

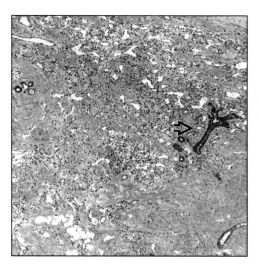 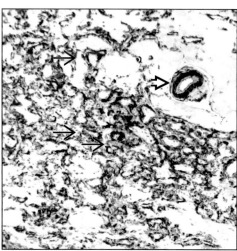

(Left) Some hemangiomas have a diffusely infiltrative pattern that can raise concern for an angiosarcoma. In this case, the vessels infiltrate around a duct and lobule ➡. Nuclear pleomorphism, tufting, and solid areas should be absent. *(Right)* The blood vessels of a hemangioma will usually be accompanied by pericytes positive for smooth muscle actin ➡, as are adjacent normal blood vessels ➡.

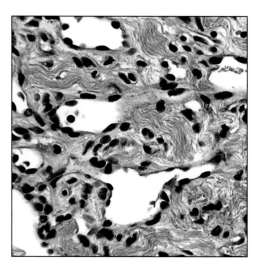 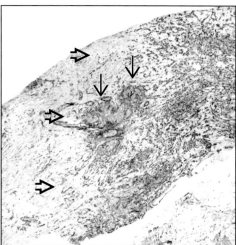

(Left) Hemangiomas may consist of thin-walled irregular anastomosing vessels as seen here. The endothelial cells are flattened and should not show significant nuclear atypia, proliferation, or solid areas. *(Right)* This hemangioma presented as a circumscribed enhancing mass on MR. Although the pattern is complex, as seen on this IHC study for CD34, and the vessels surround normal epithelial structures ➡, the lesion was small and had a histologically well-defined border ➡.

6

DDx: Angiomatosis and Angiolipoma

(Left) Hemangiomas can be detected as small masses ⊳ with smooth contours on mammography, ultrasound, and MR. By MR, they often slowly enhance as compared to malignant lesions. *(**Right**)* Unlike hemangiomas, angiosarcomas typically present as large palpable masses ⊳. The contours can be circumscribed or irregular. Enhancement is seen on MR. Primary angiosarcomas usually arise in the breast, as in this case. Angiosarcomas after radiation therapy typically involve the skin.

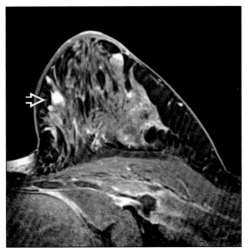
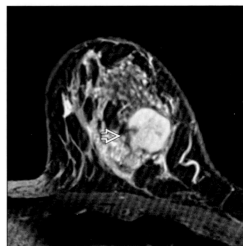

*(**Left**)* Angiomatosis is a rare benign tumor of the breast that presents as a large palpable mass. The vascular spaces have large calibers and are uniform throughout the lesion. Some of the spaces are filled with blood. Others are empty and may be abnormal lymphatic channels. *(Courtesy S. Schnitt, MD.)* *(**Right**)* Angiomatosis forms around lobules ⊳ rather than infiltrating into them. The lining cells have small bland nuclei and may be difficult to discern ⊳. *(Courtesy S. Schnitt, MD.)*

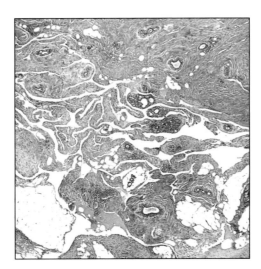
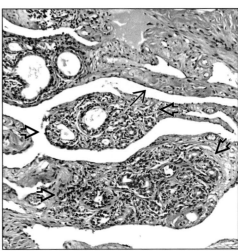

*(**Left**)* Angiolipomas are benign neoplasms consisting of adipose tissue and small rounded blood vessels. The borders are well circumscribed ⊳. They can be considered a type of hemangioma. *(**Right**)* Fibrin thrombi ⊳ are a characteristic finding in angiolipomas. Thrombi are not typically found in other types of vascular lesions. Unlike subcutaneous angiolipomas, lesions in the breast are rarely reported to be painful.

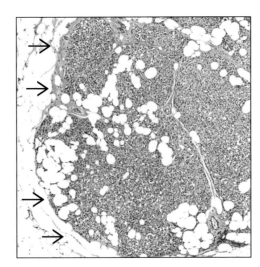
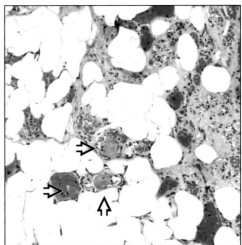

HEMANGIOMAS

Differential Diagnosis

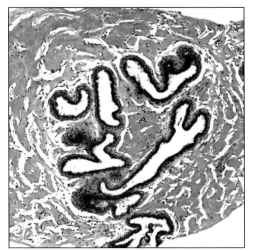
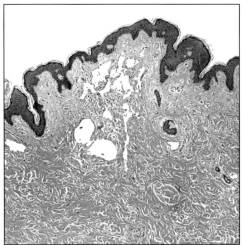

(Left) Pseudoangiomatous stromal hyperplasia consists of prominent clefts in stroma that mimic vascular channels. The spaces are empty, and the lining cells are fibroblasts rather than endothelium. *(Right)* Atypical vascular lesions may occur in the skin after radiation treatment for breast cancer. The majority consist of empty spaces and may arise from lymphatics. A subset appear to be derived from blood vessels and must be distinguished from hemangiomas and angiosarcomas.

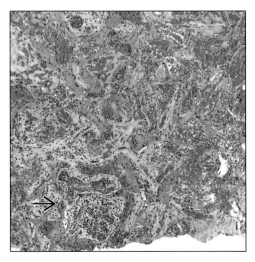
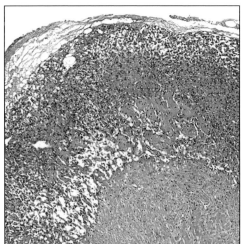

(Left) This angiosarcoma is composed of large dilated vessels filled with blood. The malignant blood vessels invade into and around lobules ➡ in a complex pattern. *(Right)* Papillary endothelial hyperplasia (PEH or Masson lesion) is an organizing thrombus. When within a vessel, it is easy to recognize. However, these lesions can closely mimic angiosarcomas (AS). The borders should be well circumscribed.

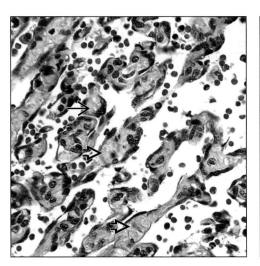
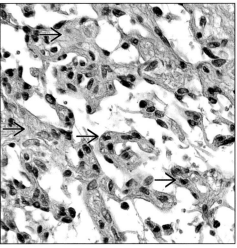

(Left) Unlike PEH, in AS the malignant vascular cells show nuclear pleomorphism ➡ and invade into stroma ➡ rather than being present within a localized area of organizing fibrin. *(Right)* In the center of PEH, the cells surrounding organizing fibrin ➡ can closely mimic anastomosing blood vessels. However, nuclear pleomorphism and solid areas should not be seen. The pseudovessels are restricted to a generally circumscribed mass and do not infiltrate into the adjacent tissue.

ATYPICAL VASCULAR LESIONS OF SKIN

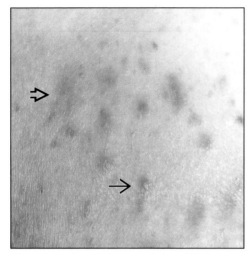

The majority of atypical vascular lesions (AVLs) present as small raised brown papules in the radiation field ⇨. The 2nd most common appearance is as an ill-defined erythematous patch ⇲.

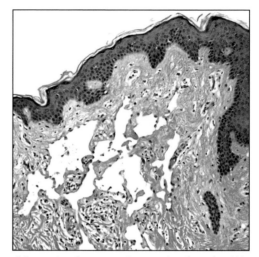

AVLs consist of anastomosing vascular channels within the dermis. The spaces usually appear empty (appearing as flesh-colored papules) but may be filled with blood (appearing as erythematous plaques).

TERMINOLOGY

Abbreviations
- Atypical vascular lesion (AVL)

Synonyms
- Benign lymphangiomatous papules
- Lymphangioma circumscriptum
- Benign lymphangioendothelioma
- Acquired progressive lymphangioma
- Acquired lymphangiectasis

Definitions
- Proliferation of endothelial-like cells within dermis of skin several years after exposure to therapeutic radiation treatment

ETIOLOGY/PATHOGENESIS

Etiology
- These lesions are only seen in clinical setting of prior radiation treatment for carcinoma
  - Young women treated with radiation therapy for Hodgkin disease are at increased risk for breast carcinoma
    - AVLs have not been reported following radiation for Hodgkin disease
  - Reason why Hodgkin disease patients are not affected is not known
    - May be related to age at exposure and dosage
- Radiation may damage cells lining lymphatics and small blood vessels
  - Radiation damage may cause abnormal proliferation
- Typical time from radiation exposure to diagnosis of AVL: 3-4 years

CLINICAL ISSUES

Epidemiology
- Gender
  - Only women have been reported to be affected

Presentation
- 2 types of AVLs
  - Lymphatic type (2/3)
    - Present as soft, flesh-colored (or pink to brown) papules, fluid-filled vesicles, or plaques
  - Vascular type (1/3)
    - Present as erythematous plaques or nodules
    - Gross appearance can closely mimic angiosarcoma
  - Patients may have lesions of both types

Treatment
- Complete excision of lesion is generally required for diagnosis and treatment
  - In some cases, diagnostic features of angiosarcoma are apparent after complete excision
  - Benign-appearing lesions may progress to angiosarcoma over period of years
    - Complete excision may reduce likelihood of this

Prognosis
- Majority of cases do not recur or develop malignancy after complete excision
  - However, 10-20% of patients experience recurrence at same site with AVL or develop new lesions
- Rare patients progress to cutaneous angiosarcomas
  - It may be difficult to determine if angiosarcoma arose from AVL or is independent lesion

MACROSCOPIC FEATURES

General Features
- Initial specimen may be incisional biopsy
  - Skin lesion is usually not discernible in these small specimens

ATYPICAL VASCULAR LESIONS OF SKIN

Key Facts

Terminology

- Proliferation of endothelial-like cells within dermis of skin several years after exposure to therapeutic radiation treatment

Etiology/Pathogenesis

- These lesions are only seen in clinical setting of prior radiation treatment

Clinical Issues

- Lesions appear as fluid-filled vesicles or soft flesh-colored papules of skin
- Complete excision of lesion is generally required for diagnosis and treatment
- Majority of cases do not recur or develop malignancy after complete excision
- Rare patients may develop angiosarcomas

Microscopic Pathology

- Lesions consist of complex anastomosing vascular channels in dermis
- Subcutaneous tissue or breast parenchyma is generally not involved
- 2 types
  - Lymphatic type (most common): Vessels are empty or filled with clear fluid
  - Vascular type (less common): Vessels are filled with blood

Top Differential Diagnoses

- Angiosarcoma
- Cutaneous hemangiomas
- Acquired progressive lymphangioma
- Reactive angioendotheliosis

- In complete excisions, raised papule or vesicular lesion should be evident

Sections to Be Submitted

- Specimens must be oriented and margins inked
  - Different colors of ink may be used to designate specific margins
  - In general, specimens are small and can be completely examined microscopically
- Sections are taken perpendicular to skin surface
  - Each margin should be identifiable by ink color or location

Size

- Lesions are generally small (0.1-2 cm) as compared to size of typical angiosarcoma (median: 7.5 cm)
- Lesions are generally solitary but may be multiple (2-4)

MICROSCOPIC PATHOLOGY

Histologic Features

- Lesions consist of large dilated vessels in dermis
- Nuclei are small and bland without prominent nucleoli
- Lumens are empty or filled with clear fluid; blood may be present in vascular type
  - If there has been prior biopsy, there may be hemorrhage from prior procedure
- Lesion is restricted to dermis
  - Involvement of subcutaneous tissue is unusual; if present, it should be very focal
- Mitoses should not be present
- Single layer of lining cells; papillary tufts or solid areas are not present

ANCILLARY TESTS

Immunohistochemistry

- Endothelial cells are positive for CD31, CD34, factor VIII, and D2-40

- Therefore, IHC is not helpful to distinguish AVL from other vascular lesions in differential diagnosis

DIFFERENTIAL DIAGNOSIS

Angiosarcoma

- Most important, and most difficult, lesion to distinguish from AVL
  - Prognosis for these 2 lesions markedly different
  - Clinical and histologic features of these 2 lesions may overlap, and it may not be possible to make definitive diagnosis
  - Complete excision and microscopic examination of AVLs is recommended to ensure areas diagnostic of angiosarcoma are not missed
- Angiosarcomas can usually be distinguished from AVL based on their histologic features
  - Marked nuclear pleomorphism
  - Red blood cells within lumens
  - Extravasated red blood cells and blood lakes
  - Mitoses
  - Tufting within lumens
  - Solid areas
  - Involvement of subcutaneous tissue and breast tissue
- Immunohistochemical studies are not helpful as both lesions are positive for vascular makers

Cutaneous Hemangiomas

- Lesions also consist of dilated blood vessels in skin
- Vessels have round contours; complex anastomosing channels should not be present
- Lumens are filled with blood
- Lesions occur primarily in patients without history of radiation therapy

Acquired Progressive Lymphangioma (Benign Lymphangioendothelioma)

- Occurs in both men and women over wide age range
- H&N most common site, followed by limbs and trunk

ATYPICAL VASCULAR LESIONS OF SKIN

Distinguishing Atypical Vascular Lesions from Radiation-related Angiosarcomas

Feature	Atypical Vascular Lesion	Angiosarcoma
Clinical presentation	Flesh-colored or brown papule or vesicle of skin or erythematous plaque	Red or violaceous skin lesion, often with palpable mass
Size	Generally small (0.5-1 cm)	Generally large (median: 7-8 cm)
Location	Restricted to dermis; rarely may involve subcutis	Dermis with frequent involvement of subcutaneous adipose tissue and breast tissue
Anastomosing vessels	Present	Present
Content of vessels	Empty or clear fluid; blood may be present in a subset or may be present after trauma (biopsy)	Blood; extravasation and blood lakes may be present
Nuclear pleomorphism	Absent	Usually present
Mitoses	Absent	May be present
Solid areas	Absent	May be present
Chronic inflammation	Often present	Not typical
Circumscription	Generally circumscribed, symmetrical, and wedge-shaped	Typically has raggedly infiltrative borders
Papillary endothelial hyperplasia	Absent	Usually present
Prominent nucleoli	Usually absent	Usually present
Blood lakes	Absent	Often present
Hyperchromatic nuclei	Present	Present

- Usually single affected site; skin lesions may be macular or papular and are pigmented
- Microscopically, anastomosing dilated vessels lined by flattened endothelium are present in superficial dermis
- Spaces may be empty or contain red blood cells
- Cytologic atypia and mitoses are absent
- Local recurrence has been reported

Reactive Angioendotheliosis
- Occurs in both men and women from ages 40-90
- Majority of patients have systemic disease (e.g., renal failure, valvular cardiac disease, malignancy, autoimmune disease)
- Approximately 1/2 of patients are immunosuppressed due to treatment modalities
- Patients present with multiple erythematous skin lesions
  - Limbs are most commonly affected
  - Macules, masses, and plaques may be present
  - Ulceration may occur
- Lesions may resolve, stabilize, or progress
- Microscopically, there is proliferation of small capillaries in dermis
  - Many of vessels contain fibrin thrombi
- Some cases are reported to be positive for HHV8 latent nuclear antigen

SELECTED REFERENCES

1. Lucas DR: Angiosarcoma, radiation-associated angiosarcoma, and atypical vascular lesion. Arch Pathol Lab Med. 133(11):1804-9, 2009
2. Uchin JM et al: Radiotherapy-associated atypical vascular lesions of the breast. J Cutan Pathol. 36(1):87-8, 2009
3. Patton KT et al: Atypical vascular lesions after surgery and radiation of the breast: a clinicopathologic study of 32 cases analyzing histologic heterogeneity and association with angiosarcoma. Am J Surg Pathol. 32(6):943-50, 2008
4. Gengler C et al: Vascular proliferations of the skin after radiation therapy for breast cancer: clinicopathologic analysis of a series in favor of a benign process: a study from the French Sarcoma Group. Cancer. 109(8):1584-98, 2007
5. Mattoch IW et al: Post-radiotherapy vascular proliferations in mammary skin: a clinicopathologic study of 11 cases. J Am Acad Dermatol. 57(1):126-33, 2007
6. Brenn T et al: Postradiation vascular proliferations: an increasing problem. Histopathology. 48(1):106-14, 2006
7. Brenn T et al: Radiation-associated cutaneous atypical vascular lesions and angiosarcoma: clinicopathologic analysis of 42 cases. Am J Surg Pathol. 29(8):983-96, 2005
8. Di Tommaso L et al: The capillary lobule: a deceptively benign feature of post-radiation angiosarcoma of the skin: report of three cases. Am J Dermatopathol. 27(4):301-5, 2005
9. McMenamin ME et al: Reactive angioendotheliomatosis: a study of 15 cases demonstrating a wide clinicopathologic spectrum. Am J Surg Pathol. 26(6):685-97, 2002
10. Requena L et al: Benign vascular proliferations in irradiated skin. Am J Surg Pathol. 26(3):328-37, 2002
11. Guillou L et al: Benign lymphangioendothelioma (acquired progressive lymphangioma): a lesion not to be confused with well-differentiated angiosarcoma and patch stage Kaposi's sarcoma: clinicopathologic analysis of a series. Am J Surg Pathol. 24(8):1047-57, 2000
12. Fineberg S et al: Cutaneous angiosarcoma and atypical vascular lesions of the skin and breast after radiation therapy for breast carcinoma. Am J Clin Pathol. 102(6):757-63, 1994

ATYPICAL VASCULAR LESIONS OF SKIN

Microscopic Features

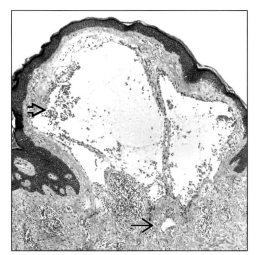

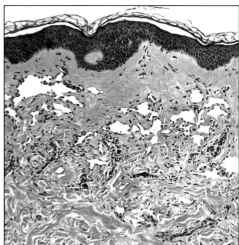

(Left) The most common type of AVL consists of markedly dilated vessels in the dermis forming a flesh-colored papule. In this case, some blood is present within the lumens due to prior trauma ⇗, but blood is not seen in the smaller vessels ➡. *(Right)* The anastomosing vascular channels infiltrate within the dermis but should not extend into the subcutaneous tissue.

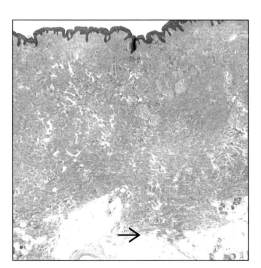

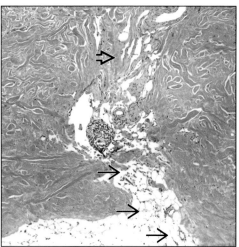

(Left) This is a large AVL presenting as a macular skin lesion with abnormal vessels involving the full thickness of the dermis. The vessels very focally involve the adipose tissue of the breast ➡. *(Right)* The majority of the vessels are present in the dermis ⇗. A few of the vessels extend into the adipose tissue of the breast ➡, an unusual feature for an AVL. In this case, no other feature suggesting a diagnosis of angiosarcoma was present.

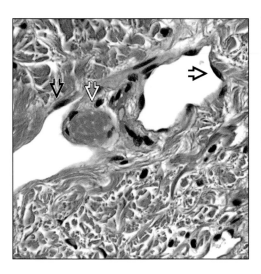

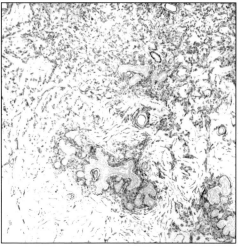

(Left) The cells lining the spaces in AVLs may be hyperchromatic, but they show minimal nuclear atypia and do not form papillary tufts or solid areas ⇗. The spaces are generally empty. In this case, the vessels surround a normal capillary filled with blood ⇗. *(Right)* The endothelial cells of AVL are positive for CD31, CD34, factor VIII, and D2-40. This is a case of a very unusual benign vascular lesion involving deeper breast tissue. The cells are positive for CD34.

ANGIOSARCOMA

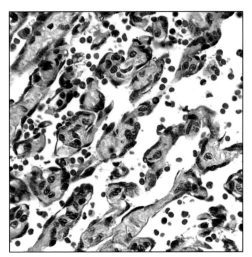

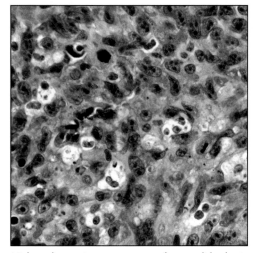

Angiosarcomas are composed of a malignant population of endothelial-type cells forming complex anastomosing channels. The lumens are filled with red blood cells.

High-grade angiosarcomas can form solid sheets of epithelioid-appearing cells. Immunohistochemical studies may be necessary to distinguish recurrent carcinoma from radiation-induced angiosarcoma.

TERMINOLOGY

Abbreviations
- Angiosarcoma (AS)

Definitions
- Malignant neoplasm arising from endothelial cells or their precursors

ETIOLOGY/PATHOGENESIS

Idiopathic
- Breast is most common site of origin of AS
  - However, AS are rare tumors compared to carcinomas (< 0.1% of all breast malignancies)

Radiation
- Women who have received radiation treatment for breast cancer have 9x increased risk of AS
  - However, absolute number of affected women is small: Approximately 3 in 1,000 women will develop AS after treatment at 15 years
  - Women who received chest wall radiation for Hodgkin disease are at increased risk for developing breast cancer, but AS has not been reported
    - Reason for this is unknown; probably related to age when radiated &/or radiation doses
- Incidence of tumors peaks from 5-10 years after treatment and is elevated out to 30 years

Edema
- Women with markedly edematous arms after breast and axillary surgery for cancer are at increased risk for AS of skin (Stewart-Treves syndrome)
- With more limited axillary surgery and better surgical techniques, this type of AS has become exceedingly uncommon

CLINICAL ISSUES

Epidemiology
- Age
  - Average age of women diagnosed with idiopathic AS: 40s
  - Average age of women diagnosed with radiation-related or edema-related AS: 60s
- Gender
  - Almost all patients are female; male breast AS is very rare

Site
- Idiopathic AS generally arises deep in the breast
  - Large tumors may also involve the skin
- Radiation-related AS arises in the skin
  - Tumors involve deeper breast tissue if large
  - Atypical vascular lesions (AVLs) also occur in the skin in this group of patients
  - Distinguishing AS from AVL may be difficult in some cases
- Edema-related AS arises in the skin of edematous area
  - Arm is most common site

Presentation
- Patients with radiation-related or edema-related AS present with dark red or violaceous discoloration of skin
  - Palpable mass may be associated with skin changes
- Patients with idiopathic angiosarcoma present with ill-defined palpable mass in the breast

Treatment
- Most effective treatment is surgical removal of tumor with wide margins
  - Most patients will require mastectomy to achieve this goal
- Chemotherapy and radiation therapy are also used but have uncertain benefit

ANGIOSARCOMA

Key Facts

Terminology
- Malignant neoplasm arising from endothelial cells or their precursors

Etiology/Pathogenesis
- Breast is most common site of origin of angiosarcomas; however, they comprise < 0.1% of breast malignancies
- 3 groups of women who develop breast angiosarcomas
  - Idiopathic cases with no known cause
  - Women with history of breast cancer who have received radiation therapy
  - Women with markedly edematous arms after breast and axillary surgery for cancer (Stewart-Treves syndrome)

Clinical Issues
- Idiopathic AS presents as ill-defined palpable mass in the breast
- Radiation-related or edema-related AS presents with dark red or violaceous discoloration of skin
- Most effective treatment is surgical removal of tumor with wide margins
- Median survival: 3 years

Top Differential Diagnoses
- Perilobular hemangioma
- Proliferative endothelial hyperplasia
- Atypical vascular lesion (AVL)
- Pseudoangiomatous stromal hyperplasia (PASH)
- Carcinoma
- Angiolipoma

Prognosis
- Many patients develop distant metastases
  - Most common sites are lung, liver, bone, and contralateral breast
  - Metastasis to regional lymph nodes is rare
- Median survival: 3 years
  - Same for idiopathic and treatment-related AS
- Larger tumors have poorer prognosis
  - Tumor grade has not been consistently linked to prognosis

IMAGE FINDINGS

Mammographic Findings
- Tumors may be difficult to image as desmoplastic response commonly associated with carcinomas is not present

Ultrasonographic Findings
- Tumors may appear lobulated, irregular, or ill defined
- Echogenicity may be variable
  - May have hyperechoic areas if AS invades into adipose tissue

MACROSCOPIC FEATURES

Size
- Tumors vary in size
  - Range: 1-20 cm
  - Average: 5 cm
  - Majority > 2 cm
    - Almost all vascular lesions of the breast > 2 cm in size will be malignant
- Size can be difficult to determine grossly both visually and by palpation
  - Central portion of the tumor is usually hemorrhagic and firm to palpation
  - Infiltrative periphery of the tumor can blend into surrounding tissue and may not be visible

MICROSCOPIC PATHOLOGY

Histologic Features
- Tumor consists of abnormal blood vessels
  - Blood vessels are increased in number
  - Vessels may be present in dermis &/or breast stroma and may invade into lobules
  - Borders are infiltrative and not well circumscribed
  - Vessels form complex anastomosing channels
  - In high-grade tumors, solid areas without evident vessel formation may be present
    - Blood lakes due to massive extravasation from tumor vessels are helpful diagnostic feature
    - Necrosis may be present
    - These features need to be distinguished from the possible effects of prior diagnostic biopsy
- Tumor cells are abnormal in appearance
  - Nuclei may be enlarged and pleomorphic
  - Frequent mitotic figures may be seen
  - Number of endothelial cells may be increased to form papillary tufts within vessel lumens

ANCILLARY TESTS

Immunohistochemistry
- Tumor cells will be immunoreactive for markers of endothelial cells
  - Factor VIII is very specific but may not be positive in all tumors
  - CD34 is very sensitive but is also positive in fibroblastic lesions and in other types of sarcomas
  - CD31 is sensitive marker
- Tumor cells can also be immunoreactive for cytokeratin
  - Usually focal or weak as compared to carcinomas
  - Panels to distinguish carcinoma from AS should include both epithelial and endothelial markers

ANGIOSARCOMA

Grading of Angiosarcomas

Feature	Low Grade	Intermediate Grade	High Grade
Nuclear pleomorphism	Minimal	Intermediate	Marked
Blood lakes	Absent	Absent	Present
Necrosis	Absent	Absent	Present
Solid foci	Absent	Absent/focal	Present
Endothelial tufting	May be focal	Present	Frequent
Mitoses	Absent or rare	Present	Frequent

DIFFERENTIAL DIAGNOSIS

Hemangioma
- Benign proliferations of blood vessels; almost all < 2 cm in size
  - Small (perilobular or capillary) hemangiomas are almost always small incidental findings (0.1-0.2 cm)
  - Larger (cavernous or venous) hemangiomas may be palpable or present as mass on imaging
- Borders are circumscribed or lobulated, but some vessels may extend into adjacent stroma
- There is no or minimal nuclear pleomorphism; mitoses are absent

Proliferative Endothelial Hyperplasia (PEH, Masson Lesion, Organizing Thrombus)
- These lesions of reactive endothelial cells can closely mimic AS
- There may be history of prior trauma or surgery
- Borders are usually circumscribed; pseudovascular spaces should not infiltrate into surrounding breast tissue
  - Some lesions occur within blood vessels
- Areas of thrombus without ingrowth of endothelial cells or fibroblasts can be mistaken for blood lake
- Lesion is very rare in the breast; much less common than AS
- Majority of cases are much smaller than 2 cm in size

Atypical Vascular Lesion (AVL)
- Occurs in skin after therapeutic radiation exposure
- Lesions usually are seen clinically as flesh-colored raised papules or flat erythematous plaques
- Vascular proliferation is confined to dermis
- Spaces appear empty, and majority do not contain red blood cells
  - If there has been prior diagnostic biopsy, hemorrhage from surgery may be present
- These lesions should be completely excised
  - Some cases are difficult to distinguish from AS until entire lesion is completely examined
  - In rare cases, it is possible AVL could progress to AS

Pseudoangiomatous Stromal Hyperplasia (PASH)
- Presents as palpable mass or radiologic density
  - Not associated with hemorrhage and does not involve skin or cause hemorrhagic skin lesions
- Proliferation of myofibroblasts is associated with stromal clefting that mimics anastomosing blood vessels
  - Because proliferation is "pseudoangiomatous," spaces are empty without red blood cells
- Stromal clefting can dissect into lobules, simulating the invasive pattern of angiosarcoma
- Nuclear pleomorphism, mitoses, and solid areas (or tufting) are absent

Carcinoma
- Women with history of breast cancer and radiation therapy are at risk for both recurrent carcinoma and treatment-related AS
- Poorly differentiated carcinoma and poorly differentiated AS can be similar in histologic appearance
- Some carcinomas have pseudovascular pattern
- In some cases, IHC for epithelial and endothelial markers may be necessary for diagnosis

Angiolipoma
- Benign lesions composed of adipose tissue and small round capillary-sized blood vessels
- Lesions are well circumscribed and usually small (< 2 cm)
- Cellular pleomorphism and mitoses are absent

REPORTING CRITERIA

Tumor Grade and Stage
- Angiosarcomas can be divided into 3 groups according to grade
  - Some studies have shown that grade correlates with clinical outcome
  - However, in a recent study grade did not predict outcome
- There is no AJCC staging system for AS of the breast

SELECTED REFERENCES

1. Mobini N: Cutaneous epithelioid angiosarcoma: a neoplasm with potential pitfalls in diagnosis. J Cutan Pathol. 36(3):362-9, 2009
2. Nascimento AF et al: Primary angiosarcoma of the breast: clinicopathologic analysis of 49 cases, suggesting that grade is not prognostic. Am J Surg Pathol. 32(12):1896-904, 2008
3. Branton PA et al: Papillary endothelial hyperplasia of the breast: the great impostor for angiosarcoma: a clinicopathologic review of 17 cases. Int J Surg Pathol. 11(2):83-7, 2003

ANGIOSARCOMA

Gross and Microscopic Features

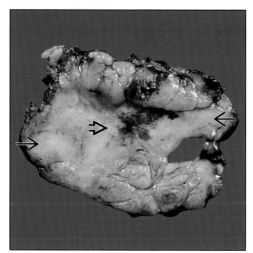
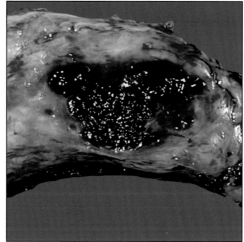

(Left) This is an idiopathic intermediate-grade AS arising deep in the breast. The central area of the tumor can be seen grossly as areas of hemorrhage ⟐. However, the tumor also extends into the adjacent fibrous tissue where it could not be seen or palpated grossly ⟐. *(Right)* This idiopathic AS is within the breast parenchyma, and the skin is not involved. Blood lakes and cystic degeneration are grossly evident.

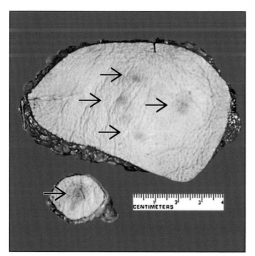
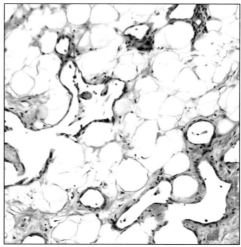

(Left) Angiosarcoma is seen as red-tan flat lesions in these 2 excisions ⟐ from a patient who developed multiple ASs of the upper arm due to chronic lymphedema after a radical mastectomy for breast cancer (Stewart-Treves syndrome). *(Right)* This low-grade AS is composed of deceptively bland-appearing blood vessels infiltrating in fat without a stromal response. However, note the complex branching pattern and tufting of endothelial cells that are not seen in benign vascular lesions.

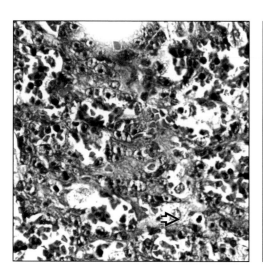
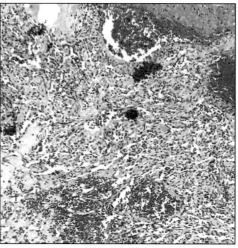

(Left) This high-grade AS forms blood vessels, but solid nests of tumor cells are also present. The nuclei are large and pleomorphic, and mitoses are frequent ⟐. Some high-grade ASs resemble poorly differentiated carcinomas. *(Right)* In this high-grade AS, blood lakes and extravasated red blood cells are present.

ANGIOSARCOMA

Microscopic Features

(Left) This low-grade AS would be difficult to identify based on this image. Although the blood vessels are increased in number, the branching is not complex and the endothelial cells are bland. The periphery of higher grade AS can have this deceptively benign appearance. *(Right)* This high-grade AS has a predominant spindle cell appearance. The vascular spaces are poorly formed. This type of AS may be difficult to distinguish from other types of sarcomas or a spindle cell carcinoma.

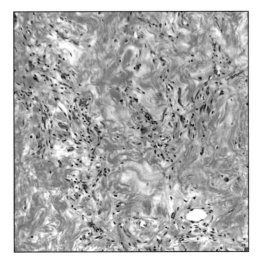
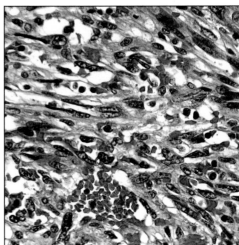

(Left) This is a post-radiation AS. The malignant cells are proliferating within the dermis. In most cases, the subcutaneous tissue will also be involved. This can be a helpful feature as atypical vascular lesions should not extend deeper than the dermis. *(Right)* The endothelial cells of AS can proliferate to form solid areas or papillary tufts ⊟ within the lumens of the neoplastic vessels.

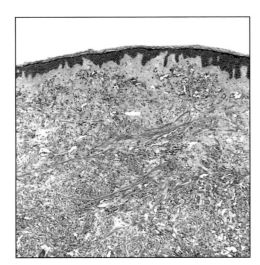
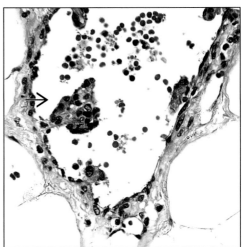

(Left) The malignant vessels of this AS invade into a benign lobule. Benign vascular lesions usually do not involve lobules. However, the myofibroblasts of PASH can mimic this appearance. *(Right)* Most women with AS eventually develop distant metastases. A common metastatic site for AS is the lung. In this case, tumor emboli are also readily apparent in adjacent lymph-vascular spaces ⊡.

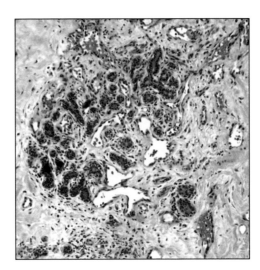
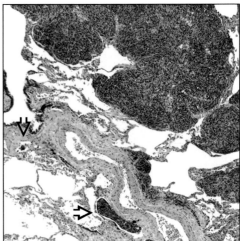

ANGIOSARCOMA

Differential Diagnosis

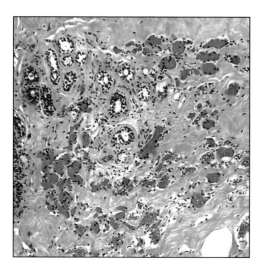

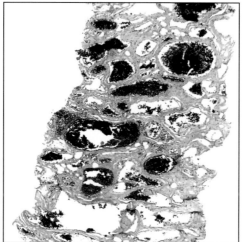

(Left) Perilobular hemangiomas are usually small (0.1-0.2 cm) incidental findings. They are composed of minute round blood vessels, often surrounding or within a lobule. *(Right)* Larger hemangiomas may present as palpable masses or densities by imaging. The lesions consist of dilated thin-walled vessels filled with blood and thromboses, as seen in this core needle biopsy.

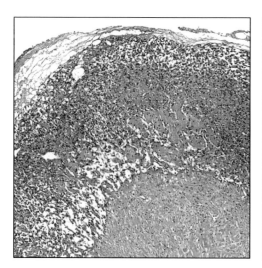

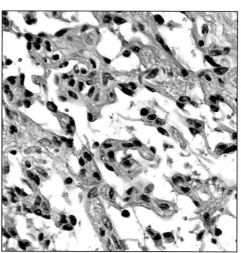

(Left) Papillary endothelial hyperplasia (PEH) is an organizing thrombus. Most cases have a circumscribed border, and some are confined within a blood vessel. The majority are larger than 2 cm in size. *(Right)* On high power, the reactive fibroblasts and fibrin in the center of PEH can closely mimic the anastomosing channels of AS. Correct diagnosis requires examination of the edges of the lesion.

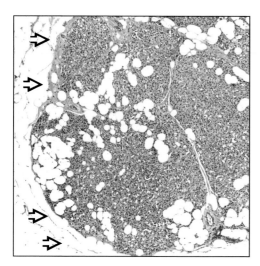

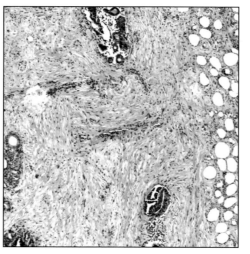

(Left) Angiolipomas are composed of adipose tissue and a proliferation of small capillary-sized blood vessels. The margins are well circumscribed ⧐. If the entire lesion were removed, it would be unlikely to be confused with AS. Diagnosis on core needle biopsy may be more difficult. *(Right)* Some AS have an epithelioid appearance, and some carcinomas have a spindle cell pattern (as in this case) or a pseudovascular appearance. IHC may be necessary for the correct classification.

SARCOMAS

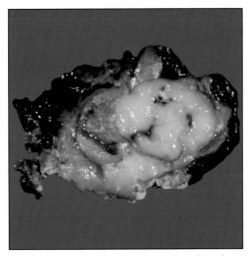

A 19-year old female patient presented with a circumscribed palpable mass lesion thought to be a fibroadenoma based on clinical exam and imaging. Needle biopsy showed an undifferentiated malignancy.

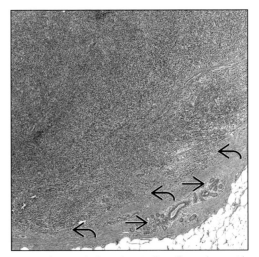

Section shows a high-grade spindle cell neoplasm with pushing borders ⇗, compressing adjacent breast tissue ⇨. Further work-up showed this tumor to be a rhabdomyosarcoma. Staging studies were negative.

TERMINOLOGY

Definitions

- Malignant mesenchymal neoplasm derived from connective tissue elements of the breast
  - Sarcomas of the breast are rare
  - Sarcomatous-appearing tumors more likely to be metaplastic carcinoma or malignant phyllodes
  - Mammary sarcoma should be diagnosis of exclusion
- Sarcoma involving breast tissue can be broadly divided into 3 categories
  - Idiopathic (de novo) sporadic cases (primary)
  - Post therapy (secondary)
  - Metastatic
- Any sarcoma that occurs elsewhere can occur in the beast as a primary tumor
  - Angiosarcoma is most common primary sarcoma followed by liposarcoma

ETIOLOGY/PATHOGENESIS

Environmental Exposure

- Etiology of most soft tissue sarcomas remains unknown
- Primary mammary sarcoma of the breast can be de novo or secondary to prior treatment for carcinoma
  - Sporadic sarcomas tend to occur in younger age group
  - Sarcomas associated with prior use of breast external beam radiation therapy
    - Most common: Angiosarcoma, malignant fibrous histiocytoma, fibrosarcoma
  - Sarcomas association with chronic lymphedema that occurs after surgery with or without radiation treatment
    - Stewart-Treves syndrome
    - Lymphedema-associated lymphangiosarcoma

CLINICAL ISSUES

Epidemiology

- Incidence
  - Mammary sarcomas: < 0.1% of breast malignancies
    - Primary sarcomas (other than angiosarcoma) are exceedingly rare
    - Annual incidence of breast sarcomas: 4.6 cases per 1,000,000 women

Presentation

- Most common presentation: Palpable mass
  - Often rapidly enlarging

Natural History

- Based on histologic type of tumor, grade, and stage at presentation
- May show aggressive behavior with high likelihood for local/systemic recurrence
  - Hematogenous dissemination
    - Metastases to lungs, bone marrow, and liver are most common
    - Metastases to axillary lymph node are exceedingly rare

Treatment

- Surgical approaches
  - Surgical excision with clean margins
    - Total mastectomy is most common
    - Smaller lesion may be treated with breast-conserving therapy
  - Axillary dissection is not indicated given the rarity of lymph node involvement
- Adjuvant therapy
  - Any role for adjuvant chemotherapy &/or radiation therapy is unclear

Prognosis

- Primary mammary sarcomas have prognosis similar to that of their soft tissue counterparts

SARCOMAS

Key Facts

Terminology
- Malignant mesenchymal neoplasm derived from connective tissue elements of the breast

Etiology/Pathogenesis
- Mammary sarcoma can be de novo or secondary to prior treatment for carcinoma

Clinical Issues
- Most common presentation: Palpable mass
- Prognosis depends on histologic type of tumor, grade, and stage at presentation
  - May show aggressive behavior with local/systemic recurrence
  - Metastases to lungs, bone marrow, and liver most common
  - Metastases to lymph nodes are rare
  - Tumor size is significantly associated with survival

Microscopic Pathology
- Virtually any type of sarcoma described elsewhere may occur rarely as primary lesion in the breast
  - Liposarcoma, leiomyosarcoma, osteosarcoma, and pleomorphic spindle cell sarcoma most common

Top Differential Diagnoses
- **Metaplastic carcinoma**
  - Can show prominent sarcomatous differentiation
  - Immunostains for cytokeratin important to help confirm diagnosis
- **Phyllodes tumor of breast**
  - May demonstrate extensive areas of overt sarcomatous overgrowth of stromal component
  - Look for biphasic pattern and epithelial component

- Based on histologic type, grade, and stage of tumor
- Tumor size is significantly associated with overall survival (risk ratio = 1.3 per 1 cm increase)
- Tumor grade is prognostically significant in some but not all reports

Post-Irradiation Sarcoma
- Radiation therapy (RT) is important in adjuvant treatment of breast cancer
  - Complications include development of post-irradiation malignancy
- Criteria for defining a post-irradiation sarcoma
  - Histological confirmation of sarcoma
  - Prior history of RT
    - Latency periods of several years until development of sarcoma
    - Development of sarcoma within previously irradiated field
  - Risk for development of post-irradiation sarcoma
    - 0.03-0.8% with long-term follow-up (15 years)

IMAGE FINDINGS

Mammographic Findings
- Lobulated or ill-defined mass
  - Architectural distortion

Ultrasonographic Findings
- Circumscribed or spiculated mass
  - Ultrasound is generally better for delineating size of lesion

MACROSCOPIC FEATURES

Size
- Superficial lesions tend to be smaller than those located deep in the breast
  - Larger lesions may show areas of hemorrhage and necrosis
- Mean: 5.7 cm (range: 0.3–12.0 cm)

MICROSCOPIC PATHOLOGY

Histologic Features
- Virtually any type of sarcoma described elsewhere may occur rarely as primary lesion in the breast
- **Leiomyosarcoma (LMS)**
  - May arise from smooth muscle of nipple-areolar complex or vasculature
  - Morphologic and immunohistochemical findings are similar to LMS arising in other sites
    - Intersecting bundles of spindle cells with eosinophilic cytoplasm
    - Elongated nuclei with blunt ends and varying degrees of pleomorphism and mitotic activity
- **Liposarcoma (LS)**
  - All grades of LS have been reported arising in the breast as a primary tumor
    - Low-grade tumors and myxoid variant more common than pleomorphic variant in most series
    - Low-grade tumors have more favorable outcome compared with pleomorphic variants
  - Morphologic findings are similar to LS arising in other sites
    - Malignant soft tissue tumor containing lipoblasts and other typical features
  - Liposarcomatous heterologous differentiation can be seen in metaplastic carcinoma and phyllodes tumor
    - Diagnosis of primary liposarcoma of the breast is one of exclusion
- **Osteogenic sarcoma (OGS)**
  - Extraskeletal OGS can rarely arise in a number of soft tissue sites, including the breast
    - All histologic variants, including fibroblastic, osteoblastic, chondroblastic, and telangiectatic, have been reported
    - High-grade, mitotically active tumors tend to have worse outcome
  - Extraskeletal primary OGS of the breast is diagnosis of exclusion

- Osteogenic differentiation can be seen in metaplastic carcinoma and phyllodes tumor and may be prominent
- Extensive sampling of lesion and immunohistochemistry for cytokeratin is helpful in making distinction
- **Pleomorphic spindle cell sarcoma**
  o Some tumors in this category may be considered fibrosarcomas or malignant fibrous histiocytomas
    - Malignant spindle cell proliferation arranged in herringbone or storiform patterns
    - Tumors tend to be high grade with frequent mitotic activity and areas of necrosis
    - May arise at site of prior breast irradiation
  o Important to exclude metaplastic carcinoma and malignant phyllodes tumor
    - Tumor cells should be cytokeratin negative
- **Sarcomas in adolescents and children**
  o Rarely rhabdomyosarcomas and synovial sarcomas can involve the breast in younger patients
    - May represent primary neoplasm or metastatic disease
    - Clinical evaluation and staging studies are needed to make this distinction

ANCILLARY TESTS

Immunohistochemistry
- Careful clinical, morphologic, and immunohistochemical evaluation is important for potential mammary sarcomas
  o Prior history, patient age, and morphologic findings important in formulating differential diagnosis
- Panel of immunostains should be performed to help support &/or confirm diagnosis
  o Panel of multiple immunostains for cytokeratins can help exclude metaplastic carcinoma
    - Synovial sarcoma will usually show foci of cytokeratin expression
    - Morphologic context for cytokeratin expression should be considered
- Other immunohistochemical markers may be indicated based on specific histologic features
  o LMS is positive for vimentin, smooth muscle actin, desmin, caldesmon
    - Typically negative for cytokeratin
  o S100 staining can be used for suspected neural differentiation
  o Rhabdomyosarcoma shows expression of desmin, myogenin, myoglobin

Cytogenetics
- Availability of tissue for cytogenetic analysis may be helpful in cases of suspected primary mammary sarcoma
  o Number of sarcomas have characteristic translocations that can be evaluated in specific cases

DIFFERENTIAL DIAGNOSIS

Metaplastic Carcinoma
- Can show prominent sarcomatous differentiation
  o May present as pure spindle cell tumor or show heterologous morphology
- Extensively sampling the lesion looking for epithelial differentiation &/or DCIS can to help exclude metaplastic carcinoma
  o Panel of immunostains for cytokeratin (particularly high molecular weight) important to help confirm diagnosis

Phyllodes Tumor of Breast
- Malignant phyllodes tumor can show areas of overt sarcomatous overgrowth of stromal component
  o May be extensive
    - Heterologous areas of liposarcoma or osteogenic sarcoma may be seen
  o Extensively sample lesion looking for biphasic pattern and epithelial component to help exclude phyllodes tumor

Metastatic Sarcoma
- Breast involvement usually part of widespread disseminated disease
  o Important to look for prior history

DIAGNOSTIC CHECKLIST

Pathologic Interpretation Pearls
- Diagnosis of primary mammary sarcoma is one of exclusion
  o Sarcoma diagnosis can be established only after excluding metaplastic carcinoma and phyllodes tumor
    - Extensive sampling of lesion looking for epithelial or biphasic component should be undertaken
    - Immunohistochemical analysis using multiple antibodies against cytokeratin is also warranted

SELECTED REFERENCES

1. des Guetz G et al: Postirradiation sarcoma: clinicopathologic features and role of chemotherapy in the treatment strategy. Sarcoma. 2009:764379, 2009
2. Kijima Y et al: Stromal sarcoma with features of giant cell malignant fibrous histiocytoma. Breast Cancer. 14(2):239-44, 2007
3. Adem C et al: Primary breast sarcoma: clinicopathologic series from the Mayo Clinic and review of the literature. Br J Cancer. 91(2):237-41, 2004
4. McGowan TS et al: An analysis of 78 breast sarcoma patients without distant metastases at presentation. Int J Radiat Oncol Biol Phys. 46(2):383-90, 2000
5. Callery CD et al: Sarcoma of the breast. A study of 32 patients with reappraisal of classification and therapy. Ann Surg. 201(4):527-32, 1985

SARCOMAS

Microscopic Features

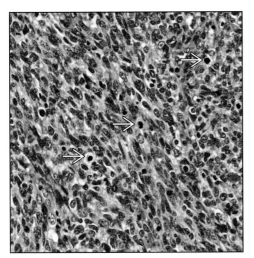 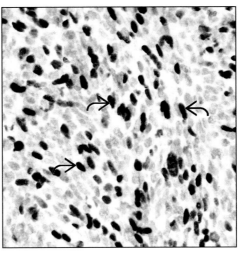

(Left) Embryonal rhabdomyosarcoma can involve the breast as either a primary tumor or as metastatic disease. This high-grade tumor shows pleomorphic spindle cells with frequent mitotic figures ➡. **(Right)** Immunohistochemistry for myogenin shows strong nuclear staining in tumor cells ➡. The myogenin gene codes for a phosphoprotein that induces skeletal muscle differentiation in mesenchymal cells and is a good marker for rhabdomyosarcoma.

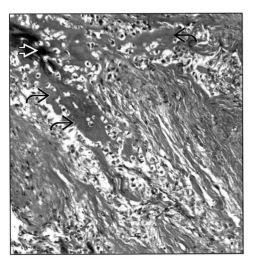 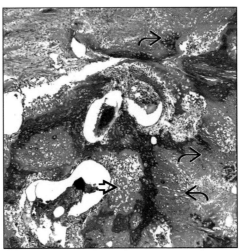

(Left) Osteosarcoma of the breast is shown with evidence of neoplastic osteoid matrix production ➡ and calcification ➡. Extensive sampling failed to show a biphasic pattern or evidence of epithelial differentiation within the tumor and cytokeratin stains were negative, supporting the diagnosis of primary mammary sarcoma. **(Right)** Primary osteogenic sarcomas can show abundant matrix production with osteoid production ➡ and evidence of cartilaginous differentiation ➡.

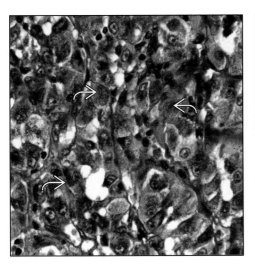 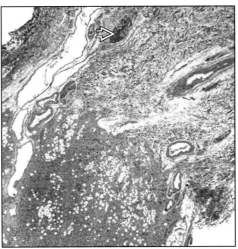

(Left) Alveolar soft part sarcoma shows PAS-positive cytoplasmic granules ➡. These tumors are exceedingly rare and may mimic a carcinoma morphologically. Careful consideration of the clinical features and IHC evaluation are necessary for accurate diagnosis. **(Right)** Dermatofibrosarcoma protuberans may arise in the superficial subcutaneous tissue of the breast and infiltrate into the underlying normal breast tissue ➡. These tumors may mimic spindle cell carcinomas.

SARCOMAS

Differential Diagnosis: Metaplastic Carcinoma

(Left) High-grade malignant spindle cell tumors of the breast may be metaplastic carcinoma, a malignant phyllodes tumor, a primary sarcoma, or a metastasis. Examination of multiple sections looking for diagnostic clues and correlation with history and imaging is important for a correct diagnosis. *(Right)* On higher magnification, spindle cells invade normal breast tissue ➱. This tumor showed staining with p63 and cytokeratin, supporting a diagnosis of metaplastic carcinoma.

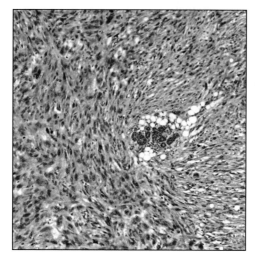 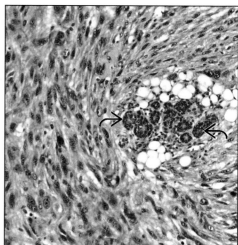

(Left) This 46-year-old woman presented with a rapidly enlarging palpable mass. A needle biopsy showed a pleomorphic spindle cell tumor with no morphologic evidence of epithelial differentiation or of biphasic pattern. *(Right)* Immunostains for cytokeratin show strong cytoplasmic reactivity ➱ in scattered tumor cells supporting a diagnosis of a high-grade metaplastic carcinoma of the breast. The tumor was negative for ER, PR, and HER2.

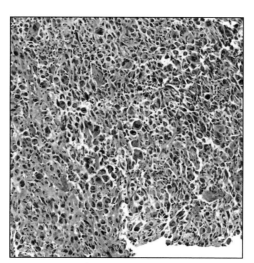 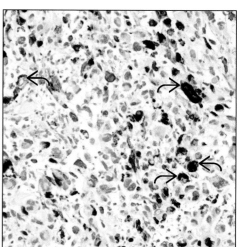

(Left) A 58-year-old woman presented with a well-circumscribed density within breast parenchyma detected by screening mammography. Sections of the tumor show neoplastic cells with abundant extracellular cartilage matrix production ➱. *(Right)* Examination of the periphery of the mass shows epithelial differentiation with nests of tumor cells ➱ diagnostic of infiltrating ductal carcinoma. Final diagnosis was metaplastic carcinoma with extracellular matrix production.

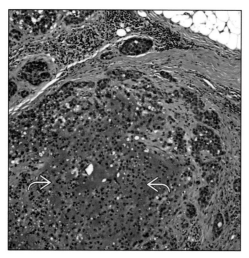 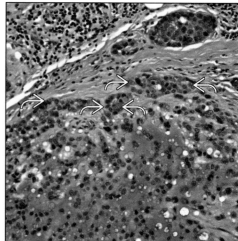

SARCOMAS

Differential Diagnosis: Malignant Phyllodes Tumor

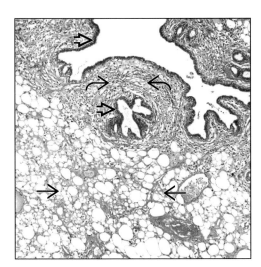

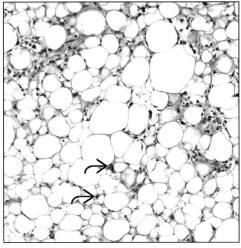

(Left) In this phyllodes tumor with liposarcoma, the diagnostic biphasic glandular ⬧ and stromal ➔ elements can be seen in upper portion of image. The lower portion shows sarcomatous overgrowth of the stroma with liposarcomatous differentiation ➔. (Right) On higher magnification, the liposarcomatous stromal component shows adipocytes with atypia and numerous lipoblasts ➔. A limited sample, such as a needle biopsy, may miss the biphasic component of the tumor.

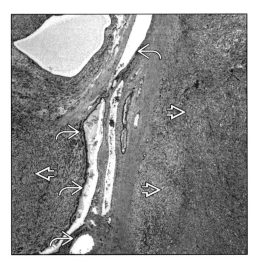

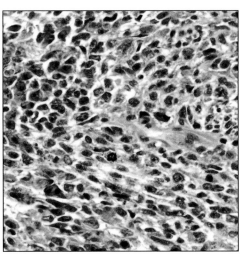

(Left) A malignant phyllodes tumor with a diagnostic biphasic pattern shows admixed glandular ➔ and stromal elements with an overt sarcomatous stromal overgrowth ⬧. For such cases, examination of multiple sections looking for the biphasic areas would be key in establishing the correct diagnosis. (Right) Higher magnification shows a pleomorphic sarcomatous stromal component. On a limited biopsy sample, diagnosis of malignant phyllodes tumor may not be possible.

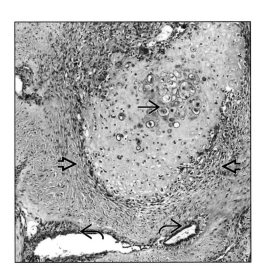

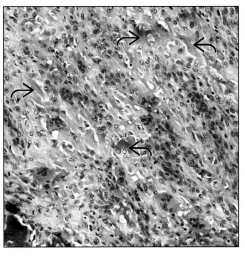

(Left) Malignant phyllodes tumor shows a biphasic area ➔, which is diagnostic with sarcomatous overgrowth ⬧. The tumor shows heterologous differentiation with neoplastic cartilage ➔ & osteoid matrix production. (Right) On higher magnification, osteoid matrix production ➔ by sarcomatous elements is seen. The correct diagnosis of heterologous osteosarcomatous differentiation in a malignant phyllodes tumor requires identification of the biphasic component of the tumor.

Inflammatory Lesions

LACTATIONAL ABSCESS

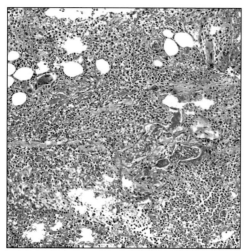

Abscesses occurring during lactation are due to the introduction of skin bacteria into the breast via breaks in the nipple skin. An acute inflammatory infiltrate obscures the normal breast tissue.

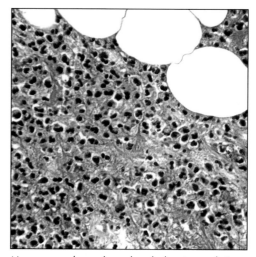

Numerous polymorphonuclear leukocytes and tissue necrosis are present. Special stains may show the causative bacteria. The most commonly cultured bacteria is Staphylococcus aureus.

TERMINOLOGY

Definitions
- Bacterial infection occurring during lactational period

ETIOLOGY/PATHOGENESIS

Etiology/Pathogenesis
- Breaks in nipple skin during breastfeeding are common
- Skin bacteria can be introduced into breast tissue
  - Most abscesses are due to *Staphylococcus* species
  - Streptococcal infections are less common
- Bacterial growth is supported by presence of milk

CLINICAL ISSUES

Presentation
- Breast is focally swollen, painful, and erythematous

Treatment
- Breastfeeding or mechanical expression of milk should continue
- Antibiotics targeting *Staphylococcus* species are effective in most cases
- In rare cases, surgical incision and drainage may be necessary

Prognosis
- Most abscesses resolve with treatment, and breastfeeding can continue

MACROSCOPIC FEATURES

Macroscopic Appearance
- Most specimens will be from an incision and drainage procedure and will consist of multiple small fragments

MICROSCOPIC PATHOLOGY

Histologic Features
- Acute inflammatory infiltrate in breast tissue; tissue necrosis may be present
- Special stains for microorganisms may reveal bacterial forms

DIFFERENTIAL DIAGNOSIS

Inflammatory Breast Carcinoma
- Obstruction of dermal lymphatics by tumor cells causes erythema and edema resulting in marked swelling of breast
- No true inflammation is present
- Inflammatory breast carcinoma should be suspected in women presenting with swollen red breast, particularly if outside lactational period
  - Inflammatory carcinoma presenting during lactation is very rare and difficult to diagnose
- Skin biopsy often reveals dermal lymph-vascular invasion by carcinoma
  - However, lymphatic involvement may be focal and can be missed if only small punch biopsy is performed

Squamous Metaplasia of Lactiferous Ducts (SMOLD)
- Due to abnormal keratin production deep in lactiferous sinuses
  - Therefore, occurs only in subareolar tissue
- If duct ruptures, intense inflammatory reaction to keratin debris ensues
  - Patients typically present with painful erythematous subareolar mass
  - Initial presentation is frequently mistaken for bacterial infection
- Treatment with incision and drainage does not remove causative ducts with squamous metaplasia

LACTATIONAL ABSCESS

Key Facts

Terminology
- Bacterial infection occurring during lactational period

Etiology/Pathogenesis
- Skin bacteria can be introduced into breast tissue
  - Most abscesses are due to *Staphylococcus*
  - Streptococcal infections are less common
- Bacterial growth is supported by presence of milk

Clinical Issues
- Breast is focally swollen, painful, and erythematous
- Most abscesses resolve with treatment, and breastfeeding can continue

Macroscopic Features
- Most specimens will be from an incision and drainage procedure and will consist of multiple fragments

Microscopic Pathology
- Acute inflammatory infiltrate in breast tissue; tissue necrosis may be present

Top Differential Diagnoses
- Inflammatory breast carcinoma
- Squamous metaplasia of lactiferous ducts ("recurrent subareolar abscess")
- Other bacterial infections
- Fungal infections
- Parasitic infections
- Granulomatous lobular mastitis

  - Recurrences are common if treated as lactational abscess
  - Therefore, condition is also termed "recurrent subareolar abscess"
- Recurrent lesions may be infected by bacteria, typically mixed anaerobes
  - Fistula may form
    - Opens at the edge of the areola, just beyond supporting smooth muscle
- Majority of patients use tobacco
- Effective treatment requires surgical removal of involved duct(s) and effective antibiotic treatment directed toward specific infecting bacteria

Other Bacterial Infections
- Very unusual; noninfectious diseases are more common
- Tuberculosis (TB) of breast is rare, even in countries with high rates of TB
  - Some cases in USA have occurred in women with AIDS
  - Granulomas are scattered in breast tissue and have central caseating necrosis

Fungal Infections
- Candidiasis of nipple may occur during breastfeeding
- All other fungal infections of breast are very rare
  - Rare cases of aspergillosis have been associated with breast implants
  - Isolated cases of infection with *Cryptococcus*, *Blastomyces*, *Coccidioides*, and *Mucor* species have been reported
  - Affected patients are often immunocompromised due to steroid use, organ transplantation, AIDS, or other reasons

Parasitic Infections
- Can closely mimic breast carcinoma
  - Inflammation forms superficial, hard, nontender mass that may retract skin
  - Regional lymph nodes may be enlarged
- Inflammatory reaction consists of necrotic center and prominent infiltrate of eosinophils

  - Portions of viable and degenerating worms may be present within area of necrosis
- Filarial diseases are seen worldwide
  - *Wuchereria bancrofti*: South America, China, India
  - *Dirofilaria repens* (or *D. tenuis*): North America, Europe, Asia
    - More commonly infects dogs and cats but can also infect humans
  - *Onchocerca volvulus*: Latin America, sub-Saharan Africa
  - Other types of mammary parasitic infections have been reported but are very rare

Granulomatous Lobular Mastitis
- Often presents with tender breast mass
  - Fistula tracks may form in advanced or recurrent cases
- All patients have history of pregnancy, but disease usually occurs months or years after last pregnancy
- Microscopic examination reveals well-formed granulomas centered on ducts and lobules
- Unusual types of infections should be excluded by culture and special stains

SELECTED REFERENCES

1. Bharat A et al: Predictors of primary breast abscesses and recurrence. World J Surg. 33(12):2582-6, 2009
2. da Silva BB et al: Tuberculosis of the breast: analysis of 20 cases and a literature review. Trans R Soc Trop Med Hyg. 103(6):559-63, 2009

Microscopic Features and Differential Diagnosis

(Left) The inflammatory cells diffusely infiltrate fibroadipose tissue. The majority of lactational abscesses are treated with incision and drainage with antibiotic coverage. Surgical specimens are uncommon unless the infection is quite advanced. **(Right)** After the termination of lactation, there is regression of the greatly expanded milk-producing lobules. A mild intralobular B-cell lymphocytic infiltrate ⊵ is a normal finding and is not indicative of an infectious process.

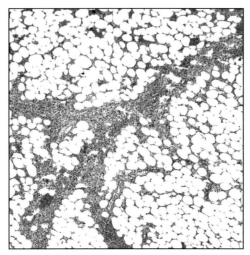
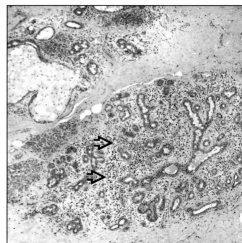

(Left) Women with squamous metaplasia of lactiferous ducts (SMOLD) are typically thought to have a bacterial infection. Surgical specimens often consist of multiple fragments of debrided tissue. The infiltrate consists of lymphocytes, plasma cells, and occasional giant cells reacting to keratin debris ⊵. Polymorphonuclear leukocytes may be present if there is a superimposed bacterial infection. SMOLD is unlikely to occur during pregnancy. **(Right)** SMOLD is due to keratin production deep within the lactiferous sinuses.

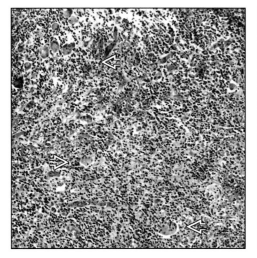
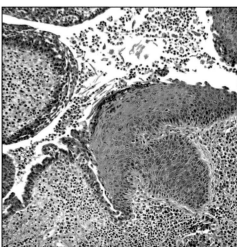

(Left) In patients with SMOLD, keratin debris in stroma causes the intense inflammatory response after a duct rupture. **(Right)** Bacterial infections may occur in the perioperative period after surgery for breast reconstruction or augmentation. In this case, necrotic debris and numerous bacterial forms are adjacent to an implant capsule ⊵. Cultures were positive for S. aureus. Very rare Aspergillus infections have also been reported in association with implants.

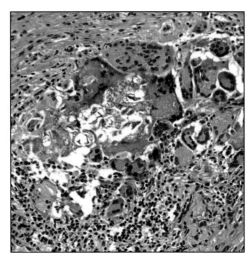
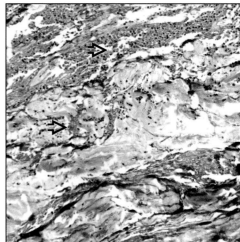

LACTATIONAL ABSCESS

Differential Diagnosis

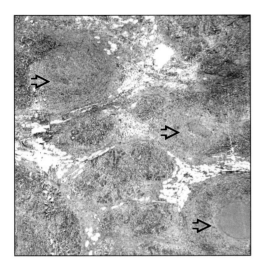

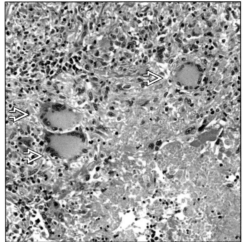

(Left) Tuberculosis is a rare infection in the breast, even in countries where the disease is common. Granulomas with central caseating necrosis ➡ are scattered throughout the breast tissue. The granulomas are not specifically associated with ducts and lobules. *(Right)* Characteristic Langhans giant cells with peripheral nuclei ➡ are present in areas of necrosis in tuberculosis. Special stains, culture, or PCR can be used to demonstrate the presence of mycobacteria.

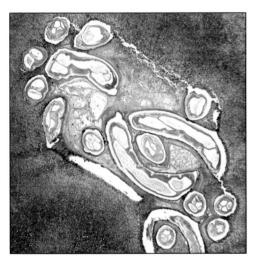

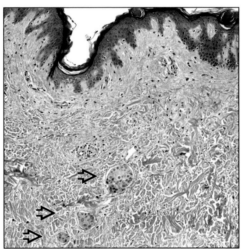

(Left) This is a case of mammary dirofilariasis. The segments of the worm are surrounded by a dense chronic inflammatory infiltrate that includes lymphocytes and numerous eosinophils. *(Right)* Inflammatory carcinoma mimics an infection, as it presents as a red swollen breast. These findings are due to tumor cells plugging dermal lymphatics ➡. No true inflammation is present. This diagnosis should always be suspected in women outside the lactational period.

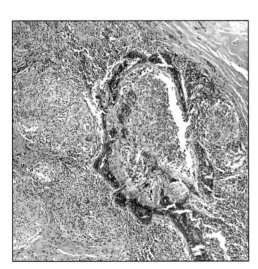

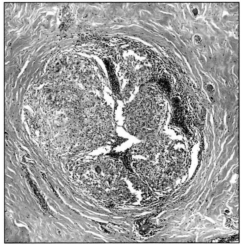

(Left) Granulomatous lobular mastitis often presents as a tender breast mass. Fistula tracts may be present. Although almost all affected women have been parous, this disease usually occurs several years after the last pregnancy. *(Right)* The characteristic histologic feature of granulomatous lobular mastitis is multiple granulomas centered on, and distorting, ducts and lobules. Infectious diseases should always be considered and excluded by appropriate special stains and cultures.

FAT NECROSIS

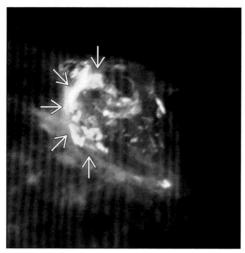

Calcifications around the edge of a central area of fat necrosis gives rise to a characteristic eggshell appearance ➡ radiographically. Fewer calcifications can appear as a suspicious cluster.

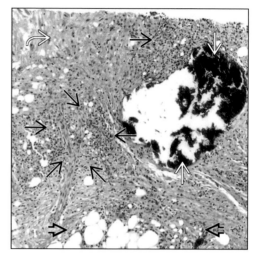

Fat necrosis includes a histiocytic infiltrate reacting to degenerating adipose tissue ⇨ with varying amounts of lymphocytic infiltrates ➡, fibrosis ➡, and calcifications ➡.

TERMINOLOGY

Abbreviations
- Fat necrosis (FN)

Definitions
- Common benign inflammatory reaction that is secondary to injury of breast connective tissue and adipose tissue

ETIOLOGY/PATHOGENESIS

Causes of Fat Necrosis
- Trauma
  - Blunt trauma to breast
  - Seat belt injury after motor vehicle crashes
    - Produces different radiologic patterns of injury in driver and passenger
- Pressure necrosis
  - Can occur in lower portion of pendulous breasts
- Radiation therapy
  - Post-radiation vascular damage (endarteritis obliterans) with subsequent ischemia
- Surgery
  - Cyst aspiration
  - Core needle biopsies
  - Excisions
  - Reduction mammoplasty
  - Implants
  - Autologous fat injection
- Other rare causes
  - Polyarteritis nodosa, Weber-Christian disease, granulomatous angiopanniculitis
  - Heparin-induced thrombocytopenia (single case report)
- In about 50% of patients, cause is unknown

CLINICAL ISSUES

Epidemiology
- Incidence
  - Estimated to be 0.6% of breast excisions
- Age
  - Broad range: 37-68 years (mean: ~ 50 years)

Presentation
- Symptomatic FN typically presents as palpable mass
  - May enlarge, remain unchanged, regress, or resolve
  - FN is typically detected in periareolar area and is often superficial in location
    - These sites are most vulnerable to trauma
  - Can be associated with skin changes
    - Bruising and tenderness (due to original trauma)
    - Skin tethering or dimpling, nipple retraction (due to fibrosis associated with healing)
- May be detected on mammographic screening
  - Forms multiple types of lesions
    - Lipid cysts, coarse calcifications, focal asymmetries, microcalcifications, or irregular masses
  - Many cases can be identified by radiographic appearance
    - Biopsy is required for cases with unusual imaging features

Prognosis
- Benign inflammatory process that should regress or resolve over time

Management
- FN must be distinguished from carcinoma
  - Physical examination and imaging findings can be similar
- Even with clear history of previous trauma, possibility of malignancy should not be overlooked
  - Patient's attention may be drawn to a palpable mass by an episode of trauma

FAT NECROSIS

Key Facts

Terminology
- Common benign inflammatory reaction secondary to injury of breast adipose tissue
  - Wide spectrum of clinical and radiologic appearances
  - May be confused with carcinoma, both clinically and radiologically

Etiology/Pathogenesis
- May be due to trauma, surgical procedures, pressure necrosis, radiation, or other rare causes

Image Findings
- Reflect histological evolution of inflammatory process
  - Common findings are dystrophic calcifications and radiolucent oil cysts

- Oil cysts may be associated with continuous eggshell calcification
- Irregular mass may be present

Microscopic Pathology
- Early changes: Hemorrhage in fat with induration
  - Followed by cystic degeneration with oily fluid secondary to necrotic fat
  - Calcifications frequently develop in cyst wall
- Later changes: Hemosiderin deposition, varying degrees of fibrosis and calcification

Top Differential Diagnoses
- Granular cell tumor
- Other inflammatory lesions
- Lupus mastitis
- Erdheim-Chester disease

- Patients who have undergone breast-conserving surgery for breast cancer may develop FN
  - FN related to treatment must be distinguished from cancer recurrence
- Management may include short-term follow-up with imaging and physical examination in selected cases
  - In specific cases with worrisome clinical/radiographic features, biopsy is required to confirm diagnosis

IMAGE FINDINGS

General Features
- Location
  - In lesions precipitated by trauma, mass typically occurs at site of injury
  - In patients with no history of trauma, lesion is most often seen in upper outer quadrant of breast
- Morphology
  - Imaging features of FN reflect histological evolution of inflammatory process

Mammographic Findings
- Variable
- Attributable to degree of fibrosis and types of calcifications changing as lesion develops
  - Early discrete round or oval radiolucent oil cyst with thin capsule
    - Oil cysts may be associated with uniform continuous eggshell calcification
  - Progressive thickening and deformity of skin and subcutaneous tissue
  - Formation of ill-defined irregular mass
  - Development of multiple clustered pleomorphic microcalcifications, possibly suspicious for malignancy
- Most common mammographic findings are dystrophic calcifications, followed by radiolucent oil cysts

Ultrasonographic Findings
- Appearance ranges from solid nodules with posterior shadowing to complex intracystic masses

- Cystic lesions may appear complex with mural nodules or with internal echogenic bands
  - Oil cysts typically show posterior acoustic shadowing, corresponding to round radiolucent lesion with curvilinear wall calcification on mammography
  - Fat-fluid level that shifts in orientation with changes in patient position is considered diagnostic of oil cysts
  - Presence of oil cyst within a spiculated mass is reassuring for diagnosis of fat necrosis
- Solid masses have well-circumscribed or ill-defined margins
  - Often associated with distortion of surrounding breast parenchyma

MR Findings
- FN produces wide spectrum of findings on MR
  - Fibrosis may be seen as architectural distortion with or without irregular margins
    - Fibrosis may appear as high, intermediate, or low signal on T1-weighted MR
  - Necrotic fat usually shows low signal intensity on T1-weighted MR
    - May be due to hemorrhagic and inflammatory infiltrate
- FN can enhance after injection of contrast material
  - Amount of enhancement depends on intensity of inflammatory process
    - Enhancement can be focal or diffuse, homogeneous or heterogeneous
    - Enhancement patterns may vary from slow gradual enhancement to rapid enhancement
    - Most avid enhancement usually occurs in early phase after initial injury
    - As inflammatory changes resolve, degree of enhancement may decrease
- FN may mimic malignancy on MR on basis of morphology or contrast kinetics

FAT NECROSIS

MACROSCOPIC FEATURES

General Features
- FN forms a demarcated mass lesion with distinct yellow-gray and focally reddish color
  - Often retracts surrounding parenchyma
  - Cystic degeneration may occur, resulting in a cavity that contains oily fluid secondary to necrotic fat

MICROSCOPIC PATHOLOGY

Histologic Features
- Varies over time from initial injury to reaction to damaged tissue and, ultimately, to resolution
  - **Early-stage lesions**
    - Early changes include hemorrhage in fat, resulting in induration and firmness on gross pathology
    - Over several weeks, affected area becomes demarcated, forming distinct yellow-gray and focally reddish mass
    - Cystic degeneration may result in a cavity that contains oily fluid secondary to necrotic fat
    - Calcifications frequently develop in cyst walls
  - **Intermediate-stage lesions**
    - Infiltration of histiocytes, lymphocytes, plasma cells, and multinucleated giant cells
    - Foamy cytoplasm of histiocytes and giant cells is due to phagocytosis of necrotic adipose cells
  - **Late-stage lesions**
    - Later changes are characterized by hemosiderin deposition and the development of varying degrees of fibrosis
    - Reactive inflammatory components gradually replaced by fibrosis lead to scar formation
    - Loculated degenerated fat may persist for months or years in a cyst surrounded by fibrosis
    - In some cases, fibrosis and calcifications are only sequelae of fat necrosis
    - Reparative fibrotic process may replace areas of necrotic fat, resulting in a suspicious irregular mass
- Histiocytes adjacent to ruptured cysts are termed "ochrocytes" when they contain brown pigment
  - Likely due to oxidized secretory lipids
- Varied appearances of FN on imaging studies is due to various amounts of histiocytic infiltration, hemorrhage, fibrosis, and calcification

Cytologic Features
- FN is characterized by a polymorphous inflammatory infiltrate in response to tissue injury
  - Lesion is characterized by admixed histiocytes, giant cells, lymphocytes, and fibroblasts
    - Cellular composition of infiltrate will vary with age of lesion
    - Cytologic atypia should not be present

DIFFERENTIAL DIAGNOSIS

Granular Cell Tumor
- Lipid-laden histiocytes in FN and cells of a granular cell tumor can be similar in appearance
  - Histiocytes should be strongly positive for CD68 and may be positive for S100
  - Granular cells are strongly S100 positive and may be CD68 positive
- Granular cell tumor lacks other inflammatory cells and fat involvement characteristic of FN

Other Inflammatory Lesions
- FN is a frequent component of other inflammatory lesions
  - Abscess, ruptured cysts, surgical procedures, needle tracks
    - Etiology is usually clinically apparent
- Correlation with clinical, imaging, and culture studies may be needed for diagnosis

Lupus Mastitis
- Rare manifestation of lupus
  - Can be presenting finding
- Average patient age: 40 years (range: 18-70 years)
- Single or multiple palpable masses
  - Subcutaneous or deep
- Lymphocytic lobular panniculitis present
  - Lymphocytic infiltration can be nodular or diffuse, periductal or perilobular
  - Germinal centers may be present
  - Mixed B- and T-cell population
  - May include plasma cells
- Hyaline fat necrosis also present
- Lymphocytic vasculitis common

Erdheim-Chester Disease
- Very rare non-Langerhans cell histiocytosis ("polyostotic sclerosing histiocytosis") that may involve breast
- Characterized by infiltration of histiocytes
  - Histiocytes are CD68 positive and negative for CD1a and S100
  - Touton-type giant cells may be present
- Mild lymphocytic infiltrate is present

SELECTED REFERENCES

1. Kinonen C et al: Lupus mastitis: an uncommon complication of systemic or discoid lupus. Am J Surg Pathol. 34(6):901-6, 2010
2. Ganau S et al: The great mimicker: fat necrosis of the breast--magnetic resonance mammography approach. Curr Probl Diagn Radiol. 38(4):189-97, 2009
3. Taboada JL et al: The many faces of fat necrosis in the breast. AJR Am J Roentgenol. 192(3):815-25, 2009
4. Tan PH et al: Fat necrosis of the breast--a review. Breast. 15(3):313-8, 2006
5. Bilgen IG et al: Fat necrosis of the breast: clinical, mammographic and sonographic features. Eur J Radiol. 39(2):92-9, 2001
6. Villeirs G et al: Heparin-induced thrombocytopenia and fat necrosis of the breast. Eur Radiol. 10(3):527-30, 2000

FAT NECROSIS

Imaging and Microscopic Features

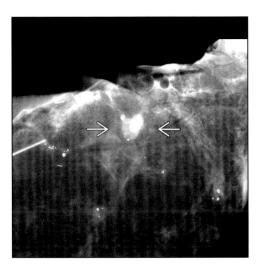

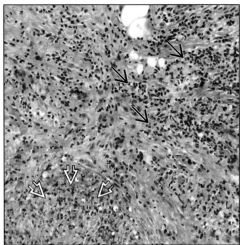

(Left) This specimen was excised due to a concern for malignancy. Specimen radiograph shows a discrete radiodense lesion with clustered microcalcifications ➡. The findings are suspicious because the calcifications do not have the diagnostic eggshell pattern that would identify this lesion as FN. *(Right)* The early stages of FN are characterized by a mixed infiltrate of lymphocytes and histiocytes ➡ in an area of fibrosis. Both fat and tissue necrosis ➡ are present.

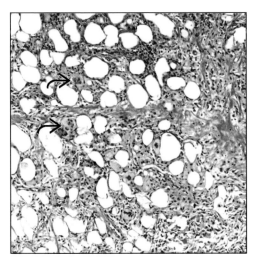

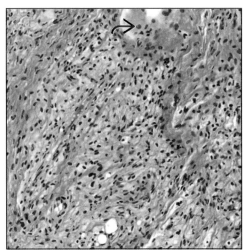

(Left) An intermediate stage of FN typically shows an abundant infiltrate of lipid-laden histocytes in response to necrotic adipose cells. Multinucleated giant cells ➡ are frequently seen at this stage. *(Right)* The infiltrate of lipid-laden histocytes in fat necrosis with their abundant eosinophilic cytoplasm can mimic a granular cell tumor. The presence of multinucleated giant cells ➡, other inflammatory cells, and calcifications favor a diagnosis of fat necrosis.

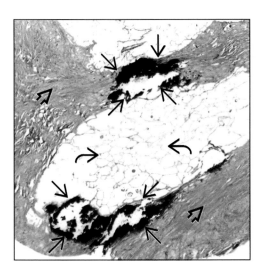

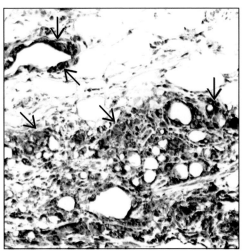

(Left) Later features of FN typically include dense fibrosis ➡, loculated necrotic fat ➡ (which may persist for months to years), and peripheral coarse calcifications ➡. *(Right)* Immunohistochemistry can be helpful in distinguishing granular cell tumor from fat necrosis. The histiocytes in fat necrosis are strongly positive for CD68 ➡ and usually S100 negative. In contrast, granular cell tumors are strongly positive for S100 and may be positive or negative for CD68.

DUCT ECTASIA

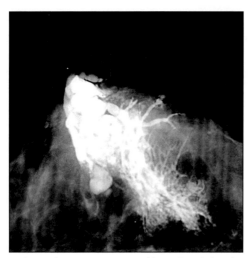

With age, the supporting tissue of large ducts below the nipple may weaken. The ducts can fill with inspissated secretions and become markedly dilated, as seen in this nipple duct injection.

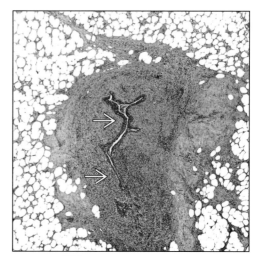

Ectatic ducts ➡ are surrounded by chronic inflammatory cells and fibrosis. The inflammatory reaction can form an irregular mass that closely mimics invasive cancer clinically and radiologically.

TERMINOLOGY

Abbreviations
- Duct ectasia (DE)

Definitions
- Benign condition characterized by ectasia (dilation) of large subareolar ducts with associated periductal inflammation and fibrosis

ETIOLOGY/PATHOGENESIS

Etiology
- Walls of large ducts weaken with age
  - Elastic fibers thin and become attenuated
- Dilated ducts fill with secretory debris
  - Inspissated secretions can result in thick white nipple discharge
- If rupture occurs, an intense chronic inflammatory response results in response to extravasated lipids
- Periductal fibrosis forms an irregular mass
  - Fibrosis can involve overlying skin causing retraction

CLINICAL ISSUES

Epidemiology
- Age
  - Perimenopausal or postmenopausal women

Presentation
- Most common: Palpable irregular subareolar mass that can be tethered to skin and nipple
- Usually not painful or erythematous
- May be associated with thick nipple discharge
- Screening mammography may show irregular mass, dilated ducts, &/or calcifications

Treatment
- No treatment is necessary after biopsy demonstrates that clinical signs and symptoms are not due to carcinoma

Prognosis
- Benign finding in breast

IMAGE FINDINGS

Mammographic Findings
- Irregular subareolar mass
- Calcifications in ductal distribution ("casting calcifications")

Ultrasonographic Findings
- Subareolar, anechoic, fluid-filled dilated ducts
- Ducts may be filled with debris
  - Inspissated secretions are often visible and may be sufficiently echogenic to mimic an intraductal tumor

MACROSCOPIC FEATURES

General Features
- Tissue is usually dense, but a discrete hard mass is not typically present
- In some cases, dilated ducts with inspissated debris may be seen grossly

MICROSCOPIC PATHOLOGY

Histologic Features
- Subareolar ducts are dilated (ectatic)
- Chronic inflammation surrounds ducts
  - Lymphocytes and plasma cells are frequently seen; giant cells and well-formed granulomas are uncommon

DUCT ECTASIA

Key Facts

Terminology
- Large subareolar ducts dilate due to loss of elastic fibers with age ("duct ectasia")
- If ducts rupture, secretions spill into surrounding tissues resulting in chronic inflammation and fibrosis

Clinical Issues
- Patients present with palpable irregular subareolar mass
  - Mass can be tethered to skin and nipple

- Thick nipple discharge may be present
- Mammography may show irregular mass, dilated ducts, &/or calcifications

Top Differential Diagnoses
- Squamous metaplasia of lactiferous ducts (SMOLD)
- Plasma cell mastitis
- Invasive carcinoma
- Lymphoma

- Hemosiderin and hemosiderin-laden macrophages may be present if there has been erosion of duct walls
- Lipids and lipid-laden macrophages ("ochrocytes") are often present due to spillage of duct contents into stroma
- Luminal cells lining ducts may be infiltrated by lymphocytes and macrophages

DIFFERENTIAL DIAGNOSIS

Squamous Metaplasia of Lactiferous Ducts (SMOLD)
- Also termed periductal mastitis, recurrent subareolar abscess, or Zuska disease
- Patients can be of any age, and both females and males are affected
  - DE usually occurs in older females
- Patients present with painful erythematous periareolar mass, usually thought to be infection
- SMOLD results from keratin being trapped deep in lactiferous ducts
  - If duct ruptures, keratin debris causes intense foreign-body-type inflammatory response
- Recurrences are common
- Periareolar fistulas may form with recurrences
  - Fistulas do not occur with duct ectasia
- SMOLD is strongly associated with history of tobacco use
  - DE is not associated with tobacco use

Plasma Cell Mastitis
- Many cases of DE are associated with plasma cells
- Some cases described as plasma cell mastitis may be DE

Invasive Carcinoma
- Invasive carcinomas can also form irregular subareolar palpable masses that retract skin &/or nipple
- Biopsy is usually necessary to distinguish invasive carcinoma from DE

Lymphoma
- Composed of solid masses of malignant lymphoid cells
  - Lymphocytic infiltrate does not center around ducts, as in DE
  - In DE, there is generally mixture of lymphocytes, plasma cells, and histiocytes

SELECTED REFERENCES
1. Da Costa D et al: Common and unusual diseases of the nipple-areolar complex. Radiographics. 27 Suppl 1:S65-77, 2007
2. Hari S et al: Bilateral severe mammary duct ectasia. Acta Radiol. 48(4):398-400, 2007
3. Dixon JM et al: Periductal mastitis and duct ectasia: different conditions with different aetiologies. Br J Surg. 83(6):820-2, 1996
4. Sweeney DJ et al: Mammographic appearances of mammary duct ectasia that mimic carcinoma in a screening programme. Australas Radiol. 39(1):18-23, 1995

IMAGE GALLERY

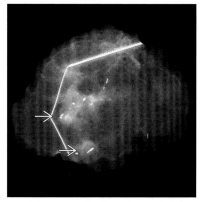 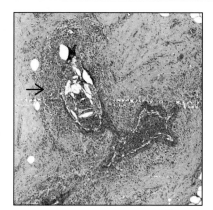 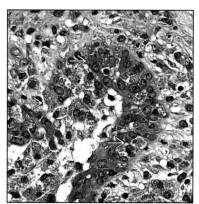

(Left) Inspissated secretions in large ducts can calcify and form casting calcifications ➡. The surrounding density is due to associated fibrosis. (Center) Secretory material spills out into the stroma from the weakened duct walls and incites an intense chronic inflammatory reaction consisting of lymphocytes and plasma cells ➡. (Right) Lymphocytes and macrophages, containing hemosiderin or lipids ("ochrocytes"), infiltrate into the duct walls ➡.

SQUAMOUS METAPLASIA OF LACTIFEROUS DUCTS

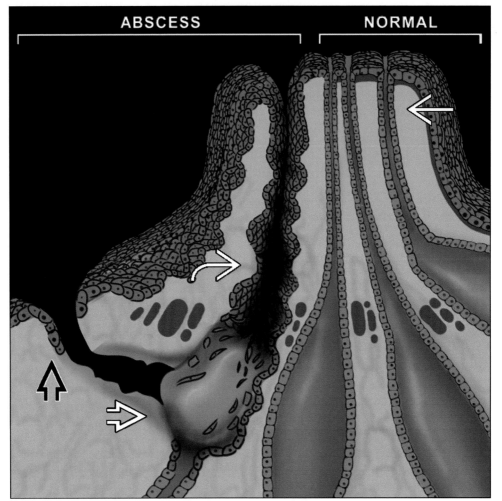

The normal keratinizing surface epithelium normally dips into the nipple orifice for only 2-3 mm ➡. If keratin production occurs deeper in the duct ➡, the keratin is trapped and causes distension of the duct. If rupture occurs, an intense foreign body inflammatory response to the keratin ensues ➡. The patient develops an erythematous painful subareolar mass, often mistaken for a bacterial infection. Incision and drainage procedure does not remove the pathologic lesion, and recurrences are common. The path of least resistance is beneath the smooth muscle of the nipple. Patients may develop a fistula track opening at the edge of the areola ➡. Definitive surgery removes the offending duct.

TERMINOLOGY

Abbreviations
- Squamous metaplasia of lactiferous ducts (SMOLD)

Synonyms
- Recurrent subareolar abscess
- Zuska disease
- Periductal mastitis

Definitions
- Abnormal keratin formation in lactiferous sinuses leads to rupture and intense inflammatory response to keratin debris

ETIOLOGY/PATHOGENESIS

Etiology
- Tobacco use

- Almost all men and women affected by SMOLD have history of tobacco use
  - It has been proposed that smoking leads to vitamin A deficiency, which results in abnormal squamous metaplasia
- Inverted nipple
  - Many patients with SMOLD have inverted nipple
  - Inversion of nipple is more likely a result of retroareolar inflammation and fibrosis rather than a cause of the condition
    - Recurrent episodes of inflammation and healing with fibrosis lead to nipple retraction
- Subareolar abscess formation
  - Keratinizing cells extend abnormally deep into lactiferous sinuses
  - Keratin becomes trapped and equivalent of an epidermal inclusion cyst is formed
  - If duct ruptures, keratin is released into surrounding tissue

SQUAMOUS METAPLASIA OF LACTIFEROUS DUCTS

Key Facts

Terminology

- Squamous metaplasia of lactiferous ducts (SMOLD) is also known as recurrent subareolar abscess, periductal mastitis, and Zuska disease

Etiology/Pathogenesis

- Keratin-producing cells extend abnormally deep into lactiferous sinuses
- "Epidermal inclusion cyst" filled with keratin forms in sinuses
- When ruptured, an intense inflammatory response ensues
- Almost all men and women affected by SMOLD have history of tobacco use
  - May reduce vitamin A levels resulting in abnormal metaplasia

Clinical Issues

- Presents with an erythematous painful subareolar mass
- Recurrences are common if the lesion is treated as a bacterial abscess
  - Fistula track may develop
- Effective surgical management reduces likelihood of recurrence
- Secondary infections, often due to mixed anaerobes, may occur after surgical intervention

Top Differential Diagnoses

- Bacterial abscess
- Duct ectasia
- Biopsy site changes
- Granulomatous lobular mastitis

  - Intense inflammatory response ensues, causing erythema, swelling, and pain
  - If involved duct is not removed, recurrences are common

CLINICAL ISSUES

Epidemiology

- Incidence
  - Rare: < 1% of all breast biopsies
- Age
  - Occurs at any adult age
- Gender
  - Occurs in both females and males

Presentation

- Patients initially present with erythematous painful subareolar mass
  - Usually mistaken for bacterial abscess
    - Initial lesions are sterile; inflammatory response is to keratin debris
  - Typical treatment is incision and drainage (I&D) and antibiotics for *Staphylococcus* species
    - Surgeons avoid surgery involving nipple due to cosmetic and functional concerns
  - Symptoms may be relieved temporarily
- Recurrences are common
  - Often mystify patient and clinicians, as adequate treatment for an infection has been provided
    - Patients have been suspected of having Munchausen syndrome
  - Subsequent treatment may again be I&D and antibiotics
  - Secondary infections may occur
- Fistula track may form after recurrences
  - Path of least resistance is below smooth muscle of areola
  - Track opens at edge of areola
  - Only 1 track is present

Treatment

- Effective treatment requires surgical removal of keratin-producing epithelium
  - Wedge resection of nipple to remove involved duct may be performed
  - If a fistula track is present, it should be removed in continuity with involved duct
- Antibiotics may be required for recurrent lesions with secondary infections
  - Secondary infections are often due to mixed anaerobic bacteria
  - Cultures are often helpful to establish type of bacteria and sensitivity to antibiotics

Prognosis

- After effective surgical management, recurrences are uncommon
- Termination of tobacco use may reduce likelihood of recurrence

IMAGE FINDINGS

Mammographic Findings

- Patient may not tolerate compression due to painful mass
- Location of lesion below nipple also makes it difficult to visualize
- In some patients, a density may be present due to inflammatory reaction

Ultrasonographic Findings

- May not be possible, as patient may not tolerate pressure from transducer
- In some patients, a mass with irregular margins is present

MR Findings

- MR may be better tolerated, as compression is not required
- In 1 study, MR was effective in imaging abscess cavity and associated fistula track

SQUAMOUS METAPLASIA OF LACTIFEROUS DUCTS

MACROSCOPIC FEATURES

General Features
- 1st specimen is often an I&D
  - Specimen consists of multiple fragments of tissue that cannot be oriented
- If a definitive procedure is performed, there should be a small fragment of nipple skin and the underlying abscess cavity
  - If possible, sections should be oriented perpendicular to nipple skin

MICROSCOPIC PATHOLOGY

Histologic Features
- I&D specimens usually consist of tissue from center of abscess
  - Findings may be nonspecific, consisting of chronic active inflammation
  - Presence of giant cells, especially if associated with keratin debris, is very suggestive of SMOLD
  - In some cases, ducts partially replaced by squamous epithelium and with entrapped keratin debris may be present
  - Because patients often have multiple prior procedures, changes due to surgery may be difficult to distinguish from primary lesion
- Definitive procedures should include nipple skin and orifice of involved duct
  - Squamous metaplasia of ductal epithelium with entrapped keratin deep to nipple is characteristic of SMOLD
- If secondary infection is present, acute inflammatory cells and bacteria will be present

DIFFERENTIAL DIAGNOSIS

Bacterial Abscess
- Acute infections are rare outside lactational period
- I&D followed by antibiotics is effective treatment
  - Specimens usually consist of acute inflammatory cells
- Causative agent is usually *Staphylococcus* species or, less commonly, *Streptococcus* species
  - Secondary infections that occur after recurrences of SMOLD are often due to mixed anaerobes
- Bacterial infections can occur anywhere in breast and are not necessarily subareolar

Duct Ectasia
- Usually occurs in older women and is not associated with tobacco use
- Typical presentation is as a palpable or radiographic mass or cheesy nipple discharge
  - Unlike SMOLD, duct ectasia is not usually painful
  - Usually treated with excision for mass rather than I&D
- In many studies, duct ectasia is not clearly distinguished from SMOLD

- Duct ectasia is associated with periductal chronic inflammation
  - Squamous metaplasia and giant cell reaction to keratin are not typical features

Biopsy Site Changes
- Also associated with squamous metaplasia, chronic inflammation, and giant cells
- Because women with SMOLD often undergo multiple surgical procedures, it can be difficult to distinguish biopsy changes from primary lesion
- Squamous metaplasia associated with surgery usually lines excisional site rather than being present in ducts
  - Not associated with extensive keratinaceous debris
  - Giant cell reaction is to foreign material and not to keratin

Granulomatous Lobular Mastitis (GLM)
- Rare disease only occurring in women who have borne children; it is not associated with tobacco use
- Women present with mass in breast; mass is usually not subareolar
  - Fistula tracts may open to skin
- Defining histologic feature is pattern of well-formed granulomas centered on ducts and lobules
- Some women have been successfully treated with steroids
  - This treatment could be harmful for patients with SMOLD and secondary bacterial infections

REPORTING CONSIDERATIONS

Key Elements to Report
- Findings from small incisional biopsies are often not diagnostic but may be very suggestive of SMOLD
- Pathologists can play important role in patient care by suggesting diagnosis in appropriate clinical setting
  - Patients with recurrent painful subareolar abscesses, particularly if there is history of tobacco use

SELECTED REFERENCES

1. Fu P et al: High-resolution MRI in detecting subareolar breast abscess. AJR Am J Roentgenol. 188(6):1568-72, 2007
2. Li S et al: Surgical management of recurrent subareolar breast abscesses: Mayo Clinic experience. Am J Surg. 192(4):528-9, 2006
3. Versluijs-Ossewaarde FN et al: Subareolar breast abscesses: characteristics and results of surgical treatment. Breast J. 11(3):179-82, 2005
4. Dixon JM et al: Periductal mastitis and duct ectasia: different conditions with different aetiologies. Br J Surg. 83(6):820-2, 1996
5. Meguid MM et al: Pathogenesis-based treatment of recurring subareolar breast abscesses. Surgery. 118(4):775-82, 1995
6. Powell BC et al: Recurrent subareolar abscess of the breast and squamous metaplasia of the lactiferous ducts: a clinical syndrome. South Med J. 70(8):935-7, 1977
7. ZUSKA JJ et al: Fistulas of lactiferous ducts. Am J Surg. 81(3):312-7, 1951

SQUAMOUS METAPLASIA OF LACTIFEROUS DUCTS

Microscopic Features

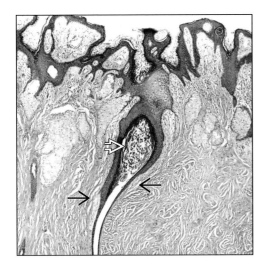

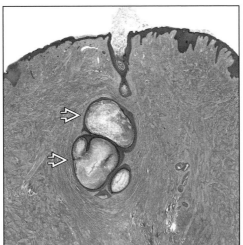

(Left) The keratin-producing squamous epithelium normally dips into the main duct orifices for 1-2 mm. There is an abrupt transition ⇨ to the normal nonkeratinizing ductal lining. A keratin plug may form ⇨ but is easily extruded onto the skin surface. *(Right)* In SMOLD, keratinizing squamous cells extend abnormally deep into ducts forming the equivalent of an epidermal inclusion cyst ⇨. If these ducts rupture, an intense inflammatory response to keratin results.

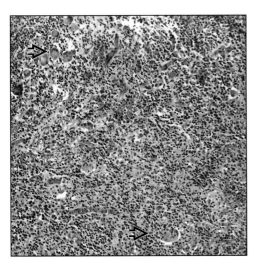

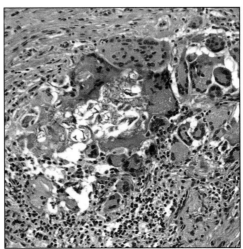

(Left) If I&D is performed, the specimen consists entirely of inflammatory debris. The presence of giant cells ⇨, particularly when associated with keratin, is very suggestive of SMOLD. In the appropriate clinical setting, the differential diagnosis includes SMOLD, even without diagnostic areas of squamous metaplasia. *(Right)* After rupture, the keratin spills into the stroma and incites an inflammatory response. In this image, multiple giant cells are engulfing keratin fragments.

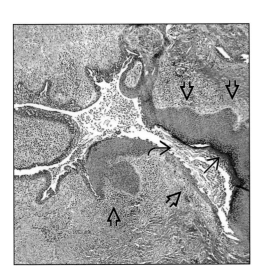

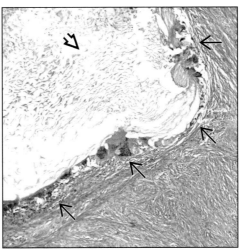

(Left) This duct is located in subareolar tissue and is partially lined by a keratinizing squamous epithelium ⇨. There is a granular cell layer ⇨, and keratin debris is present within the duct ⇨. The duct is surrounded by chronic inflammatory cells. *(Right)* This is an area of abundant keratin debris ⇨ that has been extruded from a ruptured duct. The keratin is surrounded by a foreign body giant cell response ⇨. Keratin can sometimes be identified inside the giant cells.

SQUAMOUS METAPLASIA OF LACTIFEROUS DUCTS

Imaging and Microscopic Features

(Left) In this patient with SMOLD, an ultrasound examination demonstrates a subareolar abscess cavity with an irregular shape filled with heterogeneous internal echoes ➡. However, in many patients, imaging cannot be performed due to pain and swelling around the nipple. **(Right)** With recurrences, the inflammatory mass enlarges and a fistula track forms ➡ along the path of least resistance: Below the smooth muscle of the areola to open at the skin ⇨ at the edge of the areola.

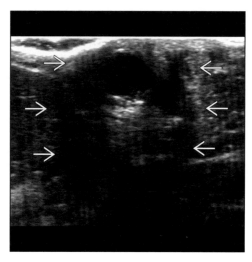
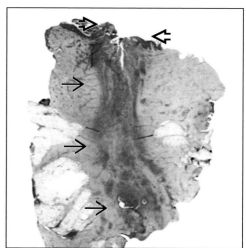

(Left) An I&D is often performed as SMOLD is mistaken for a bacterial infection. The specimen is typically received as multiple small fragments that cannot be oriented. It may be difficult to distinguish skin ➡ from squamous metaplasia ⇨. **(Right)** This duct has been almost completely replaced by squamous metaplasia. There is only a small area with normal epithelial cells ➡. In fragmented specimens, it may be difficult to distinguish skin from metaplasia within ducts.

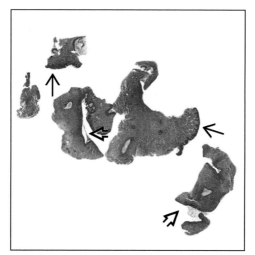
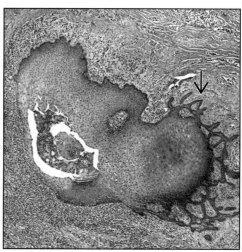

(Left) With repeated surgical interventions, secondary infections may occur. In addition to the giant cell reaction to keratin debris ⇨, an acute inflammatory reaction ➡ may also be present. **(Right)** Numerous plasma cells ➡ may be present in the inflammatory infiltrate and can be quite prominent. Some cases described as "plasma cell mastitis" occurring near the nipple may be SMOLD.

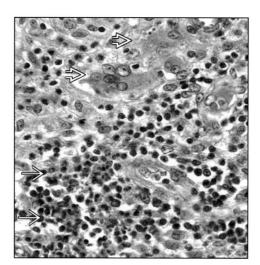
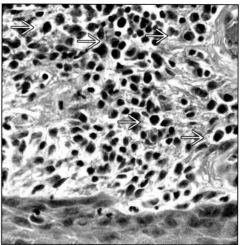

SQUAMOUS METAPLASIA OF LACTIFEROUS DUCTS

Differential Diagnosis

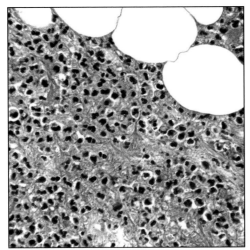
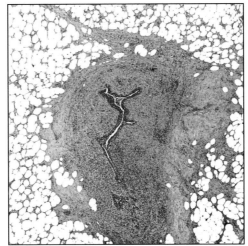

(Left) SMOLD is typically mistaken for a bacterial infection due to the erythema, swelling, and pain. Infections are characterized by an infiltrate of polymorphonuclear leukocytes. Bacteria can be identified by culture or by special stains. *(Right)* Duct ectasia and SMOLD are both inflammatory processes that involve the nipple. Duct ectasia usually presents as a mass due to periductal chronic inflammation and fibrosis involving the major ducts. Squamous metaplasia is not a feature.

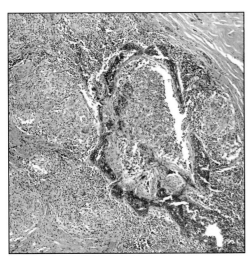
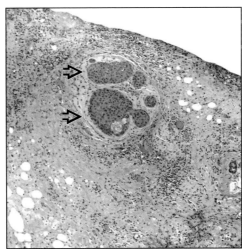

(Left) GLM can form painful masses and fistula tracks, but it occurs deep in the breast unlike the subareolar location of SMOLD. The characteristic histologic feature is the presence of well-formed granulomas impinging on ducts and lobules. *(Right)* Biopsy sites share many similar features with SMOLD, including squamous metaplasia ⊟, chronic inflammation, and a giant cell reaction. SMOLD patients often have multiple surgical procedures, which can make evaluation difficult.

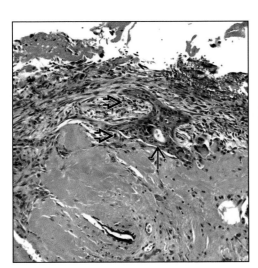
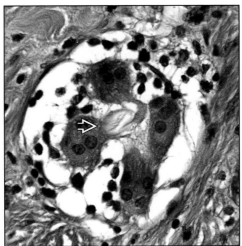

(Left) The squamous metaplasia ⊟ found in association with surgical sites is usually present lining a hematoma or seroma cavity. Foreign material ⊟ is often present. *(Right)* The giant cells within biopsy sites often form in reaction to foreign material ⊟ (surgical debris such as sutures or fibers from surgical sponges) that is both refractile and polarizable. In contrast, the giant cells associated with SMOLD are scattered and are associated with keratinaceous debris.

GRANULOMATOUS LOBULAR MASTITIS

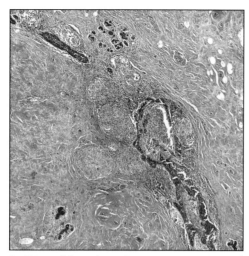

In GLM, well formed granulomas are present, centered on ducts and lobules. The epithelium appears distorted or engulfed by the inflammatory cells. A scattering of lymphocytes is also present.

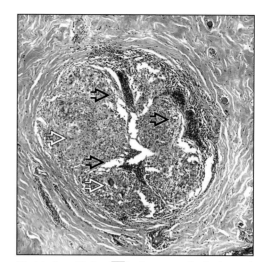

The lobular epithelium ⊟ is almost completely obscured by multiple granulomas. Scattered giant cells are present ⊟. Granulomas are not seen in the adjacent stroma, away from epithelium.

TERMINOLOGY

Abbreviations
- Granulomatous lobular mastitis (GLM)

Synonyms
- Postlactational granulomatous mastitis
- Idiopathic granulomatous mastitis
- Lobular granulomatous mastitis

Definitions
- Specific disease of breast occurring only in parous women and characterized by lobulocentric granulomas

ETIOLOGY/PATHOGENESIS

Etiology
- Association with prior childbirth suggests cell-mediated response to antigen within lobules arising during or after pregnancy
- Many women have used oral contraceptives after pregnancy, but causal relationship has not been established
- No infectious agents have been identified by special stains or by culture

CLINICAL ISSUES

Presentation
- Occurs in women up to 15 years after a pregnancy
  - Average length of time between pregnancy and presentation: 2 years
- Age range: Late teens to 40s; average age: 30s
- Patients present with firm discrete palpable breast mass ranging in size from 1-8 cm
  - Mass can occur anywhere in breast and typically does not involve nipple
    - Nipple discharge is not characteristic
  - Mass may be tender

- In advanced cases, multiple sinus tracts can open onto skin

Treatment
- Excisional biopsy is generally performed to exclude malignancy
  - In some patients, surgery is curative
- If inflammation persists, patients have been treated successfully with corticosteroids
  - Microorganisms must 1st be excluded as primary cause or as secondary infection

Prognosis
- Majority of patients are treated successfully with combination of surgery and corticosteroids

IMAGE FINDINGS

Mammographic Findings
- May show multiple small masses or ill-defined masses
- Calcifications are not associated with GLM

Ultrasonographic Findings
- May show multiple adjacent hypoechoic masses
- Dilated ducts (tubular structures) may also be present

MICROSCOPIC PATHOLOGY

Histologic Features
- Well-formed granulomas are present
  - Located within lobules or next to ducts
  - Epithelium appears to be distorted or obscured by granulomas
  - Microabscesses may be present in granulomas
    - Empty spaces (possibly due to lipids) surrounded by acute inflammatory cells are typical
- Special stains for microorganisms will be negative

GRANULOMATOUS LOBULAR MASTITIS

Key Facts

Terminology
- Specific disease of breast occurring only in parous women and characterized by lobulocentric granulomas

Etiology/Pathogenesis
- Association with prior childbirth suggests cell-mediated response to antigen within lobules arising during or after pregnancy

Clinical Issues
- Average length of time between pregnancy and presentation: 2 years
- Patients present with sometimes tender firm discrete palpable breast mass ranging in size from 1-8 cm
- Mass can occur anywhere in breast and typically does not involve nipple

- In advanced cases, multiple sinus tracts can open onto skin
- Excisional biopsy is generally performed to exclude malignancy
- If inflammation persists, patients have been treated successfully with corticosteroids

Top Differential Diagnoses
- Squamous metaplasia of lactiferous ducts (SMOLD)
- Sarcoidosis
- Wegener granulomatosis (WG)
- Infections with granulomas
  ○ TB and fungal infections must be excluded before making a diagnosis of GLM
- Duct ectasia

GLM vs. SMOLD

Feature	GLM	SMOLD
Factors increasing risk	Prior pregnancy	Tobacco use
Presentation	Tender erythematous mass in women	Tender erythematous mass in men or women
Location	Breast (rarely nipple)	Nipple
Sinus tracts	Empty onto skin	Empty at edge of areola
Microscopic appearance	Well-formed granulomas centered on ducts and lobules	Mixed inflammatory infiltrate, including giant cells
Treatment	Local excision and steroids	Surgery to remove offending duct

DIFFERENTIAL DIAGNOSIS

Squamous Metaplasia of Lactiferous Ducts (SMOLD)
- SMOLD can be described as "granulomatous mastitis," but this is not synonymous with GLM

Sarcoidosis
- Breast may be affected in patients with sarcoidosis
  ○ In rare cases, breast may be 1st or only site of involvement
- Granulomas are well formed and scattered throughout breast tissue
  ○ Granulomas are not specifically located adjacent to breast epithelium
- Necrosis is rarely, if ever, present
- Sinus tracts would be very unusual

Wegener Granulomatosis (WG)
- WG can involve breast primarily (rare) or as part of systemic involvement (lung and kidney)
- Necrotizing vasculitis is present
- Generally an area of chronic-active inflammation with fat necrosis; granulomas may be present but are not predominant feature

Infections with Granulomas
- Infections with mycobacteria (principally tuberculosis) or fungi are characterized by granulomas in breast

- Granulomas are scattered in breast tissue and not specifically associated with breast epithelium
- TB is characterized by granulomas with large areas of central caseating necrosis
- Possibility of infection should always be excluded in GLM by performing special stains &/or cultures
  ○ This is particularly important as some patients may be treated with corticosteroids

Duct Ectasia
- Inflammation involves large lactiferous ducts of nipple
- Well-formed granulomas are not typical

SELECTED REFERENCES

1. Hovanessian Larsen LJ et al: Granulomatous lobular mastitis: imaging, diagnosis, and treatment. AJR Am J Roentgenol. 193(2):574-81, 2009
2. Kuba S et al: Vacuum-assisted biopsy and steroid therapy for granulomatous lobular mastitis: report of three cases. Surg Today. 39(8):695-9, 2009
3. Baslaim MM et al: Idiopathic granulomatous mastitis: a heterogeneous disease with variable clinical presentation. World J Surg. 31(8):1677-81, 2007
4. Khamapirad T et al: Granulomatous lobular mastitis: two case reports with focus on radiologic and histopathologic features. Ann Diagn Pathol. 11(2):109-12, 2007
5. Wilson JP et al: Idiopathic granulomatous mastitis: in search of a therapeutic paradigm. Am Surg. 73(8):798-802, 2007

GRANULOMATOUS LOBULAR MASTITIS

Microscopic Features and Differential Diagnosis

(Left) A defining feature of GLM is that the granulomas are lobulocentric and appear to push against and distort the associated lobular epithelium. Here, the center of the lobule is replaced by granulomas. *(Right)* Central caseating necrosis, such as would be seen in tuberculosis, is not typical. However, focal necrosis in the center of granulomas, as seen here ⊵, may be present. Special stains for microorganisms should be performed and must be negative before making a diagnosis of GLM.

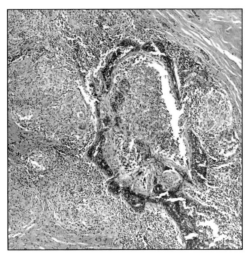
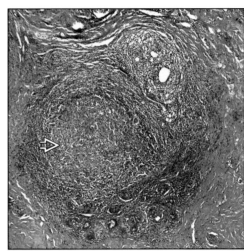

(Left) It is common to find spaces within necrotic foci that appear to be empty ⊵. The spaces are typically lined by neutrophils. The holes may represent collections of lipids that are dissolved during tissue processing. *(Right)* Similar to GLM, SMOLD can mimic an infectious process by presenting with a painful mass & sinus tract. Unlike GLM, SMOLD only occurs in a subareolar location, is associated with tobacco use, & may occur in men.

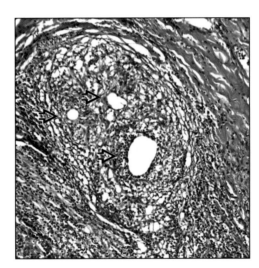
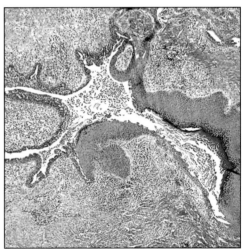

(Left) SMOLD is associated with a mixed inflammatory infiltrate consisting of lymphocytes, histiocytes, plasma cells, & neutrophils. Although scattered giant cells associated with keratin debris may be present, well-formed granulomas would be an unusual finding. *(Right)* In this case of sarcoidosis, the granulomas are located randomly in stroma ⊵. There is no specific association with ducts or lobules, and the normal architecture of the breast is not distorted.

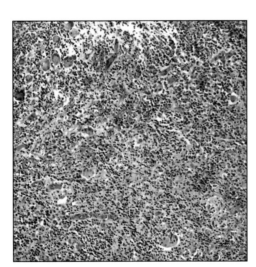
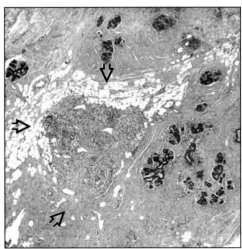

GRANULOMATOUS LOBULAR MASTITIS

Differential Diagnosis

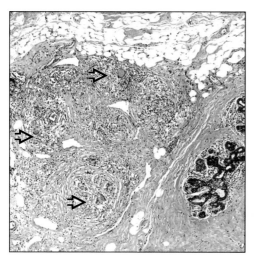
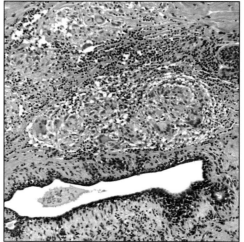

(Left) The granulomas of sarcoidosis of the breast tend to be smaller than those seen in GLM. Scattered Langhans giant cells are present ⮞. Asteroid or Schaumann bodies may be seen but are not specific for sarcoidosis. Necrosis is not a typical feature. (Right) This is another case of sarcoidosis showing a typical granuloma adjacent to, but not involving, a duct.

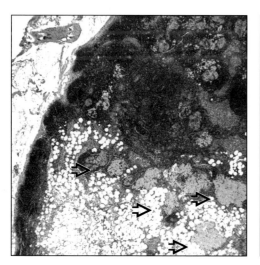
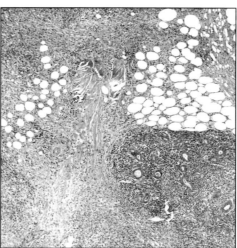

(Left) In sarcoidosis, granulomas ⮞ are often present in lymph nodes as well as other organ sites throughout the body. The granulomas of GLM are restricted to the breast parenchyma. (Right) Wegener granulomatosis is a form of necrotizing vasculitis that rarely affects the breast. A chronic active inflammatory infiltrate involves the breast tissue. Granulomatous inflammation, consisting of scattered giant cells, may be present. Well-formed granulomas are not typical.

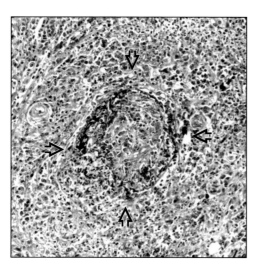
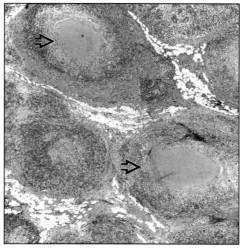

(Left) The vasculitis of Wegener granulomatosis is shown by this reticulin stain demonstrating a blood vessel completely engulfed by inflammatory cells ⮞. (Right) TB of the breast is a rare diagnosis worldwide. In the USA, it has been reported in patients with AIDS. The granulomas are scattered in the breast without a specific relationship to ducts or lobules. Large areas of caseous necrosis are present ⮞. Special stains should reveal mycobacteria.

IMPLANT PATHOLOGY

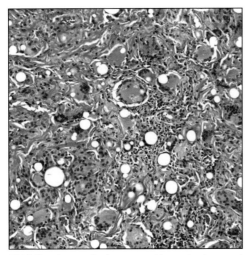

Thick fibrotic capsules form around breast implants and are associated with various types of foreign material. It may not be possible to determine the composition of many implants.

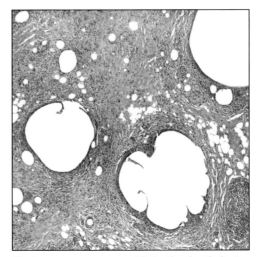

The large empty spaces are filled with refractile foreign material of uncertain type. There is a surrounding lymphocytic infiltrate.

TERMINOLOGY

Synonyms
- Silicone implant
- Saline implant
- Tissue expanders

Definitions
- Foreign material placed within chest wall to replace or enhance breast tissue
  - Some implants are placed between breast tissue and pectoral muscle
  - Subpectoral implants are placed between pectoral muscle and chest wall

ETIOLOGY/PATHOGENESIS

Types of Implants
- Direct injection of substances has been used to augment breast size
  - Substances used have included organic oils, silicone, paraffin, and others
  - These substances usually migrate over time and result in a poor cosmetic appearance
  - This is not an accepted medical procedure
  - Foreign material can closely mimic a malignancy on breast imaging
    - Material may cause skin or nipple retraction and migrate to lymph nodes causing lymphadenopathy
- Saline implants
  - These implants have thin silicone outer shell that is filled with saline
  - Some are intended for permanent use
  - Tissue expanders are temporary saline implants used prior to definitive breast reconstruction
    - Usually have a port that can be used to inject more saline

- Implant is eventually replaced by permanent implant or by tissue reconstruction
  - If saline implant ruptures, there is immediate deflation and saline is quickly resorbed by surrounding tissue
- Silicone implants
  - Silicone implants have thin silicone outer shell and are filled with silicone gel
  - These implants are intended for permanent use
  - If silicone implant ruptures, silicone is usually confined within surrounding fibrotic capsule
    - Imaging studies may be necessary to detect ruptured implant
- Implants with polyurethane patches
  - Rough surfaced patches were used on some older implants to reduce effects of fibrotic response
  - Polyurethane has specific histologic appearance in capsular tissue

History of Breast Implants
- 1st silicone shell implant was used in 1961
- From 1992-2006, use of silicone implants was restricted to FDA-approved research projects due to safety concerns
  - Many well-publicized lawsuits were based on claims that implants were associated with autoimmune-type diseases
- In 1999, National Institute of Medicine released a report stating that connective tissue disease was not more common in women with implants
- In 2006, FDA lifted the moratorium on implants but did require follow-up studies of patients
- In 1992, 32,000 women underwent augmentation procedures
- In 2007, 347,000 underwent augmentation procedures
- There are likely 2,000,000-5,000,000 women in USA currently with breast implants

IMPLANT PATHOLOGY

Key Facts

Terminology

- Breasts may be augmented or replaced by foreign material for cosmetic reasons or for reconstruction after surgery
- Foreign material (such as silicone, paraffin, or organic oils) may be directly injected into breast tissue
  - This procedure is associated with high rate of complications
- Majority of implants consist of thin silicone shell filled with saline or silicone gel
  - Tissue expanders are saline implants that are placed temporarily before tissue reconstruction
- Implants may be placed within the breast anterior to pectoralis muscle or below the muscle

Clinical Issues

- Implants are associated with a variety of complications
  - Capsular contracture is most common complication and may require surgery to correct
  - Silicone shell thins and may rupture; silicone can migrate to lymph nodes and distant sites
  - Infection may occur, usually during perioperative period
  - Capsule may calcify; this, and a thin delicate shell, can make mammographic screening more difficult
  - Rare cases of fibromatosis have been associated with implants
  - Very rare cases of T-cell lymphomas are reported in association with implants

CLINICAL ISSUES

Presentation

- Infections associated with implants are rare
  - Most cases occur in perioperative period and are due to skin bacteria
  - In very rare cases, unusual organisms have been reported (fungi or mycobacteria)

Treatment

- If contracture is pronounced, implant may need to be replaced to achieve acceptable cosmetic result
  - In the past, contractures were treated with pressure to "break" the capsule
  - This technique is no longer used as it may result in leakage of silicone into adjacent breast tissue
- If infection occurs, implant must be removed

Complications and Treatment

- Silicone implant rupture and migration of silicone
  - Silicone can "bleed" through intact implant shell and may be present in surrounding capsule
    - Silicone is usually restricted to capsule when implant is intact
  - If both implant and capsule are ruptured, silicone can migrate to distant sites
    - Most common site is regional lymph nodes
    - Silicone has also been reported to migrate to distant subcutaneous tissue and lung
- Implant-associated lymphoma
  - May occur with both saline and silicone implants
  - Usually presents as implant complication, such as seroma or presumed infection
  - Presents 1-23 years after surgery
  - About 1/2 of patients have had cosmetic surgery and 1/2 breast reconstruction after breast cancer
  - Majority of implant-associated lymphomas arise from T cells
    - Only 10% of all primary breast lymphomas are T-cell lymphomas

- 22 of 30 cases of primary breast anaplastic large cell lymphomas have been associated with implants
- Implant-associated mesenchymal tumors
  - Most common type of soft tissue tumor occurring in breasts with implants (either silicone or saline filled) is fibromatosis
  - Tumor is generally detected with 2-3 years of surgery
  - These women are not known to have mutations in adenomatosis polyposis coli gene or to have Gardner syndrome
  - Sarcomas occurring in women with implants are extremely rare and are of diverse types
  - Specific etiologic relationship between tumor formation and implants has not been established
- Capsular contracture
  - Most common complication associated with implants
  - Additional surgery to remove implant &/or capsule may be necessary to achieve acceptable cosmetic result
  - In the past, capsule was compressed to "break" the capsule
    - This technique is no longer used as it can lead to migration of silicone to other sites
  - Thick area of fibrosis forms around the implant
    - Pseudosynovial lining consisting of histiocytes and inflammatory cells often forms
- Infection
  - Most infections occur during perisurgical period and are due to common bacteria
  - In very rare cases, unusual organisms have been reported (i.e., fungi or mycobacteria)

IMAGE FINDINGS

Mammographic Findings

- Presence of implant complicates mammographic examination
  - Special views are available to visualize breast tissue around implant

o Care must be taken to not rupture the implant with compression

o Calcification of implant shell can obscure breast calcifications

Ultrasonographic Findings

- Free silicone is highly echogenic and has "snowstorm" appearance

MR Findings

- Best imaging technique to detect rupture of silicone-filled implant
  o Silicone shell can be seen floating within silicone gel ("linguine" sign)
  o Intracapsular and extracapsular rupture can be detected
  o Silicone in adjacent tissue and in axillary lymph nodes can also be imaged

MACROSCOPIC FEATURES

General Features

- Documentation of implants
  o Gross description includes appearance and identifying marks
  o Intact implants: May not be possible to distinguish saline from silicone implant
  o Ruptured implants
    ▪ Saline implants will be empty and usually dry
    ▪ Silicone implants will consist of portions of shell within viscous silicone gel
    ▪ Rupture can occur during surgery for explantation; pathologist cannot determine when rupture occurred
- Documentation of surrounding tissue
  o Capsule is usually received in multiple fragments
  o Silicone granulomas can have gross appearance of hard, irregular, gritty masses
    ▪ Gross appearance can closely mimic invasive carcinoma
  o Capsule should be sectioned perpendicular to capsule surface, if possible
  o All grossly evident masses should be sampled

MICROSCOPIC PATHOLOGY

Histologic Features

- All implants
  o Capsule consists of dense fibrosis
  o Chronic inflammatory cells may be present
  o Acute inflammation, eosinophils, or granulomas are unusual and suggest another pathologic process
    ▪ Secondary infections should be suspected and tissue sent for culture, if possible
  o Inner surface of capsule is lined by pseudosynovium consisting of histiocytes
- Silicone implants
  o All silicone implants "bleed" silicone gel through the shell
    ▪ This occurs in the absence of frank rupture of the shell

o Silicone has a number of appearances
  ▪ Silicone may be refractile but is not polarizable
  ▪ Much of silicone is dissolved during tissue processing
  ▪ Intracellular silicone has appearance of multiple vacuoles of varying sizes within histiocytes
  ▪ Vacuoles can cause notching of nucleus and mimic appearance of lipoblasts
  ▪ Extracellular silicone has appearance of clear spaces partially occupied by refractile material and surrounded by macrophages, giant cells, and lymphocytes
  ▪ Other organic oils can have same histologic appearance
  ▪ Special techniques (e.g., x-ray analysis or Raman spectroscopy) can be used to specifically identify foreign material as silicone

- Implants with polyurethane patches
  o Polyurethane has structure of a sponge
  o In cross section, interstices of the sponge have triangular shape
  o Polyurethane will be found within fibrotic capsule
- Directly injected materials
  o Wide variety of materials have been injected into breasts for augmentation
  o Histologic appearance and tissue response depend on type of material

SELECTED REFERENCES

1. Balzer BL et al: Do biomaterials cause implant-associated mesenchymal tumors of the breast? Analysis of 8 new cases and review of the literature. Hum Pathol. 40(11):1564-70, 2009
2. Dragu A et al: Intrapulmonary and cutaneous siliconomas after silent silicone breast implant failure. Breast J. 15(5):496-9, 2009
3. Gonçales ES et al: Silicone implant for chin augmentation mimicking a low-grade liposarcoma. Oral Surg Oral Med Oral Pathol Oral Radiol Endod. 107(4):e21-3, 2009
4. Li S et al: Silicone implant and primary breast ALK1-negative anaplastic large cell lymphoma, fact or fiction? Int J Clin Exp Pathol. 3(1):117-27, 2009
5. Miranda RN et al: Anaplastic large cell lymphoma involving the breast: a clinicopathologic study of 6 cases and review of the literature. Arch Pathol Lab Med. 133(9):1383-90, 2009
6. Sagi L et al: Silicone breast implant rupture presenting as bilateral leg nodules. Clin Exp Dermatol. 34(5):e99-101, 2009
7. Bar-Meir E et al: Silicone gel breast implants and connective tissue disease--a comprehensive review. Autoimmunity. 36(4):193-7, 2003
8. Abbondanzo SL et al: Silicone gel-filled breast and testicular implant capsules: a histologic and immunophenotypic study. Mod Pathol. 12(7):706-13, 1999
9. van Diest PJ et al: Pathology of silicone leakage from breast implants. J Clin Pathol. 51(7):493-7, 1998
10. Raso DS et al: Silicone breast implants: pathology. Ultrastruct Pathol. 21(3):263-71, 1997

IMPLANT PATHOLOGY

Microscopic Features

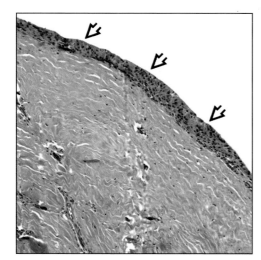

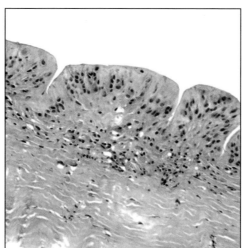

(Left) A densely fibrous capsule forms around all types of implants. The most common implant complication is contracture of this capsule, which causes cosmetic deformity. Chronic inflammatory cells, calcifications, and silicone that has bled through the shell are often present. A pseudosynovial lining forms at the interface between the fibrous capsule and the implant ⮞. *(Right)* The pseudosynovium ("synovial metaplasia") consists of a layer of macrophages that may appear oriented.

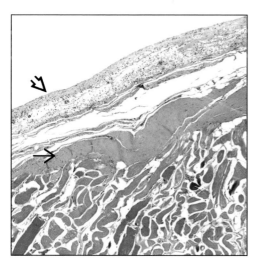

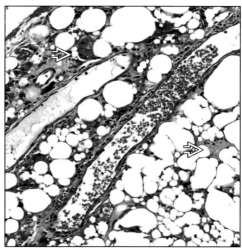

(Left) Subpectoral implants are placed below the pectoralis muscle. In this case, the fibrotic implant capsule ⮞ is located above skeletal muscle ➡. *(Right)* Silicone can fill cells and mimic adipocytes. The variety of cell sizes and the presence of occasional pleomorphic nuclei can mimic the appearance of liposarcoma. In such cases, it is important to note the presence of giant cells ⮞, foreign material, and the clinical setting.

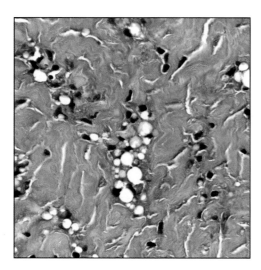

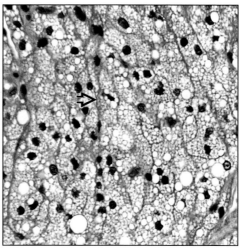

(Left) Silicone is found in the capsules of silicone implants even in the absence of rupture, as the silicone gel can "bleed" through the longer silicone polymers making up the implant envelope. Silicone can be extracellular or appear as fine vacuoles within histiocytes. *(Right)* When histiocytes are filled with silicone, the vacuoles can indent the nucleus ⮞ and mimic the appearance of lipoblasts.

Microscopic Features

(Left) Some older implants had patches made of polyurethane in an attempt to reduce capsular contracture. The polyurethane has a sponge-like structure. Cross sections are angular in shape ⊡. *(Right)* Polyurethane is identified in this capsule as refractile triangular fragments.

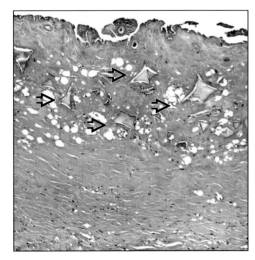

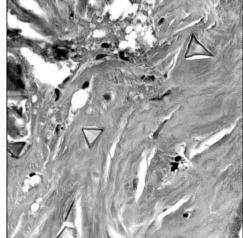

(Left) This implant has larger areas of foreign material surrounded by giant cells. *(Right)* The lymphocytes adjacent to implant capsules are predominantly T cells, as demonstrated in this case with an antibody to the T-cell marker CD3. The most common type of lymphoma associated with implants is anaplastic T-cell lymphoma.

CD 3

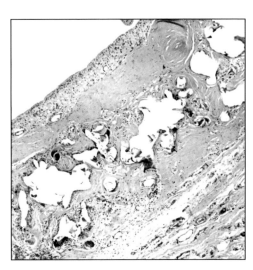

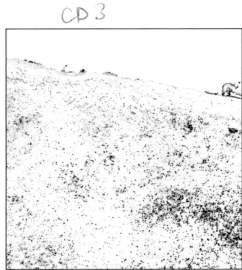

(Left) Over time, an implant capsule can become calcified ⊡. The presence of these calcifications can complicate the detection of cancer-associated calcifications during mammographic screening. *(Right)* Infections are a rare complication of implants and usually occur in the perioperative period. This was postoperative S. aureus infection. Numerous polymorphonuclear leukocytes are present. In rare cases, fungal or mycobacterial infections are reported.

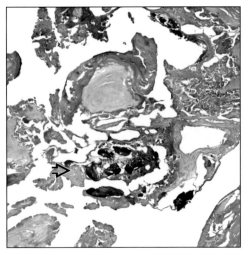

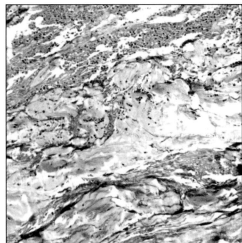

IMPLANT PATHOLOGY

Complications

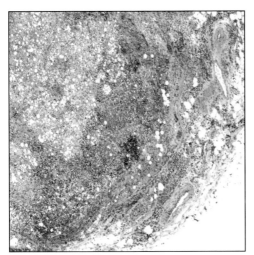 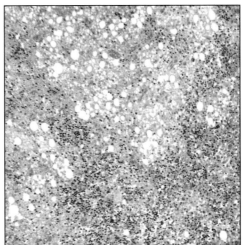

(Left) After a silicone implant ruptures, silicone can migrate to other sites in the body. The most common site is the regional lymph nodes, as in this case. (Right) The silicone is present in histiocytes in the lymph node. Silicone has also been reported to migrate to distant skin sites and the lung.

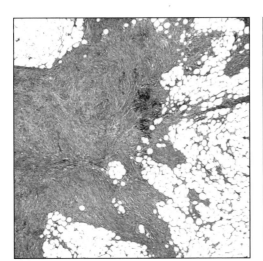 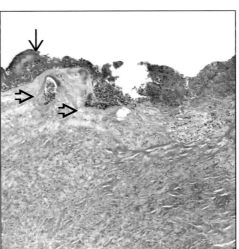

(Left) In rare cases, fibromatosis has been associated with the presence of an implant or other foreign material in the breast. (Right) This patient presented with a clinical seroma adjacent to a breast implant. An anaplastic lymphoma was present in the fluid around the implant ➡ and within the capsule ➡.

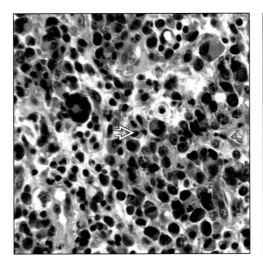 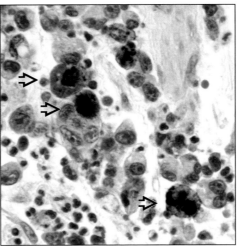

(Left) Anaplastic large cell lymphoma is characterized by cells with pleomorphic nuclei, some of them horseshoe-shaped ➡. Mitotic figures and areas of necrosis are common. (Right) Anaplastic large cell lymphomas associated with breast implants are characteristically immunoreactive for CD30 and CD43 and may be reactive for some T cell markers. The cells can also be focally positive for EMA ➡ but are keratin negative and should not be mistaken for carcinoma.

IATROGENIC CHANGES

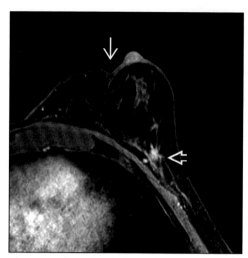

This patient has a history of breast cancer. The prior excisional site caused retraction of the skin ➡. A subsequent cancer ➡ is located at a different site and is likely a new primary.

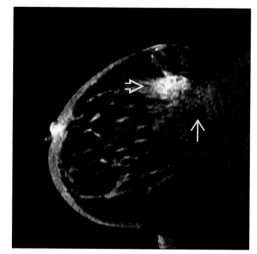

This is a recurrent invasive carcinoma ➡ at the site of a prior excision for cancer ➡. Therefore, this is most likely a treatment-resistant cancer and is associated with a very poor prognosis.

TERMINOLOGY

Definitions
- Pathologic changes in breast due to prior treatment (surgery, radiation, or medical treatment)

ETIOLOGY/PATHOGENESIS

Treatment-related Changes
- Breast is unusual organ in that entire organ is typically not removed and multiple surgical procedures are often performed over short period of time
  - Thus, recent biopsy sites and excisional sites as well as older excisional sites are common findings in breast specimens
- Medical treatments and radiation therapy can also result in pathologic changes
- Recognition of changes associated with prior treatment is important to understand relationship of breast lesions to these prior procedures and to avoid misinterpretation of iatrogenic changes as malignancy

Documentation of Removal of Targeted Lesion
- Excisions after core needle biopsy must include prior biopsy site
  - Specimen radiography should document removal of any residual lesion &/or clips marking site
  - In some cases, clip may not have been deployed at site of lesion
  - In other cases, clip may be lost if biopsy site is transected during procedure
  - Histologic findings of core biopsy site must be documented
    - However, if excision occurs > 1 month after biopsy, inflammatory changes may have resolved
- Margin excisions should include a portion of prior biopsy cavity

- Biopsy site changes at margin may indicate incomplete removal of a lesion

Indication of Important Clinical History
- Results of any prior excision should be available
  - Interpretation of residual lesions may be altered with respect to prior history
- If there is prior history of cancer, patient may have received treatment
  - Radiation therapy can cause nuclear atypia
  - These changes could be mistaken for neoplasia if pathologist is unaware of this history

Recurrence vs. New Primary Invasive Cancers
- Recurrent invasive cancers have poor prognosis as they are treatment resistant
  - These cancers usually occur at site of original cancer
  - New primary carcinomas have a better prognosis as they may be sensitive to treatment
- Prior biopsy sites can sometimes be recognized by dense fibrosis &/or suture material
  - If present, it is important to document location of 2nd carcinoma with respect to 1st

Treatment-associated Tumors
- Some types of treatment can cause tumors
- Fibromatosis associated with surgery (or breast implant)
  - May occur at site of prior surgery
- Radiation-associated sarcoma
  - Most commonly, angiosarcoma of skin after radiation therapy for breast carcinoma
- Radiation-associated carcinoma
  - Occurs in women undergoing radiation to breasts during late teens and early 20s
    - Radiation at later ages does not markedly increase cancer risk
- Implant-associated lymphoma

IATROGENIC CHANGES

Key Facts

Etiology/Pathogenesis
- Pathologic changes occur in breast due to prior surgery, radiation therapy, and medical treatment
- Treatment-related changes are important to recognize

Clinical Issues
- Excisions after core needle biopsy must document prior biopsy site
- Biopsy site changes must be correlated with prior clinical history and treatment
- Recurrent carcinomas should be distinguished from new primary carcinomas
- Tumors caused by treatment should be recognized
  - Biopsy-associated fibromatosis
  - Radiation-associated sarcoma
  - Radiation-associated carcinoma
  - Implant-associated lymphoma

- Fibroadenomas associated with cyclosporine
- Carcinomas associated with hormone replacement therapy
- Iatrogenic changes can mimic malignancy
  - Squamous metaplasia
  - Radiation atypia
  - Epithelial displacement
  - Degenerating skeletal muscle
  - Neuromas

Image Findings
- May be difficult to detect recurrent carcinoma

Top Differential Diagnoses
- Ruptured cysts
- Fat necrosis
- Tumors mimicking inflammatory lesions

- Very rare form of T-cell lymphoma has been reported in ~ 30 cases of women with breast implants
- Lymphoma is found in a seroma cavity surrounding implant
- Cyclosporine-associated fibroadenomas
  - Renal transplant patients treated with cyclosporine may develop fibroadenomas
  - Fibroadenomas can regress when cyclosporine is withdrawn
- Hormone replacement treatment-related carcinomas
  - Women taking hormonal therapy after menopause are at increased risk for estrogen receptor-positive cancers
  - It is unknown if estrogen acts as a carcinogen to cause cancers or if it stimulates growth (and therefore detection) of already existing carcinomas

IMAGE FINDINGS

Mammographic Findings
- Prior surgical sites generally have an irregular appearance
  - May be difficult to detect recurrent carcinoma
- Radiodense debris can be present due to surgical procedure (e.g., metallic fragments)
- Associated fat necrosis can calcify
- For excisional sites, skin scar will be present

MACROSCOPIC FEATURES

Core Needle Biopsy Sites
- Site usually has small central area of hemorrhage (~ 0.5 cm) surrounded by ill-defined area of firm tissue and fat necrosis
- Clip is very small (1-2 mm) but may be seen with careful examination
- Some clip deployment systems place gelatin foam pledgets within biopsy site
  - These are often color and shape of rice
    - May be mistaken for calcifications or papilloma

- Usually fall out of tissue
- Some systems use larger rectangular-shaped gel
  - May be surrounded by pseudocapsule with minimal inflammatory response
  - If gel falls out of tissue, site can be difficult to identify
- If core biopsy was of small invasive carcinoma, size of carcinoma may be difficult to ascertain grossly
  - Correlation with imaging studies prior to biopsy may be necessary to determine best size for AJCC T classification

Excisional Sites
- There is generally bleeding at center of excisional site and loss of tissue
- Surrounding tissue is firm but not hard and may extend for several millimeters into surrounding breast
- Fat necrosis appears as chalky white or yellowish streaks
- Residual invasive cancer may be present as areas hard to palpation adjacent to cavity

MICROSCOPIC PATHOLOGY

Core Needle Biopsy Sites
- Usually linear track of fibrosis with increased cellularity and hemosiderin-laden macrophages
- If gelatin foam pledgets are present, they appear as acellular amphophilic material in center of biopsy site
  - There is chronic inflammatory response with giant cells around gelatin

Recent Excisional Sites
- Usually easily identified due to fibrosis, hemorrhage, fat necrosis, and chronic inflammation
- Cautery artifact is often present due to common use of electrocautery (e.g., Bovie™) to excise breast tissue
  - Electric field is generated in tissue
  - Cells and nuclei become elongated due to electrical potential across the cell membrane
  - Tissue with extensive cauterization loses recognizable histologic features and antigenicity

o Other types of heat (e.g., ultrasonic coagulation or ablation) result in coagulative necrosis
- Suture material is often present
  o Biodegradable suture ("catgut" suture) is monofilament made of strands of collagen
  o Usually ovoid in shape and brightly eosinophilic
  o Sutures are resorbed by exuberant chronic inflammatory infiltrate with foreign body giant cells
  o Collagen can have jagged edges, and elongated nuclei may be present
    ▪ May be mistaken for heterotopic bone formation
  o Polyfilament sutures may also be present
- Seromas and postoperative infections are possible complications

Remote Excisional Sites

- Extent of healing varies greatly from patient to patient in terms of degree of response and time course
- In some patients, there will not be any histologic evidence of a prior site
- In majority of patients, an area of fibrosis will mark prior site
  o It is often difficult to distinguish this area with certainty from normal dense breast tissue
- In a few patients, suture material and other types of foreign material may remain for many years
  o In rare cases, these sites can appear to increase in size
- Traumatic neuromas may form
  o May cause masses increasing in size at prior biopsy sites

Iatrogenic Changes Mimicking Malignancy

- Squamous metaplasia
  o Frequently occurs in epithelial cells next to sites of trauma and inflammation
  o Changes can mimic carcinoma due to monomorphic appearance of cells, nuclear enlargement and irregularity, and associated stromal reaction
  o Spindle cell carcinomas can occur in this setting
    ▪ Atypical-appearing spindle cell proliferations should be evaluated by IHC
    ▪ Basal keratins and p63 are often positive in tumor cells
- Radiation atypia
  o Prior radiation therapy can cause nuclear enlargement
  o Atypical cells are typically scattered in atrophic lobules
  o Cells should not be proliferative (i.e., have mitotic figures or form architecturally complex patterns)
  o Diagnosis of malignancy should be made with great caution
    ▪ After radiation therapy, mastectomy may be only option for recurrent carcinoma
- Epithelial displacement
  o Normal or malignant cells can be pushed into stroma, vascular channels, or lymph nodes by palpation, biopsy, or pathology processing
    ▪ Increased number of isolated tumor cells is found after breast massage prior to sentinel node biopsy

▪ Benign epithelial cells associated with myoepithelial cells may be identified in lymph nodes after breast surgery
    ▪ Normal epithelial cells can be found in needle tracks or vascular spaces; most commonly seen related to papillary lesions
  o Clinical significance of displacement of malignant cells is unknown
    ▪ Finding of epithelial cells in needle tracks diminishes with length of time between needle biopsy and excision
    ▪ Suggests that displaced cells may not survive
  o Diagnosis of invasive carcinoma should be made with great caution if the only areas of "invasion" are in biopsy site changes
- Degenerating or regenerating skeletal muscle
  o Cells become rounded, and nuclei move to center of cells
  o Nuclei appear enlarged and hyperchromatic

DIFFERENTIAL DIAGNOSIS

Ruptured Cysts

- Cysts can rupture spontaneously or due to trauma
- Secretory material dispersed into the surrounding tissue can incite an intense chronic active inflammatory response

Fat Necrosis

- Can occur due to trauma or be present in absence of trauma
- Foreign material and cautery changes are absent

Tumors

- Some tumors can mimic inflammatory cells
  o Granular cell tumors (histiocytes), invasive lobular carcinoma (lymphocytes, histiocytes, or hematopoietic cells in bone marrow), histiocytoid carcinoma (histiocytes), lymphomas (lymphocytes)
- Generally lack mixed inflammatory cell infiltrate typical of true inflammatory lesions

SELECTED REFERENCES

1. Reynolds C et al: Displaced epithelium after liposuction in gynecomastia. Int J Surg Pathol. Epub ahead of print, 2010
2. Gatta G et al: Clinical, mammographic and ultrasonographic features of blunt breast trauma. Eur J Radiol. 59(3):327-30, 2006
3. Nagi C et al: Epithelial displacement in breast lesions: a papillary phenomenon. Arch Pathol Lab Med. 129(11):1465-9, 2005
4. Deurloo EE et al: Displacement of breast tissue and needle deviations during stereotactic procedures. Invest Radiol. 36(6):347-53, 2001
5. Korbin CD et al: Metallic particles on mammography after wire localization. AJR Am J Roentgenol. 169(6):1637-8, 1997

IATROGENIC CHANGES

Foreign Material at Biopsy Sites

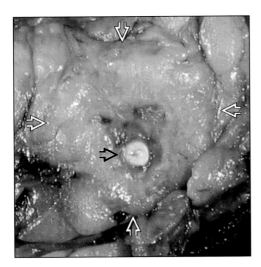 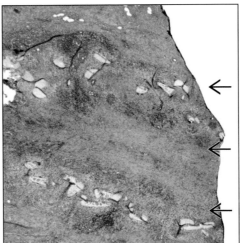

(Left) This invasive carcinoma ⮕ was previously sampled by core needle biopsy. The gel pledget and clip ⮕ mark the site of the prior biopsy. Clip placement is particularly important to mark the site of cancers prior to neoadjuvant therapy. **(Right)** A prior core needle biopsy showed ADH, and excision was recommended. In this excision, the biopsy site containing gel pledgets has been transected ⮕. The patient later recurred with calcifications and was diagnosed with DCIS.

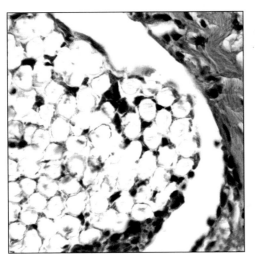 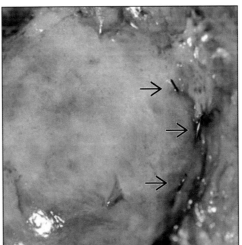

(Left) Polyfilament nonabsorbable sutures are often used to approximate the skin and are later removed. There is a mild inflammatory infiltrate associated with this suture. **(Right)** This patient developed fibromatosis in the deep breast near the chest wall at the site of prior surgery. A blue synthetic suture ⮕ left from the prior procedure confirms the location of the tumor at the previous surgical site.

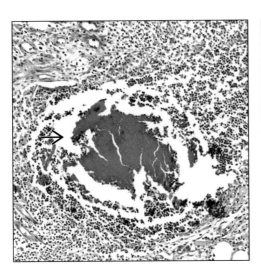 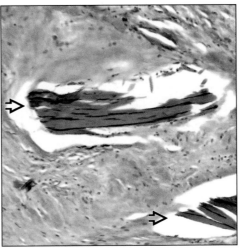

(Left) Resorbable sutures ⮕ may be made of collagen and are designed to be biodegradable. They are usually surrounded by chronic inflammatory cells and show fragmentation and dissolution. **(Right)** Sutures can be intensely eosinophilic and have jagged edges and linear nuclei (due to the sterilization procedure) ⮕. In some cases they become walled off rather than completely resorbed. They can be mistaken for heterotopic bone formation.

IATROGENIC CHANGES

Common Features of Biopsy Sites

(Left) Biopsy sites can be recognized by areas of increased stromal cellularity, hemorrhage, and hemosiderin-laden macrophages ➡. Foreign material, often with a giant cell response, mark areas of prior surgery. *(Right)* There is generally a zone of cautery &/or coagulative necrosis several millimeters in width around the center of an excisional site ➡. This is one reason why focally positive margins for invasive carcinomas usually do not correlate with residual disease.

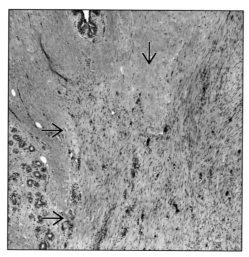

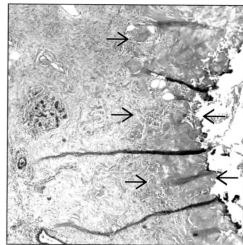

(Left) Cautery causes streaming of cell nuclei ➨ due to the application of an electric field across the cell membrane. It is helpful evidence that tissue is close to the true surgical margin. This artifact can preclude the accurate evaluation of epithelial lesions at the margin of a specimen. *(Right)* Traumatic neuromas may grow in size over time at the sites of excisions. They may present as an enlarging mass that can be worrisome for recurrent carcinoma in a scar.

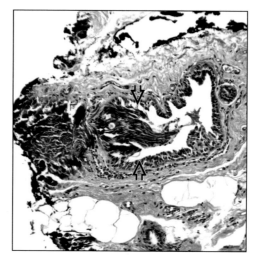

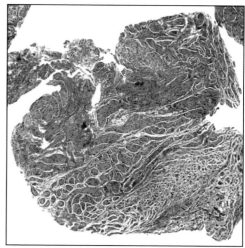

(Left) Old excisional sites may heal as large areas of dense collagenous fibrosis. Scattered clusters of hemosiderin-laden macrophages ➡ support identification of this area as a prior surgical site. *(Right)* This intermediate-grade phyllodes tumor ➨ is invasive into the adjacent tissue. An important part of the history is evident from the presence of an adjacent surgical site ➡. A low-grade phyllodes tumor was excised 3 years previously and has now recurred at a higher grade.

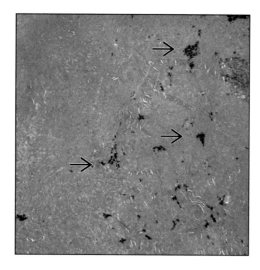

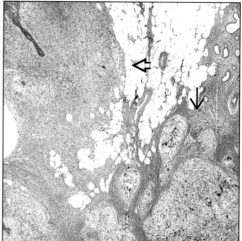

IATROGENIC CHANGES

Iatrogenic Mimics of Malignancy

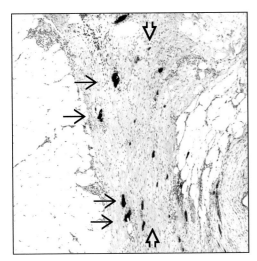 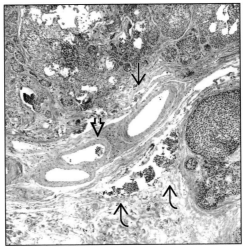

(Left) Multiple areas of displaced keratin-positive epithelium ⮕ have been pushed into the stroma of a needle track ⮎ in a case of DCIS. *(Right)* In this excisional specimen with DCIS after a core needle biopsy, tumor cells are present in blood vessels ⮎ and lymphatics ⮕. This was interpreted as artifactual displacement, as tumor cells were also present in tissue clefts ⮎ and no invasive carcinoma was identified in the breast nor metastatic carcinoma in the lymph nodes.

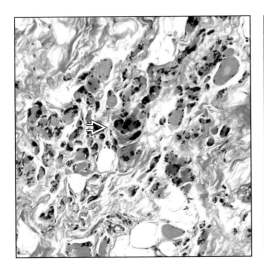 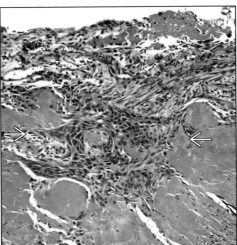

(Left) Regenerating skeletal muscle cells have centrally located nuclei ⮎ and a more rounded shape. This is a common finding in deep excisional sites that involve the pectoralis muscle. These cells should not be mistaken for tumor cells. *(Right)* Squamous metaplasia is a frequent response to trauma or inflammation of epithelium. It is often seen in the walls of biopsy site cavities ⮕. The nuclei can appear atypical but should not be overinterpreted as residual carcinoma.

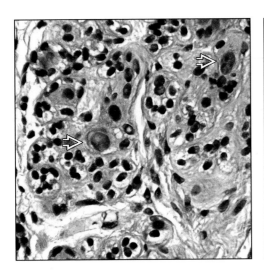 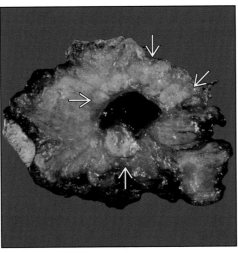

(Left) Radiation therapy can cause marked nuclear atypia ⮎ in atrophic lobules. The cells should not form solid masses or proliferate. In some cases, it can be difficult to distinguish these changes from carcinoma in situ. *(Right)* This seroma cavity marks the site of an excision for an invasive carcinoma. Areas of adjacent fat necrosis form firm tan areas ⮕ that could be mistaken for residual carcinoma grossly. No residual invasive carcinoma was present.

IATROGENIC CHANGES

Tumors Mimicking Inflammatory Lesions

(Left) The cells of histiocytoid carcinomas have abundant amphophilic foamy cytoplasm and resemble histiocytes. The majority are lobular carcinomas and are positive for keratin and GCDFP-15. However, this type of cancer may also express E-cadherin. *(Right)* A histiocytoid carcinoma can usually be distinguished from true histiocytes due to nuclear pleomorphism ⊟ and mitotic figures ➡. In some cases, an immunoperoxidase study may be necessary to confirm the presence of cytokeratin.

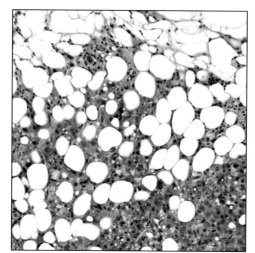 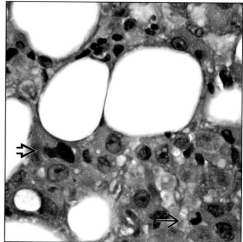

S100

(Left) The cells of a granular cell tumor have abundant foamy cytoplasm and inconspicuous nuclei. Although the cells can resemble histiocytes, the other cells usually present in inflammatory lesions such as lymphocytes and plasma cells are absent. *(Right)* It is important to note that both granular cells and histiocytes are positive for CD68. A better marker is S100, which is strongly and diffusely positive in the granular cells ➡ and generally absent or focal in histiocytes.

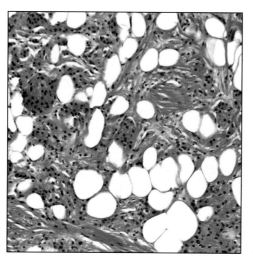 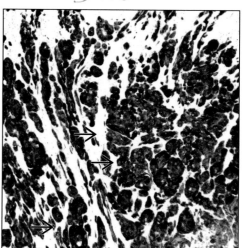

(Left) The cells of grade 1 invasive lobular carcinomas can resemble lymphocytes, and the cells of grade 2 lobular carcinomas can mimic histiocytes. Metastatic lobular carcinoma ➡ in this hernia sac was mistaken for an inflammatory reaction and reactive mesothelial cells. *(Right)* Low-grade lymphomas can be difficult to distinguish from benign inflammatory infiltrates in small biopsies. Usually, lymphomas form solid masses although they may on occasion involve lobules ⊟.

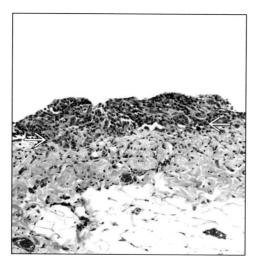 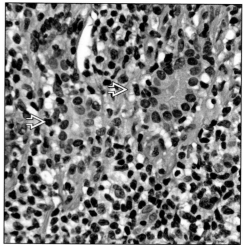

IATROGENIC CHANGES

Iatrogenic Tumors

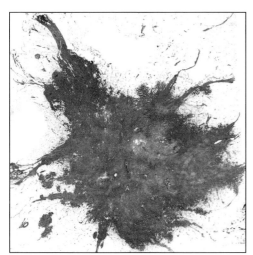

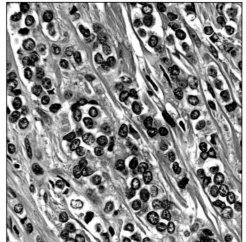

(Left) Chest wall radiation at a young age increases the risk of developing breast carcinomas of no special type. Many of these patients are young women who were treated for Hodgkin disease. They should undergo increased surveillance. (Right) Women taking postmenopausal hormones are at increased risk for developing estrogen receptor-positive carcinomas, such as lobular carcinoma. It is unknown if estrogen acts as a carcinogen or if it stimulates growth of preexisting carcinomas.

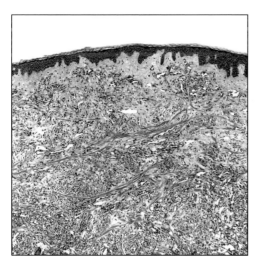

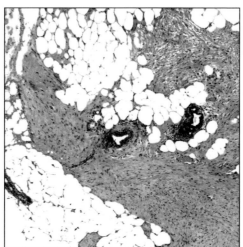

(Left) Radiation treatment for breast cancer increases the risk of developing sarcomas, particularly angiosarcoma, usually 5-10 years later. Radiation-related tumors occur in the skin. The incidence is also increased in arms with edema after lymphadenectomy (Stewart-Treves syndrome). (Right) A minority of cases of fibromatosis of the breast arise at the site of prior surgery or trauma. There are no special features associated with these tumors.

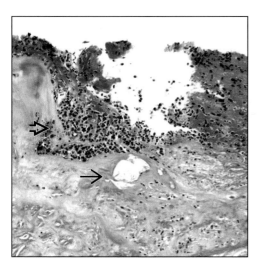

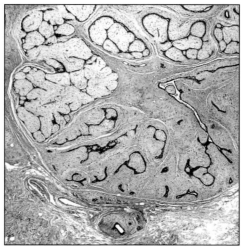

(Left) ALK1-negative anaplastic large T-cell lymphoma ⇨ is a very rare malignancy of the breast. More than 1/2 of the cases have been diagnosed in the seroma fluid and capsules surrounding breast implants, both silicone ⇨ and saline-filled implants. (Right) Multiple fibroadenomas may develop in the breasts of patients treated with cyclosporine after renal transplantation. The tumors can regress after the type of therapy is changed.

Other Types of Malignancies

METASTASES TO THE BREAST

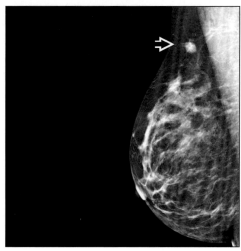

This patient with lung cancer developed a palpable mass corresponding to a mammographic density ⊃ in an area of adipose tissue. A core needle biopsy confirmed metastatic lung carcinoma.

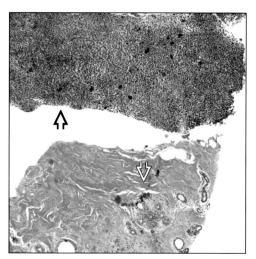

The most common metastatic tumor to the breast is melanoma. In this core needle biopsy, the melanoma ⊃ is present in adipose tissue and is detached from adjacent areas of breast tissue ⊃.

TERMINOLOGY

Definitions
- Metastatic tumors to the breast from different primary sites

CLINICAL ISSUES

Presentation
- Metastases to the breast comprise < 3% of all breast malignancies
- Most common presentation is palpable breast mass
  - Less common presentations are mass on imaging (about 10% with calcifications) or inflammatory carcinoma
  - Axillary and other regional lymph nodes are often enlarged
- In 70-80% of cases, patient is known to have another malignancy
  - Metastases to the breast typically occur about 1 year after initial diagnosis
- In 20-30% of cases, breast metastasis is 1st indication the patient has cancer
  - Many types of metastases are difficult to distinguish from primary breast cancer
  - Metastasis should be considered if cancer is negative for ER, PR, and HER2 and lacks in situ component
    - However, majority of such cancers will prove to be primary breast carcinomas

Treatment
- Breast surgery to remove metastasis and lymph node evaluation generally do not improve outcome and are not performed
  - Therefore, it is very important to distinguish metastases from primary breast carcinomas
- Systemic treatment depends on type of metastatic cancer

Prognosis
- Outcome is generally poor, as metastasis to the breast is manifestation of disseminated systemic disease

IMAGE FINDINGS

General Features
- Most metastases present as circumscribed or ill-defined masses
  - A few present as irregular masses
  - Calcifications may be present (e.g., in papillary serous carcinomas)
- Metastases may be present in adipose tissue near chest wall
- Multiple masses may be present in 1 or both breasts
- No specific features to distinguish primary carcinoma from metastasis

MACROSCOPIC FEATURES

General Features
- Majority of metastases are diagnosed by core needle biopsy and not excised
- Only gross feature that would identify metastatic cancer would be black pigmentation in melanoma

MICROSCOPIC PATHOLOGY

Histologic Features
- Vary with primary site
- In children, metastatic embryonal rhabdomyosarcoma is most common type of metastasis
  - Some children will have Li-Fraumeni syndrome
  - Primary rhabdomyosarcoma of the breast occurs primarily in adults but can also occur in children
  - Approximately 6% of patients with rhabdomyosarcoma will develop breast metastasis

METASTASES TO THE BREAST

Key Facts

Clinical Issues

- Metastases to the breast are < 3% of all breast malignancies
- Most common presentation is as palpable breast mass
- In 70-80% of cases, patient is known to have another malignancy
- In 20-30% of cases, breast metastasis is 1st indication the patient has cancer
- In majority of cases, breast surgery and lymph node evaluation are not necessary
- Therefore, it is very important not to mistake metastasis for primary breast carcinoma
- Outcome is generally poor, as metastasis to the breast is manifestation of disseminated systemic disease

Microscopic Pathology

- Embryonal rhabdomyosarcoma is most common type of metastasis to the breast in children
  - Some affected children will have Li-Fraumeni syndrome
- Malignant melanoma is most common type of metastasis to the breast in adults
  - Prostate carcinoma is most common type of metastasis in men
  - Wide variety of other tumor types have been reported, including lung, ovarian, gastric, colon, and carcinoid tumor

Top Differential Diagnoses

- Primary breast carcinoma
- Lymphoma

- In some cases, breast metastasis was present with occult primary site
  - Histologic appearance of tumor is generally sufficient for diagnosis
    - IHC studies for muscle markers may be used to support the diagnosis
- In adults, wide variety of cancers may metastasize to the breast; the following types have specific considerations
  - Malignant melanoma: Most common type of metastasis to the breast in adult women
    - Melanomas, lymphomas, and high-grade discohesive breast carcinomas can have similar histologic appearance
    - IHC studies will be positive for melanoma markers (e.g., S100 and HMB-45) and negative for epithelial markers (e.g., cytokeratin)
    - Primary site may be occult or diagnosed in distant past
    - Median time between diagnosis of primary melanoma and detection of breast metastasis is 5 years
  - Lung carcinoma: 2nd most common type of metastasis to the breast
    - Histologic appearance in lung (e.g., squamous cell carcinoma, adenocarcinoma, small cell carcinoma) should match appearance of metastasis in the breast
    - Histologic comparison of carcinoma in the lung to carcinoma in the breast is best method for identification
    - TTF-1 can be helpful to identify lung adenocarcinomas as 2/3 will be positive for this marker
    - TTF-1 positivity in breast carcinomas is very rare and may be limited to breast cancers with neuroendocrine features
    - Some lung carcinomas are positive for ER (primarily ER-β) and PR; frequency varies with antibody used
  - Prostatic carcinoma: Most common type of metastasis to the breast in men
    - Men with prostatic carcinoma undergoing hormonal treatments are at increased risk for primary breast carcinoma
    - Metastatic prostatic carcinoma can closely mimic low-grade breast carcinoma or metastatic carcinoid tumor
    - Some (10-20%) of breast carcinomas are positive for PSA; PSAP may be more specific for prostatic carcinoma
    - Pattern of PSA/PSAP(+), ER/PR(-), GCDFP-15(-), and cytokeratin 7(-) strongly favors prostatic carcinoma
    - Pattern of PSA/PSAP(-), ER/PR(+), GCDFP-15(+), and cytokeratin 7(+) strongly favors breast carcinoma
    - Mixed patterns may be difficult to interpret and may require clinical correlation
    - Prostatic carcinomas (and breast carcinomas) can be strongly positive for neuroendocrine markers (including chromogranin)
  - Gastric carcinoma
    - Signet ring cell carcinomas are histologically similar (or identical) to some invasive lobular carcinomas
    - Signet ring cells with foamy cytoplasm are more common in gastric carcinomas; cells with vacuole and distinct mucin dot are more common in lobular carcinomas
    - Both tumors occur in patients with germline mutations of E-cadherin; however, gastric carcinomas are more common
    - Gastric signet ring cell carcinomas are generally positive for CDX-2 and negative for ER and PR
    - Breast lobular carcinomas are generally positive for ER and PR and negative for CDX-2
  - Gynecologic carcinomas
    - Women with gynecologic carcinomas are at higher risk for developing primary breast carcinoma
    - In these women, it would be unusual for gynecologic malignancy to not be apparent clinically

- Gynecologic carcinomas can be positive for breast markers
- Breast carcinomas can be positive for gynecologic carcinoma markers
- Pax-8 is positive in almost all papillary serous carcinomas and has not been reported in breast carcinoma
- WT1 (nuclear positivity) is more commonly positive in gynecologic carcinomas but is also present in some breast carcinomas
- Ovarian serous carcinomas more commonly metastasize to the breast than mucinous or clear cell carcinomas
- Metastatic ovarian carcinomas may present as mammographic mass with calcifications
- Psammoma bodies may be frequent in ovarian serous carcinomas but would be unusual in breast carcinomas
- Carcinoid tumor
  - Existence of primary carcinoid tumor of the breast is controversial
  - Many breast carcinomas can express neuroendocrine markers, including chromogranin and synaptophysin
  - Metastatic carcinoid may be suspected when low-grade nested tumor is negative for ER and PR
  - Myoepithelial markers can be helpful to distinguish circumscribed tumor nests from carcinoma in situ
  - Carcinoid can also resemble LCIS; carcinoid should be positive for E-cadherin and lack myoepithelial cells
- Contralateral breast carcinoma
  - Women with breast carcinoma are at increased risk for developing 2nd primary carcinoma in contralateral breast
  - In absence of in situ carcinoma, it is often difficult or impossible to distinguish metastasis from 2nd carcinoma
  - In majority of these cases, there will be extensive lymph-vascular invasion and involved axillary lymph nodes

DIFFERENTIAL DIAGNOSIS

Primary Breast Carcinoma
- Metastasis to the breast should be considered in cases of breast carcinoma that are negative for ER, PR, and HER2 and that lack in situ carcinoma
  - Majority of these cancers (> 95%) will be primary breast carcinomas
  - Rare metastases may be positive for ER, PR, or HER2; additional markers may be required for diagnosis
  - Metastatic carcinomas may be present as multiple foci
    - However, multiple primary breast carcinomas can be present if there is extensive carcinoma in situ, intramammary metastasis due to lymph-vascular invasion, or in high-risk women
- History of another malignancy should prompt histologic comparison between the 2 tumors

- In difficult cases, immunohistochemical studies are generally of value
- Myoepithelial markers may be helpful to document presence of carcinoma in situ
- If there is no history of another malignancy and histologic appearance is compatible with breast primary, additional studies are rarely helpful

Lymphoma
- May be primary in the breast or can involve the breast as part of systemic disease
- Do not require local surgery and nodal evaluation
- High-grade (anaplastic) lymphomas can mimic breast carcinoma and melanoma
- Immunohistochemical markers are useful to identify the type of lymphoma and to exclude carcinoma and melanoma

SELECTED REFERENCES

1. Ersahin C et al: Thyroid transcription factor-1 and "basal marker"--expressing small cell carcinoma of the breast. Int J Surg Pathol. 17(5):368-72, 2009
2. Klingen TA et al: Secondary breast cancer: a 5-year population-based study with review of the literature. APMIS. 117(10):762-7, 2009
3. Vollmer RT: Primary lung cancer vs metastatic breast cancer: a probabilistic approach. Am J Clin Pathol. 132(3):391-5, 2009
4. Canda AE et al: Metastatic tumors in the breast: a report of 5 cases and review of the literature. Clin Breast Cancer. 7(8):638-43, 2007
5. Lee AH: The histological diagnosis of metastases to the breast from extramammary malignancies. J Clin Pathol. 60(12):1333-41, 2007
6. Cheng CW et al: Breast metastasis from prostate cancer and interpretation of immunoreactivity to prostate-specific antigen. Int J Urol. 13(4):463-5, 2006
7. Upalakalin JN et al: Carcinoid tumors in the breast. Am J Surg. 191(6):799-805, 2006
8. Carder PJ et al: Expression of prostate specific antigen in male breast cancer. J Clin Pathol. 58(1):69-71, 2005
9. Loffeld A et al: Management of melanoma metastasis to the breast: case series and review of the literature. Br J Dermatol. 152(6):1206-10, 2005
10. Recine MA et al: Serous carcinoma of the ovary and peritoneum with metastases to the breast and axillary lymph nodes: a potential pitfall. Am J Surg Pathol. 28(12):1646-51, 2004
11. Bartella L et al: Metastases to the breast revisited: radiological-histopathological correlation. Clin Radiol. 58(7):524-31, 2003
12. Gupta D et al: Metastases to breast simulating ductal carcinoma in situ: report of two cases and review of the literature. Ann Diagn Pathol. 5(1):15-20, 2001
13. Hall RE et al: Prostate-specific antigen and gross cystic disease fluid protein-15 are co-expressed in androgen receptor-positive breast tumours. Br J Cancer. 78(3):360-5, 1998

METASTASES TO THE BREAST

Microscopic Features

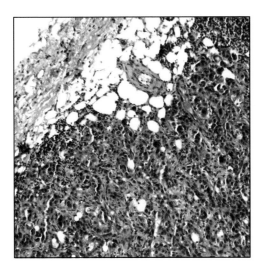
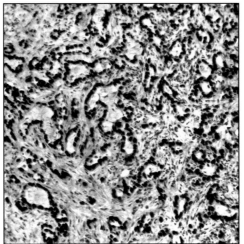

(Left) This metastatic lung carcinoma invades as small tubules or nests of cells. The carcinoma was negative for ER and PR and lacked an in situ carcinoma. The differential diagnosis includes primary breast cancer and metastatic adenocarcinoma. *(Right)* TTF-1 shows strong nuclear positivity, strongly supporting a diagnosis of metastatic lung carcinoma. Only rare breast cancers have been reported to be TTF-1 positive, and these carcinomas have a neuroendocrine appearance.

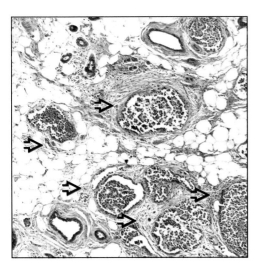
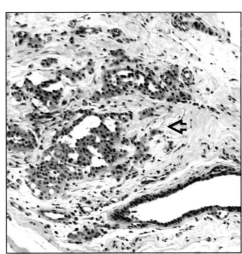

(Left) This metastatic lung carcinoma has papillary and micropapillary patterns and extensively involves lymphatic spaces ⊳. This carcinoma could easily be mistaken for DCIS. *(Right)* Men with prostate carcinoma are at increased risk for breast carcinoma as well as metastatic breast carcinoma. A panel of IHC markers is often necessary to identify the carcinoma. This metastatic prostatic carcinoma ⊳ could easily be confused with a breast carcinoma with apocrine features.

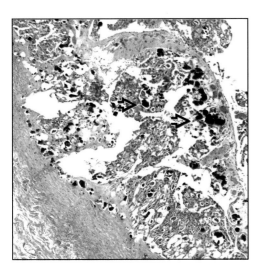
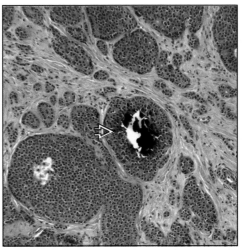

(Left) The most common metastatic gynecologic carcinoma is serous ovarian carcinoma. This case shows numerous psammomatous calcifications ⊳ identified on mammography. This appearance would be unusual for a primary breast carcinoma. *(Right)* Metastatic carcinoid tumor can closely resemble an invasive ductal carcinoma, DCIS, or LCIS. This case was detected due to the associated calcifications ⊳. Multiple IHC markers may be necessary to confirm the diagnosis.

LYMPHOMA

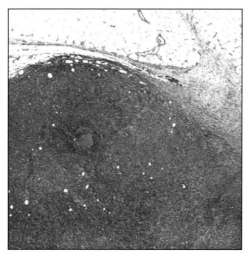

Lymphomas of the breast usually present as circumscribed masses by palpation or by imaging. This lymphoma consists of a solid proliferation of malignant lymphoid cells with a rounded border.

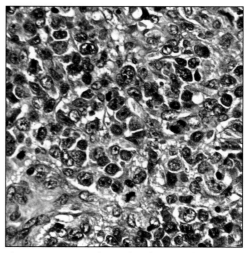

The most common breast lymphoma is large B-cell lymphoma, as seen here. The cells have pleomorphic nuclei and are discohesive. The differential diagnosis can include melanoma and carcinoma.

TERMINOLOGY

Definitions
- Clonal population of malignant lymphocytes involving the breast
  - Primary breast lymphoma: Restricted to breast parenchyma and axillary nodes when initially diagnosed
    - Should not be prior history of lymphoma with involvement of other sites
  - Secondary breast lymphoma: Breast involvement in patient with systemic disease
    - In some cases, intramammary lymph node is involved by the lymphoma

CLINICAL ISSUES

Presentation
- Most patients present with palpable breast mass
- Rare cases present as mammographic density; associated calcifications may be present in areas of necrosis but are unusual
- Borders may be circumscribed or irregular
- Lymphomas of breast are rare; < 0.5% of all breast malignancies
- Unusual presentation mimics inflammatory breast carcinoma
  - Breast becomes edematous and enlarged due to lymphatic blockage by involved axillary lymph nodes
- Age range is from 12-90 years with bimodal peaks in mid-30s and mid-60s

Treatment
- Appropriate treatment is dependent on type of lymphoma

Prognosis
- Prognosis is dependent on type of lymphoma

IMAGE FINDINGS

Mammographic Findings
- Unusual cases present as mammographic density
  - Borders may be irregular or circumscribed
  - No specific imaging findings to identify a mass as lymphoma
  - Calcifications would be unusual but are rarely associated with foci of necrosis
- If patient has systemic lymphoma, bilateral lymph node enlargement may be present
- Rare cases present as diffuse breast involvement with trabecular pattern and skin thickening

MACROSCOPIC FEATURES

General Features
- Gross mass is usually white to gray with fleshy appearance
- Many cases are diagnosed by core needle biopsy
  - Surgical excision is usually not performed if diagnosis of lymphoma is known

MICROSCOPIC PATHOLOGY

Histologic Features
- Majority of breast lymphomas are non-Hodgkin B-cell lymphomas
  - Hodgkin disease of the breast is very rare and is usually accompanied by nodal involvement
  - Women who have been treated for Hodgkin disease with mantle radiation are at increased risk for developing breast carcinoma
- Majority of breast lymphomas are B-cell lymphomas
  - Most common type is diffuse large B-cell lymphoma (approximately 60% of cases)
  - Lymphoplasmacytic lymphoma, extranodal marginal zone B-cell lymphoma, follicle center cell

LYMPHOMA

Key Facts

Terminology

- Malignancy consisting of clonal population of lymphocytes involving breast
  - Primary breast lymphoma: Restricted to breast parenchyma and axillary nodes when initially diagnosed
  - Secondary breast lymphoma: Breast involvement in a patient with systemic disease

Clinical Issues

- Lymphomas of the breast are rare; < 0.5% of all breast malignances
- Majority of patients present with palpable breast mass
- Unusual presentation mimics inflammatory breast carcinoma due to enlarged axillary lymph nodes

Microscopic Pathology

- Majority of breast lymphomas are non-Hodgkin B-cell lymphomas
  - Hodgkin disease of the breast is very rare
- T-cell lymphomas account for < 10%

Top Differential Diagnoses

- Inflammatory myofibroblastic tumor (pseudo-lymphoma, plasma cell granuloma)
- Lymphocytic mastopathy (diabetic mastopathy)
- Carcinoma
- Leukemic breast involvement (granulocytic sarcoma)
- Chronic inflammation associated with benign breast conditions
- T-cell lymphocytic lobulitis
- Intramammary lymph node

---

lymphoma, and lymphoblastic lymphoma have also been reported
- Burkitt lymphoma has been reported in young pregnant or lactating women and may be bilateral
  - These cases occur predominantly in Africa
- Only 3 cases of B-cell lymphomas have been reported in association with breast implant
  - Follicular lymphoma, primary effusion lymphoma, and lymphoplasmacytic lymphoma
- T-cell lymphomas are less common (< 10% of all primary breast lymphomas)
  - ALK1-negative anaplastic large cell lymphoma (ALCL) is rare peripheral T-cell lymphoma
    - Over 1/2 of cases in the breast have been reported arising adjacent to implant (22 of 30 cases)
    - Presenting symptom is usually thought to be related to implant, seroma, or infection
    - Cells are immunoreactive for CD30 (membrane and Golgi) and usually at least 1 T-cell marker
    - Both silicone and saline implants are associated with cases; used for both cosmetic and reconstructive purposes
    - Diagnosed 1-23 years after placement of implant
    - Some cases can be positive for EMA and negative for typical T-cell markers
    - Molecular studies may be used to demonstrate rearrangement of T-cell receptor gene
    - Majority of patients undergo chemotherapy, and recurrences are rare
  - Cutaneous T-cell lymphomas have also been reported in association with breast implants
    - Presenting symptoms may be exfoliative erythrodermia, erythematous plaques, and skin irritation over implant

DIFFERENTIAL DIAGNOSIS

Inflammatory Myofibroblastic Tumor (IMT)

- Synonyms (or closely related lesions) include pseudolymphoma, inflammatory pseudotumor, plasma cell granuloma, xanthomatous pseudotumor,

and pseudosarcomatous myofibrohistiocytic proliferation
- Consist of infiltrate of mixed inflammatory cells, often with prominent component of plasma cells
  - Rare cases show preponderance of IgG4 plasma cells and have been termed IgG4-related sclerosing mastitis
  - Normal germinal centers are often present
- Stromal sclerosis with collagen deposition and myofibroblastic proliferation is constant feature
  - Clonality of stromal cells has been demonstrated in some IMTs
- A few cases of IMT have recurred locally
  - Reports of IMT behaving in malignant fashion may reflect difficulty of distinguishing these lesions from malignant tumors or indicate low probability of progression to malignant neoplasm
- IMT is less common than lymphoma in the breast

Lymphocytic (or Diabetic) Mastopathy

- Predominant component is very dense collagenized stroma
  - Tissue on slides typically looks uniformly pink
  - In contrast, slides from lymphomas typically have "blue" tissue due to dense lymphocytic infiltrate
- Lymphocytic infiltrate consists predominantly of small round lymphocytes and clusters around ducts, lobules, and blood vessels
- Ducts and lobules typically appear atrophic with thickened basement membranes

Carcinoma

- Low-grade lymphomas can mimic lobular carcinomas
  - Some lymphomas have cells that mimic signet ring cells; however, mucin is not present
  - Important features to support a diagnosis of carcinoma are the presence of LCIS and immunoreactivity for keratin
  - ER and PR positivity may be unreliable; some lymphocytes are positive for these markers

- Absence of ER and PR in carcinoma that appears lobular in type would be a clue that malignancy might be lymphoma
  - Lymphomas can infiltrate in concentric pattern around ducts, similar to lobular carcinomas
- High-grade lymphomas can mimic poorly differentiated ductal carcinomas
  - Lymphoma should be suspected if cells are discohesive and there is no DCIS
  - Some high-grade lymphomas are immunoreactive for EMA; keratin is more reliable marker to identify carcinomas
  - Some triple negative carcinomas (e.g., basal-like, medullary, and *BRCA1* associated) are associated with dense lymphocytic infiltrate
    - Infiltrate may obscure epithelial cells, and lesion could be mistaken for lymphoma
    - Lymphocytic infiltrate consists predominantly of T cells

Leukemic Breast Involvement ("Granulocytic Sarcoma," Chloroma)

- Solid tumors composed of myeloid leukemia cells rarely present as breast mass without systemic AML
  - At least half of patients will eventually develop systemic leukemia
  - Very rare diagnosis in breast; only 19 reported cases
- Misdiagnosis as lymphoma or sarcoma is common
  - Leukemia should be considered when B- and T-cell markers are negative in a case suspected to be lymphoma

Chronic Inflammation Associated with Benign Breast Conditions

- Lymphocytic infiltrates can be seen in many benign conditions
  - Regression after pregnancy and breastfeeding
  - Adjacent to ruptured cysts
  - Adjacent to ectatic &/or rupture lactiferous sinuses (as part of "duct ectasia")
- Lymphocytic infiltrate should be incidental to clinically or radiologically evident lesion
- Infiltrate is generally a mixture of small lymphocytes and occasional plasma cells

T-cell Lymphocytic Lobulitis

- Perilobular infiltrate of T cells has been described in patients with *BRCA1* mutations
- This is generally an incidental finding; would be unusual for this finding to present as a clinically/ radiologically evident mass
- T-cell infiltrate can also be present in association with carcinomas (e.g., medullary carcinoma)

Intramammary Lymph Node

- Most common in upper outer quadrant but may be present at other locations
- Imaging features are usually characteristic for lymph node; fatty hilum should be present
- These nodes may be biopsied if unusual in size or appearance

- On core needle biopsy, it is important to identify lymph node capsule and normal germinal centers
- Immunohistochemical studies may be helpful to document that a normal complement of lymphocytes is present

SELECTED REFERENCES

1. Cordeiro A et al: Burkitt's lymphoma related to Epstein-Barr virus infection during pregnancy. Arch Gynecol Obstet. 280(2):297-300, 2009
2. Jeanneret-Sozzi W et al: Primary breast lymphoma: patient profile, outcome and prognostic factors. A multicentre Rare Cancer Network study. BMC Cancer. 8:86, 2008
3. Karbasian-Esfahani M et al: Leukemic infiltration of the breast in acute lymphocytic leukemia (ALL). Hematology. 13(2):101-6, 2008
4. Cao YB et al: [Primary breast lymphoma--a report of 27 cases with literature review.] Ai Zheng. 26(1):84-9, 2007
5. Cunningham I: A clinical review of breast involvement in acute leukemia. Leuk Lymphoma. 47(12):2517-26, 2006
6. Shim GJ et al: Differential expression of oestrogen receptors in human secondary lymphoid tissues. J Pathol. 208(3):408-14, 2006
7. Hermsen BB et al: Lobulitis is a frequent finding in prophylactically removed breast tissue from women at hereditary high risk of breast cancer. J Pathol. 206(2):220-3, 2005
8. Ilvan S et al: Inflammatory myofibroblastic tumor (inflammatory pseudotumor) of the breast. APMIS. 113(1):66-9, 2005
9. Khanafshar E et al: Inflammatory myofibroblastic tumor of the breast. Ann Diagn Pathol. 9(3):123-9, 2005
10. Vignot S et al: Non-Hodgkin's lymphoma of the breast: a report of 19 cases and a review of the literature. Clin Lymphoma. 6(1):37-42, 2005
11. Zen Y et al: Inflammatory pseudotumor of the breast in a patient with a high serum IgG4 level: histologic similarity to sclerosing pancreatitis. Am J Surg Pathol. 29(2):275-8, 2005
12. Chugh R et al: Nonepithelial malignancies of the breast. Oncology (Williston Park). 18(5):665-73; discussion 673-6, 2004
13. Shea B et al: Granulocytic sarcoma (chloroma) of the breast: a diagnostic dilemma and review of the literature. Breast J. 10(1):48-53, 2004
14. Gholam D et al: Primary breast lymphoma. Leuk Lymphoma. 44(7):1173-8, 2003
15. Haj M et al: Inflammatory pseudotumor of the breast: case report and literature review. Breast J. 9(5):423-5, 2003
16. Wong WW et al: Primary non-Hodgkin lymphoma of the breast: The Mayo Clinic Experience. J Surg Oncol. 80(1):19-25; discussion 26, 2002
17. Brogi E et al: Lymphomas of the breast: pathology and clinical behavior. Semin Oncol. 26(3):357-64, 1999

LYMPHOMA

Microscopic Features

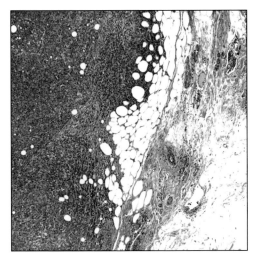 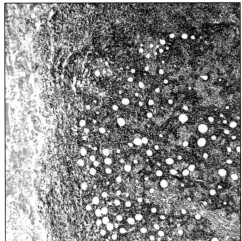

(Left) Although the majority of lymphomas have circumscribed borders, lymphoma may less commonly present as an irregular mass (as seen in this case of a large B-cell lymphoma) or as diffuse infiltration of breast tissue. (Right) Low-grade B-cell lymphomas are the 2nd most common group of breast lymphomas. This follicular center cell lymphoma (FCC) consists of sheets of lymphocytes in fibroadipose tissue.

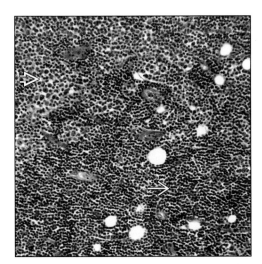 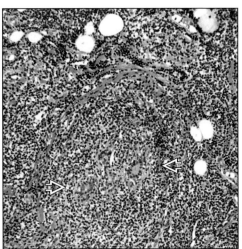

(Left) This FCC consists of monocytoid B-cells with irregular nuclei and abundant cytoplasm ➡ intermingled with smaller lymphocytes ➡. The majority of FCC lymphomas have a characteristic t(14;18). (Right) This is a marginal zone B-cell lymphoma (MZL) of mucosa-associated lymphoid tissue (MALT) type surrounding a small lobule ➡. A t(11;18) is typical for this type of lymphoma.

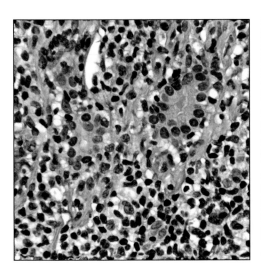 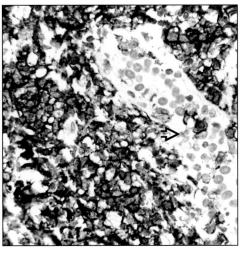

(Left) This MZL consists of small to intermediated-sized lymphocytes with round indistinct nucleoli and scant cytoplasm completely surrounding the epithelium. The lymphocytic infiltrate can sometimes mimic low-grade invasive lobular carcinoma. (Right) Lympho-epithelial lesions are present in this MZL, as seen in this CD20 study identifying B cells within the epithelium of the lobule ➡. In some cases, the intraepithelial lymphocytes can mimic Paget disease or carcinoma in situ.

LYMPHOMA

Microscopic Features

(Left) Anaplastic large cell lymphomas (ALCL) are the most common lymphomas associated with breast implants. The clinical presentation is often as an implant seroma ➡. **(Right)** The malignant cells of ALCL are often present in the seroma fluid ⊡, as well as within the implant capsule. In this case, foreign material consistent with silicone bleed is adjacent to the malignant cells ⊡.

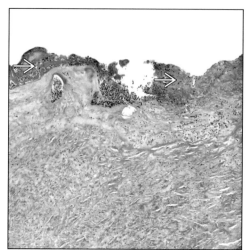
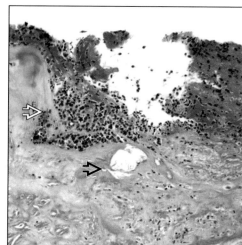

(Left) This ALCL ⊡ is present within an implant capsule and is associated with refractile foreign material ➡ from a ruptured implant. **(Right)** In ALCL, the lymphocytes are large, and anaplastic nuclei with reniform and horseshoe shapes are common ⊡.

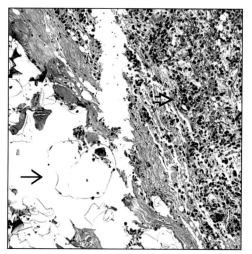
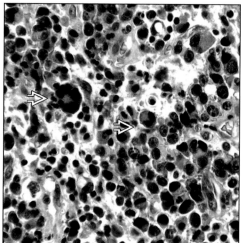

(Left) ALCL is generally immunoreactive for CD30 and at least 1 T-cell marker. However, molecular studies may be necessary to demonstrate a rearrangement of the T-cell receptor. Lymphomas associated with implants are usually negative for ALK. **(Right)** ALCL can show focal immunoreactivity for EMA, and this may cause confusion with breast cancer, particularly in patients undergoing reconstruction after a cancer diagnosis. Cytokeratins are better markers for epithelial differentiation.

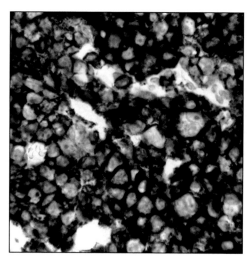
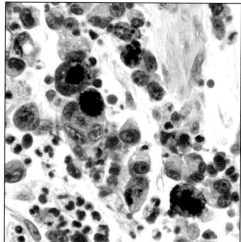

Differential Diagnosis

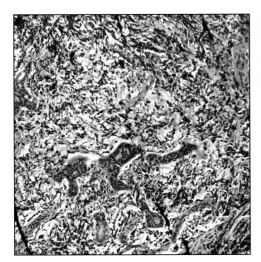
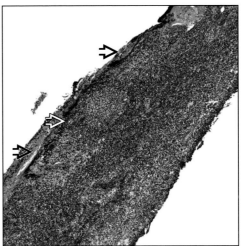

(Left) This biopsy shows a cellular infiltrate surrounding a lobular unit with extensive crush artifact. The differential diagnosis includes melanoma, carcinoma, and lymphoma. IHC studies confirmed that this was a lymphoma. (Right) Normal or reactive intramammary lymph nodes are sometimes biopsied if the imaging findings are atypical. It is important to identify normal germinal centers ➡ and a lymph node capsule ➡.

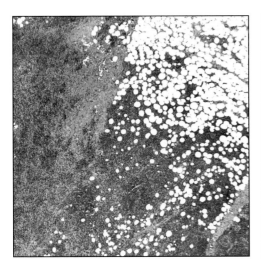
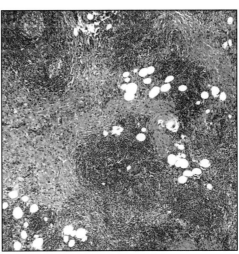

(Left) Pseudolymphomas form masses consisting of a dense proliferation of lymphocytes and plasma cells. Immunohistochemical studies can be used to demonstrate the polyclonal nature of the lymphocytes. (Right) The stroma associated with pseudolymphomas is usually sclerotic and forms only a small portion of the clinical or radiologic mass. Normal breast ducts and lobules are generally absent or only seen at the periphery.

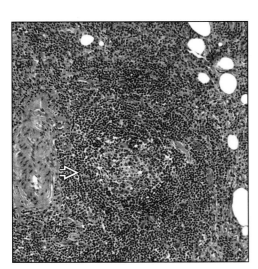
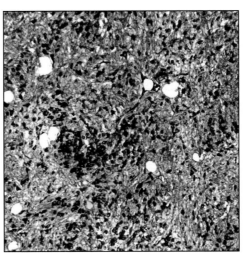

(Left) The infiltrate in pseudolymphomas consists of a mixture of normal cells, and small germinal centers may be present ➡. (Right) The infiltrate of this pseudolymphoma contains numerous plasma cells, as shown by their immunoreactivity for IgG. Polyclonal B cells are also present, as well as T cells.

Reference

Antibodies Discussed

Antibody Name/ Symbol	Antibody Description	Clones/Alternative Names	Chapters
β-catenin	beta catenin; involved in regulation of cell adhesion and in signal transduction through Wnt pathway	B-catenin, CLONE 14, E-5, RB-9035Po, 17C2, 5H10	Fibromatosis; Granular Cell Tumor; Medullary Carcinoma; Nodular Fasciitis; Phyllodes Tumor; Tubulolobular Carcinoma;
β-catenin cytoplasm		B-caten-cyt	Granular Cell Tumor Basal-like Carcinomas
1A6	progesterone receptor protein	PR, 10A9, PGR-1A6, KD68, PGR-ICA, PRP-P, PRI, 1A6, 1AR, HPRA3, PGR-636, 636, PR88, NCL-PGR	Hormone Receptors (ER/PR)
1D5	estrogen receptor protein	1D5, 6F11, SP1, 15D, H222, TE111, ERP, ER1D5, NCLER611, NCL-ER-LH2, PGP-1A6	Hormone Receptors (ER/PR)
34bE12	cytokeratin, high molecular weight (34bE12- CK 1, 5, 10, 14)	MA-903, CK903	Basal-like Carcinomas; Lobular Carcinoma In Situ;
3B5	v-erb-b2 erythroblastic leukemia viral gene protein, human epidermal growth factor receptor 2	Her2/neu, NEU, Her2, NCL-CBE1, 10A7, 9G6.10, SP3, 4B5, P185, 9G6.20, A0485, C-ERBB-2, CB11, ERBB-2, 3B5, TAB250, HERCEPTEST, E2-4001, HER-2_NEU	HER2
4B5	v-erb-b2 erythroblastic leukemia viral gene protein, human epidermal growth factor receptor 2	Her2/neu, NEU, Her2, NCL-CBE1, 10A7, 9G6.10, SP3, 3B5, P185, 9G6.20, A0485, C-ERBB-2, CB11, ERBB-2, 3B5, TAB250, HERCEPTEST, E2-4001, HER-2_NEU	HER2
6F11	estrogen receptor protein	1D5, SP1, 15D, H222, TE111, ERP, ER1D5, NCLER611, NCL-ER-LH2, PGP-1A6	Hormone Receptors (ER/PR)
Actin-sm	smooth muscle actin	SMA, ASM-1, CGA7, IA4, HUC-1	Anatomic Structure and Lifecycle Changes; Ductal Carcinoma In Situ with Microinvasion; Ductal Carcinoma In Situ; Encapsulated Papillary Carcinoma; Hemangiomas; Invasive Papillary Carcinoma; Myofibroblastoma; Nodular Fasciitis; Papilloma, Large Duct and Small Duct Sclerosing Adenosis; Tubular/ Cribriform Carcinoma
AE1/AE3	AE1/AE3; mixture of 2 anticytokeratin clones that detect a variety of both high- and low- molecular weight cytokeratins		Invasive Lobular Carcinoma; Collagenous Spherulosis; Secretory Carcinoma; Neoadjuvant Therapy; Metaplastic Carcinoma; Lymph Node Metastases; Myofibroblastoma; HER2
ALK1	anaplastic lymphoma kinase-1	5A4, ALK, ALKC	Iatrogenic Changes
Androgen receptor		AR441, F39.4.1, AR-N20, ANDROGEN RE, AR27	Invasive Apocrine Carcinoma; Epidemiology: Lesions Conferring Increased Risk of Breast Carcinoma; Gynecomastia; HER2; Lobular Carcinoma In Situ; Metastases to the Breast; Myofibroblastoma; Myofibroblastoma; Nonproliferative Changes;
Aromatase	key enzyme in the byosynthesis of estrogen		Expression Profiling, mRNA; Expression Profiling, Oncotype DX Assay; Expression Profiling, Protein; Gynecomastia; Hormone Receptors (ER/PR); Invasive Ductal Carcinoma (Adenocarcinomas of No Special Type); Locally Recurrent Carcinoma
Bcl-2	B-cell lymphoma 2; suppresses apoptosis in a variety of cell systems	ONCL2, BCL2/100/D5, 124, 124.3	Epidemiology: Lesions Conferring Increased Risk of Breast Carcinoma; Myofibroblastoma
Bombesin	tumor marker for small cell carcinoma of the lung		Neuroendocrine/Small Cell Carcinoma
BRCA1	breast and ovarian cancer susceptibility protein 1; DNA repair protein	MS110	Basal-like Carcinomas; Diabetic Mastopathy/Lymphocytic Mastopathy; Epidemiology: Lesions Conferring Increased Risk of Breast Carcinoma; Expression Profiling, mRNA; HER2 Positive Carcinoma; Hereditary Cancer; Hormone Receptors (ER/PR); Lobular Carcinoma In Situ; Lymphoma; Mastectomies; Medullary Carcinoma;

			Risk Factors for Developing Breast Carcinoma
BRCA2	breast and ovarian cancer susceptibility protein 2; protein involved in chromosome repair	3E6	Gynecomastia; HER2 Positive Carcinoma Hereditary Cancer; Hormone Receptors (ER/PR); Lobular Carcinoma In Situ; Mastectomies; Medullary Carcinoma; Risk Factors for Developing Breast Carcinoma
Calcitonin	polypeptide hormone produced by parafollicular cells (C cells) of the thyroid	CALBINDIN28	Neuroendocrine/Small Cell Carcinoma
Caldesmon	actin interacting and calmodulin binding protein found in smooth muscle and other cell types		Sarcomas
Calponin	thin filament-associated protein that is implicated in regulation and modulation of smooth muscle contraction	N3, 26A11, CALP, CNN1, SMCC, Sm Calp	Adenoid Cystic Carcinoma; Anatomic Structure and Lifecycle Changes; Invasive Apocrine Carcinoma; Ductal Carcinoma In Situ with Microinvasion; Ductal Carcinoma In Situ; Fibromatosis; Hamartoma (Fibroadenolipoma); Nipple Adenoma; Nodular Fasciitis; Papilloma, Large Duct and Small Duct; Radial Sclerosing Lesion/Radial Scar Sclerosing Adenosis
Calretinin	29 kDa calcium binding protein that is expressed in central and peripheral nervous system and in many normal and pathological tissues	DAK-CALRET, 5A5, CAL 3F5, DC8, AB149	Granular Cell Tumor
Carcinoembryonic antigen, monoclonal		CEA-M, mCEA, CEA-B18, CEA-D14, CEAGOLD 1, T84.6, CEA-GOLD 2, CEA 11, CEA-GOLD 3, CEA 27, CEAGOLD 4, CEA 41, CEA-GOLD 5, T84.1, CEA-M, A5B7, CEJO65, IL-7, T84.66, TF3H8-1, 0062, D14, alpha-7, PARLAM 1, ZC23, CEM010, A115, COL-1, AF4, 12.140.10, 11-7, M773, CEA-M431_31, CEJO65	Apocrine Carcinoma
Carcinoembryonic antigen, polyclonal		CEA-P	Apocrine Carcinoma
Cathepsin-D	lysosomal aspartic protease over-expressed and hyper-secreted by epithelial breast cancer cells		Microglandular Adenosis
CB11	HER2/neu	NCL-CBE1, 10A7, 9G6.10, SP3, 4B5, P185, 9G6.20, A0485, C-ERBB-2, ERBB-2, 3B5, TAB250, HERCEPTEST, E2-4001, HER-2_NEU	HER2
CD1a	T-cell surface glycoprotein	JPM30, CD1A, O10, NA1/34	Fat Necrosis
CD2	T-cell surface antigen, LFA2	271, MT910, AB75, LFA-2	Expression Profiling, mRNA; Histologic Grade;
CD3	T-cell receptor	F7238, A0452, CD3-P, CD3-M, SP7, PS1	Implant Pathology
CD4	T-cell surface glycoprotein, L3T4	IF6, 1290, 4B12, CD4, 1F6, CD04	Diabetic Mastopathy/Lymphocytic Mastopathy
CD10	neutral endopeptidase	CALLA, neprilysin, NEP	Anatomic Structure and Lifecycle Changes; Lipoma and Angiolipoma; Metaplastic Carcinoma
CD20	membrane spanning 4 domains of B lymphocytes	FB1, B1, L26, MS4A1	Diabetic Mastopathy/Lymphocytic Mastopathy; Lymphoma
CD30	tumor necrosis factor SF8	BER-H2, KI-1, TNFRSF8	Implant Pathology; Lymphoma
CD31	platelet endothelial cell adhesion molecule	JC/70, JC/70A, PECAM-1	Angiosarcoma; Atypical Vascular Lesions of Skin; Ductal Carcinoma In Situ; Hemangiomas; Inflammatory Carcinoma; Lymph-Vascular Invasion; Pseudoangiomatous Stromal Hyperplasia
CD34	hematopoietic progenitor cell antigen	MY10, IOM34, QBEND10, 8G12, 1309, HPCA-1, NU-4A1, TUK4, clone 581, BI-3c5	Anatomic Structure and Lifecycle Changes; Angiosarcoma; Atypical Vascular Lesions of Skin; Diabetic Mastopathy/Lymphocytic Mastopathy; Fibroadenoma; Fibromatosis; Hemangiomas; Lipoma and Angiolipoma; Lymph-Vascular Invasion; Metaplastic Carcinoma; Myofibroblastoma; Nodular Fasciitis; Phyllodes Tumor; Pseudoangiomatous Stromal Hyperplasia;

9

ANTIBODY INDEX

CD43	major sialoglycoprotein on surface of human T lymphocytes, monocytes, granulocytes, and some B lymphocytes	LEU-22, DF-T1, L60, MT1, sialophorin, leukosialin, SPN	Implant Pathology
CD45	leukocyte common antigen	LCA, PD7/26, 1.22/4.14, T29/33, RP2/18, PD7, 2D1, 2B11+PD7/26	Circulating Tumor Cells
CD56	NCAM (neutral cellular adhesion molecule)	MAB735, ERIC-1, 25-KD11, 123C3, 24- MB2, BC56C04, 1B6, 14- MAB735, NCCLU- 243, MOC-1, NCAM	Mucinous (Colloid) Carcinoma
CD68	cytoplasmic granule protein of monocytes, macrophages	PG-M1, KP-1, LN5	Expression Profiling, Oncotype DX Assay; Fat Necrosis; Granular Cell Tumor; Nodular Fasciitis
CD117	C-kit; tyrosine protein kinase activity	C-19 (C-KIT), 104D2, 2E4, C-KIT, A4502, H300, CMA-767	Adenoid Cystic Carcinoma; Basal-like Carcinomas; Phyllodes Tumor; Secretory Carcinoma
CDC2	cell division cycle 2 kinase		Histologic Grade
CDH1	epithelial calcium dependent adhesion molecule	36B5, ECH-6, ECCD-2, 5H9, NCH 38, CLONE 36, 4A2 C7, E9, 67A4, HECD-1, SC-8426	Hereditary Cancer; Invasive Lobular Carcinoma Variants; Invasive Lobular Carcinoma; Lobular Carcinoma In Situ
CDX-2	caudal-type homeobox transcription factor 2	AMT28, 7C7/D4, CDX-2-88	Invasive Lobular Carcinoma; Metastases to the Breast
CEA-M	carcinoembryonic antigen, monoclonal	mCEA, CEA-B18, CEA-D14, CEAGOLD 1, T84.6, CEA-GOLD 2, CEA 11, CEA-GOLD 3, CEA 27, CEAGOLD 4, CEA 41, CEA-GOLD 5, T84.1, CEA-M, A5B7, CEJ065, IL-7, T84.66, TF3H8-1, 0062, D14, alpha-7, PARLAM 1, ZC23, CEM010, A115, COL-1, AF4, 12.140.10, 11-7, M773, CEA-M431_31, CEJO65	Expression Profiling, Protein
CEA-P	carcinoembryonic antigen, polyclonal		Ductal Carcinoma In Situ, Paget Disease
Chromogranin-A	pituitary secretory protein 1	PHE-5, PHE5, E001, DAK-A3	Neuroendocrine/Small Cell Carcinoma
CK5	cytokeratin 5	CK 05, XM26, RCK103, 34BEH12	Invasive Apocrine Carcinoma Expression Profiling, mRNA; Expression Profiling, Protein; HER2 Positive Carcinoma
CK5/6	cytokeratin 5/6	CK 05_06, D5/16 B4	Anatomic Structure and Lifecycle Changes; Invasive Apocrine Carcinoma; Basal-like Carcinomas; Ductal Carcinoma In Situ, Paget Disease; Epithelial Hyperplasia; Expression Profiling, mRNA; Expression Profiling, Protein; Hamartoma (Fibroadenolipoma); HER2 Positive Carcinoma; Hereditary Cancer; Invasive Ductal Carcinoma (Adenocarcinomas of No Special Type); Lobular Carcinoma In Situ; Medullary Carcinoma; Metaplastic Carcinoma; Nipple Adenoma; Papilloma, Large Duct and Small Duct; Risk Factors for Developing Breast Carcinoma; Sclerosing Adenosis; Tubular/Cribriform Carcinoma
CK7	cytokeratin 7	CK 7, K72.7, KS7.18, OVTL 12/30, LDS-68, CK 07	Anatomic Structure and Lifecycle Changes; Ductal Carcinoma In Situ, Paget Disease; Neuroendocrine/Small Cell Carcinoma
CK8	cytokeratin 8	K8.8, 4.1.18, TS1, C-51, M20, CK 08, 35BH11, MA-902	Anatomic Structure and Lifecycle Changes; Atypical Ductal Hyperplasia Medullary Carcinoma;
CK14	cytokeratin 14, high molecular weight cytokeratin	LL002	Expression Profiling, Protein; Fibromatosis; Medullary Carcinoma; Metaplastic Carcinoma
CK17	cytokeratin 17	E3	Expression Profiling, Protein
CK18	cytokeratin 18	M9, DC-10, CY-90, KS18.04	Anatomic Structure and Lifecycle Changes; Expression Profiling, Protein; Lobular Carcinoma In Situ; Medullary Carcinoma; Papilloma, Large Duct and Small Duct; Risk Factors for Developing Breast Carcinoma
CK19	cytokeratin 19, low molecular weight cytokeratin	BA17, RCK108, LP2K, B170, A53-BA2, KS19.1, 170.2.14	Circulating Tumor Cells
CK20	cytokeratin 20, low molecular weight cytokeratin	KS20.8	Ductal Carcinoma In Situ, Paget Disease; Invasive Micropapillary Carcinoma

ANTIBODY INDEX

CK-HMW-NOS	cytokeratin, high molecular weight, not otherwise specified	keratin-HMW	Atypical Ductal Hyperplasia; Ductal Carcinoma In Situ
C-Kit	tyrosine protein kinase activity	C-19 (C-KIT), 104D2, 2E4, CD117, A4502, H300, CMA-767	Adenoid Cystic Carcinoma; Basal-like Carcinomas
CK-PAN	cytokeratin-pan (AE1/AE3/LP34); cocktail of high and low molecular weight cytokeratins	keratin pan, MAK-6, K576, LU-5, KL-1, KC-8, MNF 116, pankeratin, pancytokeratin	Core Needle Biopsies; Ductal Carcinoma In Situ with Microinvasion; Ductal Carcinoma In Situ, Paget Disease; Fibromatosis; Granular Cell Tumor; Iatrogenic Changes; Invasive Lobular Carcinoma; Lymph Node Metastases; Metaplastic Carcinoma; Myofibroblastoma; Phyllodes Tumor
Collagen IV	major constituent of the basement membranes along with laminins, proteoglycans, and enactins	CIV22, COL4A [1-5], collagen α-1(IV) chain	Ductal Carcinoma In Situ with Microinvasion; Microglandular Adenosis;
CTSL2		Cathespin L	Expression Profiling, Oncotype DX Assay
Cytokeratin			Adenoid Cystic Carcinoma; Anatomic Structure and Lifecycle Changes; Angiosarcoma; Invasive Apocrine Carcinoma; Atypical Ductal Hyperplasia; Atypical Lobular Hyperplasia; Basal-like Carcinomas; Circulating Tumor Cells; Collagenous Spherulosis; Ductal Carcinoma In Situ with Microinvasion; Ductal Carcinoma In Situ, Paget Disease; Ductal Carcinoma In Situ; Encapsulated Papillary Carcinoma; Epithelial Hyperplasia; Expression Profiling, mRNA; Expression Profiling, Protein; Fibromatosis; Granular Cell Tumor; Gynecomastia; HER2 Positive Carcinoma; HER2; Hereditary Cancer; Invasive Ductal Carcinoma (Adenocarcinomas of No Special Type); Invasive Lobular Carcinoma Variants Invasive Lobular Carcinoma; Invasive Papillary Carcinoma; Lobular Carcinoma In Situ; Locally Recurrent Carcinoma; Lymph Node Metastases; Medullary Carcinoma; Metaplastic Carcinoma; Metastases to the Breast; Microglandular Adenosis; Myofibroblastoma; Neoadjuvant Therapy; Papilloma, Large Duct and Small Duct; Radial Sclerosing Lesion/Radial Scar; Risk Factors for Developing Breast Carcinoma; Sarcomas; Sclerosing Adenosis; Secretory Carcinoma
Cytokeratin 1		CK1, CK 01, 34BB4	Basal-like Carcinomas Circulating Tumor Cells; Ductal Carcinoma In Situ with Microinvasion; Fibromatosis; Hereditary Cancer; Secretory Carcinoma;
Cytokeratin 4		215B8, 6B10	Basal-like Carcinomas
Cytokeratin 5		CK5, CK 05, XM26, RCK103, 34BEH12	Adenoid Cystic Carcinoma; Atypical Ductal Hyperplasia; Basal-like Carcinomas; Ductal Carcinoma In Situ, Paget Disease; Epithelial Hyperplasia; Expression Profiling, Protein; Hereditary Cancer; Locally Recurrent Carcinoma; Metaplastic Carcinoma; Papilloma, Large Duct and Small Duct; Secretory Carcinoma
Cytokeratin 5/6		CK5/6, CK 05_06, D5/16 B4	Papilloma, Large Duct and Small Duct; Basal-like Carcinomas
Cytokeratin 7		CK7, CK 7, K72.7, KS7.18, OVTL 12/30, LDS-68, CK 07	Ductal Carcinoma In Situ, Paget Disease; Basal-like Carcinomas
Cytokeratin 8		CK8, K8.8, 4.1.18, TS1, C-51, M20, CK 08, 35BH11, MA-902	Adenoid Cystic Carcinoma; Basal-like Carcinomas; Papilloma, Large Duct and Small Duct
Cytokeratin 8/18	cytokeratin 8/18; simple epithelial-type cytokeratins	5D3, Zym5.2, CAM 5.2, KER 10.11, NCL-5D3, cytokeratin LMW	Basal-like Carcinomas; Papilloma, Large Duct and Small Duct

9

Cytokeratin 14	high molecular weight cytokeratin	CK14, LL002	Basal-like Carcinomas; Hereditary Cancer; Fibromatosis; Secretory Carcinoma
Cytokeratin 17		E3, CK17	Basal-like Carcinomas
Cytokeratin 18		CK18, M9, DC-10, CY-90, KS18.04	Ductal Carcinoma In Situ with Microinvasion
Cytokeratin 19	low molecular weight cytokeratin	CK19, BA17, RCK108, LP2K, B170, A53-BA2, KS19.1, 170.2.14	Circulating Tumor Cells
D2-40	marker for reactive follicular dendritic cells and follicular dendritic cell sarcomas	Podoplanin, M2A	Atypical Vascular Lesions of Skin; Lymph-Vascular Invasion
Desmin	class III intermediate filaments found in muscle cells	M760, DE-R-11, D33, DE5, DE-U-10, ZC18	Diabetic Mastopathy/Lymphocytic Mastopathy; Fibromatosis; Granular Cell Tumor; Lipoma and Angiolipoma; Myofibroblastoma; Nodular Fasciitis; Sarcomas
E-cadherin	epithelial calcium dependent adhesion molecule	36B5, ECH-6, ECCD-2, CDH1, 5H9, NCH 38, CLONE 36, 4A2 C7, E9, 67A4, HECD-1, SC-8426	Anatomic Structure and Lifecycle Changes; Invasive Apocrine Carcinoma; Atypical Ductal Hyperplasia; Atypical Lobular Hyperplasia; Collagenous Spherulosis; Ductal Carcinoma In Situ; Epidemiology: Lesions Conferring Increased Risk of Breast Carcinoma; Epithelial Hyperplasia; HER2 Positive Carcinoma; Hereditary Cancer; Invasive Lobular Carcinoma Variants; Invasive Lobular Carcinoma; Invasive Micropapillary Carcinoma; Lobular Carcinoma In Situ; Medullary Carcinoma; Metaplastic Carcinoma; Metastases to the Breast; Neuroendocrine/Small Cell Carcinoma; Risk Factors for Developing Breast Carcinoma; Sclerosing Adenosis; Secretory Carcinoma; Tubulolobular Carcinoma
EGFR	v-erb-b1 erythroblastic leukemia viral gene,epidermal growth factor receptor	2-18C9, EGFR1, EGFR PHRMDX, NCL-R1, H11, C-ERBB-1, E30, EGFR, EGFR.113, 31G7, 3C6, HER1, ERBB1, c-erb-B1	Invasive Apocrine Carcinoma; Basal-like Carcinomas; Expression Profiling, mRNA; Expression Profiling, Protein; HER2; Hereditary Cancer; Invasive Ductal Carcinoma (Adenocarcinomas of No Special Type); Locally Recurrent Carcinoma; Low-Grade Adenosquamous Carcinoma; Metaplastic Carcinoma; Mucinous (Colloid) Carcinoma; Secretory Carcinoma
EMA	epithelial membrane antigen	GP1.4, 214D4, MC5, E29	Ductal Carcinoma In Situ, Paget Disease; Implant Pathology; Invasive Micropapillary Carcinoma; Lymphoma; Tubular/Cribriform Carcinoma
Epidermal growth factor	v-erb-b1 erythroblastic leukemia viral gene,epidermal growth factor receptor	2-18C9, EGFR1, EGFR PHRMDX, NCL-R1, H11, C-ERBB-1, E30, EGFR, EGFR.113, 31G7, 3C6, HER1, ERBB1, c-erb-B1	Medullary Carcinoma
Epithelial membrane antigen		EMA, GP1.4, 214D4, MC5, E29	Lymph Node Metastases; Microglandular Adenosis
ER	estrogen receptor protein	1D5, 6F11, SP1, 15D, H222, TE111, ERP, ER1D5, NCLER611, NCL-ERLH2, PGP-1A6	Adenoid Cystic Carcinoma; Anatomic Structure and Lifecycle Changes; Invasive Apocrine Carcinoma; Atypical Ductal Hyperplasia; Atypical Lobular Hyperplasia; Basal-like Carcinomas; Carcinomas with Extensive Intraductal Component; Checklist for the Reporting of Invasive Breast Carcinoma; Core Needle Biopsies; Ductal Carcinoma In Situ with Microinvasion; Ductal Carcinoma In Situ; Epidemiology: Lesions Conferring Increased Risk of Breast Carcinoma; Epithelial Hyperplasia; Expression Profiling, Mammaprint Assay; Expression Profiling, mRNA; Expression Profiling, Oncotype DX Assay; Expression Profiling, Protein; Fibromatosis; General Considerations; Gynecomastia; Hamartoma (Fibroadenolipoma); HER2 Positive Carcinoma; HER2;

			Histologic Grade; Hormone Receptors (ER/PR); Inflammatory Carcinoma; Introduction: Prognostic and Predictive Factors; Invasive Ductal Carcinoma (Adenocarcinomas of No Special Type); Invasive Lobular Carcinoma Variants; Invasive Lobular Carcinoma; Invasive Micropapillary Carcinoma; Invasive Papillary Carcinoma; Lobular Carcinoma In Situ; Locally Recurrent Carcinoma; Lymph Node Metastases; Lymphoma; Medullary Carcinoma; Metaplastic Carcinoma; Metastases to the Breast; Mucinous (Colloid) Carcinoma; Myofibroblastoma; Neoadjuvant Therapy; Neuroendocrine/Small Cell Carcinoma; Risk Factors for Developing Breast Carcinoma; Sclerosing Adenosis; Secretory Carcinoma; Size and Multiple Foci; Syringomatous Adenoma of the Nipple; Tubular/Cribriform Carcinoma; Tubulolobular Carcinoma
ER-α	estrogen receptor protein α	ER-ALPHA, ERP-α	Anatomic Structure and Lifecycle Changes; Apocrine Carcinoma; Hormone Receptors (ER/PR)
ER-β	estrogen receptor protein β	ER-BETA, 14C8, 57/3, PPG5/10	Apocrine Carcinoma; Hormone Receptors (ER/PR)
ERP	estrogen receptor protein	1D5, 6F11, SP1, 15D, H222, TE111, ER, ER1D5, NCLER611, NCL-ERLH2, PGP-1A6	Anatomic Structure and Lifecycle Changes; Atypical Ductal Hyperplasia; Ductal Carcinoma In Situ, Paget Disease; Ductal Carcinoma In Situ; Expression Profiling, Protein; Hormone Receptors (ER/PR); Introduction: Prognostic and Predictive Factors; Invasive Ductal Carcinoma (Adenocarcinomas of No Special Type); Invasive Lobular Carcinoma; Invasive Micropapillary Carcinoma; Lobular Carcinoma In Situ; Microglandular Adenosis; Mucinous (Colloid) Carcinoma; Myofibroblastoma; Neoadjuvant Therapy; Neuroendocrine/Small Cell Carcinoma; Risk Factors for Developing Breast Carcinoma; Secretory Carcinoma; Syringomatous Adenoma of the Nipple; Tubular/Cribriform Carcinoma
ERP-α	estrogen receptor protein α	ER-ALPHA, ERP-α	Ductal Carcinoma In Situ, Paget Disease; Expression Profiling, mRNA; Hormone Receptors (ER/PR)
Fascin	marker for Reed-Sternberg cells of Hodgkin disease	55K2	Basal-like Carcinomas
GCDFP-15	gross cystic fluid protein 15	SABP, GPIP4, Gp17, 23A3, BRST-2, D6 (GROSS CYSTIC DISEASE FLUID PROTEIN)	Encapsulated Papillary Carcinoma; Invasive Apocrine Carcinoma; Invasive Lobular Carcinoma Variants; Invasive Lobular Carcinoma; Lobular Carcinoma In Situ; Nonproliferative Changes; Papilloma, Large Duct and Small Duct; Secretory Carcinoma
GH	growth hormone	HGH, hGH	Ductal Carcinoma In Situ; Gynecomastoid Hyperplasia; HER2; Fibroadenoma
Hep-Par1	hepatocyte paraffin 1	OCH1E5.2.10, HEPPAR1	Invasive Lobular Carcinoma
HER2	v-erb-b2 erythroblastic leukemia viral gene protein, human epidermal growth factor receptor 2	c-erb-B2, HER2/neu, NEU, HER-2, NCL-CBE1, 10A7, 9G6.10, SP3, 4B5, Epidermal Growth Factor Receptor 2, P185, 9G6.20, A0485, C-ERBB-2, CB11, ERBB-2, 3B5, TAB250, HERCEPTEST, E2-4001, HER-2_NEU	Basal-like Carcinomas; Carcinomas with Extensive Intraductal Component; Checklist for the Reporting of Invasive Breast Carcinoma; Circulating Tumor Cells; Core Needle Biopsies; DNA Analysis; Ductal Carcinoma In Situ; Ductal Carcinoma In Situ with Microinvasion; Ductal Carcinoma In Situ, Paget Disease; Encapsulated Papillary Carcinoma; Epidemiology: Lesions Conferring Increased Risk of Breast Carcinoma; Expression Profiling, Mammaprint Assay; Expression Profiling, mRNA;

Reference

			Expression Profiling, Oncotype DX Assay; Expression Profiling, Protein; General Considerations; Hamartoma (Fibroadenolipoma); HER2; HER2 Positive Carcinoma; Hereditary Cancer; Histologic Grade; Hormone Receptors (ER/PR); Inflammatory Carcinoma; Introduction: Prognostic and Predictive Factors; Invasive Apocrine Carcinoma; Invasive Ductal Carcinoma (Adenocarcinomas of No Special Type); Invasive Lobular Carcinoma; Invasive Lobular Carcinoma Variants; Invasive Micropapillary Carcinoma; Invasive Papillary Carcinoma; Lobular Carcinoma In Situ; Locally Recurrent Carcinoma; Low-Grade Adenosquamous Carcinoma; Lymph Node Metastases; Margins and Reexcisions; Medullary Carcinoma; Metaplastic Carcinoma; Metastases to the Breast; Mucinous (Colloid) Carcinoma; Neoadjuvant Therapy; Neuroendocrine/Small Cell Carcinoma; Nipple Adenoma; Nonproliferative Changes; Secretory Carcinoma; Size and Multiple Foci; Tubular/Cribriform Carcinoma; Tubulolobular Carcinoma
HER-2_NEU	v-erb-b2 erythroblastic leukemia viral gene protein, human epidermal growth factor receptor 2	c-erb-B2, HER2/neu, NEU, HER-2, NCL-CBE1, 10A7, 9G6.10, SP3, 4B5, epidermal growth factor receptor 2, P185, 9G6.20, A0485, C-ERBB-2, CB11, ERBB-2, 3B5, TAB250, HERCEPTEST, E2-4001, HER-2_NEU	HER2
HER3	v-erb-b3 erythroblastic leukemia viral gene protein, human epidermal growth factor receptor 3	HER-3 AB-8, ERBB3, C-ERBBB-3	HER2
HER4	v-erb-4 erythroblastic leukemia viral gene protein, human epidermal growth factor receptor 4	HFR-1, ERBB-4, HER-4 AB-4	HER2
HMB-45	antigen present in melanocytic tumors such as melanomas	LB39 AA, CMM1, CMM, DNS, FAMMM, Mart1, Melan-A, MLM, tyrosinase	Ductal Carcinoma In Situ, Paget Disease; Granular Cell Tumor
IgG	immunoglobulin G	IGG	Lymphoma
Ki-67	marker of cell proliferation	MMI, KI88, IVAK-2, MIB1	Anatomic Structure and Lifecycle Changes; Basal-like Carcinomas; Ductal Carcinoma In Situ, Paget Disease; Epidemiology: Lesions Conferring Increased Risk of Breast Carcinoma; Epithelial Hyperplasia; Expression Profiling, mRNA; Expression Profiling, Oncotype DX Assay; Expression Profiling, Protein; Fibroadenoma; Hemangiomas; HER2 Positive Carcinoma; Hereditary Cancer; Histologic Grade; Introduction: Prognostic and Predictive Factors; Invasive Ductal Carcinoma (Adenocarcinomas of No Special Type); Lymph-Vascular Invasion; Phyllodes Tumor; Sclerosing Adenosis; Tubular/Cribriform Carcinoma; Expression Profiling, Protein; Histologic Grade; Introduction: Prognostic and Predictive Factors; Invasive Ductal Carcinoma (Adenocarcinomas of No Special Type)
Laminin	major protein in basal lamina	LAMININ-4C7, 4C12.8, LAM-89	Adenoid Cystic Carcinoma; Anatomic Structure and Lifecycle Changes; Collagenous Spherulosis; Ductal Carcinoma In Situ with Microinvasion; Microglandular Adenosis
Mammaglobin	breast tissue-specific glycoprotein	304-1A5	Anatomic Structure and Lifecycle Changes; Circulating Tumor Cells; Introduction: Prognostic and Predictive Factors; Invasive Micropapillary Carcinoma
Mart-1	mart-1 clone of Melan A		Ductal Carcinoma In Situ, Paget Disease

ANTIBODY INDEX

Melan-A	melanoma antigen recognized by T cells 1 (MART-1); protein found on melanocytes; melanocyte differentiation antigen	M2-7C10, CK-MM	Ductal Carcinoma In Situ, Paget Disease
Melan-A-103	clone of Melan-A	A103	Ductal Carcinoma In Situ, Paget Disease
MNF 116	cytokeratin-pan (AE1/AE3/LP34); cocktail of high and low molecular weight cytokeratins	keratin pan, MAK-6, K576, LU-5, KL-1, KC-8, MNF 116, pankeratin, pancytokeratin	Metaplastic Carcinoma
MUC1	epithelial membrane antigen	LICR-LON-M8, BC3, DF3, VU3D1, MUSEII, RD-1, MA695, MA552, PS2P446, 115D8	Circulating Tumor Cells; Invasive Lobular Carcinoma; Invasive Micropapillary Carcinoma; Mucinous (Colloid) Carcinoma
MUC2	mucin 1, intestinal	CCP58, MUC2-P, M53, MRP, LUM2-3, LDQ10	Mucinous (Colloid) Carcinoma; Mucocele-like Lesions
MUC5AC	mucin 5AC, tracheobronchial, gastric	CLH2 2, 45M1, CLH2	Mucinous (Colloid) Carcinoma
MUC6	mucin 6, gastric	CLH5	Mucinous (Colloid) Carcinoma; Mucocele-like Lesions
Myogenin	myogenic factor 4; class C basic helix-loophelix protein 3	F5D, MYF3, MYF4, LO26, bHLHc3, cb553, MYF4, MYOG	Sarcomas
Myoglobin	iron and oxygen-building protein found in muscle tissue	MG-1	Granular Cell Tumor; Sarcomas
Myosin	motor proteins responsible for actin-based motility in striated and smooth muscle cells		Adenoid Cystic Carcinoma; Collagenous Spherulosis; Ductal Carcinoma In Situ with Microinvasion; Pseudoangiomatous Stromal Hyperplasia; Sclerosing Adenosis
NDRG1	n-myc downstream-regulated gene 1		Expression Profiling, Protein
neuron specific enolase		BSS/H14, NSE	Granular Cell Tumor
NTRK3	neurotrophic tyrosine kinase receptor 3	TRKC	Secretory Carcinoma
p21	cyclin dependent kinase inhibitor 1A	WAF1, DCS-60.2, EA10, 6B6, 4D10, SX118, P21, P21_WAF1, WAFT	Introduction: Prognostic and Predictive Factors
p27	cyclin dependent kinase inhibitor 1B	P27_KIP1, 57, 1B4, DCS-72.F6, SX53G8, P27, K25020, DCS72, KIP-1	Introduction: Prognostic and Predictive Factors
p53	p53 tumor suppressor gene protein	DO7, 21N, BP53-12-1, AB6, CM1, PAB1801, DO1, BP53-11, PAB240, RSP53, MU195, P53	Basal-like Carcinomas; DNA Analysis; Encapsulated Papillary Carcinoma; Epidemiology: Lesions Conferring Increased Risk of Breast Carcinoma; Expression Profiling, Protein; Hamartoma (Fibroadenolipoma); HER2 Positive Carcinoma; Hereditary Cancer; Inflammatory Carcinoma; Invasive Apocrine Carcinoma; Invasive Lobular Carcinoma Variants; Medullary Carcinoma; Metaplastic Carcinoma; Phyllodes Tumor
p63	tumor protein p63	H-137, 7JUL	Anatomic Structure and Lifecycle Changes; Atypical Lobular Hyperplasia; Basal-like Carcinomas; Collagenous Spherulosis; Ductal Carcinoma In Situ; Ductal Carcinoma In Situ with Microinvasion; Ductal Carcinoma In Situ, Paget Disease; Encapsulated Papillary Carcinoma; Fibromatosis; Hamartoma (Fibroadenolipoma); HER2; Iatrogenic Changes; Invasive Ductal Carcinoma (Adenocarcinomas of No Special Type); Invasive Papillary Carcinoma; Lobular Carcinoma In Situ; Locally Recurrent Carcinoma; Low-Grade Adenosquamous Carcinoma; Lymph-Vascular Invasion; Metaplastic Carcinoma; Microglandular Adenosis; Mucinous (Colloid) Carcinoma; Neuroendocrine/Small Cell Carcinoma; Nipple Adenoma; Nodular Fasciitis; Papilloma, Large Duct and Small Duct; Phyllodes Tumor; Radial Sclerosing Lesion/Radial Scar; Risk Factors for Developing Breast Carcinoma; Sarcomas; Sclerosing Adenosis; Secretory Carcinoma; Syringomatous Adenoma of the Nipple; Tubular/Cribriform Carcinoma

ANTIBODY INDEX

p120 catenin	cell adhesion molecule		Invasive Lobular Carcinoma; Tubulolobular Carcinoma
pax-8	paired box gene 8	PAX-8	Metastases to the Breast
P-cadherin	placental dependent adhesion protein	56, clone 56	Anatomic Structure and Lifecycle Changes; Invasive Lobular Carcinoma; Metaplastic Carcinoma
Podoplanin	marker for reactive follicular dendritic cells and follicular dendritic cell sarcomas	D2-40, M2A	Anatomic Structure and Lifecycle Changes; Ductal Carcinoma In Situ; Inflammatory Carcinoma; Invasive Ductal Carcinoma (Adenocarcinomas of No Special Type); Locally Recurrent Carcinoma; Lymph-Vascular Invasion
PR	progesterone receptor protein	10A9, PGR-1A6, KD68, PGR-ICA, PRP-P, PRP, PRI, 1A6, 1AR, HPRA3, PGR-636, 636, PR88, NCL-PGR	Adenoid Cystic Carcinoma; Anatomic Structure and Lifecycle Changes; Basal-like Carcinomas; Checklist for the Reporting of Invasive Breast Carcinoma; Core Needle Biopsies; Ductal Carcinoma In Situ; Ductal Carcinoma In Situ with Microinvasion; Epithelial Hyperplasia; Expression Profiling, mRNA; Expression Profiling, Oncotype DX Assay; Expression Profiling, Protein; General Considerations; Gynecomastia; Hamartoma (Fibroadenolipoma); HER2; HER2 Positive Carcinoma; Histologic Grade; Hormone Receptors (ER/PR); Inflammatory Carcinoma; Introduction: Prognostic and Predictive Factors; Invasive Apocrine Carcinoma; Invasive Ductal Carcinoma (Adenocarcinomas of No Special Type); Invasive Lobular Carcinoma; Invasive Lobular Carcinoma Variants; Invasive Micropapillary Carcinoma; Lobular Carcinoma In Situ; Locally Recurrent Carcinoma; Lymph Node Metastases; Lymphoma; Margins and Reexcisions; Medullary Carcinoma; Metaplastic Carcinoma; Metastases to the Breast; Mucinous (Colloid) Carcinoma; Myofibroblastoma; Neoadjuvant Therapy; Neuroendocrine/Small Cell Carcinoma; Risk Factors for Developing Breast Carcinoma; Secretory Carcinoma; Size and Multiple Foci; Syringomatous Adenoma of the Nipple; Tubular/Cribriform Carcinoma; Tubulolobular Carcinoma
Prostate specific antigen		PSA, PSA-M, PSA, ER-PR8, PSA-P, F5	Gynecomastia
Prostatic acid phosphatase		PAP, PASE/4LJ, PAP-P	Gynecomastia
PRP	progesterone receptor protein	10A9, PGR-1A6, KD68, PGR-ICA, PRP-P, PRI, 1A6, 1AR, HPRA3, PGR-636, 636, PR88, NCL-PGR	Hormone Receptors (ER/PR); Invasive Micropapillary Carcinoma Medullary Carcinoma
PSAP			Metastases to the Breast
PTEN	phosphatase and tensin homolog	PN37	Hamartoma (Fibroadenolipoma); Hereditary Cancer; Invasive Apocrine Carcinoma; Risk Factors for Developing Breast Carcinoma
S100	Low molecular weight protein normally present in cells derived from neural crest (Schwann cells, melanocytes, and glial cells), chondrocytes, adipocytes, myoepithelial cells, macrophages, Langerhans cells, dendritic cells, and keratinocytes	S-100, A6, 15E2E2, Z311, 4C4.9	Ductal Carcinoma In Situ, Paget Disease; Fat Necrosis; Granular Cell Tumor; Hamartoma (Fibroadenolipoma); Iatrogenic Changes; Invasive Apocrine Carcinoma; Invasive Ductal Carcinoma (Adenocarcinomas of No Special Type); Invasive Lobular Carcinoma Variants; Lymph Node Metastases; Metastases to the Breast; Microglandular Adenosis; Sarcomas; Secretory Carcinoma; Tubular/Cribriform Carcinoma; Sclerosing Adenosis
SMHC	myosin heavy chain smooth muscle	ID8, SM_MYOSIN_H, HSM-V, SMMS-1	Anatomic Structure and Lifecycle Changes; Ductal Carcinoma In Situ with

ANTIBODY INDEX

			Microinvasion; Pseudoangiomatous Stromal Hyperplasia
SP1	estrogen receptor protein	1D5, 6F11, 15D, H222, TE111, ERP, ER1D5, NCLER611, NCL-ER-LH2 PGP-1A6	Hormone Receptors (ER/PR)
SP3	v-erb-b2 erythroblastic leukemia viral gene protein, human epidermal growth factor receptor 2	c-erb-B2, HER2/neu, NEU, HER2, HER-2, NCL-CBE1, 10A7, 9G6.10, 4B5, Epidermal Growth Factor Receptor 2, P185, 9G6.20, A0485, C-ERBB-2, CB11, ERBB-2, 3B5, TAB250, HERCEPTEST, E2-4001, HER-2_NEU	HER2
Survivin	inhibitor of apoptosis	AB469, SURVIVIN, FL-142, D8, 8E12	Expression Profiling, Oncotype DX Assay
Synaptophysin	major synaptic vesicle protein p38 antibody	SVP38, SY38, SNP-88, SYP, SYPH, Sypl, Syn p38	Encapsulated Papillary Carcinoma; Invasive Papillary Carcinoma; Metastases to the Breast; Mucinous (Colloid) Carcinoma; Neuroendocrine/Small Cell Carcinoma
TFE3	transcription factor E3		Granular Cell Tumor
TTF-1	transcription termination factor	8G7G3/1, SPT-24, SC-13040	Invasive Micropapillary Carcinoma; Metastases to the Breast; Neuroendocrine/Small Cell Carcinoma
VEGF	Vascular endothelial growth factor	JH121, 26503.11, VPF, VPF/ VEGF, VEGF-A, VEGF-C, RP 077, VEGFR-1, RP 076, VEGFR-2, 9D9, VEGFR-3, FLT-4	Basal-like Carcinomas; Inflammatory Carcinoma
Vimentin	major subunit protein of intermediate filaments of mesenchymal cells	43BE8, 3B4, V10, V9, VIM-B34, VIM	Granular Cell Tumor; Lipoma and Angiolipoma; Myofibromatoma; Pseudoangiomatous Stromal Hyperplasia; Sarcomas
WT1	Wilms tumor gene-1	6F-H2, C-19	Invasive Ductal Carcinoma (Adenocarcinomas of No Special Type); Invasive Micropapillary Carcinoma; Lymph Node Metastases; Metastases to the Breast

Molecular Factors Discussed

Molecular Factor	Chromosomal Location	Alternative Names/Terms	Chapters
β-actin			Expression Profiling, Oncotype DX Assay
10p12, loss of	10p12		Phyllodes Tumor
10q, loss of	10q		Epidemiology: Lesions Conferring Increased Risk of Breast Carcinoma
11q, gain of	11q		DNA Analysis
11q, loss of	11q		DNA Analysis; Epidemiology: Lesions Conferring Increased Risk of Breast Carcinoma
13, loss of	13		Phyllodes Tumor
13q, gain of	13q		Epidemiology: Lesions Conferring Increased Risk of Breast Carcinoma
13q, loss of	13q		DNA Analysis; Epidemiology: Lesions Conferring Increased Risk of Breast Carcinoma; Myofibroblastoma
13q, rearrangements of	13q		Lipoma and Angiolipoma
13q14, loss of	13q14		Myofibroblastoma
14q, loss of	14q		Epidemiology: Lesions Conferring Increased Risk of Breast Carcinoma
15q, gain of	15q		Epidemiology: Lesions Conferring Increased Risk of Breast Carcinoma
16p, gain of	16p		DNA Analysis; Invasive Lobular Carcinoma
16p, loss of	16p		Epidemiology: Lesions Conferring Increased Risk of Breast Carcinoma
16q, loss of	16q		Atypical Ductal Hyperplasia; Columnar Cell Change with or without Flat Atypia; DNA Analysis; Epidemiology: Lesions Conferring Increased Risk of Breast Carcinoma; Invasive Lobular Carcinoma; Lobular Carcinoma In Situ; Myofibroblastoma; Risk Factors for Developing Breast Carcinoma; Tubular/Cribriform Carcinoma
16q, rearrangements of	16q		Lipoma and Angiolipoma
17p, loss of	17p		DNA Analysis; Epidemiology: Lesions Conferring Increased Risk of Breast Carcinoma
17p13.1	17p13.1		Invasive Micropapillary Carcinoma
17q, gain of	17q		DNA Analysis; Epidemiology: Lesions Conferring Increased Risk of Breast Carcinoma
17q12	17q12		HER2; HER2 Positive Carcinoma
19p, loss of	19p		DNA Analysis
19q, gain of	19q		Epidemiology: Lesions Conferring Increased Risk of Breast Carcinoma; DNA Analysis
19q, loss of	19q		DNA Analysis
1p, gain of	1p		Epidemiology: Lesions Conferring Increased Risk of Breast Carcinoma; Lobular Carcinoma In Situ
1p, loss of	1p		DNA Analysis; Epidemiology: Lesions Conferring Increased Risk of Breast Carcinoma
1q, gain of	1q		Atypical Ductal Hyperplasia; DNA Analysis; Epidemiology: Lesions Conferring Increased Risk of Breast Carcinoma; Fibroadenoma; Invasive Lobular Carcinoma; Lobular Carcinoma In Situ; Phyllodes Tumor; Secretory Carcinoma; Tubular/Cribriform Carcinoma
1q, loss of	1q		Epidemiology: Lesions Conferring Increased Risk of Breast Carcinoma
20q, gain of	20q		DNA Analysis; Epidemiology: Lesions Conferring Increased Risk of Breast Carcinoma
22q, loss of	22q		DNA Analysis; Secretory Carcinoma
2p16	2p16		Fibroadenoma
2q, gain of	2q		Epidemiology: Lesions Conferring Increased Risk of Breast Carcinoma
3p24, loss of	3p24		Phyllodes Tumor

MOLECULAR FACTOR INDEX

			Carcinoma; Hereditary Cancer; Invasive Apocrine Carcinoma; Invasive Lobular Carcinoma; Invasive Lobular Carcinoma Variants; Invasive Micropapillary Carcinoma; Lobular Carcinoma In Situ; Medullary Carcinoma; Metaplastic Carcinoma; Metastases to the Breast; Neuroendocrine/Small Cell Carcinoma; Risk Factors for Developing Breast Carcinoma; Sclerosing Adenosis; Secretory Carcinoma; Tubulolobular Carcinoma
EGFR	7p12	Epidermal growth factor receptor; ERBB1; HER1	Basal-like Carcinomas; Expression Profiling, mRNA; Expression Profiling, Protein; HER2; Hereditary Cancer; Invasive Apocrine Carcinoma; Invasive Ductal Carcinoma (Adenocarcinomas of No Special Type); Locally Recurrent Carcinoma; Low-Grade Adenosquamous Carcinoma; Metaplastic Carcinoma; Mucinous (Colloid) Carcinoma; Secretory Carcinoma
ER	6q25.1	estrogen receptor	Adenoid Cystic Carcinoma; Anatomic Structure and Lifecycle Changes; Atypical Ductal Hyperplasia; Atypical Lobular Hyperplasia; Basal-like Carcinomas; Carcinomas with Extensive Intraductal Component; Checklist for the Reporting of Invasive Breast Carcinoma; Core Needle Biopsies; Ductal Carcinoma In Situ; Ductal Carcinoma In Situ with Microinvasion; Epidemiology: Lesions Conferring Increased Risk of Breast Carcinoma; Epithelial Hyperplasia; Expression Profiling, mRNA; Expression Profiling, Oncotype DX Assay; Expression Profiling, Protein; Fibromatosis; General Considerations; Gynecomastia; Hamartoma (Fibroadenolipoma); HER2; HER2 Positive Carcinoma; Histologic Grade; Hormone Receptors (ER/PR); Inflammatory Carcinoma; Introduction: Prognostic and Predictive Factors; Invasive Apocrine Carcinoma; Invasive Ductal Carcinoma (Adenocarcinomas of No Special Type); Invasive Lobular Carcinoma; Invasive Lobular Carcinoma Variants; Invasive Micropapillary Carcinoma; Invasive Papillary Carcinoma; Lobular Carcinoma In Situ; Locally Recurrent Carcinoma; Lymph Node Metastases; Lymphoma; Medullary Carcinoma; Metaplastic Carcinoma; Metastases to the Breast; Mucinous (Colloid) Carcinoma; Myofibroblastoma Neoadjuvant Therapy; Neuroendocrine/Small Cell Carcinoma; Risk Factors for Developing Breast Carcinoma; Sclerosing Adenosis; Secretory Carcinoma; Size and Multiple Foci; Syringomatous Adenoma of the Nipple; Tubular/Cribriform Carcinoma; Tubulolobular Carcinoma
ESR2	14q23.2	estrogen receptor 2 (ER beta)	Hormone Receptors (ER/PR)
Estrogen receptor	6q25.1	ER	Anatomic Structure and Lifecycle Changes; Basal-like Carcinomas; Carcinomas with Extensive Intraductal Component; Checklist for the Reporting of Invasive Breast Carcinoma; Ductal Carcinoma In Situ; Ductal Carcinoma In Situ, Paget Disease; Epidemiology: Lesions Conferring Increased Risk of Breast Carcinoma; Expression Profiling, mRNA; Expression Profiling, Oncotype DX Assay; Expression Profiling, Protein; Fibroadenoma; Granular Cell Tumor; Gynecomastia; HER2 Positive Carcinoma; Hereditary Cancer; Hormone Receptors (ER/PR); Iatrogenic Changes; Invasive Apocrine Carcinoma; Invasive Micropapillary Carcinoma; Invasive Papillary Carcinoma; Locally Recurrent Carcinoma; Lymphoma; Microglandular Adenosis; Neoadjuvant Therapy; Risk Factors for Developing Breast Carcinoma; Sclerosing Adenosis
ETV6	12p13	ets variant 6	Secretory Carcinoma
ETV6-NTRK3	t(12;15)(p13;q25)		Secretory Carcinoma
GAPDH	12p13	glyceraldehyde-3-phosphate dehydrogenase	Expression Profiling, Oncotype DX Assay
GRB7	17q12	growth factor receptor-bound protein 7	Expression Profiling, mRNA
GSTM1	1p13.3	glutathione S-transferase mu 1	Expression Profiling, Oncotype DX Assay
GUS			Expression Profiling, Oncotype DX Assay
HER2	17q12	c-erbB-2	Basal-like Carcinomas; Carcinomas with Extensive Intraductal Component; Checklist for the Reporting of Invasive Breast Carcinoma; Circulating Tumor Cells; Core Needle Biopsies; DNA Analysis; Ductal Carcinoma In Situ; Ductal Carcinoma In Situ with Microinvasion;

			Ductal Carcinoma In Situ, Paget Disease; Encapsulated Papillary Carcinoma; Epidemiology: Lesions Conferring Increased Risk of Breast Carcinoma; Expression Profiling, mRNA; Expression Profiling, Oncotype DX Assay; Expression Profiling, Protein; General Considerations; Hamartoma (Fibroadenolipoma) HER2; HER2 Positive Carcinoma; Hereditary Cancer; Histologic Grade; Hormone Receptors (ER/PR); Inflammatory Carcinoma; Introduction: Prognostic and Predictive Factors; Invasive Apocrine Carcinoma; Invasive Ductal Carcinoma (Adenocarcinomas of No Special Type); Invasive Lobular Carcinoma; Invasive Lobular Carcinoma Variants; Invasive Micropapillary Carcinoma; Invasive Papillary Carcinoma; Lobular Carcinoma In Situ Locally Recurrent Carcinoma; Low-Grade Adenosquamous Carcinoma; Lymph Node Metastases; Margins and Reexcisions Medullary Carcinoma; Metaplastic Carcinoma; Metastases to the Breast; Mucinous (Colloid) Carcinoma; Neoadjuvant Therapy; Neuroendocrine/Small Cell Carcinoma; Nipple Adenoma; Nonproliferative Changes; Secretory Carcinoma; Size and Multiple Foci; Tubular/Cribriform Carcinoma; Tubulolobular Carcinoma
HER2-type			Invasive Ductal Carcinoma (Adenocarcinomas of No Special Type)
HOXB13	17q21.2	homeobox B13	Expression Profiling, mRNA
IL17BR			Expression Profiling, mRNA
Ki-67	10q26.2		Anatomic Structure and Lifecycle Changes; Basal-like Carcinomas; Ductal Carcinoma In Situ, Paget Disease; Epidemiology: Lesions Conferring Increased Risk of Breast Carcinoma; Epithelial Hyperplasia; Expression Profiling, mRNA; Expression Profiling, Oncotype DX Assay; Expression Profiling, Protein; Fibroadenoma; Hemangiomas; HER2 Positive Carcinoma; Hereditary Cancer; Histologic Grade; Introduction: Prognostic and Predictive Factors; Invasive Ductal Carcinoma (Adenocarcinomas of No Special Type); Lymph-Vascular Invasion; Phyllodes Tumor; Sclerosing Adenosis; Tubular/Cribriform Carcinoma
KIT	4q11-q12	v-kit Hardy-Zuckerman 4 feline sarcoma viral oncogene homolog; c-Kit; CD117	Adenoid Cystic Carcinoma
KPNA2	17q24.2	karyopherin alpha 2 (RAG cohort 1, importin alpha 1)	Expression Profiling, mRNA; Histologic Grade
Luminal A			Basal-like Carcinomas; Ductal Carcinoma In Situ; Expression Profiling, mRNA; Expression Profiling, Protein; Introduction: Prognostic and Predictive Factors; Invasive Ductal Carcinoma (Adenocarcinomas of No Special Type); Locally Recurrent Carcinoma; Margins and Reexcisions
Luminal B			Ductal Carcinoma In Situ; Expression Profiling, mRNA; Expression Profiling, Protein; Introduction: Prognostic and Predictive Factors; Invasive Ductal Carcinoma (Adenocarcinomas of No Special Type); Margins and Reexcisions
Luminal type A			Mucinous (Colloid) Carcinoma
MLL	11q23	HRX;ALL1	Mucocele-like Lesions
MMP11	22q11.2	matrix metallopeptidase 11 (stromelysin 3)	Expression Profiling, Oncotype DX Assay
MUC2	11p15.5	mucin 2, oligomeric mucus/gel-forming	Mucinous (Colloid) Carcinoma
MUC6	11p15.5	mucin 6, oligomeric mucus/gel-forming	Mucinous (Colloid) Carcinoma; Mucocele-like Lesions
MYB	6q22-q23	v-myb myeloblastosis viral oncogene homolog (avian)	Adenoid Cystic Carcinoma
MYBL2	20q13.1	v-myb myeloblastosis viral oncogene homolog (avian)-like 2	Expression Profiling, mRNA; Expression Profiling, Oncotype DX Assay
MYC	c-myc		Invasive Micropapillary Carcinoma
MZL			Lymphoma
NFIB	9p24.1	nuclear factor I/B	Adenoid Cystic Carcinoma
P53	17p13.1	TP53	Basal-like Carcinomas; HER2 Positive Carcinoma; Hereditary Cancer; Metaplastic Carcinoma; Risk Factors for Developing Breast Carcinoma; Secretory Carcinoma

MOLECULAR FACTOR INDEX

PAX3	2q35	Paired-box (PAX) gene 3	Phyllodes Tumor
PR	11q22-q23	progesterone receptor	Adenoid Cystic Carcinoma; Anatomic Structure and Lifecycle Changes; Basal-like Carcinomas; Checklist for the Reporting of Invasive Breast Carcinoma; Core Needle Biopsies; Ductal Carcinoma In Situ; Ductal Carcinoma In Situ with Microinvasion; Epithelial Hyperplasia; Expression Profiling, mRNA; Expression Profiling, Oncotype DX Assay; Expression Profiling, Protein; General Considerations; Gynecomastia; Hamartoma (Fibroadenolipoma); HER2; HER2 Positive Carcinoma; Histologic Grade; Hormone Receptors (ER/PR); Inflammatory Carcinoma; Introduction: Prognostic and Predictive Factors; Invasive Apocrine Carcinoma; Invasive Ductal Carcinoma (Adenocarcinomas of No Special Type); Invasive Lobular Carcinoma; Invasive Lobular Carcinoma Variants; Invasive Micropapillary Carcinoma; Lobular Carcinoma In Situ; Locally Recurrent Carcinoma; Lymph Node Metastases; Lymphoma; Margins and Reexcisions; Medullary Carcinoma; Metaplastic Carcinoma; Metastases to the Breast; Mucinous (Colloid) Carcinoma; Myofibroblastoma; Neoadjuvant Therapy; Neuroendocrine/Small Cell Carcinoma; Risk Factors for Developing Breast Carcinoma; Secretory Carcinoma; Size and Multiple Foci; Syringomatous Adenoma of the Nipple; Tubular/Cribriform Carcinoma; Tubulolobular Carcinoma
PRKAR1A	17q23-q24	protein kinase, cAMP-dependent, regulatory, type I, alpha (tissue specific extinguisher 1)	Fibroadenoma
Progesterone receptor	11q22-q23	PR	Anatomic Structure and Lifecycle Changes; Atypical Lobular Hyperplasia; Checklist for the Reporting of Invasive Breast Carcinoma; Ductal Carcinoma In Situ, Paget Disease; Encapsulated Papillary Carcinoma; Epidemiology: Lesions Conferring Increased Risk of Breast Carcinoma; Fibroadenoma; Fibromatosis; Granular Cell Tumor; Gynecomastia; Hormone Receptors (ER/PR); Introduction: Prognostic and Predictive Factors; Invasive Apocrine Carcinoma; Invasive Micropapillary Carcinoma; Invasive Papillary Carcinoma; Lobular Carcinoma In Situ; Low-Grade Adenosquamous Carcinoma; Microglandular Adenosis; Myofibroblastoma; Neuroendocrine/Small Cell Carcinoma; Pseudoangiomatous Stromal Hyperplasia; Risk Factors for Developing Breast Carcinoma; Syringomatous Adenoma of the Nipple; Tubulolobular Carcinoma
PTEN	10q23.3	phosphatase and tensin homolog	Hamartoma (Fibroadenolipoma); Hereditary Cancer; Invasive Apocrine Carcinoma; Risk Factors for Developing Breast Carcinoma
RPLPO			Expression Profiling, Oncotype DX Assay
SCUBE2	11p15.3	signal peptide, CUB domain, EGF-like 2	Expression Profiling, Oncotype DX Assay
SIX1	14q23.1	SIX homeobox 1	Phyllodes Tumor
STK11/LKB1	19p13.3	serine/threonine kinase 11	Hereditary Cancer
STK15	20q13	aurora kinase A (AURKA)	Expression Profiling, Oncotype DX Assay
TFE3	Xp11.2	transcription factor E3	Granular Cell Tumor
TFRC	3q29	transferrin receptor; CD71; p90	Expression Profiling, Oncotype DX Assay
TOP2A	17q21-q22	topoisomerase (DNA) II alpha 170kDa	HER2 Positive Carcinoma
TP53	17p13.1	P53	Basal-like Carcinomas; Hereditary Cancer; Invasive Ductal Carcinoma (Adenocarcinomas of No Special Type); Medullary Carcinoma
Triple negative			Basal-like Carcinomas; Carcinomas with Extensive Intraductal Component; Ductal Carcinoma In Situ; Expression Profiling, mRNA; Expression Profiling, Protein; HER2 Positive Carcinoma; Introduction: Prognostic and Predictive Factors; Margins and Reexcisions; Basal-like Carcinomas
VEGF	6p12	vascular endothelial growth factor A (VEGFA)	Basal-like Carcinomas; Inflammatory Carcinoma

MOLECULAR FACTOR INDEX

WISP3	6q21	WNT1 inducible signaling pathway protein 3	Inflammatory Carcinoma
WT1	11p13	Wilms tumor 1	Invasive Ductal Carcinoma (Adenocarcinomas of No Special Type); Invasive Micropapillary Carcinoma; Lymph Node Metastases; Metastases to the Breast
X, loss of	X		Epidemiology: Lesions Conferring Increased Risk of Breast Carcinoma

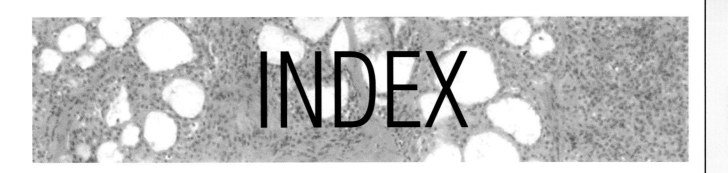

INDEX

A

INDEX

INDEX

INDEX

INDEX

INDEX

INDEX

INDEX

INDEX

INDEX

INDEX

INDEX

INDEX

INDEX

INDEX

INDEX

INDEX

INDEX

INDEX

INDEX

INDEX